Commissioning Editor: Jonathan Gregory
Project Development Manager: Louise Cook
Project Manager: Katharine Eyston
Designer: Jayne Jones
Illustration Manager: Mick Ruddy
Illustrator: Robin Dean

Canine Ophthalmology
An Atlas and Text

Keith C Barnett
OBE, MA, PhD, BSc, DVOphthal, FRCVS, DipECVO
Consultant Ophthalmologist, Comparative Ophthalmology Unit,
Centre for Small Animal Studies, Animal Health Trust, Newmarket, UK

Christine Heinrich
DVOphthal, MRCVS
Willows Referral Service, Shirley, Solihull, West Midlands, UK

Jane Sansom
BVSc, DVOphthal, MRCVS, DipECVO
Head, Comparative Ophthalmology Unit, Centre for Small Animal Studies,
Animal Health Trust, Newmarket, UK

W.B. SAUNDERS

Edinburgh London New York Oxford Philadelphia St Louis Sydney Toronto 2002

SAUNDERS
An imprint of Elsevier Science Limited

© Harcourt Publishers Limited 2002
© Elsevier Science Limited 2002. All rights reserved.

The right of Keith C. Barnett, C. Heinrich and J. Sansom to be identified as authors of this work has been asserted by them in accordance with the Copyright, Designs and Patents Act 1988

No part of this publication may be reproduced, stored in a retrieval system, or transmitted in any form or by any means, electronic, mechanical, photocopying, recording or otherwise, without either the prior permission of the publishers or a licence permitting restricted copying in the United Kingdom issued by the Copyright Licensing Agency, 90 Tottenham Court Road, London W1T 4LP. Permissions may be sought directly from Elsevier's Health Sciences Rights Department in Philadelphia, USA: phone: (+1) 215 238 7869, fax: (+1) 215 238 2239, e-mail: healthpermissions@elsevier.com. You may also complete your request on-line via the Elsevier Science homepage (http://www.elsevier.com), by selecting 'Customer Support' and then 'Obtaining Permissions'.

First published 2002
Reprinted 2002, 2003

ISBN 0 7020 1997 6

British Library Cataloguing in Publication Data
A catalogue record for this book is available from the British Library

Library of Congress Cataloging in Publication Data
A catalog record for this book is available from the Library of Congress

Note
Medical knowledge is constantly changing. As new information becomes available, changes in treatment, procedures, equipment and the use of drugs become necessary. The authors and the publishers have taken care to ensure that the information given in this text is accurate and up to date. However, readers are strongly advised to confirm that the information, especially with regard to drug usage, complies with the latest legislation and standards of practice.

Existing UK nomenclature is changing to the system of Recommended International Nonproprietary Names (rINNs). Until the UK names are no longer in use, these more familiar names are used in this book in preference to rINNs, details of which may be obtained from the British National Formulary.

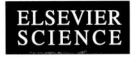

ELSEVIER SCIENCE
your source for books, journals and multimedia in the health sciences

www.elsevierhealth.com

The publisher's policy is to use **paper manufactured from sustainable forests**

Printed in China
C/03

Contents

Contributors vii
Preface ix
Acknowledgements x

1 Examination of the eye and adnexa 1

2 Postnatal development of the eye 9

3 Ocular emergencies and trauma 15
   Heidi J. Featherstone and Robin G. Stanley

4 Globe and orbit 37
   Keith Barnett with Ruth Dennis

5 Upper and lower eyelids 49

6 Third eyelid 61

7 Lacrimal system 67

8 Conjunctiva and sclera 75

9 Cornea 85

10 Glaucoma 99

11 Lens 109

12 Uveal tract 127

13 Vitreous 149

14 Fundus 155

15 Neuro-ophthalmology 181
   Jacques Penderis

Appendices 197
Further reading 205
Index 207

CONTRIBUTORS

Ruth Dennis
MA, VetMB, DVR, MRCVS, DipECVDI
RCVS-Recognised Specialist in Radiology,
Centre for Small Animal Studies, Animal Health Trust,
Newmarket, UK

Heidi J Featherstone
BVetMed, CertVOphthal, MRCVS
Clinical Ophthalmologist,
Centre for Small Animal Studies, Animal Health Trust,
Newmarket, UK

Jacques Penderis
BVSc, MVM, CVR, DipECVN, MRCVS
European Specialist in Veterinary Neurology,
Centre for Small Animal Studies, Animal Health Trust,
Newmarket, UK

Robin G Stanley
BVSc(HONS), FACVSc (OPHTHALMOLOGY), MRCVS
Veterinary Ophthalmologist,
Animal Eye Care, Melbourne,
Victoria, Australia

Preface

Canine Ophthalmology: An Atlas and Text is intended as a companion volume to *Feline Ophthalmology* published in 1998. This original intention was made more difficult to follow because of the much greater quantity of knowledge and number of publications for the dog compared with the cat. This is particularly the case in the number and complexity and breeds involved for hereditary eye diseases.

Canine Ophthalmology is primarily intended for veterinary surgeons in small animal practice and for veterinary students in their clinical years, particularly those in the United Kingdom. Books on canine ophthalmology have been published recently in the United States, Europe and Australia and give details of certain breeds and conditions not seen in the UK: these texts are included in the list of further reading at the end of the book.

The format we have followed is an opening chapter on methods of examination followed by a chapter on *postnatal development of the eye* from a clinical perspective. The third chapter, *ocular emergencies and trauma*, is by two authors different from those who wrote the rest of the book, thereby introducing different opinions, and a little overlap and duplication, which we trust will prove interesting and useful. The chapter on the *globe and orbit* includes a table on the globe size of the adult dog in different breeds. The following 10 chapters deal with parts of the eye divided anatomically. Each chapter gives very brief details of anatomy, histology, physiology and embryology in its introduction together with separate paragraphs on congenital anomalies, diseases or disorders, hereditary abnormalities and neoplasia, which are also collected together and summarised in Appendices I–III. Each chapter ends with a few selected references in addition to the books listed under further reading. There are over 570 new colour illustrations which we believe is the strength of the book, the main aim of which is in diagnosis, brief details only being included on both medical and surgical treatment.

We trust that this *Atlas and Text* will also be enjoyable to consult and to assist in the accurate diagnosis and successful treatment of eye disease in this species, which is always likely to occupy the premier position in veterinary ophthalmology.

Keith Barnett
C Heinrich
J Sansom
2001

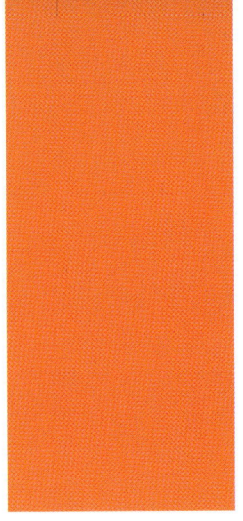

ACKNOWLEDGEMENTS

We wish to acknowledge the colleagues who kindly loaned certain illustrations, all of whom have been individually named in the text. We are particularly grateful to Ruth Dennis for her contribution 'Diagnostic imaging of globe and orbit' in Chapter 4 and the ultrasound measurements for the postnatal growth of the globe; to Jacques Penderis for Chapter 15 *Neuro-ophthalmology* and to Heidi Featherstone and Robin Stanley for Chapter 3 *Ocular emergencies and trauma*.

All illustrations, except for those mentioned above, are from the collections at the Comparative Ophthalmology Unit, Animal Health Trust and Willows Referral Service, and we readily acknowledge the assistance of past and present members of staff including Roger Curtis, Arnold Leon, Tony Read and Heidi Featherstone in contributing to this collection.

1 Examination of the Eye and Adnexa

Introduction

To gain the maximum benefit from every ocular examination a strict routine should be established and the results should be recorded on specifically designed patient charts. Ophthalmology is an especially rewarding discipline as the eye is easily accessible for examination and the majority of diagnoses can be made at the time of ocular examination. In order to distinguish ocular disease from normal variation a solid knowledge of the normal canine eye is required. Both eyes should always be examined even in cases where the other eye is normal or apparently normal.

Patient handling

To carry out a detailed ocular examination minimal patient restraint should be used (Fig. 1.1). Specifically trained personnel to hold the patient during the ocular examination is helpful but not always available and it may be necessary to instruct the owner how best to restrain the patient. Most canine patients are amenable to ocular examination, especially if a calm approach with minimal restraint is taken. Throughout the examination consideration should be given to the degree of illumination that is used with different parts of equipment, so that lighting levels are chosen that allow adequate examination but also cause minimal patient discomfort and resistance.

If required, a sedative can be given to allow examination of difficult canine patients. Alpha$_2$ agonists such as medetomidine are suitable drugs as the eye remains in a central position whereas enophthalmos and third eyelid protrusion are commonly seen if phenothiazines such as acepromazine are used.

Equipment

The ocular examination should take place in a quiet room that can be darkened. Ideally, consulting room lights should be controlled with a dimmer switch. A height-adjustable table suitable for all sizes of dog is required and hydraulic models are especially suitable for this purpose. A focal light source such as a pen torch or a Finhoff transilluminator, a hand-held direct ophthalmoscope (Figs 1.2 and 1.3) and a 20 dioptre (D) lens are essential for the ocular examination and are the minimum equipment that should be available in every general practice.

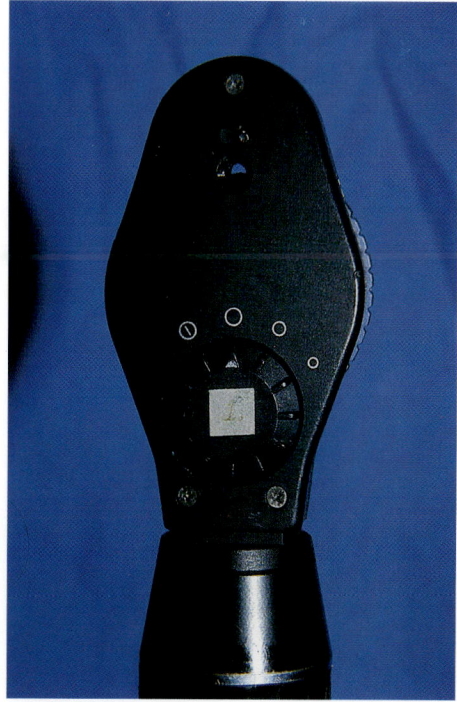

Fig. 1.2 Hand-held direct ophthalmoscope – patient side with viewhole and mirror, dial for different beam sizes, a grid for the documentation of lesions, and red free light.

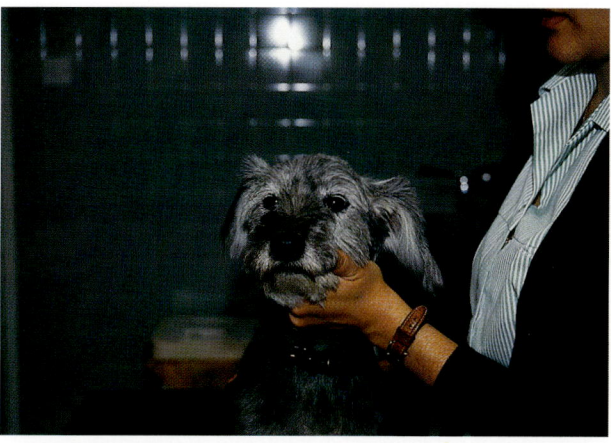

Fig. 1.1 Canine patient held for ocular examination with minimal restraint.

EXAMINATION OF THE EYE AND ADNEXA

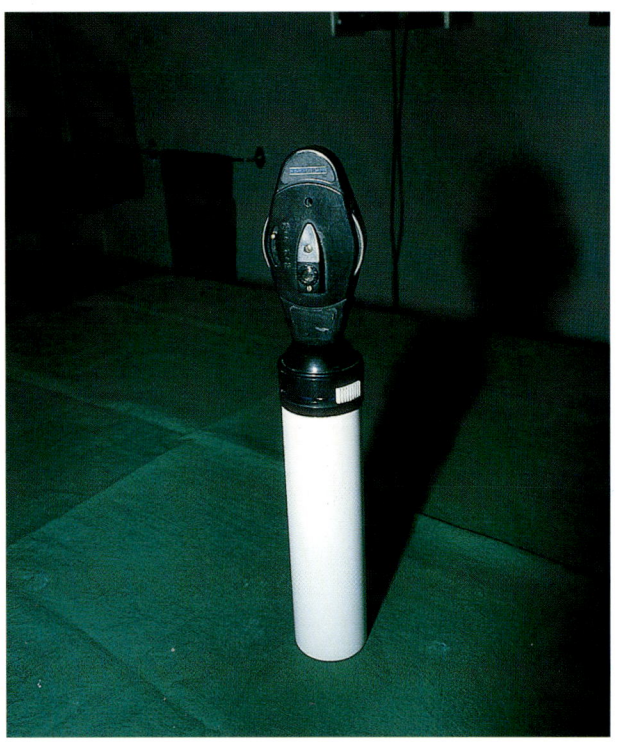

Fig. 1.3 Hand-held direct ophthalmoscope – examiner's side with dial for change of dioptres.

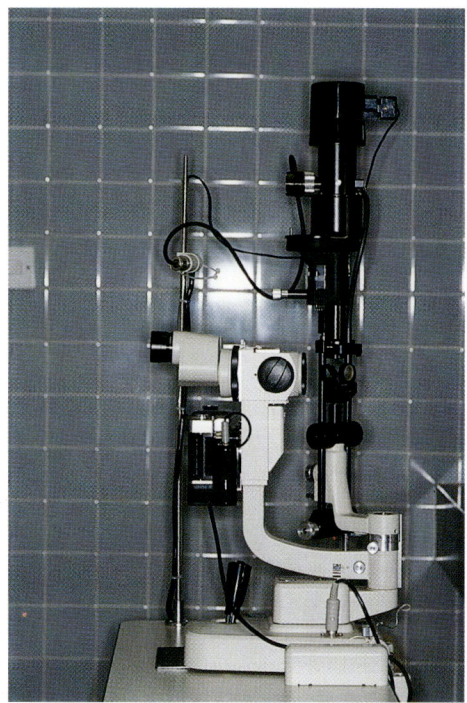

Fig. 1.5 Table-mounted slit-lamp biomicroscope with photographic attachment.

Further requirements are a topical anaesthetic solution for ocular use, such as 0.5% proxymetacaine hydrochloride (proparacaine), forceps suitable to hold and elevate the third eyelid (von Graefe's forceps or Bennett's distichia forceps) and nasolacrimal cannulae. Instruments that are usually only found in specialist practice are the slit-lamp biomicroscope (Figs 1.4 and 1.5), the head-mounted indirect ophthalmoscope (Fig. 1.6) with a large variety of fundus lenses (15, 30

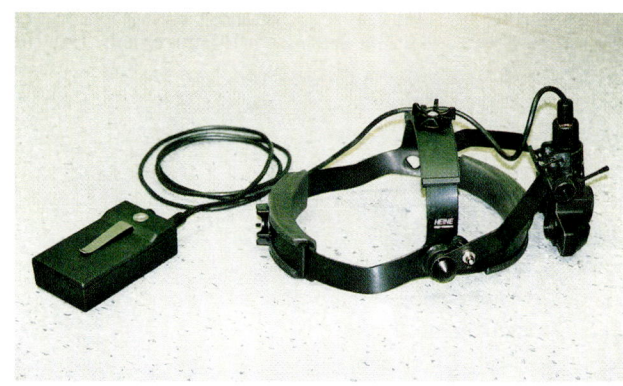

Fig. 1.6 Head-mounted indirect ophthalmoscope.

and 90 D as well as pan-retinal lenses) and the fundus camera.

HISTORY/SIGNALMENT/ANAMNESIS

The age, sex and breed of the patient must be established as they can give vital clues to diagnosis; this is of particular importance in veterinary ophthalmology because of the many hereditary eye diseases. Consideration of breed and coat colour is helpful to direct the clinician as to the appearance of iris or fundus to be expected and may help to distinguish normal variation from pathological presentation.

A brief but detailed history should be taken. This should address the patient's general health, previous illnesses and

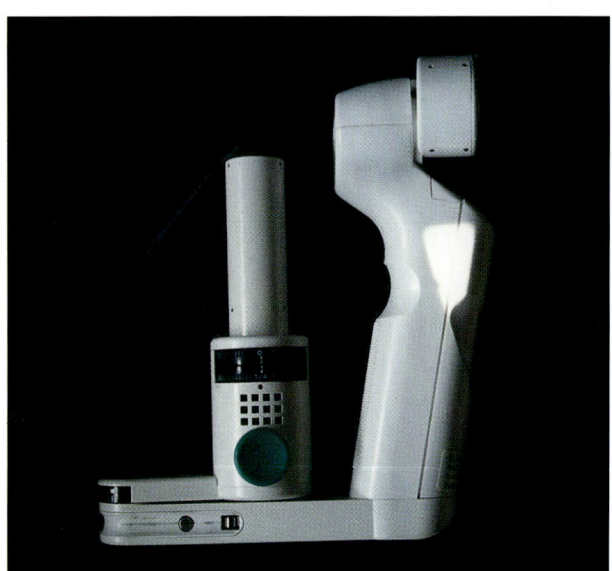

Fig. 1.4 Hand-held slit-lamp biomicroscope.

concurrent medications. Only then should the history be directed at the ocular problem and the clinician should establish the signs of ocular disease the dog is presented for, the time of onset and the rate of progression. It is essential to assess whether one or both eyes are affected, whether the patient is showing any signs of ocular discomfort or whether the owner has noticed any deterioration in sight.

DISTANCE INSPECTION

The next step is examination of the globe and its adnexa in daylight and with the help of a focal light source. It is important that a 'hands off' approach is chosen to begin with as any handling of the patient is likely to disturb the usual eyelid conformation. The patient should be assessed for facial asymmetry, the position of the globes within the orbit and the relationship of the globe to its adnexa. The blink rate should be noted as well as signs of ocular pain, and the quality and amount of discharges present should be recorded. Examination of the head from above may help to detect subtle cases of exophthalmos.

Following this initial assessment from a distance, a closer examination of the globe and adnexa is carried out. The lid conformation is assessed and the completeness of lid closure is noted. This part of the examination can be combined with the assessment of the menace and the corneal reflex (see Chapter 15). Especially in brachycephalic breeds, attention must be directed to the degree of lid movement and the possible presence of lagophthalmos.

SCHIRMER TEAR TEST

Before a closer examination of the globe and adnexa is performed, tear production is assessed with the Schirmer tear test. This test should be carried out in the conscious, unsedated dog and before tear production is falsely increased through manipulation of eye or adnexa. A strip of specifically designed filter paper is folded at the marked site approximately 5 mm from the tip and introduced into the ventral conjunctival fornix (Fig. 1.7). The paper strip is removed after 1 minute and the value of wetting is immediately read off the scale on the strip. Some manufacturers employ an indicator in their tear strips that changes colour when in contact with tears and makes easier reading of the value. The Schirmer tear test carried out routinely in the dog is performed without the application of local anaesthetic or other topical medications (Schirmer Tear Test 1) and represents both basal and reflex tear production. The Schirmer Tear Test 2, which is commonly carried out in people following topical anaesthesia, has not become popular in the dog, although studies have been carried out to establish mean values for the basal tear production in this species (Gelatt et al., 1975). A number of studies have been undertaken to evaluate mean Schirmer tear test readings for the dog and different Schirmer tear test strips from various manufacturers have been compared. In general it can be said that

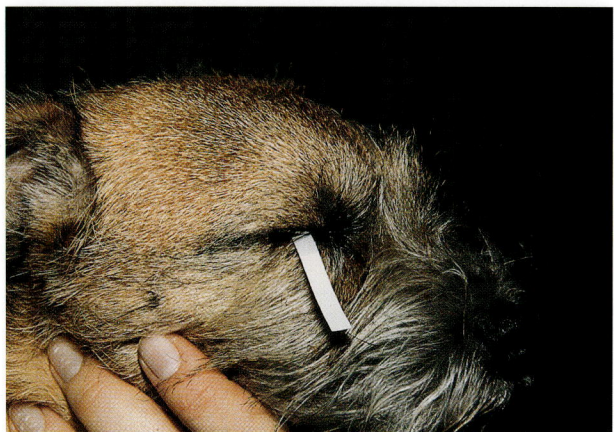

Fig. 1.7 Schirmer tear test carried out.

normal values for the Schirmer Tear Test 1 for the dog range from 15 to 25 mm of wetting (Strubbe and Gelatt, 1999). Schirmer tear test readings between 10 and 15 mm/min of wetting should raise concerns about the possible presence of insufficient tear production, whereas readings below 10 mm/min of wetting are considered pathognomonic for the presence of keratoconjunctivitis sicca.

CLOSE INSPECTION

Globe and adnexa are then closely examined with a focal light source. Care is taken to assess not only the outer lid surfaces but the lids are everted allowing inspection of the palpebral conjunctiva, meibomian glands and the conjunctival fornices (Fig. 1.8). The third eyelid can usually be protruded by gentle retropulsion of the globe through the upper eyelid. If required, a more detailed inspection of the posterior surface of the third eyelid can be carried out, following application of a topical anaesthetic, by grasping and elevating the third eyelid with the help of a pair of specially designed, atraumatic forceps such as the von Graefe's or Bennett's cilia forceps (Fig. 1.9).

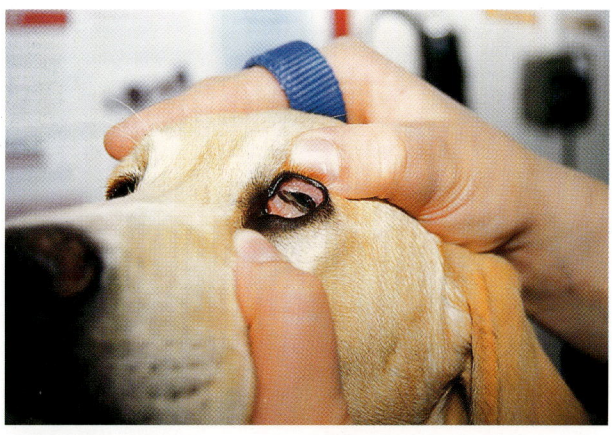

Fig. 1.8 Lid everted to allow inspection of palpebral conjunctiva, note meibomian glands visible through conjunctiva.

EXAMINATION OF THE EYE AND ADNEXA

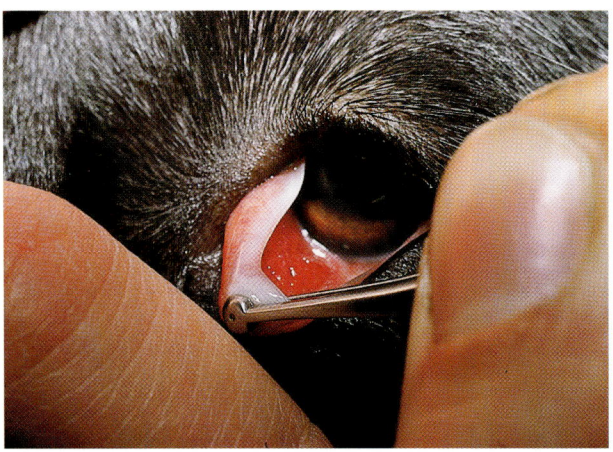

Fig. 1.9 Elevation of third eyelid with distichiasis forceps to allow inspection of the bulbar surface for inflammation or foreign bodies.

To check for a retrobulbar space-occupying lesion, both globes should be very gently retropulsed into the orbits and any resistance present should be noted. It is important to remember that retropulsion is usually restricted in brachycephalic animals due to the very shallow orbits in these breeds.

Focal light source

A focal light source is used to examine the adnexa and the cornea. The reflection of the light source on the cornea is called the Purkinje image and should present as a clear and bright mirror image of the light source itself (Fig. 1.10). In cases of ocular surface disease such as keratoconjunctivitis sicca or chronic superficial keratitis or ulceration, the image is blurred or broken (see Fig. 10.13). Further reflections of the light source can be seen on the anterior and posterior lens surface. These so-called parallax images can help to localise the depth of opacities within the eye. Both the image on the corneal surface, as well as the image on the anterior lens capsule, are upright and move with the light source as it is moved across the eye, whereas the image on the posterior lens capsule is inverted and moves in the opposite direction.

Direct and consensual light reflexes as well as the swinging flashlight test are assessed next. These tests are discussed in more detail in Chapter 15.

Examination in a darkened room

Direct ophthalmoscopy

For the following part of the ocular examination the room is darkened and the direct ophthalmoscope used on a setting of 0 D. At approximately an arm's length distance both fundus reflexes can be picked up in the normal patient (Fig. 1.11). With the help of the usually greenish yellow fundus reflection, anisocoria or opacities in the clear ocular media anterior to the retina can be detected (Fig. 1.12). The examination is continued as the examiner moves towards the patient as closely as possible (Fig. 1.13). Beginning with the optic nerve head, the entire fundus is scanned using a routine pattern, so ensuring that the whole area of fundus accessible with the ophthalmoscope is examined.

The direct ophthalmoscope allows examination of the fundus by giving a real, erect, upright and magnified image (approximately 15× magnification). Due to the small field of view examination of the peripheral retina is difficult.

Whilst the fundus in the emmetropic eye is in focus on a setting of 0 D, the lens will be in focus between 8 and 12 D and the cornea and adnexa with a setting of 20 D.

Indirect ophthalmoscopy

Indirect ophthalmoscopy can be carried out with the help of a bright, hand-held light source and a magnifying lens (Fig. 1.14) or with a head-mounted indirect binocular ophthalmoscope (Fig. 1.15). The latter technique not only allows the examiner to use both hands but also provides improved depth perception with binocular vision.

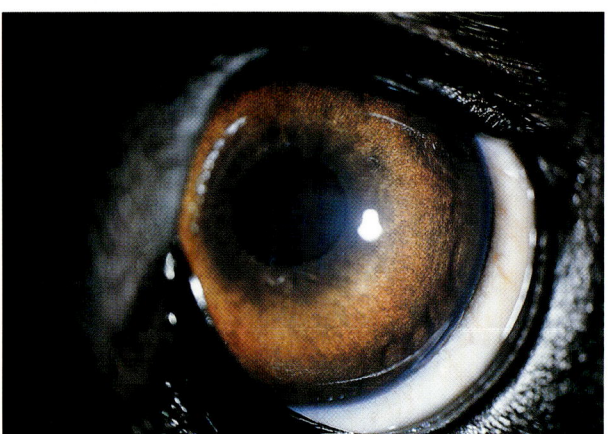

Fig. 1.10 Clear and sharp corneal Purkinje image.

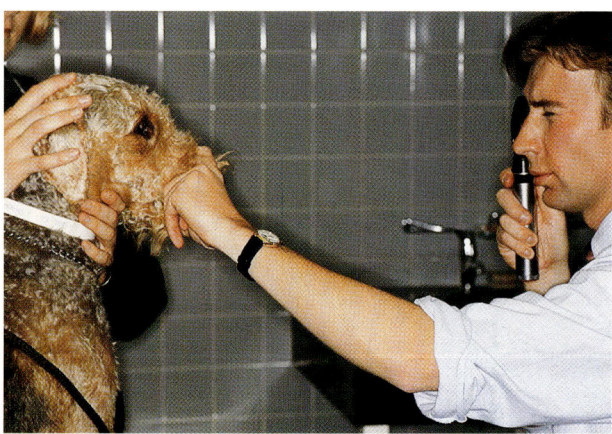

Fig. 1.11 Distant direct ophthalmoscopy – the fundus reflection is picked up from arm's length distance.

SLIT-LAMP EXAMINATION

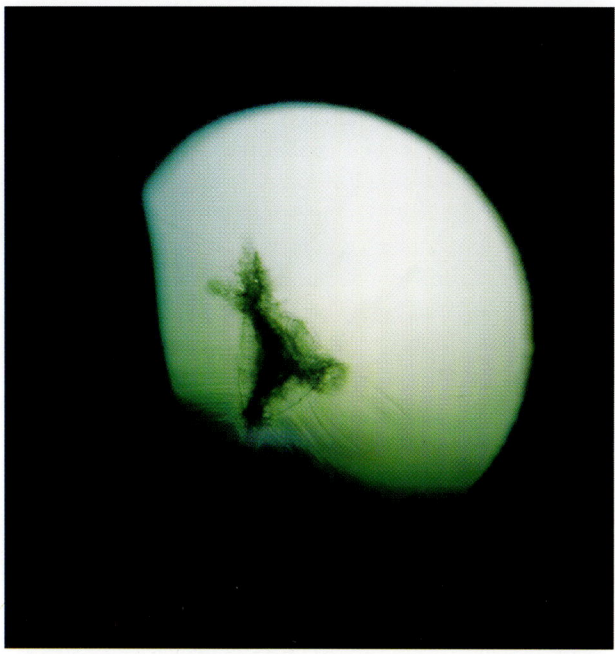

Fig. 1.12   Distant direct ophthalmoscopy – posterior polar cataract partially obscuring the fundus reflection.

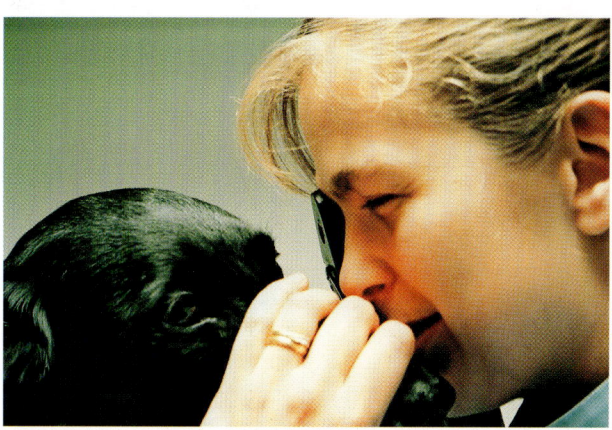

Fig. 1.13   Close direct ophthalmoscopy.

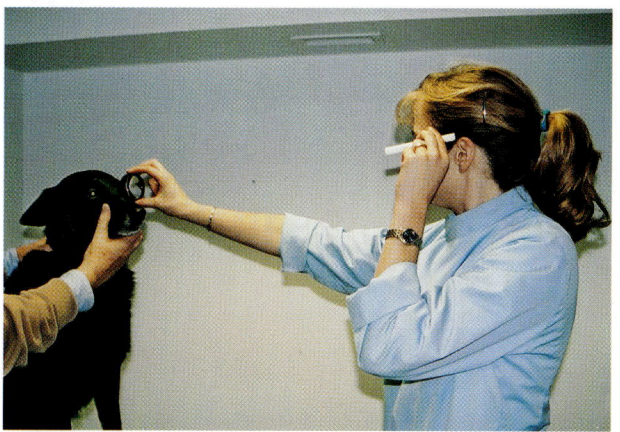

Fig. 1.14   Indirect ophthalmoscopy with pen torch and lens.

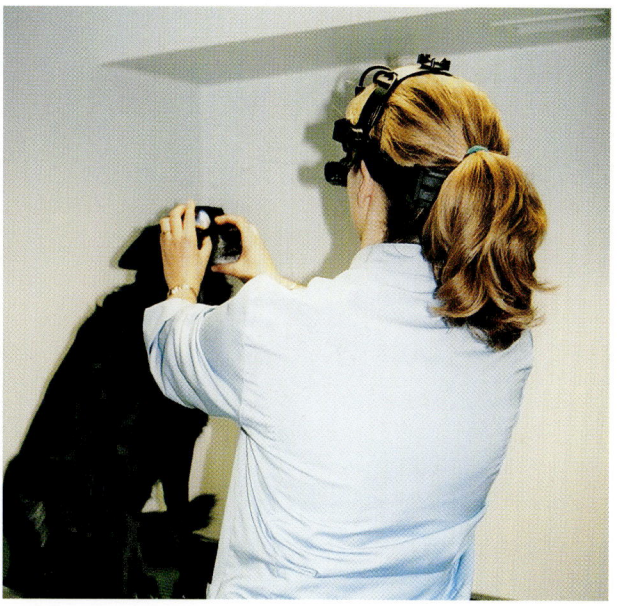

Fig. 1.15   Indirect ophthalmoscopy with the head-mounted indirect ophthalmoscope.

Indirect ophthalmoscopy should generally be carried out with the patient in mydriasis, although some of the newer head-mounted ophthalmoscopes employ special optics to allow examination through a small pupil. The application of a short-acting mydriatic (tropicamide, 1% Mydriacyl) should be considered but requires a 15-min delay before the examination can commence.

The picture seen with the indirect ophthalmoscope is virtual, inverted and upside down, which can present the inexperienced examiner with difficulties in localisation of a fundus lesion. The area of fundus shown is larger than with the direct ophthalmoscope and generally dependent on the type of magnifying lens used. The degree of magnification provided by a lens is inversely related to the area of field shown and the strength of the lens. A 15 D lens provides an approximately 5× magnified view of the fundus whereas a 30 D lens only provides approximately 2× magnification. This means that whereas the periphery of the fundus is easier to examine with indirect ophthalmoscopy, small lesions may be missed due to poorer detail caused by lower magnification.

A further instrument available for fundus examination is the monocular hand-held ophthalmoscope (Fig. 1.16) which, through an additional in-built lens, allows assessment of the fundus with an upright picture.

SLIT-LAMP EXAMINATION

The slit-lamp biomicroscope (see Fig. 1.4) is a versatile instrument consisting of a biomicroscope and a bright light source. Both are co-pivotal and con-focal and thus provide the examiner with a tool to examine ocular structures magnified and brightly illuminated (Martin, 1969a,b,c). Adnexal irregularities such as absent nasolacrimal punctae (see

EXAMINATION OF THE EYE AND ADNEXA

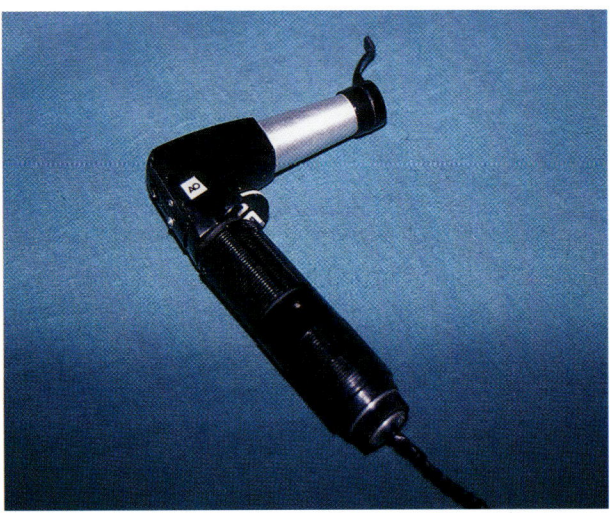

Fig. 1.16 Monocular hand-held indirect ophthalmoscope.

Fig. 7.2), micropuncta (see Fig. 7.4), distichia (see Fig. 5.30) or ectopic cilia (see Figs 5.31 and 5.32) can more easily be diagnosed. The slit lamp also allows the use of a slit beam to assess corneal thickness, depth of the anterior chamber and the localisation of lesions within cornea, anterior chamber and lens. An increased concentration of protein within the anterior chamber can be detected with the help of the slit beam producing Tyndall's phenomenon. With the help of a 90 D lens the slit-lamp biomicroscope can also be used for fundus examination.

Retinal camera

The hand-held fundus camera (Kowa) is used to document fundus lesions and is essential in fluorescein angiography (Bellhorn, 1973). In this test, fundus circulation can be observed following the injection of an intravenous dye, sodium fluorescein. The different phases of fluorescein circulation in the retinal and choroidal vasculature are documented with the help of specifically developed retinal cameras and filters and can aid in characterisation of both normal and abnormal vascular circulation (Gelatt *et al.*, 1976).

Tonometry

Assessment of the intraocular pressure should be a routine part of any ocular examination. Digital assessment of the intraocular pressure is unreliable and should be avoided. The Schiotz tonometer (see Fig. 10.1) represents an affordable instrument that, with some practice, provides the examiner with reliable readings (Gelatt, 1994). The Schiotz tonometer estimates the intraocular pressure by indentation tonometry and the reading obtained must be translated into an actual intraocular pressure value with the help of a conversion table. Care should be taken that the Schiotz tonometer is only placed onto the cornea in a horizontal position and that the jugular veins are not occluded during head elevation as this would result in falsely high readings.

Various instruments have been designed to allow assessment of the intraocular pressure by applanation tonometry. The most commonly used applanation tonometer in veterinary practice is the TonoPen (see Fig. 10.2), which is easy to use and provides exact readings for the intraocular pressure even in hydrophthalmic globes. A series of readings is obtained with the TonoPen and averaged electronically to display a mean intraocular pressure reading together with a coefficient of variance. Although a desirable instrument for every veterinary practice, the use of this instrument is restricted due its cost. Reference values for normal ranges of intraocular pressure in the dog have been established and range from 11 to 29 mmHg depending on the type of tonometer used.

Tonography is tonometry over an extended period of time. Tonography can be carried out as a non-invasive diagnostic procedure to estimate the coefficient of aqueous humour outflow, a value that gives information about the response to medication and decreases in aqueous humour outflow in glaucomatous patients.

Gonioscopy

Assessment of the ciliary cleft entrance is essential in the diagnosis, treatment and prevention of glaucoma. Visual inspection of this area is only possible in the dog (but not the cat) after a specifically designed contact lens is applied to the cornea (see Fig. 10.3). The test can usually be carried out in the conscious dog after the application of a topical anaesthetic. Structures assessed on gonioscopy are the pectinate ligaments and the width of the entrance to the ciliary cleft (Bedford, 1977).

Topical ophthalmic stains

Fluorescein sodium is the most commonly used topical ophthalmic stain. Presented as a bright orange solution in single use vials or as a coating on impregnated ocular strips, fluorescein changes colour to green once in contact with alkaline solutions. Fluorescein is a highly hydrophilic molecule and cannot penetrate the intact corneal epithelium. However, in the presence of epithelial defects, fluorescein is absorbed by the hydrophilic stroma and is thus used for the detection of corneal ulcers (Fig. 1.17). The area that has taken up fluorescein stain can be highlighted by the use of a cobalt blue light (Fig. 1.18). Care should be taken to flush superfluous amounts of fluorescein out of the eye as pooling of the stain in small depressions on the ocular surface could otherwise lead to falsely positive results. Fluorescein staining can also help to assess the depth of a corneal ulcer as Descemet's membrane is hydrophobic and does not take up stain.

Fluorescein is also used for the assessment of the nasolacrimal drainage and the tear break-up time.

SAMPLING TECHNIQUES FOR FURTHER INVESTIGATIVE TESTS

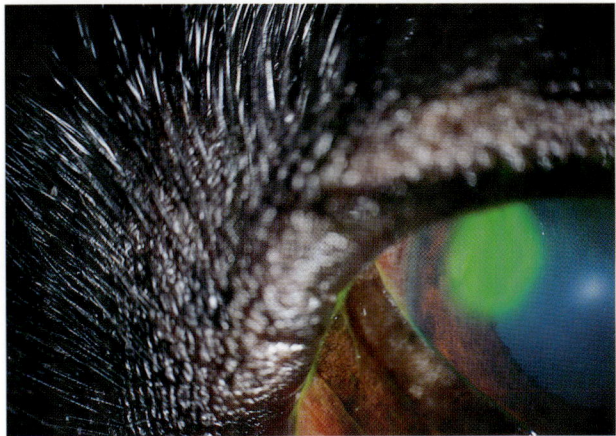

Fig. 1.17 Fluorescein staining a corneal ulcer.

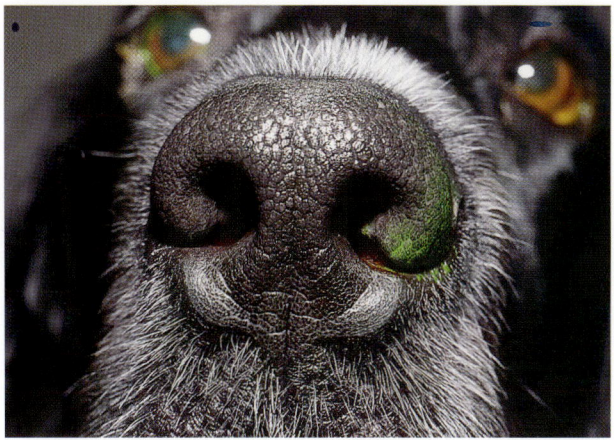

Fig. 1.19 Fluorescein drainage through the nasolacrimal duct.

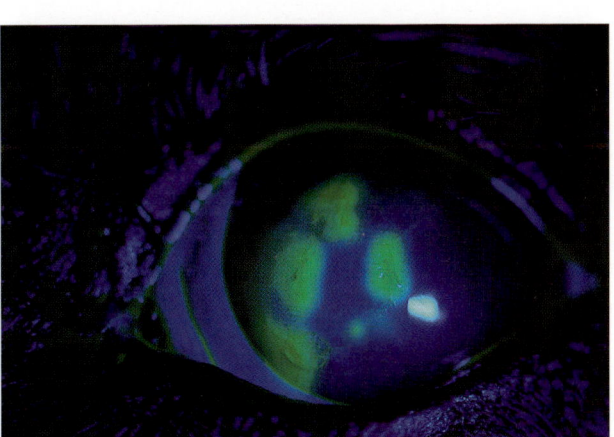

Fig. 1.18 Fluorescein uptake enhanced by cobalt blue light.

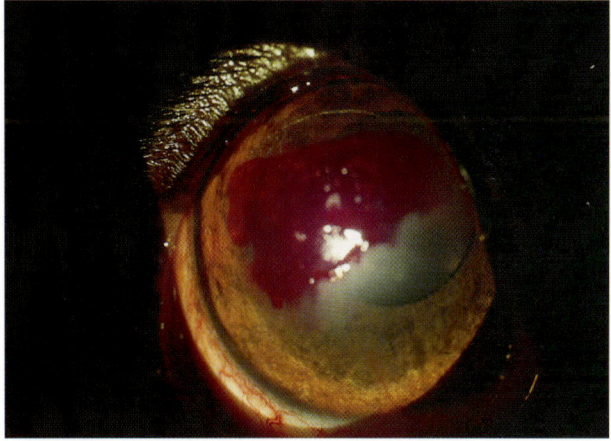

Fig. 1.20 Rose Bengal stained devitalised cells.

Following application of a generous amount of fluorescein into the conjunctival sac, stain is drained from the ocular surface through the nasolacrimal system. If stain can be detected up to 5 min after the application onto the corneal surface, a positive statement about the patency of the nasolacrimal system can be made (Fig. 1.19). However, absence of nasal staining is not diagnostic of an obstruction of the nasolacrimal system as in some dogs, the nasolacrimal duct drains into the oropharynx. Examination of the oral cavity may aid diagnosis in these patients.

The tear break-up time is a measurement for the integrity of the mucin layer of the precorneal tear film. After fluorescein has been applied to the eye, the patient is allowed to perform one blink before the lids are held open. The time that elapses until the tear film dissociates is recorded and should be around 20 seconds (Moore *et al.*, 1987).

Rose Bengal is another ophthalmic stain for topical use to assist in the diagnosis of preocular tear film disorders in the dog. At low doses, Rose Bengal will stain devitalised cells (Fig. 1.20) that are still contained within the epithelial context and mucins and may thus be a more sensitive indicator for tear film abnormalities than fluorescein. However, Rose Bengal causes local irritation and pain on instillation and its clinical applications are limited.

SAMPLING TECHNIQUES FOR FURTHER INVESTIGATIVE TESTS

Swabs for bacterial and mycological culture can be taken from the conjunctival fornix if infectious ocular disease is suspected. Previous suggestions that swabs should be taken prior to the application of local anaesthetic have proved to be unfounded. The instillation of a suitable local anaesthetic, such as 0.5% proxymetacaine hydrochloride, is not only acceptable prior to sampling (Champagne and Pickett, 1995; Massa *et al.*, 1999), but may also allow a more precise sampling technique. Samples for culture should be taken from the edge of the lesion in cases of ulcerative keratitis and, especially for fungal culture samples, must not be taken too superficially.

Samples for conjunctival cytology should be collected with a cytobrush (Bauer *et al.*, 1996; Wills *et al.*, 1997). A topical ocular anaesthetic, such as proxymetacaine hydrochloride, should be applied prior to sample collection, which is generally possible in the unsedated patient. Cytology of the corneal surface can be carried out on samples collected with the help of a Kimura spatula or the blunt end of a Bard Parker disposable scalpel blade. Smears are prepared directly onto the surface of a glass slide. The glass slide is air dried and fixed in methanol, and Diff-Quik, Gram and Giemsa stains can easily be carried out in general practice. Further slides may be submitted to commercial laboratories for special stains such as fungal or acid-fast stains.

Conjunctival or lid biopsies are easy to perform and can help to define further the disease process in cases of chronic inflammatory or proliferative conditions. Biopsies should generally be taken with the patient either lightly sedated or under general anaesthesia. Conjunctival biopsies can also be collected in the conscious patient following the repeated application of a local anaesthetic, but it should be remembered that the conjunctiva is heavily vascularised and bleeding is likely to follow surgical sampling.

Fine needle aspirates can be obtained from proliferative lesions of the adnexa or the retrobulbar area (Fig. 1.21) (Boydell, 1991). Careful interpretation is required of the samples obtained as they may not always be representative of the lesion and an experienced histopathologist should always be consulted (Strubbe and Gelatt, 1999).

Fine needle aspirates of uveal lesions, the aqueous humour and the vitreous can also be carried out. However, these procedures should be performed only in ophthalmic specialist practice.

Every enucleated eye should be forwarded for pathological examination. Histology of the ocular tissues may be valuable in confirmation of the clinical diagnosis and may help to give a clearer prognosis for the patient. It may also aid in the modification of treatment protocols in cases of neoplasia or in cases where the second eye may become involved. Enucleated eyes should be freed from all adnexa and immersed in an adequate amount of 10% formalin or glutaraldehyde.

References

Bauer GA, Spiess BM, Lutz H (1996) Exfoliative cytology of conjunctiva and cornea in domestic animals: A comparison of four collecting techniques. *Veterinary and Comparative Ophthalmology* **6**: 181–186.

Bedford PGC (1997) Gonioscopy in the dog. *Journal of Small Animal Practice* **18**: 615–629.

Bellhorn RW (1973) Fluorescein fundus photography in veterinary ophthalmology. *Journal of the American Animal Hospital Association* **9**: 227–233.

Boydell P (1991) Fine needle aspiration biopsy in the diagnosis of exophthalmos. *Journal of Small Animal Practice* **32**: 542–546.

Champagne ES, Pickett JP (1995) The effect of topical 0.5% proparacaine HCl on topical and conjunctival culture results. *Transactions of the American College of Veterinary Ophthalmologists* **26**: 144–145.

Gelatt KN (1994) Which tonometer? *Veterinary and Comparative Ophthalmology* **4**: 167–169.

Gelatt KN, Peiffer RL, Erickson JL, Gum GG (1975) Evaluation of tear formation in the dog, using a modification of the Schirmer tear test. *Journal of the American Veterinary Medical Association* **166**: 368–370.

Gelatt KN, Henderson JD, Steffen JR (1976) Fluorescein angiography of the normal and the diseased ocular fundi of the laboratory dog. *Journal of the American Veterinary Medical Association* **169**: 980–984.

Martin CL (1969a) Slit lamp examination of the normal canine anterior ocular segment. Part 1: Introduction and technique. *Journal of Small Animal Practice* **10**: 143–149.

Martin CL (1969b) Slit lamp examination of the normal canine anterior ocular segment. Part 2: Description. *Journal of Small Animal Practice* **10**: 151–162.

Martin CL (1969c) Slit lamp examination of the normal canine anterior ocular segment. Part 3: Discussion and summary. *Journal of Small Animal Practice* **10**: 163–169.

Massa KL, Murphy CJ, Hartmann FA, Miller PE, Korsower CS, Young KM (1999) Usefulness of aerobic microbial culture and cytologic evaluation of corneal specimens in the diagnosis of infectious ulcerative keratitis in animals. *Journal of the American Veterinary Medical Association* **11**: 1671–1674.

Moore CP, Wilsman NJ, Nordheim EV, Majors LJ, Collier LL (1987) Density and distribution of canine conjunctival goblet cells. *Investigative Ophthalmic and Visual Sciences* **28**: 1925–1932.

Strubbe DH and Gelatt KN (1999) Ophthalmic Examination and Diagnostic Procedures. In KN Gelatt (Endothelial dystrophy): Veterinary Ophthalmology. Lippincott, Williams and Wilkins, Baltimore, Maryland: 427–466.

Wills M, Bounous DI, Hirsh S, et al. (1997) Conjunctival brush cytology: Evaluation of a new cytological collection technique in dogs and cats with a comparison to conjunctival scraping. *Veterinary and Comparative Ophthalmology* **7**: 74–81.

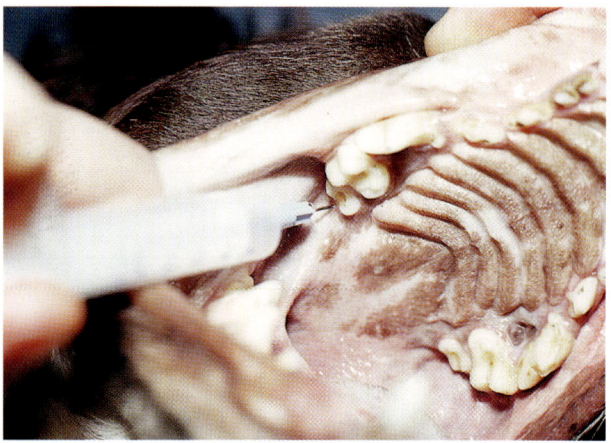

Fig. 1.21 Fine needle aspirate taken from the retrobulbar area – needle placement behind the last molar tooth.

2 Postnatal development of the eye

Introduction

The period of gestation in the dog is 60–63 days for all breeds, there being no difference between toy and giant breeds. Puppies are born with the eyes (and ears) closed and in a relatively early stage of development, similar to the kitten, but quite unlike the foal, calf and lamb where the eye is open at birth, the cornea is clear, there is no persistence of the pupillary membrane and an adult appearance of the fundus.

The following descriptions of the postnatal development of the canine eye have been compiled from the examination of several litters of Border Collie, Cavalier King Charles Spaniel, Miniature Longhaired Dachshund, Golden Retriever and Greyhound puppies. There is some variation in the timing of all the developmental changes that occur. These differences in timing may be found in different litters and also in individuals in the same litter and even between the two eyes of the same puppy. Often, as might be expected, the runt of the litter is not so well developed in its fundus as its littermates. In spite of these differences there is always a regular development of all parts of the eye and it is important that these changes are recognised, particularly tapetal development in the fundus, for the early diagnosis of such congenital and hereditary abnormalities as collie eye anomaly and retinal dysplasia.

Clinical description

Normally at birth the eyelids are fused together (Fig. 2.1), the eyes opening at anything from 1 to 2 weeks and usually 7–10 days. On opening, the cornea is cloudy because of corneal oedema (Fig. 2.2) and it is difficult to examine any detail of the interior of the globe. Clearing takes place slowly, the cornea being still a little hazy as late as 21 days of age, final clearing occurring at between 3 and 4 weeks.

At 21 days the iris is a pale grey-blue in colour and steadily darkens and slowly changes to the adult dark brown colour by 6 to 8 weeks. As soon as the cornea has cleared the pupillary membrane is visible as a spider's web-like structure within the whole pupil. At about 18–21 days the pupillary membrane appears well developed, covering most of the pupil (Fig. 2.3) but sometimes with a clear central region where atrophy first occurs (Fig. 2.4). Further loss of membrane from the centre takes place by 28–35 days, only fine filaments remaining around the periphery of the pupil (Figs 2.5–2.7),

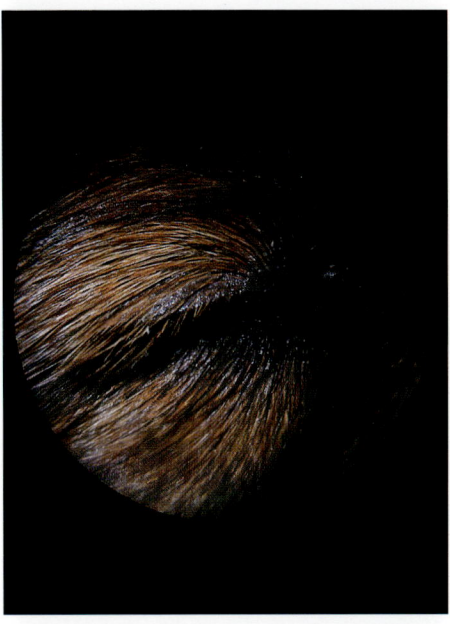

Fig. 2.1 Eyelids still fused in a 10-day-old Miniature Longhaired Dachshund.

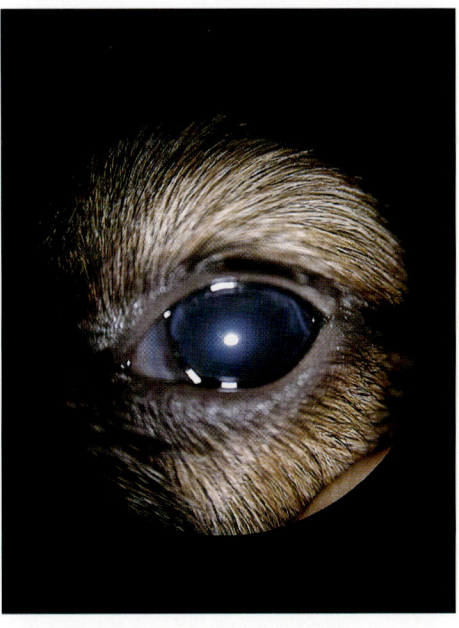

Fig. 2.2 Eyes just open in a 15-day-old Miniature Longhaired Dachshund. Note corneal oedema.

POSTNATAL DEVELOPMENT OF THE EYE

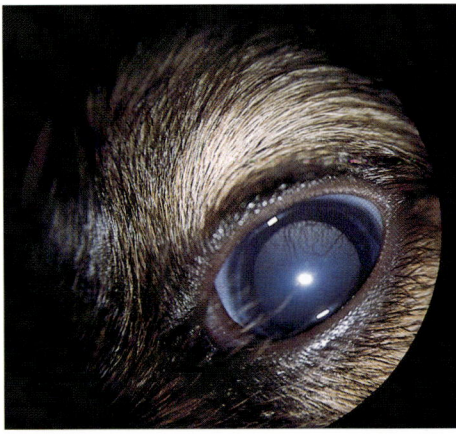

Fig. 2.3 Eye open in an 18-day-old Miniature Longhaired Dachshund. Note mild cloudiness of cornea, grey-brown iris and pupillary membrane covering most of pupil.

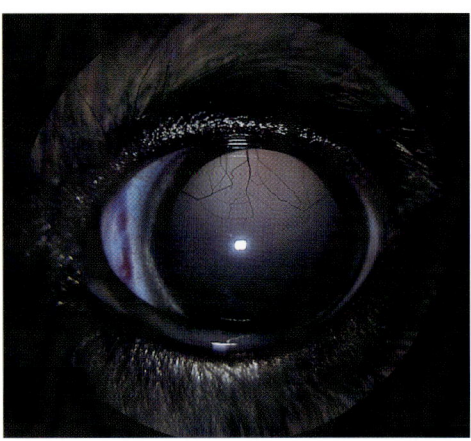

Fig. 2.6 Pupillary membranes fine and sparse in upper part of pupil in a 42-day-old Miniature Longhaired Dachshund.

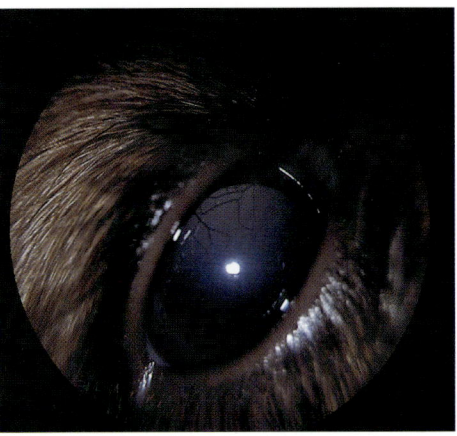

Fig. 2.4 Cornea now almost clear but pupillary membrane visible in most of pupil in a 21-day-old Miniature Longhaired Dachshund.

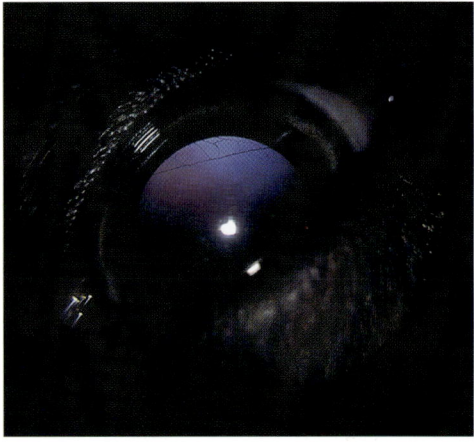

Fig. 2.7 Few remnants of pupillary membrane in superior pupil in a 45-day-old Border Collie. Note lilac colour of developing tapetal fundus.

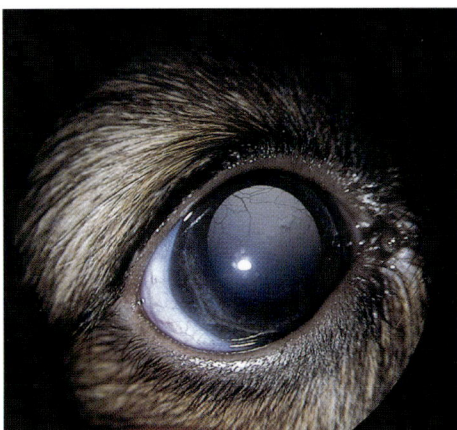

Fig. 2.5 Pupillary membrane still visible at the edge of the pupil in a 28-day-old Miniature Longhaired Dachshund. Note future tapetal fundus appearing paler above darker non tapetal fundus.

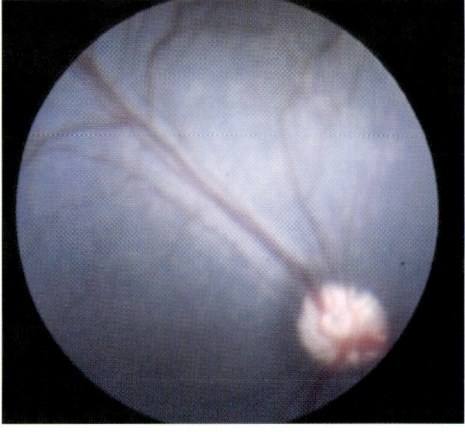

Fig. 2.8 Very early fundus appearance showing no differentiation between tapetal and non-tapetal regions in a 28-day-old Miniature Longhaired Dachshund.

CLINICAL DESCRIPTION

and by 5 to 8 weeks the whole pupillary membrane has disappeared and the pupil is clear.

Ophthalmoscopic examination of the fundus is difficult before 21 days because of the corneal oedema, pupillary membrane and lack of fundus details. At 3 weeks it is just possible to see large blood vessels, but no differentiation between future tapetal and non-tapetal areas (Fig. 2.8) and absolutely no tapetal development. From about 28 days the non-tapetal fundus takes on a darker grey-brown colour than the future tapetum lucidum (Fig. 2.9), which by 5 to 8 weeks of age appears a homogeneous lilac or violet colour (Figs 2.10–2.14). Darkening of the non-tapetal fundus continues and from 6 to 8 weeks onwards the developing tapetal fundus takes on its adult appearance with a mosaic pattern

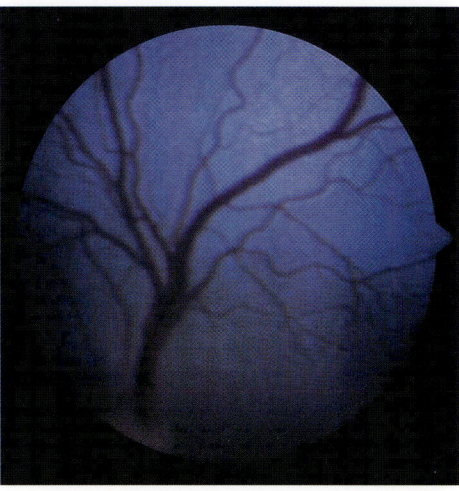

Fig. 2.11 Early lilac tapetal fundus in a 43-day-old Border Collie.

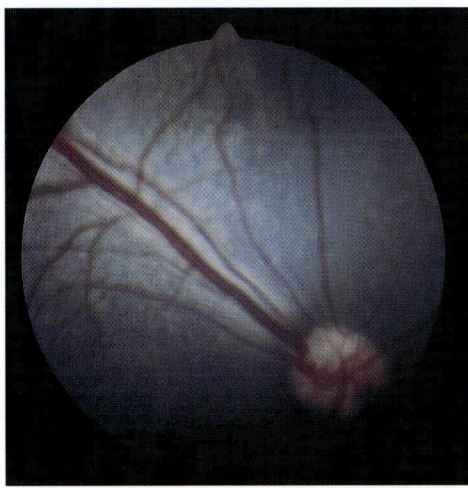

Fig. 2.9 Clear distinction between tapetal and non-tapetal fundus regions but no tapetal development so far in a 33-day-old Miniature Longhaired Dachshund.

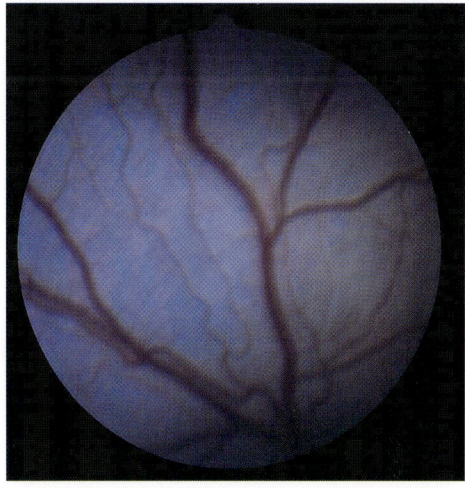

Fig. 2.12 Lilac tapetal region and darkening of non-tapetal region in a 44-day-old Border Collie.

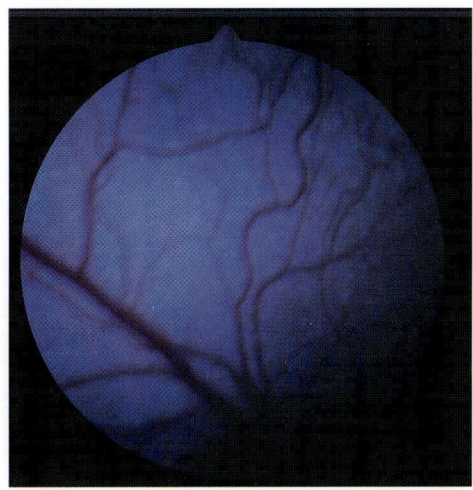

Fig. 2.10 Early violet colour of future tapetal fundus in a 36-day-old Miniature Longhaired Dachshund.

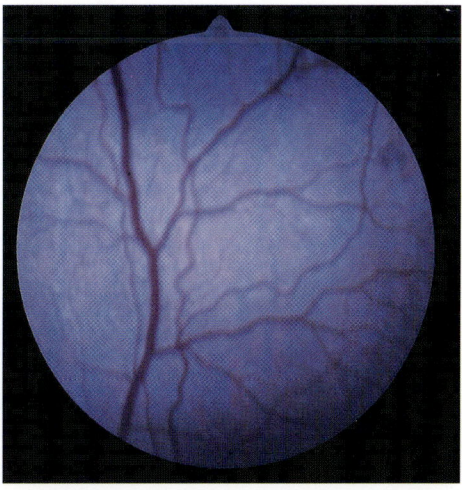

Fig. 2.13 Darker lilac tapetal region with normal choroidal vessels still visible in a 44-day-old Border Collie (littermate of puppy in Fig. 2.12).

POSTNATAL DEVELOPMENT OF THE EYE

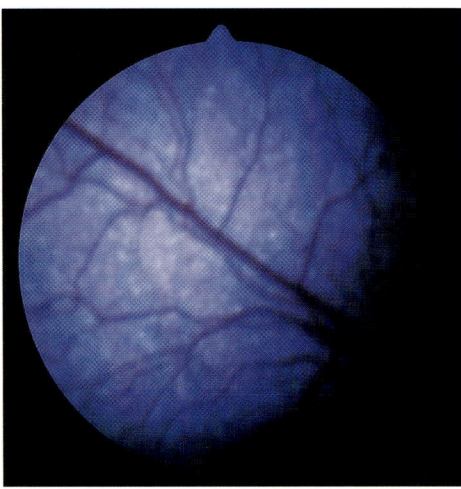

Fig. 2.14 Violet tapetal region with early mosaic pattern in a 44-day-old Miniature Longhaired Dachshund.

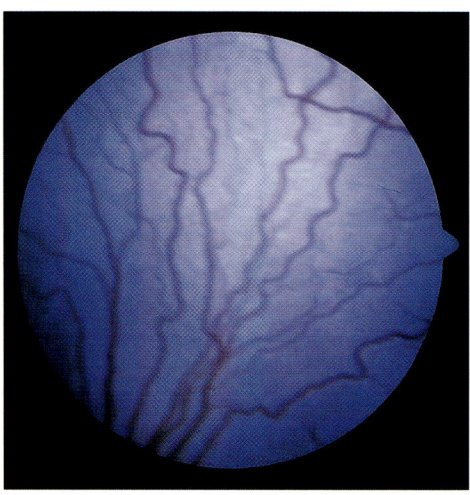

Fig. 2.16 Very early lilac colour in tapetal fundus in a 52-day-old Miniature Longhaired Dachshund.

and green coloration (Figs 2.15–2.21); by 12 to 16 weeks of age the fundus exhibits its adult form with full tapetal development (Fig. 2.22). The early diagnosis of chorioretinal dysplasia and the presence of retinal folds in multifocal retinal dysplasia, both of which are congenital and hereditary canine eye abnormalities (see Chapter 14), are related to tapetal development; for the accurate diagnosis of mild cases of both these conditions the appearance of the developing fundus must be understood and the minor variations in timing between individuals recognised.

Suture-line opacities, by definition cataracts although only temporary, are not uncommon in puppies. They are usually bilateral, although not necessarily symmetrical, and commonly occur between 3 and 4 months of age (Figs 2.23 and 2.24). They are to be found as arrowhead-like opacities at the ends of the suture lines at 12, 4 and 8 o'clock anteriorly and 2, 6

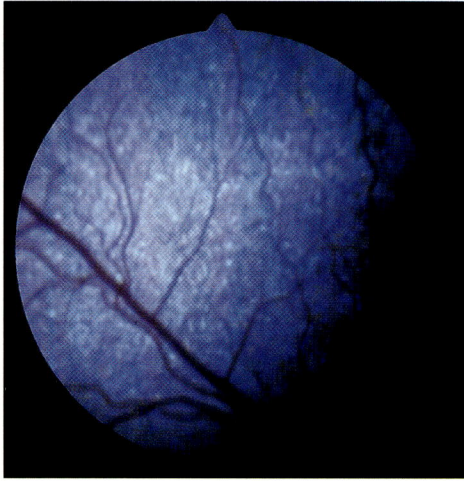

Fig. 2.17 Early tapetal colours in a 49-day-old Miniature Longhaired Dachshund (different litter from puppy in Fig. 2.16).

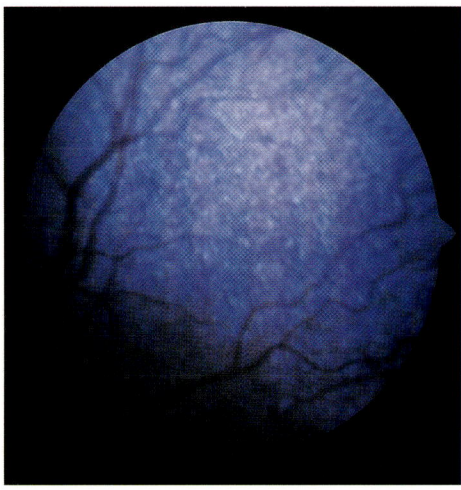

Fig. 2.15 Early tapetal colours in a 44-day-old Border Collie.

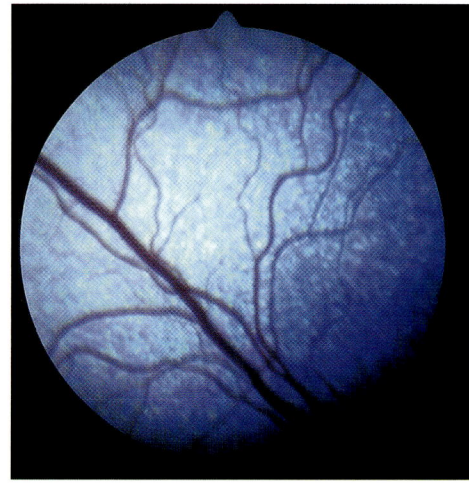

Fig. 2.18 More advanced tapetal colours in a 52-day-old Miniature Longhaired Dachshund.

CLINICAL DESCRIPTION

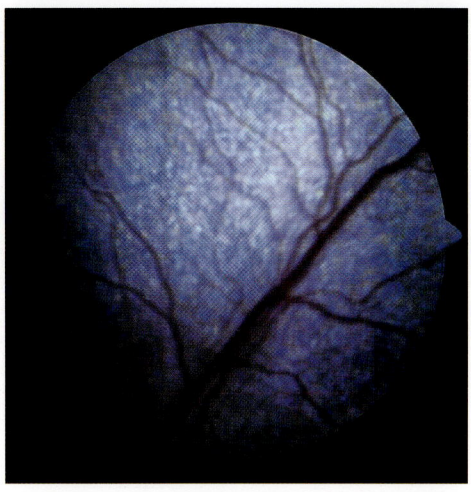

Fig. 2.19 Adult tapetal pattern now obvious in an 8-week-old Miniature Longhaired Dachshund.

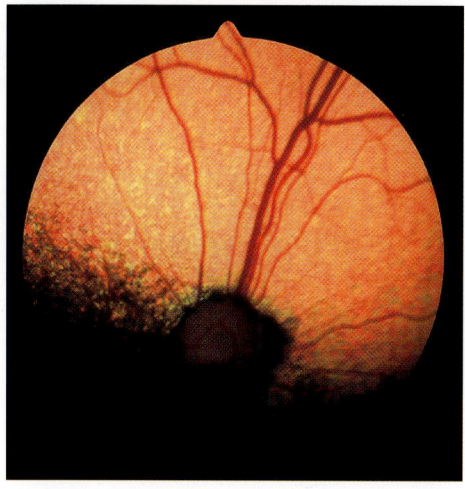

Fig. 2.22 Full tapetal development in a 16-week-old Miniature Longhaired Dachshund.

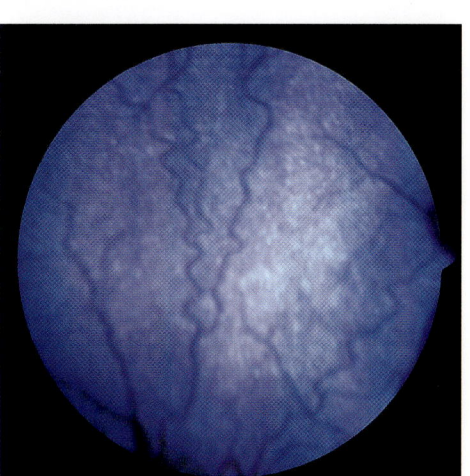

Fig. 2.20 Tapetal region not as advanced as Fig. 2.19 in an 8-week-old Cavalier King Charles Spaniel.

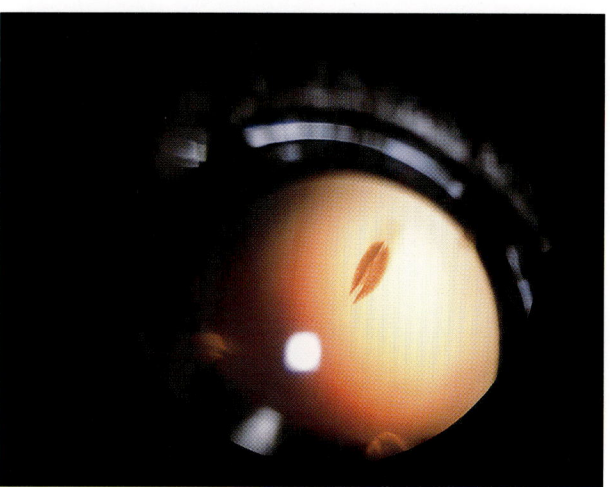

Fig. 2.23 Suture line opacities in posterior cortex at 12, 4 and 8 o'clock in a 4-month-old Miniature Longhaired Dachshund.

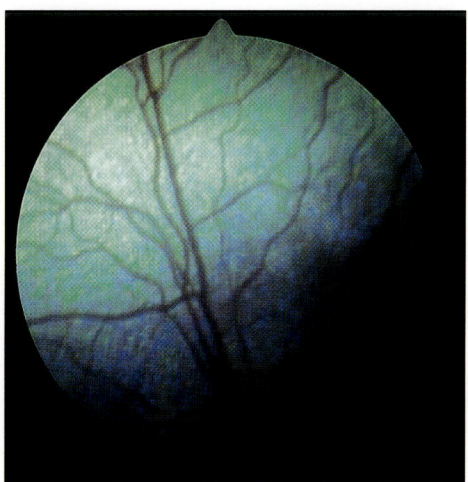

Fig. 2.21 Good development of tapetal region in an 8-week-old Miniature Longhaired Dachshund.

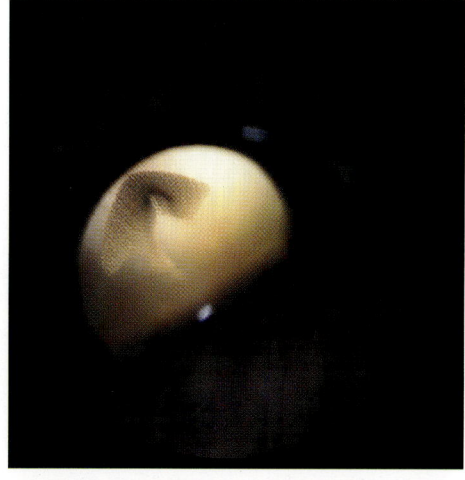

Fig. 2.24 Large arrowhead opacity in a 3-month-old Miniature Longhaired Dachshund (different litter from Fig. 2.23).

and 10 o'clock posteriorly. It is more usual to find three than six separate opacities in a lens and they seem to be more common in some breeds than others. They have been confused with congenital and early onset hereditary cataracts but this confusion should not occur if their position and form are taken into account. These opacities invariably disappear by about 9 to 12 months of age.

For descriptions of the histological development of the canine eye and retina see Aguirre *et al.* (1972) and Parry (1953).

The postnatal growth of the globe, as measured by B-mode ultrasonography, is described in Chapter 4.

References

Aguirre GD, Rubin LF, Bistner SI (1972) Development of the canine eye. *American Journal of Veterinary Research* **33**: 2399–2414.

Parry HB (1953) Degeneration of the dog retina. I Structure and development of the retina of the normal dog. *British Journal of Ophthalmology* **37**: 385–403.

3 Ocular emergencies and trauma

Blunt trauma (orbit and globe)

Blunt trauma to the orbit and globe is often associated with head trauma as in road traffic accidents, but can also occur after being kicked or, for example, being hit by a ball or golf club (Figs 3.1–3.4). Some of these may be multitraumatised patients and their overall condition must be stabilised before the eyes and the orbit can be properly assessed. Analgesia,

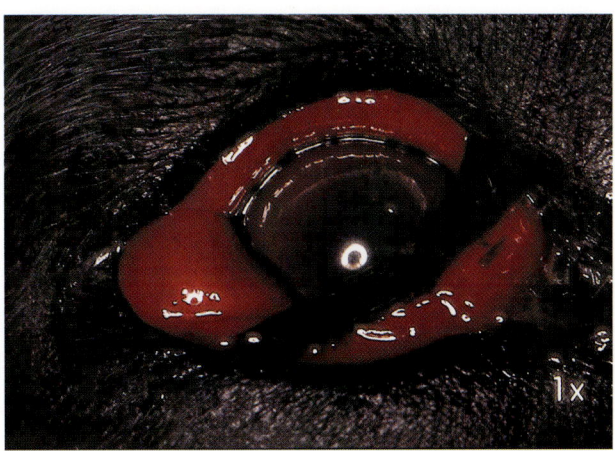

Fig. 3.1 Blunt trauma to the eye of a young Labrador accidentally hit with a golf club. Note severe subconjunctival haemorrhage and miotic pupil due to concurrent uveitis.

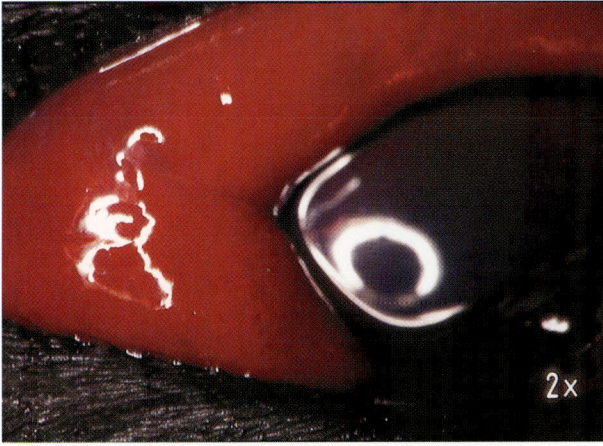

Fig. 3.2 Same case as in Fig. 3.1. Note severe chemosis and mild corneal oedema.

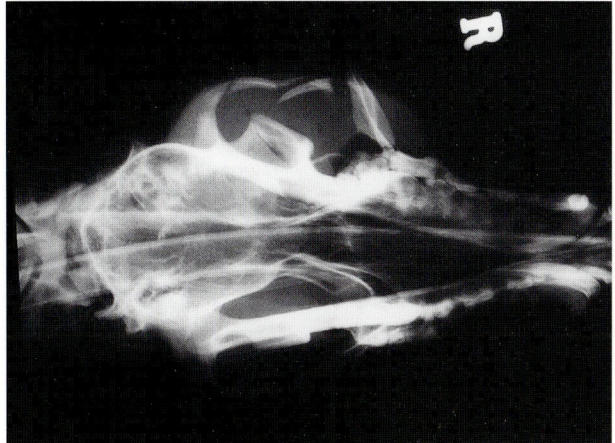

Fig. 3.3 Comminuted fracture of the right zygomatic arch in a German Shorthaired Pointer kicked by a horse. Ultrasound examination revealed no retrobulbar haematoma.

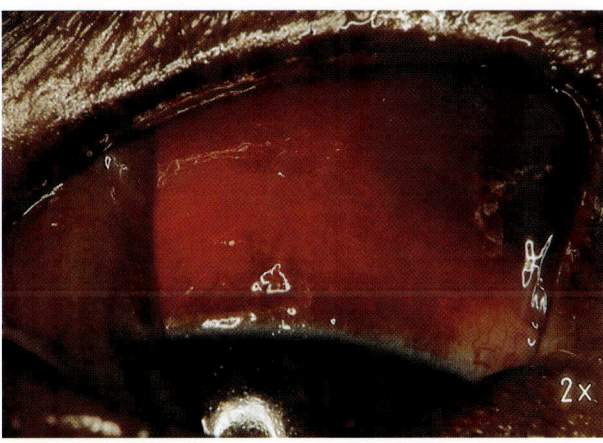

Fig. 3.4 Bulbar conjunctival and scleral haemorrhage in a young Rhodesian Ridgeback. Severe head trauma after falling into a quarry.

sedation and protection of the ocular surface are primary considerations.

Orbital haematomas usually cause acute exophthalmos with secondary lagophthalmos (incomplete blinking) and desiccation and ulceration of the ocular surface are potential complications. The ocular surface should be cleansed and kept moist with a bland ophthalmic ointment. A temporary tarsorraphy is helpful to prevent exposure keratitis until the

15

haematoma resorbs. Nonsteroidal anti-inflammatory drugs may increase the risk of further haemorrhage and anti-inflammatory doses of systemic corticosteroids are preferable.

Clinical signs of orbital fractures include pain, facial asymmetry, exophthalmos or enophthalmos and retrobulbar/periocular haemorrhage. Closed orbital fractures with little displacement require only cage rest, analgesia, anti-inflammatory treatment and soft food. Healing is usually uncomplicated. Internal surgical fixation and systemic antibiotic therapy are generally indicated for fractures which are open, grossly displaced, or affecting the position of the globe.

Subconjunctival haemorrhages occur when the subconjunctival vessels rupture above the relatively stiff sclera. They normally resorb of their own accord over 5–10 days.

Damage to the intraocular structures can be severe with blunt trauma. Tearing of the lens zonules results in dislocation of the lens either anteriorly or posteriorly into the vitreous. Hyphaema (blood in the anterior chamber) occurs secondary to ciliary body or iris damage and may be accompanied by large intravitreal and retinal haemorrhages. Retinal tears and detachment are not uncommon.

Rupture of the globe itself can occur with blunt as well as penetrating trauma. Although such damage may be visible in the anterior segment, posterior scleral ruptures are 'hidden' but should be suspected in eyes with marked hypotony and pain. Ocular ultrasonography is very helpful but computed tomography (CT) and magnetic resonance imaging (MRI) techniques have demonstrated excellent detail of ocular and orbital structures when ultrasonographic findings were inconclusive in patients that had suffered head trauma (Figs 3.5–3.7).

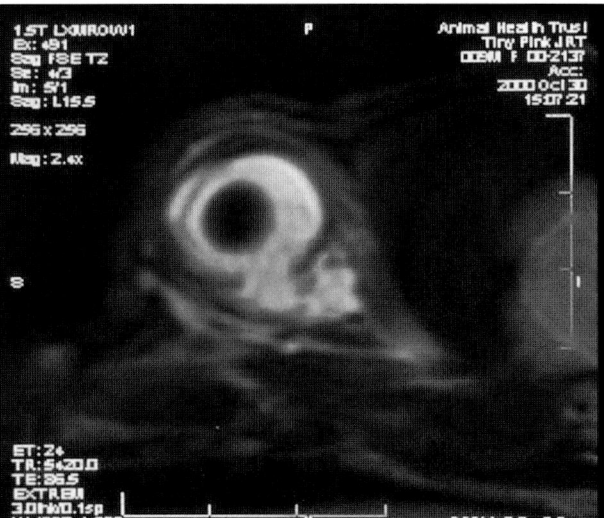

Fig. 3.6 Young Jack Russell Terrier presenting with marked ocular pain and total hyphaema following a road traffic accident. Sagittal MRI scan shows posterior scleral rupture with escape of vitreous into the retrobulbar space.

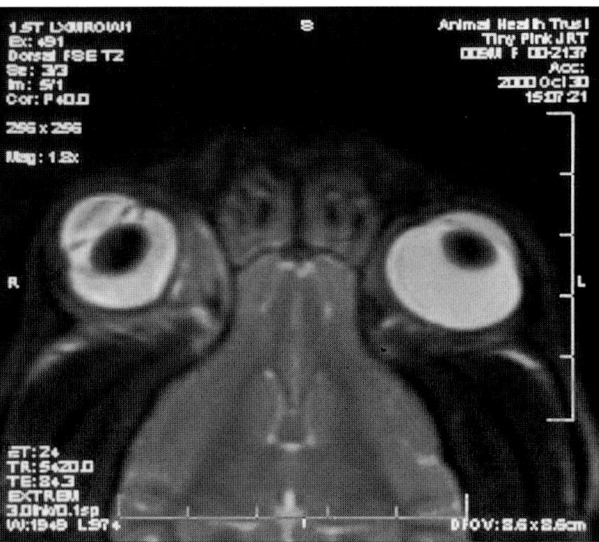

Fig. 3.7 Transverse MRI scan of the same dog as in Fig. 3.6. The scleral rupture is not evident on this view but the globe is obviously distorted and the iris leaflets displaced, together with posterior lens luxation into the vitreous.

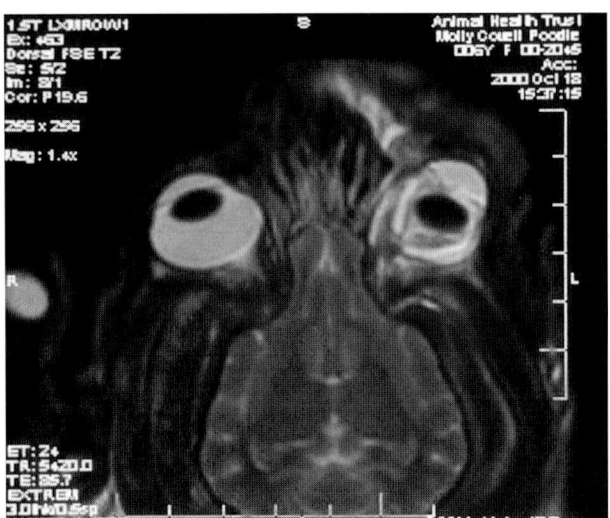

Fig. 3.5 MRI scan showing posterior globe rupture in a middle-aged Miniature Poodle presented for neurological assessment following a road traffic accident. Total hyphaema was obvious but ocular ultrasonography was inconclusive. The MRI scan was performed for suspected head trauma and revealed rupture in the posterior sclera, caudal luxation of the lens and increased depth of the anterior chamber on the right side. The left eye is normal.

Sudden changes in globe position

Changes in globe position are commonly presented as urgent cases, if not as true emergencies. Prompt diagnosis is important as some conditions, for example a retrobulbar abscess, do require immediate treatment, whereas in others, such as Horner's syndrome, treatment can be deferred until a definite diagnosis is reached.

BLUNT TRAUMA (ORBIT AND GLOBE)

SUDDEN ONSET EXOPHTHALMOS

Retrobulbar abscess/cellulitis

The typical presentation is acute onset, unilateral exophthalmos with protrusion of the third eyelid, chemosis and marked pain on opening the mouth. The eye itself is usually normal, although intraocular pressure can be raised due to the increase in intraorbital pressure and episcleral vessels are often congested due to obstructed venous drainage. Affected dogs are usually anorexic, depressed and may be pyrexic. The pupillary light reflex should be unaffected but can be slow or absent in severe cases due to optic nerve neuropraxia from the increased intraorbital pressure. Examination, which may need to be performed under general anaesthesia due to the discomfort, often reveals an area of inflammation and swelling in the pterygopalatine fossa, i.e. behind the last ipsilateral molar tooth.

These typical clinical signs are pathognomonic for orbital inflammatory disease and ocular ultrasonography is extremely useful to obtain further information. Plain skull radiography is generally unhelpful but MRI or CT imaging is beneficial in selected, difficult cases.

Management as with any abscess in the body, drainage is the most important step in appropriate management. Under general anaesthesia, an incision is made in the oral mucosa over the swollen area behind the last upper molar but should only be attempted when there is visible swelling in the pterygopalatine fossa (Fig. 3.8). A closed haemostat is gently advanced through the incision aiming towards the retrobulbar area and slowly opened slightly and then withdrawn (Fig. 3.9). Bacterial culture and sensitivity should be performed on the haemorrhagic, purulent material which is released. *Pasteurella* is a common isolate (Rühli and Spiess, 1995). The release of copious purulent material is very satisfying but does not always occur, as in cases of cellulitis, which will still subsequently improve with anti-inflammatory

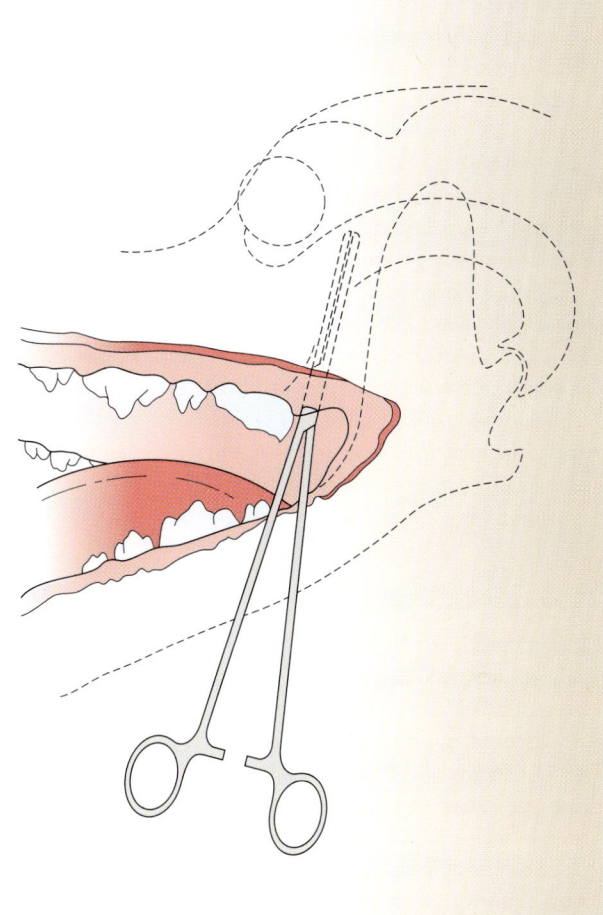

Fig. 3.9 Drainage of retrobulbar abscess.

and antibiotic therapy. Soft food is beneficial and chewing movements will 'massage' abscess contents and encourage drainage via the oropharynx. Blind probing of the retrobulbar space is not without risk as this area has a rich vascular and nerve supply and complications have been reported (Rühli and Spiess, 1995) but are fortunately unusual. Irrigation of the retrobulbar area is unnecessary.

Systemic broad spectrum antibiotics are prescribed for 10–14 days and nonsteroidal anti-inflammatory drugs are indicated until the globe returns to a normal position. An increase in the degree of exophthalmos and periorbital swelling is common after drainage, but can be alarming to the veterinarian if unexpected. Topical ophthalmic lubricants, and maybe a temporary tarsorraphy, are indicated until the swelling resolves, usually within 48–72 hours. The prognosis is very good, with most cases healing within 1 week. Recurrence is usually associated with retention of foreign material in the orbit.

Myositis

Myositis usually presents as an acute onset of bilateral exophthalmos with protrusion of the third eyelid, conjunctival and episcleral congestion and pain on opening the mouth or on

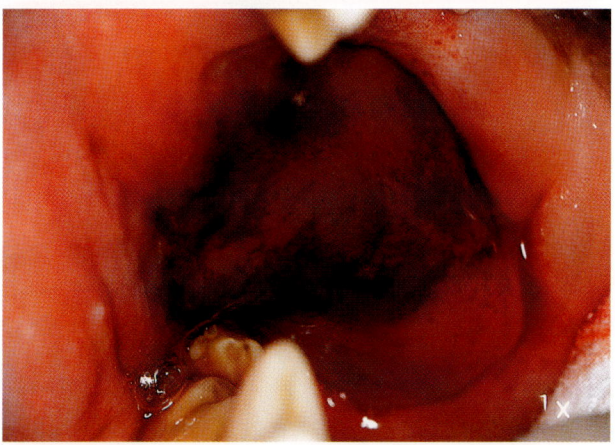

Fig. 3.8 Inflammation, swelling and discoloration of the pterygopalatine fossa in a Springer Spaniel with a large retrobulbar abscess.

OCULAR EMERGENCIES AND TRAUMA

palpation of the temporal muscles. The bilateral nature of the condition differentiates it from retrobulbar abscess/cellulitis, which is typically unilateral. Breed predisposition, eosinophilic myositis in German Shepherd dogs and Weimaraners, and extraocular polymyositis in Golden Retrievers, is also helpful (Carpenter *et al.*, 1989). Ultrasonography, CT or MRI imaging will reveal swollen extraocular muscles in cases of extraocular polymyositis. Haematology, biochemistry and muscle biopsy for histopathology can also be performed. Prednisolone at 1–2 mg/kg should be administered immediately and continued for several weeks in response to improvement of clinical signs. In refractory cases azathioprine 1–2 mg/kg may also be given in combination with the oral prednisolone.

The prognosis is guarded as recurrence is not uncommon and, if uncontrolled, atrophy of the affected muscles and associated problems such as enophthalmos, strabismus, entropion and third eyelid protrusion may occur (Whitney, 1970).

Sialoadenitis

Inflammation of the zygomatic salivary gland (Fig. 3.10), salivary retention cysts and mucocele formation can all present as sudden onset exophthalmos with third eyelid protrusion and minimal pain on opening the mouth (Simison, 1993). Diagnosis is based on clinical signs, ultrasonography and aspiration of yellow, tenacious fluid from the pterygopalatine fossa. The exophthalmos will resolve if the cyst is drained effectively. Mucoceles are managed by surgical resection. Drainage is indicated in cases of salivary retention cysts and sialoadenitis, in conjunction with systemic anti-inflammatory drugs and broad spectrum antibiotics.

Episcleritis

Diffuse inflammation of the scleral tunic with posterior and choroidal involvement is an uncommon cause of rapid onset exophthalmos (Figs 3.11 and 3.12). Referral is recommended as diagnosis and management are not straightforward (see also Chapter 8).

Pulsatile/intermittent exophthalmos

Vascular anomalies have been reported rarely in the dog. Most cases are congenital and are seen in young dogs. In older dogs they are acquired and are usually secondary to trauma. In the few reported cases dogs present with non-painful, pulsatile, intermittent exophthalmos which may be markedly exacerbated by exercise. Enophthalmos secondary to vascular anomalies has also been reported (Millichamp and Spencer, 1991). Specialist advice should be sought in suspected cases.

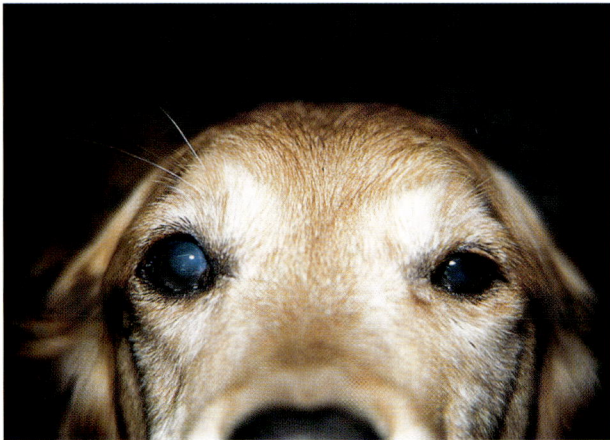

Fig. 3.11 Exophthalmos of the right eye due to episcleritis in a Golden Retriever. Note the widened palpebral fissure of the affected eye in comparison to the normal left eye.

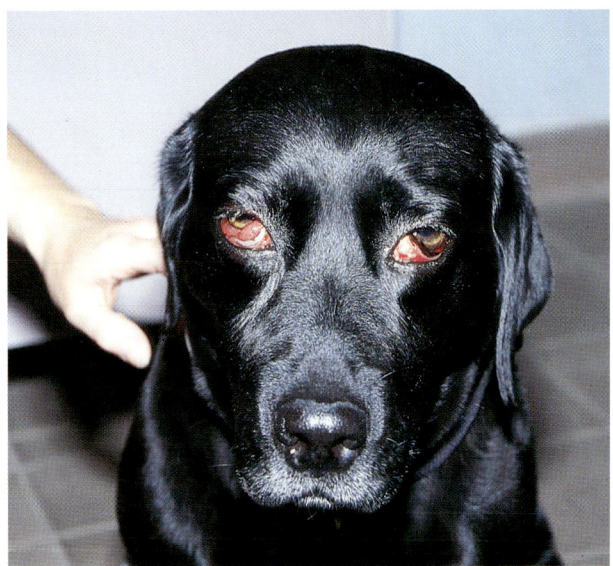

Fig. 3.10 Bilateral exophthalmos and third eyelid prominence in a middle-aged Labrador with zygomatic sialoadenitis which resolved following systemic anti-inflammatory and antibiotic therapy.

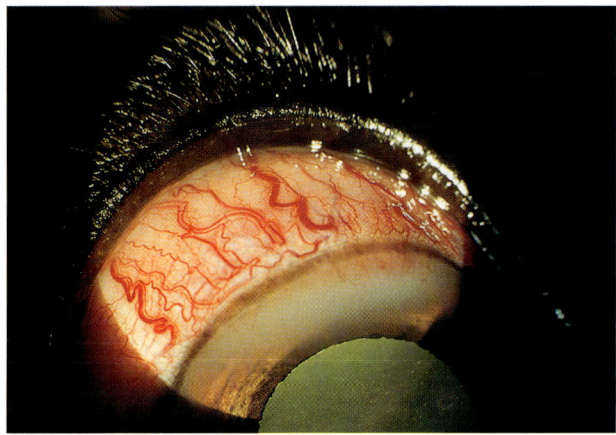

Fig. 3.12 Case of episcleritis showing marked episcleral congestion, limbal abnormality and corneal oedema.

BLUNT TRAUMA (ORBIT AND GLOBE)

Prolapse

Globe prolapse is the acute forward displacement of the eyeball beyond the bony orbital rim with resultant eyelid entrapment. It can be differentiated from exophthalmos in which the eyelids maintain a normal physiological position. Prolapse is directly vision-threatening because of traction on the optic nerve, the associated uveitis and corneal exposure. It is therefore a true ocular emergency requiring rapid assessment prior to appropriate medical and surgical management. It is often secondary to blunt trauma from road traffic accidents, or from being kicked or hit, or from dog fights (Fig. 3.13) and can even occur during excessive restraint. It can occur in any breed but brachycephalic breeds are predisposed as only minimal force is required to prolapse the eye from within a shallow orbit through a macropalpebral fissure (large eyelid opening). Chemosis, swelling of periorbital tissues and subconjunctival and retrobulbar haemorrhage represent the normal response of the injured eye. These changes are exacerbated by mechanical obstruction to venous drainage caused by the orbital swelling and the inward rolling of the eyelids behind the prolapsed globe.

Assessment replacement of the globe is generally preferable to enucleation, which can always be performed later if necessary. The dramatic clinical presentation renders the diagnosis straightforward but assessment of the globe to provide a long term prognosis is difficult at the initial emergency presentation. Less than one-third of traumatic ocular proptoses in dogs will have any functional vision, so prognosis refers primarily to salvage of a globe which is free of discomfort for the patient, cosmetically acceptable and does not require intensive long term medical treatment (Gilger *et al.*, 1995). There are several guidelines that can be used during the initial assessment:

- If only conjunctival attachments remain and the optic nerve is severed, enucleation is indicated.
- Corneal or scleral rupture (assessed by turgor and shape of globe) usually necessitates enucleation. Posterior globe ruptures may be seen with ocular ultrasonography (see Fig. 3.5).
- Severance of more than two or three extraocular muscles (assessed by degree of forward displacement and deviation) often results in impaired vascular and nerve supplies to the anterior segment and carries a poor prognosis (Fig. 3.14).
- Pupillary light reflex (PLR) is unreliable for 7–10 days following the injury (Roberts, 1985) but a positive direct PLR and a consensual PLR in the contralateral eye are both good prognostic indicators.
- Hyphaema is an unfavourable finding as it represents haemorrhage from the iris and ciliary body or choroid and phthisis bulbi often follows.
- Pupil size is unreliable (Gilger *et al.*, 1995; Spiess and Wallin-Håkanson, 1999). Many textbooks state that a miotic pupil represents the normal response of the iris sphincter muscle to trauma and therefore carries a favourable prognosis, and that a dilated pupil carries a poor prognosis as it indicates probable damage to the optic nerve and/or the oculomotor nerve and unbalanced stimulation of the sympathetic supply to the dilated smooth muscle. Current thinking is that pupil size is unreliable.
- More trauma is required to proptose the globe in dolichocephalic breeds than in brachycephalic breeds, so the prognosis is generally worse for the former.

Management the ocular surface must be immediately protected from further damage and desiccation with the liberal application of an artificial tear preparation and/or a broad-spectrum antibiotic ophthalmic ointment. After careful patient evaluation, the globe is replaced as soon as possible under general anaesthesia. The corneal surface can be stained with fluorescein to assess the presence of corneal abrasions or

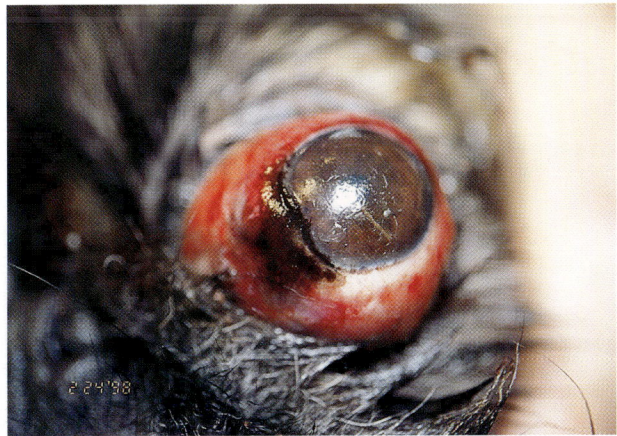

Fig. 3.13 Traumatic globe prolapse in a young Pekingese after a dog fight. Note the corneal desiccation, miotic pupil and severe anterior displacement of the globe with rupture of extraocular muscles.

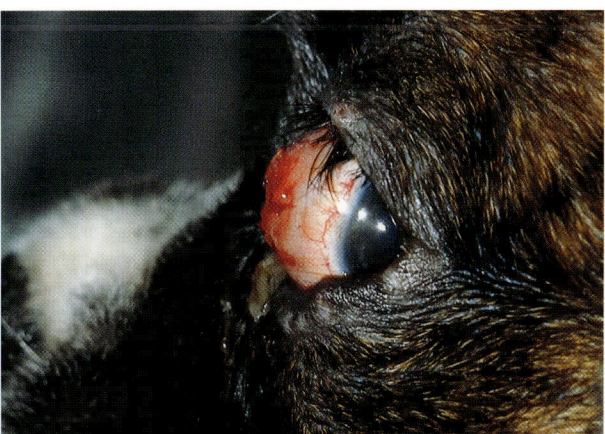

Fig. 3.14 Lateral strabismus due to rupture of the medial rectus muscle in a Boxer puppy.

ulceration. The eye and adnexal structures are irrigated with saline solution. The eyelids require only minimal clipping to prevent damage to the bruised and swollen tissues and to the globe itself.

In mild cases of proptosis the globe may be replaced simply with gentle pressure to the globe with moist cotton wool or a swab. In the majority of cases, the inwardly rolled lid margins need to be everted by a strabismus hook, although a spay hook is suitable and more readily available in most general practices (Fig. 3.15). Alternatively, a lateral canthotomy can be performed to increase the size of the palpebral fissure in order to replace the globe more easily in the orbit. A temporary tarsorraphy should be performed to prevent exposure keratitis whilst retrobulbar swelling resolves, to provide direct pressure to the globe to reduce orbital oedema and prevent re-prolapse. Two to three simple mattress sutures are placed. Each suture should only partially penetrate the lid thickness to prevent corneal damage and ideally should emerge from the meibomian gland openings on the lid margin or a few millimetres posteriorly. A 2/0 to 4/0 (depending on size of dog) monofilament non-absorbable suture material can be used, although absorbable polyglactin is soft and will cause less corneal damage if the sutures are not precisely placed. If eyelid swelling is marked, stents with intravenous tubing or wide rubber strips should be used with suture placement. The sutures are removed after 10–14 days, depending on the degree of retrobulbar swelling. It is important to check that the palpebral reflex is intact at this stage, reduced corneal sensation or eyelid function can cause severe exposure keratitis.

Postoperative medication with a systemic, broad-spectrum antibiotic such as amoxicillin clavulanate is indicated for 5–7 days. Systemic anti-inflammatory therapy with prednisolone is required to control the uveitis and to reduce the risk of phthisis bulbi in the long term. Topical medication with a broad-spectrum antibiotic ophthalmic ointment twice daily can be applied via a small opening in the temporary tarsorraphy at the medial canthus, if the clients are educated how to medicate the eye atraumatically. However, most owners find topical treatment very difficult in these cases and it is not essential. Atropine 1% ointment stabilises the blood–aqueous barrier and reduces the painful spasm of the iris in uveitis and is considered reasonably safe as no secondary glaucoma occurred in a recent study of 84 cases (Gilger *et al.*, 1995).

Sequelae deviation of the globe is one of the most common sequelae of traumatic proptosis. The globe is usually deviated in a dorsolateral direction as the medial and ventral rectus muscles insert most anteriorly and the ventral rectus is the shortest extraocular muscle and thus severed first (Samuelson, 1999). Esotropia (divergent strabismus) resulting from damage to the innervation of the medial rectus muscle usually resolves partially or completely over several months. If the esotropia is secondary to tearing of the muscle or its insertion, it may be permanent. However, there are surgical techniques that are theoretically possible, but very difficult in practice, to locate and re-appose torn ends of small strips of muscle tissue.

Exposure keratitis due to reduced corneal sensation and lagophthalmos and keratoconjunctivitis sicca may require long-term artificial tear replacement and even enucleation in severe cases. A medial canthoplasty will minimise corneal exposure, reduce the risk of repeat prolapse and cover the unsightly white sclera visible medially. Keratoconjunctivitis sicca results from compromise of the lacrimal gland and third eyelid gland function caused by the increased intraorbital pressure and damage to their vascular and nerve supply.

Blindness occurs in 20–30% of prolapse cases. Other sequelae include cataract, phthisis bulbi, glaucoma, retinal detachment/degeneration and optic nerve atrophy, the latter are later visible ophthalmoscopically.

Sudden onset enophthalmos
Orbital fracture

Displaced or depressed orbital fractures may result in enophthalmos.

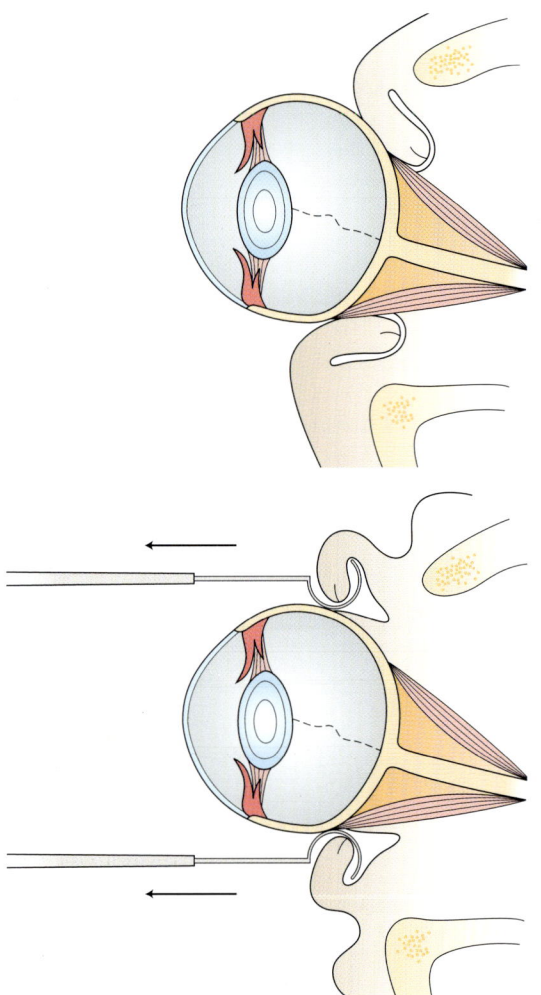

Fig. 3.15 Replacement of globe proptosis.

ADNEXAL INJURIES

Tetanus ('lock jaw')

Bilateral enophthalmos with marked third eyelid protrusion occurs in canine tetanus (Fig. 3.16). The pathognomonic 'sardonic smile' (risus sardonicus) is caused by contraction of the facial muscles, drawing the ears, eyelids and commissures of the mouth caudally. History of a recent wound, clinical signs, physical examination and positive culture from an injury site are helpful in making a diagnosis. Management includes fluid therapy and nutritional support in conjunction with penicillin and tetanus antitoxin therapy (Coleman, 1998).

Pain

Any cause of trigeminal pain (corneal sensation) may result in active retraction of the globe and subsequent third eyelid protrusion. Blepharospasm, lacrimation and photophobia make up the classic 'triad' of clinical signs associated with such corneal injury. Examples include ectopic cilium, superficial corneal ulcer and corneal foreign body. Intraocular disease such as severe uveitis and glaucoma can also result in enophthalmos.

Horner's syndrome

Interruption to the sympathetic innervation of the eye results in clinical signs which together are pathognomonic for Horner's syndrome (see Figs 6.2 and 15.13). The main clinical signs include enophthalmos, third eyelid protrusion, miosis and ptosis. Although rarely an emergency, a thorough diagnostic work-up is indicated.

ADNEXAL INJURIES

EYELID TRAUMA

Trauma to the eyelid is usually sustained as a result of a fight or road traffic accident. The profuse blood supply to the eyelids ensures that infection is rarely a major complication. Careful examination is advised to search for concurrent ocular and physical injuries.

- Abrasions, contusions and superficial wounds require simple wound lavage, systemic nonsteroidal anti-inflammatory drugs and broad-spectrum topical antibiotic ointment and should heal without complications. Always check that the eyelids can blink effectively otherwise exposure keratitis may develop.
- Full-thickness eyelid lacerations should be repaired surgically as soon as possible to restore the eyelids to their normal structure so that eyelid function is not compromised. Infection, lagophthalmos, exposure keratopathy and cicatricial entropion/ectropion can result if treatment is delayed or is inappropriate. Eyelids have an excellent vascular supply, so repair should always be attempted however necrotic and devitalised the tissue may appear. Ophthalmic lubricants should be used to protect the ocular surface, even temporarily, if there is a risk of corneal exposure due to lagophthalmos. Accurate wound apposition at the eyelid margin is essential and the lid margin should always be repaired first (Fig. 3.17). Palpebral tissue usually heals quickly and repair is generally straightforward by one- or two-layered direct closure. A carefully performed and deep one-layered closure may be adequate except in large or giant breeds in which tarsoconjunctival tissue should also be repaired as well as skin. Buried absorbable suture material should be kept to a minimum to prevent excess wound reaction. A fine absorbable suture material such as 5/0–6/0 polyglactin is used in the subcutaneous

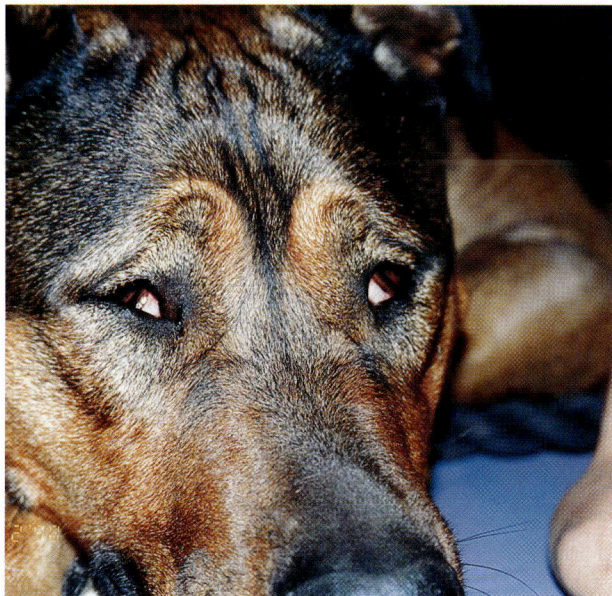

Fig. 3.16 Bilateral enophthalmos and third eyelid protrusion in a young crossbred dog with tetanus following a penetrating skin injury.

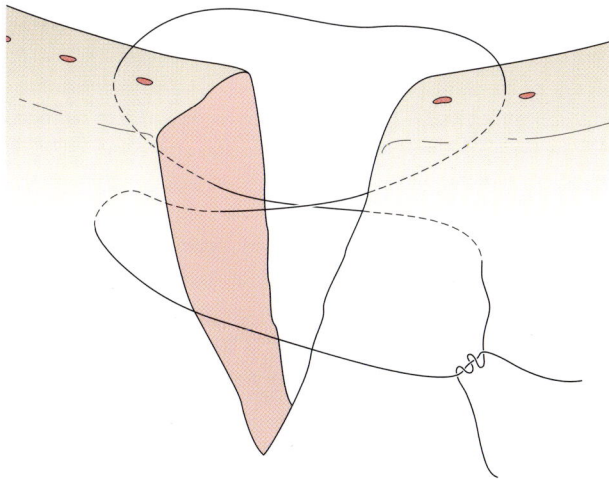

Fig. 3.17 Eyelid laceration – figure-of-eight suture.

tissues in a continuous or preferably simple interrupted pattern; 4/0–5/0 polyglactin with a cutting needle is used for a simple interrupted pattern in the skin. Great care must be taken to ensure that the knot and suture material do not contact the cornea, particularly important when less pliable suture material is used. If non-absorbable suture material is used, sedation may be required for removal at 10–14 days. A broad-spectrum systemic antibiotic and nonsteroidal anti-inflammatory drugs are administered systemically for a short period.
- Eyelid avulsion requires more challenging surgical repair with a variety of grafts and flaps which are described in the literature. These cases should be referred to a veterinary ophthalmologist.
- Injuries to the third eyelid are common. Minor wounds heal with topical broad-spectrum antibiotic ointment alone, but avulsion of the third eyelid, a large defect in the free margin, full-thickness lacerations and reduced mobility all require surgical repair. As with lid trauma, minimal debridement is required and a fine absorbable suture material such as 6/0–7/0 polyglactin is used in a continuous or simple interrupted suture pattern. Care must be taken to ensure that the nictitans cartilage is not exposed and that suture knots are buried or placed on the anterior aspect of the third eyelid to prevent corneal damage. The third eyelid has an important role in maintaining ocular surface health and extensive or malignant neoplasia is the only justification for its removal in the dog. Repair of serious injuries should always be attempted and are usually successful due to the excellent healing capacity of conjunctival tissue.
- Injuries involving the eyelid and the third eyelid may also extend to the nasolacrimal system, the superior and inferior punctal openings and the proximal duct itself. Primary repair of the nasolacrimal system requires a meticulous microsurgical technique, so referral is indicated.

Conjunctival trauma

Chemosis

Chemosis (swelling of the conjunctiva and lids) is often a dramatic and alarming clinical presentation (Fig. 3.18). It occurs as an immediate type reaction mediated by histamine and immunoglobulin E (IgE) and may be secondary to food allergy, drug allergy (topical and systemic) and insect bites. It has also been seen in cases of mast cell neoplasia (Johnson *et al.*, 1988). The loose arrangement of conjunctival stroma allows extensive oedema to develop very rapidly. Topical aminoglycosides, such as gentamicin and neomycin, and preservatives in ophthalmic preparations can cause allergic reactions of the conjunctiva but are generally associated with prolonged use rather than an acute reaction.

Management

- Parenteral administration of a short-acting corticosteroid and antihistamine.

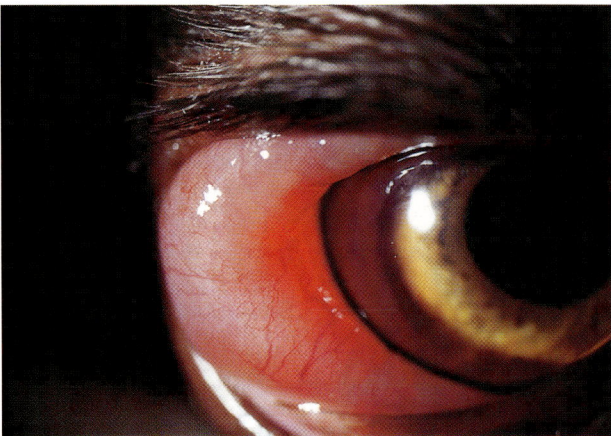

Fig. 3.18 Chemosis in a young chocolate Labrador. The chemosis in this case was intermittent, recurrent and idiopathic despite a thorough investigation for the underlying aetiology. It resolved of its own accord.

- Topical corticosteroid therapy with 1% prednisolone acetate three or four times daily or 0.1% dexamethasone acetate.
- Withdraw causal agent if identified.
- Minimise self-trauma with Elizabethan collar if necessary.

Conjunctival haemorrhage

See under 'Blunt trauma'. Acute conjunctival haemorrhage can also occur with systemic coagulopathies (Fig. 3.19).

Conjunctival lacerations

Conjunctival tissue has an excellent healing capacity due to its good vascular supply. Simple wounds will therefore heal with topical broad-spectrum antibiotic ophthalmic ointment alone. Extensive lacerations may be sutured directly with 7/0 absorbable suture material such as polyglactin in a continuous or simple interrupted pattern.

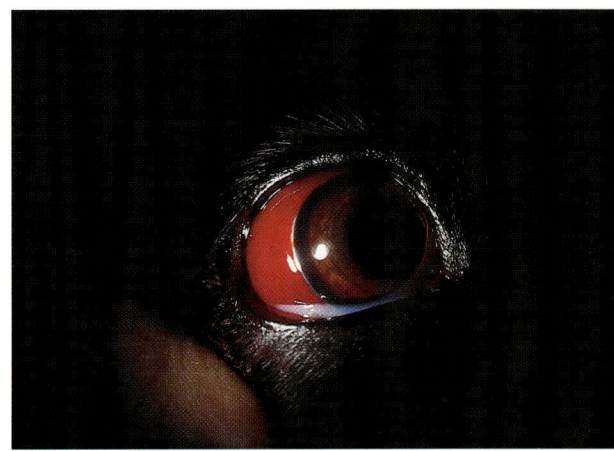

Fig. 3.19 Conjunctival haemorrhage in a case of warfarin poisoning.

CORNEAL TRAUMA

Conjunctival wounds often obscure more sinister injuries in underlying or adjacent tissues such as cornea and sclera. Careful examination under general anaesthesia is essential, particularly for apparently innocuous limbal wounds which may involve iris prolapse. A change in appearance of the intraocular structures including irregularity of the pupil, coagulated aqueous or a clear to mucoid discharge are clues for the presence of full-thickness lacerations of the ocular tunic. Do not remove coagulated aqueous until the patient can be examined under anaesthesia and primary repair can be performed immediately. Postoperative broad spectrum antibiotics are indicated systemically and/or topically, according to the extent of the injury, and a systemic non-steroidal anti-inflammatory drug when there is marked chemosis and bruising.

CORNEAL TRAUMA

CORNEAL LACERATIONS (Figs 3.20–3.25)

- A partial thickness corneal laceration may be treated as a deep ulcer if it involves less than half of the corneal thickness (see Chapter 9). The canine cornea is less than 1 mm thick and assessment of wound depth may be difficult, particularly when the wound edges are swollen and oedematous. If there is any doubt, examination with magnification under general anaesthesia should be performed.
- Small full-thickness perforations or penetrations which have sealed with fibrin do not usually require surgery, although close supervision is essential.
- Larger, full-thickness corneal lacerations must be sutured. Do not remove any coagulated aqueous, masquerading as clear to grey mucoid ocular discharge, as it is often all that is sealing the wound. Careful induction of anaesthesia is required so that any temporary wound seal does not rupture with extrusion of intraocular contents. Debridement of the wound edges is judicious and minimal, removing only necrotic tissue. Wound edges are carefully apposed with simple interrupted sutures placed to a depth of two-thirds of corneal thickness with 8/0–9/0 absorbable material. The sutures should not penetrate the full thickness of the cornea as that would provide a potential route of infection into the anterior chamber (Fig. 3.26).
- Iris prolapse visible as a black mass on the corneal surface or at the limbus is straightforward to diagnose. However, when covered with grey, coagulated aqueous and blood, it may not resemble normal iris tissue and careful examination is required. Clearly it is always associated with a full-thickness laceration of the cornea and/or sclera. Prolapsed iris tissue can usually be replaced and is only amputated if severely desiccated, necrotic or infected. Excision of prolapsed iridal tissue can result in profuse bleeding from the major arterial circle and cautery, intracameral adrenaline

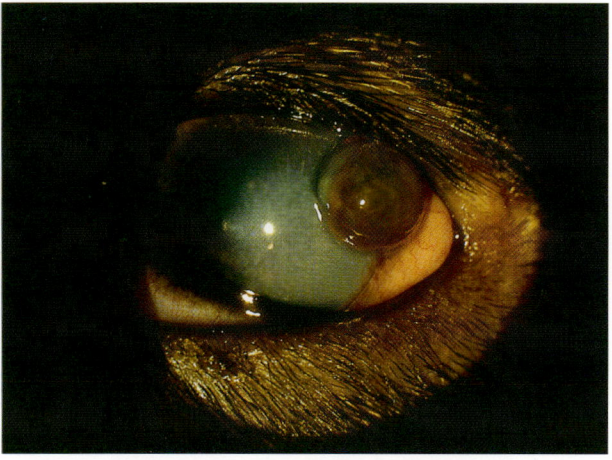

Fig. 3.21 Penetrating cat scratch corneal injury with iris prolapse at the limbus together with localised area of corneal oedema in a German Shepherd Dog puppy.

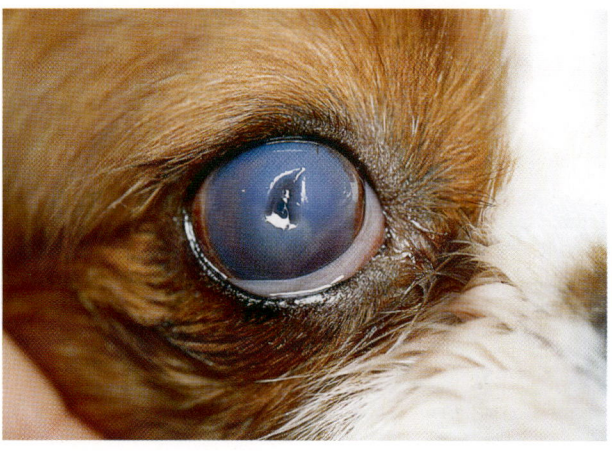

Fig. 3.22 Axial deep corneal laceration with loss of stromal tissue in a young Cavalier King Charles Spaniel.

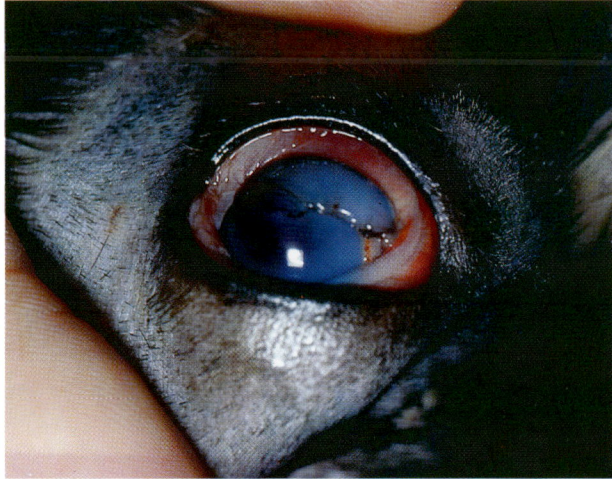

Fig. 3.20 Linear corneal laceration and associated corneal oedema and conjunctival swelling following trauma in a Pekingese (the periorbital region has been clipped and prepared for surgery).

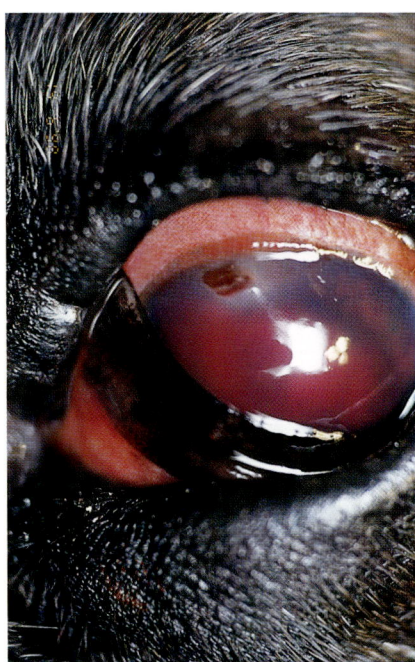

Fig. 3.23 Hyphaema following a cat scratch injury. Note focal area of intense oedema near the dorsal limbus and prominence of the nictitating membrane as evidence of ocular pain.

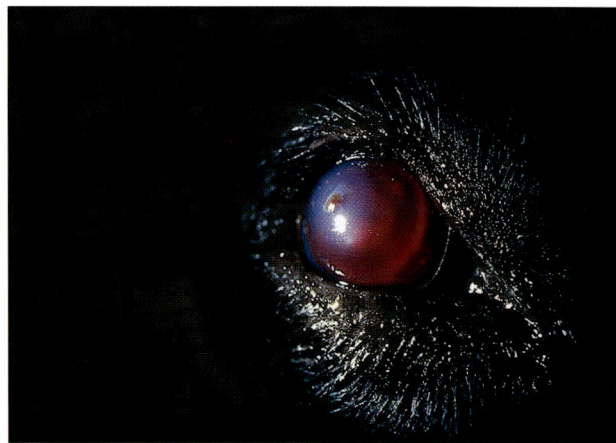

Fig. 3.25 Hyphaema and corneal penetration due to gunshot injury in a Labrador.

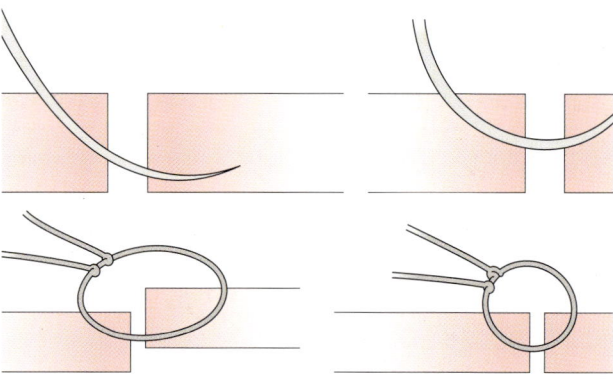

Fig. 3.26 Corneal suture.

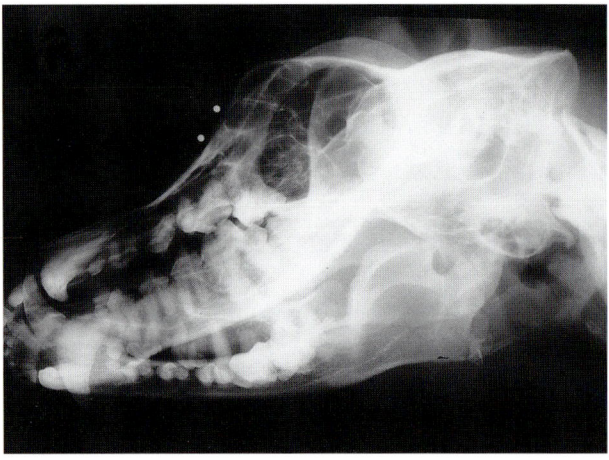

Fig. 3.24 Two lead pellets rostral to the right orbit in a young working Labrador accidentally shot in the eye and presented with total hyphaema. The most rostral pellet is probably embedded in soft tissue and the more caudal one in the lower eyelid or possibly the globe.

(epinephrine) or tamponade with a viscoelastic material (which requires subsequent removal) are helpful but often unavailable in general practice. The iris tissue is very gently dissected free from the wound edges and then replaced in the anterior chamber with an iris spatula. The anterior chamber is irrigated with lactated Ringer's solution or balanced salts solution to remove fibrin and blood clots. Distilled water is not acceptable for intraocular use.

For corneal repair 8/0 polyglactin is used in a simple interrupted pattern.

- Lacerations at the limbus must be explored carefully under general anaesthesia as simple wounds can extend a considerable distance into the sclera underneath intact conjunctiva. It is important to reflect the conjunctiva from the wound margins so that the full extent of a scleral wound can be investigated. The sclera is repaired with simple interrupted sutures using 6/0 absorbable suture material with the first suture placed carefully at the limbus to ensure good realignment.
- The anterior chamber may need to be reformed by a limbal injection with irrigating solution or an air bubble with a 25-gauge needle and syringe. This checks the integrity of the wound repair and reduces the risk of adhesion between iris and cornea (anterior synechia).
- Postoperative therapy includes broad spectrum topical and systemic antibiotic therapy together with appropriate medical treatment for uveitis, i.e. atropine and anti-inflammatory drugs. An Elizabethan collar and/or foot bandage to prevent self-trauma may also be indicated.

CORNEAL TRAUMA

DESCEMETOCOELE

A descemetocoele (Figs 3.27 and 3.28) is a true ophthalmic emergency as it is a corneal ulcer so deep that only corneal endothelium and Descemet's membrane remain as the final barrier separating the anterior chamber from the external environment. As the endothelium is a single cell layer and Descemet's membrane is 3–12 μm thick, corneal rupture is a real risk and so prompt treatment is required. Diagnosis should be straightforward as there is a characteristic 'clear area' which does not stain with fluorescein at the bottom of a descemetocoele. Pain is not always apparent as there are fewer sensory nerves in the deeper layers of the cornea than in the superficial layers.

Management

- Small (less than 1 mm) descemetocoeles can be managed medically but the patient should be hospitalised for close observation of any signs of rupture. Small lesions with healthy corneal margins can also be directly sutured but astigmatism will result.
- Large descemetocoeles and deep stromal ulcers should be managed surgically. A third eyelid flap is inadequate for such deep corneal defects and a conjunctival graft is indicated. It provides immediate mechanical support to the weakened cornea and a direct blood supply and such repairs are usually very successful (Fig. 3.29).

The eye is prepared for surgery using povidine iodine solution (not scrub) at a 1:10 dilution for periorbital skin and a 1:50 dilution to irrigate the conjunctival sac. If there is a known or suspected perforation, lactated Ringer's solution should be used in lieu of iodine solution which is toxic to the corneal endothelium. A lateral canthotomy will improve access to the conjunctiva but may not be necessary in brachycephalic breeds with large palpebral fissures. An eyelid speculum is carefully placed to apply minimal pressure to the globe. The position and size of the corneal lesion is assessed to plan the best site from which to harvest the conjunctival graft, most easily taken from the dorsolateral aspect to avoid the third eyelid. The conjunctiva at the level of the ventral graft extremity is elevated with fine-toothed forceps adjacent to the limbus and fine scissors are used to make a small incision and to dissect bluntly the conjunctiva from the underlying Tenon's capsule in a dorsal direction. The conjunctiva is then incised at the limbus for the proposed length of the graft. A second horizontal incision, corresponding to the width of the graft, is

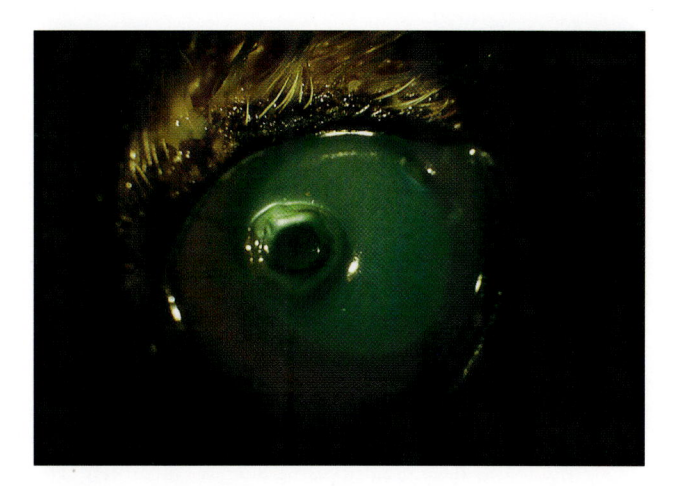

Fig. 3.27 Classic descemetocoele appearance with a clear base in a West Highland White Terrier with keratoconjunctivitis sicca.

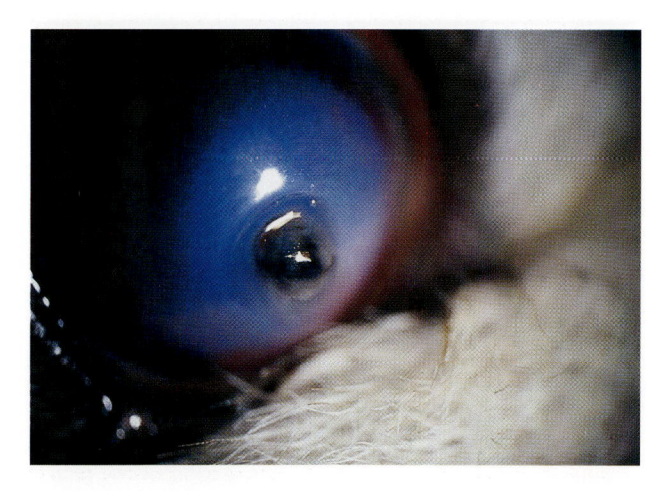

Fig. 3.28 Ruptured descemetocoele with iris prolapse in a young Shih Tzu. Note the corneal vascular fringe and obvious nasal fold trichiasis.

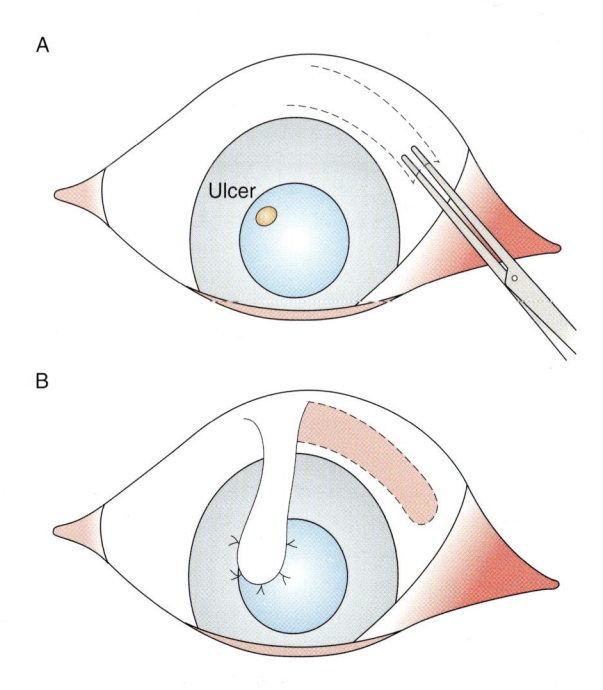

Fig. 3.29 Conjunctival pedicle flap.

made at the ventral aspect of the pedicle towards the canthus. The third and final incision is made parallel to the first but is slightly shorter. The graft should ideally be so thin that the scissor blades can be easily visualised during dissection. The pedicle graft is immobilised and manipulated to fit the corneal lesion, ensuring there is no tension along the length of the graft and that the eye can rotate ventrally without causing excessive tension on the proximal end of the graft. The recipient ulcer bed is prepared with careful debridement of necrotic or degenerate corneal tissue, which would delay healing. The edges of the graft are sutured with usually about six simple interrupted sutures using 8/0–9/0 absorbable suture material swaged to a spatulated needle. Sutures should be placed two-thirds of the corneal depth and should not penetrate the anterior chamber. Sutures can be placed either into the wall of the defect or beyond into healthy corneal tissue. Sutures are placed circumferentially to achieve a watertight seal, particularly if there is a corneal perforation. It is important not to traumatise the pedicle, which contains the vital blood supply for the graft. It is not necessary to close the conjunctival defect from where the graft was harvested. The lateral canthotomy, if performed, is closed in two layers with 6/0 and 5/0 absorbable suture material taking care to reappose the lid margins accurately. Once healing is complete, usually 6–8 weeks, the pedicle can be severed and trimmed under topical anaesthesia, leaving a small island of conjunctival tissue covering the original defect.

- Appropriate medical therapy is also indicated for the concurrent anterior uveitis which is inevitable with such corneal pathology.
- Alternative surgical techniques include corneoscleral or corneoconjunctival transposition, autogenous lamellar corneal graft and penetrating keratoplasty. Such techniques require specialist facilities. Small intestinal submucosa has also recently been used successfully as a novel graft material for corneal defects in cats (Featherstone and Sansom, 2000) but further studies are needed in the dog. Corneal gluing with tissue adhesive such as cyanoacrylate glue is not recommended for use in descemetocoeles because the heat generated during polymerisation of the glue may rupture Descemet's membrane.

MELTING ULCERS

Melting ulcers are so described as the corneal stroma is rapidly dissolved and digested so that it appears literally to liquefy or melt (see Fig. 9.32). Proteases and collagenases are enzymes that are present during normal corneal healing to remove debris and devitalised cells. If the fine balance of corneal healing is disturbed then the collagenolytic enzymatic activity becomes excessive, resulting in stromal dissolution. Such enzymes may originate from pathogenic organisms, notably *Pseudomonas* and beta-haemolytic *Streptococcus*, but also from inflammatory cells that have migrated into the diseased areas or from the cornea itself. Acute ulcerative keratitis with progressive melting requires vigorous medical therapy.

Management

- The patient should be hospitalised for observation and to ensure correct administration of an intensive regimen of topical medication.
- Corneal cytology to assess whether a gram-positive or gram-negative organism predominates assists in the choice of initial antibiotic therapy. Fusidic acid is good for gram-positive infections and a topical floroquinolone such as ofloxacin is good for gram-negative infections.
- Bacteriology for aerobic and anaerobic culture and sensitivity should be performed.
- Topical antibacterial treatment based on the cytology or with a broad-spectrum antibiotic including activity against gram-negative organisms should be started immediately. Frequency of treatment should be 1–2 hourly and then reduced to six times daily for the first 48–72 hours. Note: occasionally, topical aminoglycosides such as gentamicin can cause marked ocular irritation thus reducing patient cooperation and should be discontinued if signs of irritation occur.
- Anticollagenase therapy can be considered, although the overall efficacy in the dog is questionable. Fresh autologous serum, ethylenediamine tetra-acetic acid (EDTA) solution and parenteral tetracyclines are examples of protease inhibitors which can be used clinically. An EDTA solution can be made by mixing sterile water or saline with a sterile EDTA blood tube. Anticollagenase treatment should be administered frequently for at least the first 24 hours.
- The secondary anterior uveitis which is invariably present should be treated with 1% atropine and a systemic nonsteroidal anti-inflammatory drug such as carprofen. The atropine should be given 'to effect', i.e. to obtain and maintain pupil dilation, but care must be taken as it can lower basal tear production which further delays corneal healing.
- Systemic broad spectrum antibiotic therapy is also beneficial.
- The affected eye should be protected from self-trauma with a foot bandage or if necessary with an Elizabethan collar.
- Topical corticosteroids are contraindicated as they can potentiate collagenase activity up to 13 times. Although systemic corticosteroids have less deleterious effects on corneal healing, they should be avoided if possible in cases of serious corneal pathology. If the ulcer continues to deteriorate despite medical therapy, surgery with a conjunctival graft or flap is indicated.

THERMAL INJURIES

Thermal injuries are uncommon but may be associated with exposure to smoke, heat and hot liquids. Immediate ophthalmic first aid consists of copious irrigation of the ocular surface with cold saline or water, a topical lubricant and antibacterial ophthalmic ointment, systemic nonsteroidal anti-inflammatories and analgesia. Specialist advice should be sought for subsequent management as complications and scarring are probable.

CHEMICAL INJURIES

A variety of chemicals including those in shampoos, aerosol sprays and household cleaners can cause corneal burns. The best initial treatment is immediate copious irrigation to dilute the chemical with any available solution such as tap water, saline or eyewash solutions. Nothing, including the transportation of the dog to the veterinary surgeon, should delay immediate irrigation. Presenting clinical signs include obvious ocular pain manifested by severe blepharospasm and lacrimation.

Management

- Minor soap or detergent burns cause extensive but superficial corneal ulceration (see Fig. 9.45) and secondary anterior uveitis and should be treated with a broad spectrum topical antibiotic and atropine.
- In more serious chemical injuries, first measure the pH of the conjunctival sac (with a urinalysis dipstick) to determine whether you are dealing with an acid or alkali injury. The normal pH is slightly alkaline.
- Acids are less destructive than alkaline chemicals as they are buffered by the ocular tissues and precipitate with corneal proteins. The initial damage is therefore self-limiting. Alkaline chemicals are very destructive and remain a major challenge in ophthalmology as they cause loss of corneal epithelium and rapid dissolution of the stroma. Alkalis continue to release hydroxyl ions into the tissues and so the injury progresses. The damaged epithelial cells and polymorphonuclear cells release collagenase enzymes which digest the corneal stroma, known as a melting ulcer or keratomalacia. The situation is physiologically similar to ulcers infected with *Pseudomonas* organisms, except that the source of enzymes is the damaged cornea itself.
- Copious irrigation for approximately 30 minutes or with 1–2 litres of saline is indicated. An intravenous tubing set is useful for thorough irrigation of the ocular surfaces. If the injury is extensive, this procedure usually requires general anaesthesia.
- Topical medication consists of a broad-spectrum antibiotic ophthalmic ointment together with an anticollagenase agent such as autologous serum or EDTA solution. Atropine is indicated for the secondary uveitis.
- Systemic nonsteroidal anti-inflammatory drugs and analgesia are indicated.
- Topical corticosteroids can potentiate collagenase activity up to 13 times and are contraindicated in the acute stage but can be used with extreme caution, under specialist supervision, to minimise corneal scarring in the healing stages.
- A soft bandage contact lens can be used to minimise symblepharon (Sansom and Barnett, 1997).
- The prognosis for superficial soap burns is excellent but is always guarded for alkaline injuries depending on the concentration of the insulting chemical, area of cornea affected and the time interval between exposure and treatment.

OCULAR FOREIGN BODIES

THE ORBIT

Orbital foreign bodies and gunshot injuries usually present as acute inflammatory disease (uveitis, ophthalmitis/panophthalmitis and secondary glaucoma). The history is often an important clue in working gundogs for example and should not be ignored. Foreign bodies may enter the orbit via the conjunctival sac, oral cavity or percutaneous route; the entry wound is often not easy to identify and meticulous physical examination is indicated. Gunshot pellets are easily identified with ocular ultrasonography and plain skull radiography. It is not uncommon to identify several pellets in variable locations and a limbal metal ring, in conjunction with several radiographic views, helps to localise the foreign body. In contrast, most non-metallic foreign bodies are not recognised on plain radiographs, but ocular ultrasound is helpful in such instances. Difficult cases require CT or MRI imaging to identify and localise an orbital foreign body which may itself not be visible although the associated inflammation, abscessation or fistulation will be. Complicated orbital surgery may be indicated and referral is recommended.

NASOLACRIMAL DUCT

Foreign bodies in the nasolacrimal duct present with copious purulent discharge, epiphora, ocular discomfort and conjunctival hyperaemia. Dacryocystitis (inflammation of the nasolacrimal duct) is common in the dog and is usually secondary to a foreign body lodged in the nasolacrimal sac or duct. The foreign body is often a grass awn and there may well be more than one. Careful examination may reveal a strand of purulent material exiting from the lower punctal opening. The nasolacrimal duct system should be irrigated, often repeatedly, with saline under sedation or general anaesthesia as the procedure can be uncomfortable when there is concurrent inflammation and/or infection, and damage to the duct can occur if the dog moves suddenly. A lacrimal cannula is placed into the upper and lower punctae in turn and the canaliculae gently flushed, often resulting in a foreign body such as a grass seed emerging from the opposite punctal opening. Care must be taken not to apply excessive force as this may cause duct rupture. The nasolacrimal duct may also be flushed in a retrograde manner via the ipsilateral nasal ostium to reduce the risk of flushing a foreign body from the proximal nasolacrimal duct distally into the inaccessible intranasal portion. Good illumination and a tomcat urinary catheter are useful to cannulate the nasal ostium which is difficult. Dacryocystotomy to retrieve a foreign body from the lacrimal sac requires a microsurgical technique and specialist advice should be sought.

OCULAR EMERGENCIES AND TRAUMA

Conjunctival sac

Foreign bodies in the conjunctival sac (Figs 3.30 and 3.31) are very common in the dog and again grass awns are the usual culprit. The clinical presentation is similar to a naso-lacrimal foreign body, i.e. copious purulent discharge, discomfort and conjunctival hyperaemia. Not surprisingly, the purulent discharge persists despite a variety of topical antibacterial drugs and the conjunctival sac should be thoroughly searched with topical or general anaesthesia in all cases. The recess behind the third eyelid is easy to examine with topical anaesthesia, atraumatic forceps and a cooperative patient. A foreign body in that position can cause corneal ulceration, protrusion of the third eyelid and severe discomfort. Any focal area of conjunctival inflammation should be surgically explored as it usually leads to a fistula containing a foreign body. Once the foreign body is removed the conjunctival sac should be irrigated and a broad spectrum topical antibiotic administered for 5–7 days.

Cornea

Corneal foreign bodies (Figs 3.32–3.38) usually present as a unilateral, acute-onset problem with marked blepharospasm and a seromucoid discharge. Similar clinical signs also occur with ulcerative keratitis and corneal lacerations and so a careful examination is required. Although acute, severe ocular pain is typical, although some patients will present with a surprisingly comfortable and quiet eye, particularly if the corneal epithelium has healed over the penetrating defect. Other clinical signs include chemosis, conjunctival hyperaemia, coagulated aqueous on the ocular surface, corneal ulceration, anterior uveitis, intraocular haemorrhage and a change in appearance of the intraocular structures.

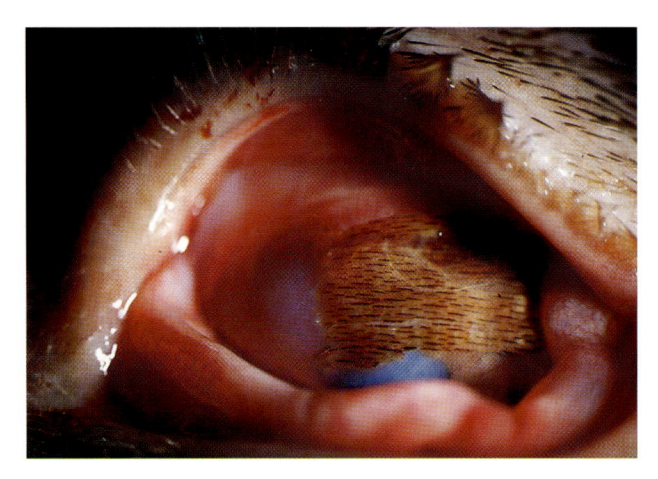

Fig. 3.32 Flat vegetative corneal foreign body, a thin piece of bark, causing intense corneal vascular reaction, corneal oedema and conjunctival inflammation in a Weimaraner. The severe corneal inflammatory response is typical for vegetative, non-penetrating foreign bodies.

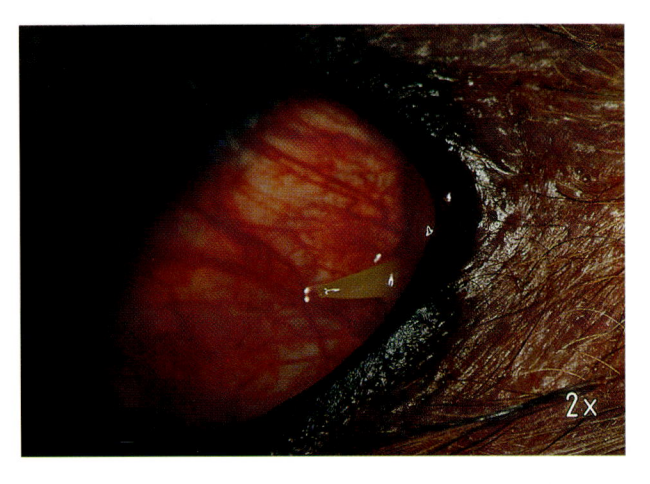

Fig. 3.30 Young Yorkshire Terrier presenting with unilateral copious purulent ocular discharge of 1 month's duration. The ocular discharge recurred after the cessation of antibiotic therapy. Under general anaesthesia the grass seed was found in a sinus in the conjunctival sac under the lateral canthus.

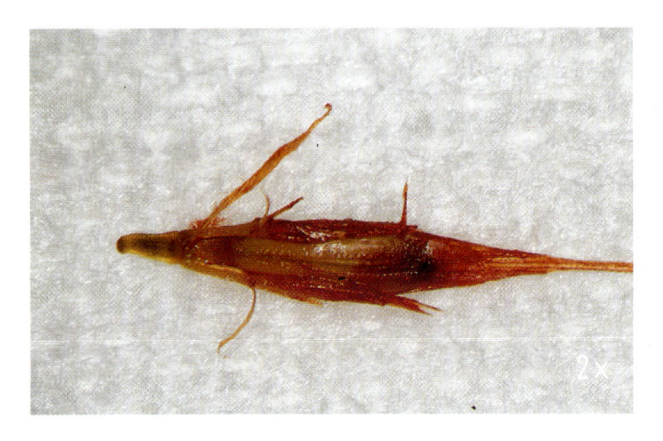

Fig. 3.31 Grass seed removed from the Yorkshire Terrier described in Fig. 3.30.

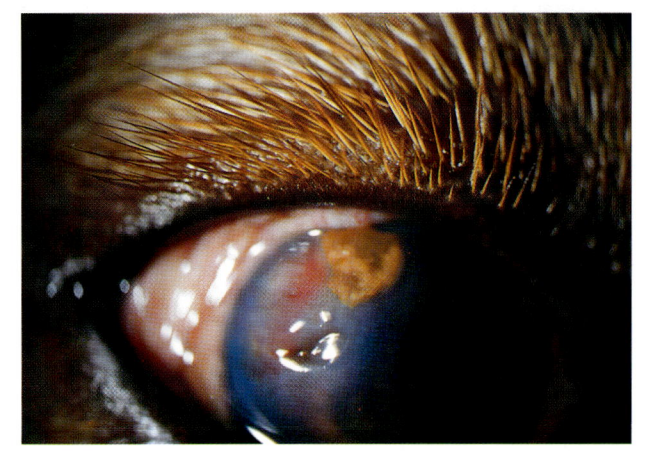

Fig. 3.33 A flake of varnish embedded within the cornea in a Labrador Retriever with a 2-week history of blepharospasm. The depression in which it lay was evident after the foreign body had been lifted away under topical anaesthesia.

OCULAR FOREIGN BODIES

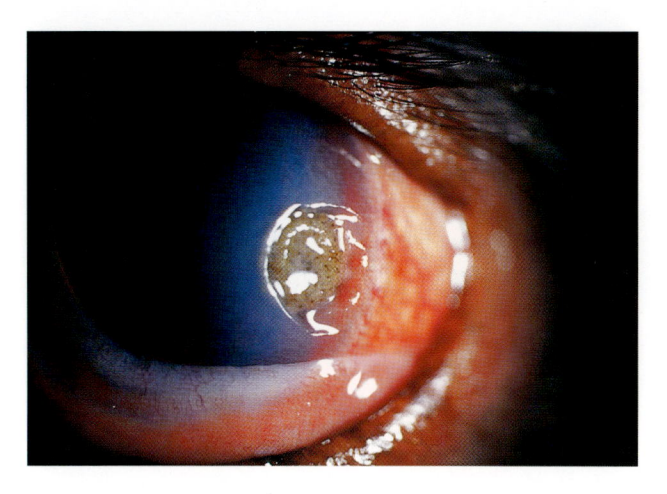

Fig. 3.34 Relatively flat circular corneal foreign body of vegetative material embedded near the limbus. Again, note the marked corneal reaction.

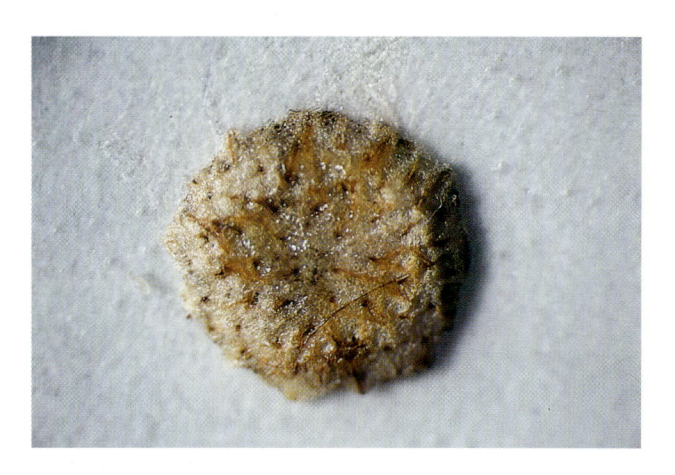

Fig. 3.35 Ragwort seed after removal from the dog described in Fig. 3.34.

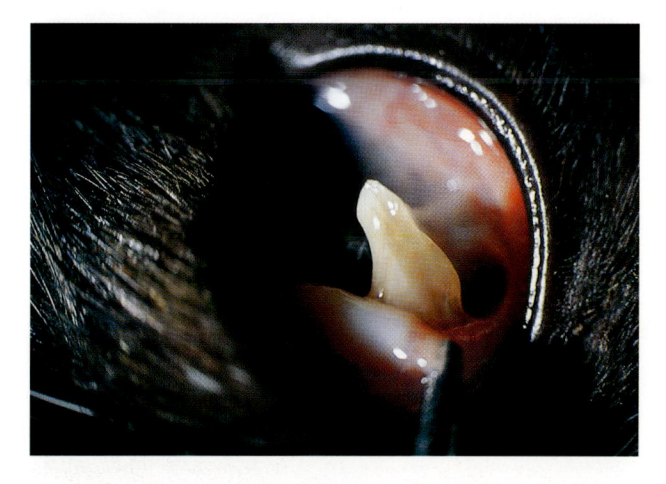

Fig. 3.36 Young crossbred dog presenting with ocular pain and dyscoria after a suspected cat fight. Examination under general anaesthesia revealed a large foreign body hidden beneath the upper eyelid and penetrating the anterior chamber at the limbus.

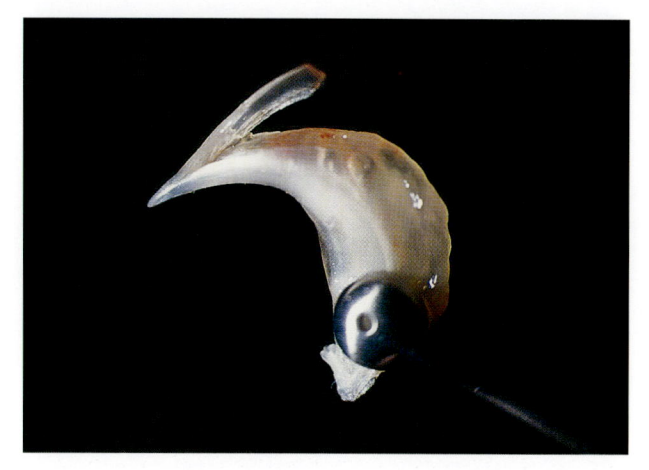

Fig. 3.37 Cat claw removed from the dog described in Fig. 3.36.

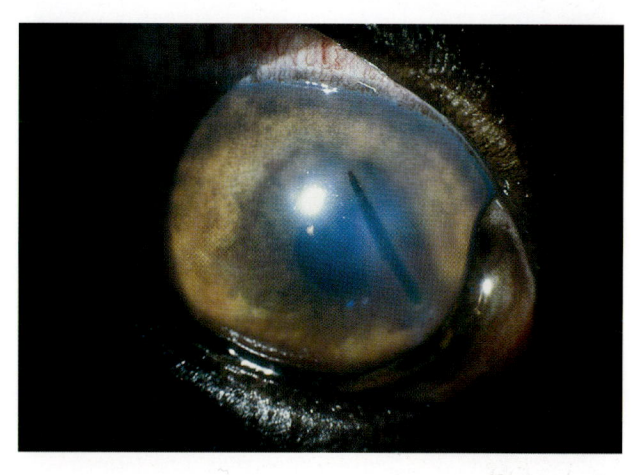

Fig. 3.38 Thorn foreign body in anterior chamber in a young Irish Setter. Note the minimal inflammatory response in this case.

Management

- Flat corneal foreign bodies such as flakes of paint or metal, plant material (bark, leaf, grass, etc.) may sit within a depression in the corneal epithelium so they are not dislodged by normal eyelid movement. A marked corneal vascular response is often associated with vegetable material (see Figs 3.32 and 3.34). Most of these foreign bodies can be removed with topical anaesthesia and a stream of saline to irrigate or flush the foreign body from the corneal surface. A moistened cotton-tipped applicator, cellulose stick swab or fine ophthalmic forceps can also be used to elevate the edge of the foreign body. Cytology and culture and sensitivity may be helpful after the removal of vegetative foreign body material as secondary bacterial or fungal infections are not uncommon.
- Intracorneal foreign bodies or those which have penetrated the anterior chamber must be removed under general anaesthesia. The observation of a fibrin 'cloud' on the endothelium adjacent to the corneal penetration is

evidence that the tip of the foreign body, usually a thorn, has penetrated the full corneal thickness and has entered the anterior chamber. The cornea surrounding the foreign body must first be carefully and gently undermined to expose a sufficient portion of the foreign body so that removal is possible. A cellulose stick swab, No. 65 Beaver blade or a 25-gauge needle can be used. Magnification and illumination is mandatory in all cases. If the foreign body is embedded lengthwise within the corneal stroma, a scalpel incision can be made over the long axis of the object so that it can be exposed for retrieval. Although very tempting, forceps should not be used to 'grab' the foreign body as the action of the forceps closing may inadvertently push it further into the anterior chamber. The tip of a protruding foreign body, or the portion made accessible after undermining, can then be impaled with one or, preferably, two 25-gauge needles placed at 90° to the foreign body. The foreign body is then removed with traction applied in a reverse direction to its line of entry (Fig. 3.39). A small amount of aqueous may leak from the site of penetration if the anterior chamber had been entered. Small wounds will seal under a soft bandage contact lens while larger wounds require direct corneal repair with 8/0–10/0 suture material or sometimes a small conjunctival pedicle graft.

■ Some foreign bodies in the anterior chamber, or those which have impaled the iris, may be more easily removed via a limbal incision, separate from the site of penetration. A viscoelastic material (which is later removed) can be injected into the anterior chamber to facilitate this. Fine intraocular forceps should be used to manipulate the foreign body. The limbal wound should be sutured with 8/0–9/0 absorbable suture material in a simple interrupted pattern. The corneal entry wound may or may not require suturing. Balanced salt solution or lactated Ringer's solution should be used to irrigate blood and fibrin from the anterior chamber if necessary.

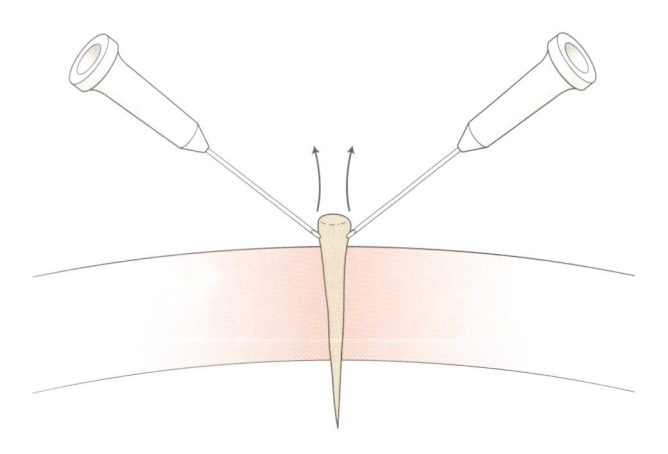

Fig. 3.39 Removal of corneal foreign body.

■ Pupil dilation with a short-acting mydriatic such as 1% tropicamide is helpful during the removal of a foreign body, which is more easily visualised when highlighted or retro-illuminated against a bright tapetal reflex. Atropine can also be used, particularly if there is a secondary uveitis.

■ Foreign bodies which have penetrated the lens are more complicated to manage. Penetration of the anterior lens capsule and subsequent release of lens protein may lead to severe phacoclastic uveitis; alternatively the lens capsular defect may seal and result in a focal traumatic cataract with little or no intraocular inflammation. Intralenticular abscess formation is also possible. Aggressive medical therapy to control the inflammation and lendectomy by phacoemulsification may be required and specialist advice should be sought.

■ Postoperative medical therapy for superficial foreign bodies that have not penetrated the anterior chamber include a topical broad spectrum antibiotic eye drop or ointment and a mydriatic/cycloplegic such as 1% atropine and systemic anti-inflammatory drugs to control the secondary uveitis.

■ When there is intraocular involvement, broad-spectrum systemic antibiotics are also required in addition to the above treatment; topical eye drops are preferable to ointment formulations.

INTRAOCULAR METALLIC FOREIGN BODIES

Intraocular metallic foreign bodies are generally associated with gunshot injuries. Assessment includes a careful history, e.g. working gundog, direct observation, plain skull radiographs and ocular ultrasonography. Ocular tolerance to a metallic foreign body depends on its inertness, size, position and the tissue in which it is lodged. In general, removal should not be attempted if the precise location of the foreign body is not known, the material is inert, the foreign body is within a non-reactive tissue site, and especially if surgical removal would cause more intraocular trauma than the presence of the foreign body itself. Small high-velocity foreign bodies, such as most gunshot injuries, are usually sterile due to the heat generated by the speed of travel, but prophylactic broad-spectrum antibiotic therapy for surface contaminants is justified. Lead, gold, silver, glass and rubber are all relatively inert within the eye. Lead shot pellets are well tolerated as they are usually covered with an insoluble carbonate that prevents diffusion of chemical reactivity. Inert metallic foreign bodies with smooth edges are well tolerated in the anterior chamber, iris, lens and vitreous (Schmidt et al., 1975). A traumatic cataract may result but removal is only indicated if it causes severe lens-induced uveitis. Conversely, copper, zinc and brass are reactive materials and will all result in severe intraocular inflammation and panophthalmitis. For example, intraocular retention of a 3 mm copper pellet in a German Shepherd dog resulted in an intravitreal abscess and endophthalmitis and necessitated enucleation (Carter and Blevins, 1970).

HYPHAEMA

Hyphaema

Hyphaema (Figs 3.40 and 3.41) can be defined as the presence of blood in the anterior chamber. The degree of hyphaema can vary from mild forms, in which a small amount of blood floats free or is trapped within fibrin, to severe cases when the anterior chamber is completely filled with blood so that the iris and pupil are obscured (total hyphaema).

The presence of hyphaema is usually straightforward to diagnose by directly observing blood in the anterior chamber. Depending on the cause, there may be associated signs of ocular inflammation such as perilimbal hyperaemia, corneal oedema and blepharospasm. If the blood persists in cases of total hyphaema for 5–7 days, it turns from a bright red to a bluish-black colour and is termed an 'eight ball haemorrhage'.

Causes

- Hyphaema in young dogs without a history or clinical signs of trauma is suggestive of a congenital anomaly such as collie eye anomaly.

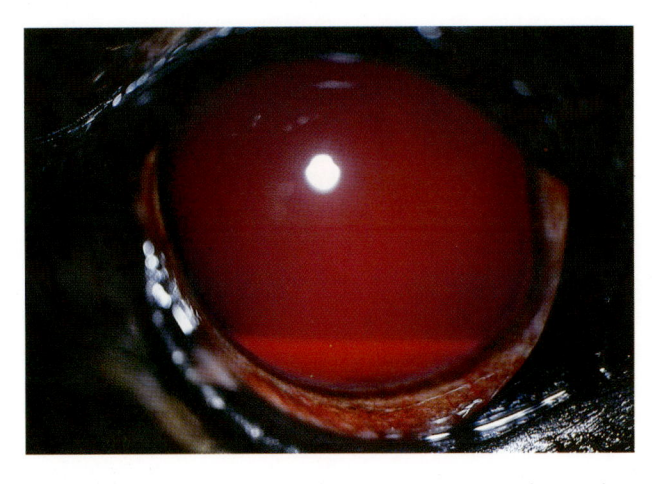

Fig. 3.40 Total hyphaema which was recurrent in this aged German Shepherd Dog with an intraocular neoplasm.

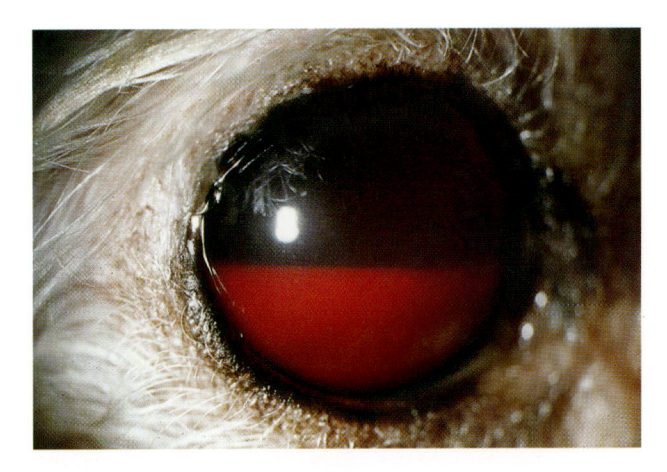

Fig. 3.41 Hyphaema with horizontal fluid line due to a systemic coagulopathy in a Shih Tzu.

- Ocular trauma can cause rupture of intraocular blood vessels and such cases are generally associated with a very poor prognosis. Hyphaema is a poor prognostic indicator in cases of traumatic proptosis of the globe.
- Hyphaema is a common finding in patients with systemic hypertension as arterioles may rupture with prolonged hypertension.
- Chronic uveitis, retinal detachment and intraocular neoplasia can also result in hyphaema due to the formation of fine blood vessels that grow across the iridal surface or in association with the retina. The former are known as 'preiridal fibrovascular membranes'. The developing blood vessels are fragile and have a tendency to 'leak', causing hyphaema.
- Acute uveitis causes a breakdown of the blood–ocular barrier allowing red blood cells to enter the eye and resulting in hyphaema.
- Hyphaema may occur if there is retrograde blood flow into the anterior chamber via the aqueous humor drainage pathways. Systemic coagulopathies may cause hyphaema in this way.
- Infectious diseases such as ehrlichiosis can cause hyphaema by causing blood hyperviscosity, vasculitis, thrombocytopaenia and platelet dysfunction.

Management

- A careful eye examination is performed initially to assess whether the aetiology of the hyphaema is primarily ocular or systemic in nature. In general, hyphaema attributable to blunt or penetrating ocular trauma is more common than that arising from endogenous causes.
- The conjunctiva of the contralateral eye, as well as the mucosal membranes, should be thoroughly examined to search for petechial haemorrhages. A careful fundic examination after pupil dilation with 1% tropicamide is necessary to check for retinal haemorrhages. The presence of haemorrhages elsewhere in addition to the hyphaema is highly suggestive of a systemic disorder and further diagnostic tests are indicated.
- Routine haematology, biochemistry, urinalysis and a clotting profile should be performed. Survey thoracic and abdominal radiographs are indicated in selected cases.
- Ocular ultrasonography is very useful to detect intraocular neoplasia, retinal detachment and disruption of the ocular tunics following ocular trauma.
- Blood pressure measurement should be performed in any dog with retinal detachment, haemorrhage or hyphaema.
- An assessment of whether the blood is clotted or unclotted helps to elucidate the cause of the hyphaema. Generally, clotted blood is found in cases of trauma and uveitis, whereas hyphaema secondary to a systemic coagulopathy is usually associated with unclotted blood. Recurrent hyphaema is suggestive of chronic retinal detachment and intraocular neoplasia (Collins and Moore, 1999).

OCULAR EMERGENCIES AND TRAUMA

Treatment
Anti-inflammatory therapy is indicated for the treatment of hyphaema.

- Topical corticosteroid therapy is indicated provided there is no corneal ulceration; 1% prednisolone acetate has excellent intraocular penetration and can be applied three to six times daily depending on the severity of the clinical signs.
- Systemic corticosteroid therapy is indicated in most cases of hyphaema. Prednisolone 1 mg/kg once daily for 5–7 days should be initially prescribed, followed by a reducing dosage until the hyphaema has resolved.
- Avoid the use of systemic nonsteroidal anti-inflammatory drugs as they can increase the risk of further haemorrhage.
- Topical 1% atropine drops or ointment is indicated if there is concurrent uveitis. Atropine can be given safely if the intraocular pressure (IOP) is reduced.
- If the IOP is increased then glaucoma therapy may be indicated; 2% dorzolamide, a topical carbonic anhydrase inhibitor, can be administered three times daily to lower the IOP. Topical pilocarpine causes miosis and the increased surface area of exposed iris facilitates the absorption of blood by phagocytosis. However, pilocarpine will potentiate uveitis and the miosis increases the risk of posterior synechiae formation and even iris bombé. The decision to use pupilloactive drugs such as atropine and pilocarpine is not always straightforward, particularly if the IOP cannot be accurately monitored.
- Tissue plasminogen activator (TPA) can be injected intracamerally to dissolve clotted blood when there is an increase in the IOP that cannot be controlled medically, or when there is extensive synechiae formation. The effects of TPA are not always straightforward and specialist advice should be sought.

Prognosis most cases of simple hyphaema will resorb within 7–14 days. However, the prognosis often cannot be fully determined until the blood has cleared sufficiently to permit fundus examination.

A number of sequelae can develop following hyphaema. Phthisis bulbi is not uncommon following severe uveitis. Secondary cataract formation can occur because the lens metabolism is altered by the surrounding blood. Corneal opacity may result from blood staining the corneal endothelium. Retinal atrophy may follow extensive intravitreal haemorrhage.

In general, the prognosis for hyphaema is very poor when there is involvement of the posterior segment such as vitreal, retinal or choroidal haemorrhages (Collins and Moore, 1999).

LIPID AQUEOUS

Dogs affected with lipid aqueous (Fig. 3.42) are often presented with an acute onset of a 'blue' or 'white' eye. Most cases are unilateral but bilateral involvement is occasionally

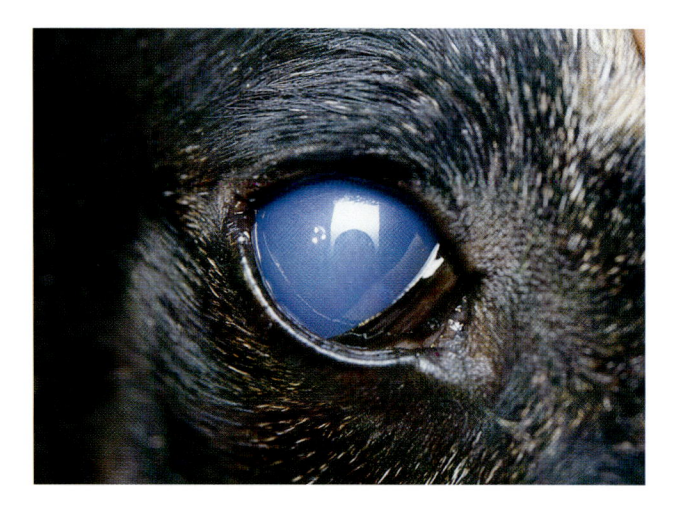

Fig. 3.42 Lipid aqueous in a middle-aged crossbred dog with hyperlipoproteinaemia secondary to Cushing's syndrome and diabetes mellitus.

seen. Lipid aqueous usually involves only the anterior chamber. Clinically an evenly distributed, light blue-white opacity, which varies in its intensity, is visible within the anterior chamber. Slit-lamp biomicroscopy confirms that the cornea is unaffected, differentiating it from corneal odema. Mild conjunctival hyperaemia may be seen in association with a mild anterior uveitis. Signs of ocular pain such as blepharospasm or lacrimation are rarely seen with this condition. Lipaemia retinalis may be recognised if the anterior segment is transparent enough to allow fundic examination. This is the term given to the abnormal 'strawberry-milkshake' appearance of the retinal vasculature which is most obvious in the non-tapetal fundus.

Lipid aqueous occurs when there is a breakdown of the blood–aqueous barrier with a concurrent hyperlipidaemia (Lane *et al.*, 1993). The most common causes of hyperlipidaemia in the dog include diabetes mellitus, pancreatitis, liver disease and postprandial effects. Lipid aqueous may also occur when there is a genetic defect that interferes with lipoprotein metabolism (Crispin, 1993; Watson and Barrie, 1993).

Management

- Treatment is directed at stabilising the blood–eye barrier by the use of a topical corticosteroid such as 1% prednisolone acetate three times daily. The lipid aqueous usually clears within 1–3 days.
- Blood tests for routine biochemistry, haematology and a lipid profile should be performed when the patient has been fasted to identify any underlying disorder that may be present.

UVEITIS

The aetiology, clinical signs and diagnosis of uveitis are discussed in detail in Chapter 12. Acute uveitis presents as a

UVEITIS

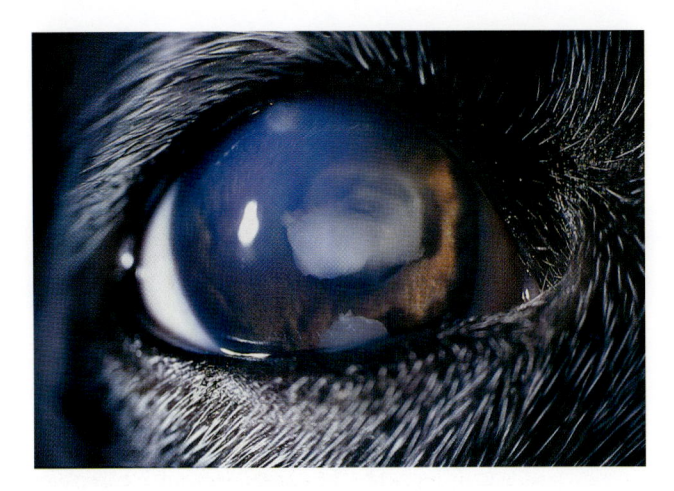

Fig. 3.43 Traumatic cataract and phacoclastic uveitis in a Dalmatian puppy following a cat scratch injury. Note site of focal corneal penetration in the dorsal peripheral cornea and the loose piece of cataractous material in the ventral anterior chamber.

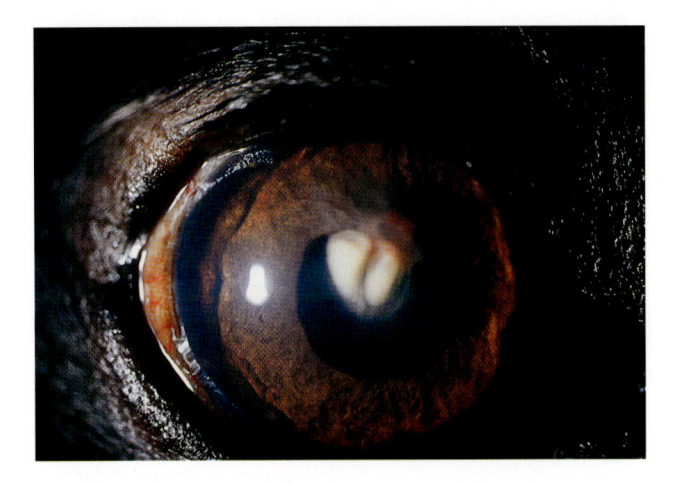

Fig. 3.44 Focal traumatic cataract and intra-lenticular abscess in a Dachshund following a foreign body penetration.

painful red eye that resembles glaucoma. Uveitis is rarely an emergency, except in cases of penetrating trauma (Figs 3.43 and 3.44) (discussed earlier) but uncontrolled inflammation can rapidly destroy the function of the globe so prompt attention is indicated.

Management

- Although the aetiology is not determined in the majority of cases, a thorough diagnostic work-up is still indicated unless the initiating cause is obvious. Physical examination, haematology, serum biochemistry and urinalysis should be performed.
- Medical treatment should be started immediately while awaiting laboratory results to avoid the potential sequelae of uveitis which can lead to loss of vision.
- 1% Atropine eye drops or ointment is used to dilate the pupil (mydriasis) to minimise the risk of posterior synechiae formation and to relax the ciliary body (cyclopegia), relieving the painful spasm associated with intense miosis. Atropine application is given 'to effect', i.e. at a frequency and/or concentration to achieve and maintain pupil dilation. Mild to moderate cases of uveitis may require once or twice daily application, whereas a severe phacoclastic uveitis with lens rupture may require a frequency of three or four times daily. Beware of the effect of lowering tear production, particularly in brachycephalic dogs with compromised tear films and eyes with a low or marginal basal tear production.
- A topical corticosteroid such as 1% prednisolone acetate eye drops with good intraocular penetration is used four to six times daily, depending on the degree of inflammation present. Treatment can initially be given hourly in severe cases if tolerated by the patient. Corneal integrity should be checked with fluorescein dye prior to the application of topical corticosteroids; 0.1% dexamethasone acetate will also penetrate the intact cornea.
- Topical nonsteroidal anti-inflammatory drugs, such as ketorolac or flurbiprofen, can be used in cases where topical corticosteroids are contraindicated, but they are generally reserved to prevent and treat inflammation associated with intraocular surgery. Such drugs should be used with caution due to their variable effects on ocular infection and possible potentiation of corneal ulceration. They are best given under the direction of an ophthalmologist.
- Systemic prednisolone at 1–2 mg/kg daily in divided doses is indicated for severe anterior uveitis and for all cases of posterior uveitis, in the absence of infection and other systemic contraindications such as diabetes mellitus. Alternatively, systemic nonsteroidal anti-inflammatory drugs such as carprofen can be given until laboratory results are received. A systemic nonsteroidal anti-inflammatory drug may offset the need for frequent atropine application to relax ciliary body spasm and can be used where systemic corticosteroids are contraindicated.
- Analgesia may be necessary in cases of severe uveitis when there is obvious ocular discomfort.
- Topical and systemic broad spectrum antibiotics should be administered in cases of penetrating trauma.
- Early and aggressive medical therapy is indicated in all cases of uveitis. It is important to continue anti-inflammatory therapy after the cessation of clinical signs, as abrupt discontinuation of treatment will result in recurrence and exacerbation of clinical signs.

GLAUCOMA

Acute glaucoma presents as a painful, 'red' (episcleral congestion) and 'blue' (diffuse corneal oedema) eye (Fig. 3.45). Vision is often impaired or absent. The pupil is unresponsive and mid to well dilated. Acute glaucoma is a true ocular emergency; it is to ophthalmology what acute intervertebral disc disease is to neurosurgery. Breed predisposition in primary glaucoma is helpful for the initial diagnosis and

OCULAR EMERGENCIES AND TRAUMA

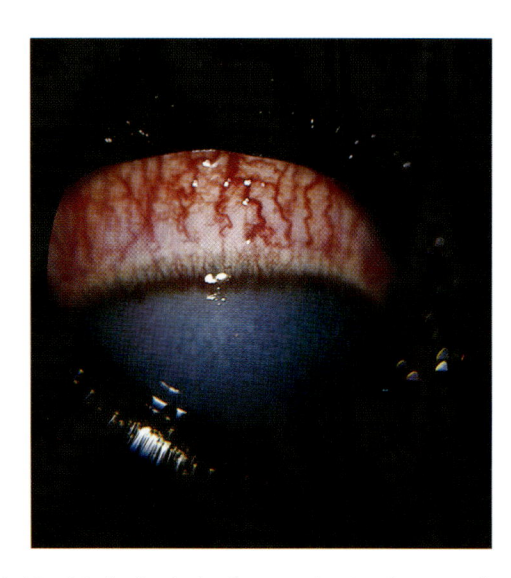

Fig. 3.45 Marked episcleral congestion ('red eye') and corneal oedema ('blue eye') in a young adult Flat-coated Retriever with acute onset primary glaucoma.

breeds such as the English and Welsh Springer Spaniel, Flat-coated Retriever, Basset Hound, Great Dane, American and English Cocker Spaniel, Siberian Husky and Dandie Dinmont should always raise concern. Ideally, referral for specialist diagnostic procedures such as tonometry and gonioscopy should be offered, but appropriate interim treatment is vital.

- Analgesia is indicated as acute glaucoma is painful, sometimes very painful; a systemic nonsteroidal anti-inflammatory drug such as carprofen in conjunction with an opioid is effective.
- The acute rise in intraocular pressure is often accompanied by marked intraocular inflammation (uveitis) and anti-inflammatory treatment is therefore indicated topically and systemically; 1% prednisolone acetate and oral prednisolone are very effective.
- Drugs to reduce intraocular pressure – a number of the more traditional antiglaucoma drugs are less commonly used as some have become unavailable in the UK (dichlorphenamide, demecarium bromide) or have been superseded (mannitol). A number of new topical agents such as latanoprost (a prostaglandin analogue) and dorzolomide (a topical carbonic anydrase inhibitor), which are successful in the human field, have been used. Unfortunately the pressure 'spikes' which occur in canine glaucoma are usually very high and drugs such as dorzolomide or timolol (a topical β-blocker) are relatively ineffective in the acute situation. Latanoprost is usually very effective at lowering the IOP quickly but will also cause an intense miosis and should be used with caution in uveitis.
- Medical therapy is often used together with surgery, such as laser trans-scleral photocoagulation and drainage implant procedures, requiring referral to an ophthalmologist.

Sudden vision loss

The most common causes of sudden vision loss in the dog are 'sudden acquired retinal degeneration' (SARD), optic neuritis and retinal detachment. Dogs cope extremely well with gradual loss of vision such as in progressive retinal atrophy (PRA) and cataract formation, in contrast to acute blindness which presents as an emergency.

Sudden acquired retinal degeneration

Dogs affected with SARD present with a loss of vision in both eyes over a period of days from 1 to 2 weeks (Mattson et al., 1992). The pupils are dilated and although pupillary light reflexes are usually present, they are slow and incomplete. The retina appears normal with fundoscopic examination. The typical signalment is middle-aged, slightly overweight, spayed female dogs. There is often a history of polydipsia/polyuria, weight gain and lethargy and the clinical features are suggestive of hyperadrenocorticism (Mattson et al., 1992). The aetiology of SARD is unknown but it has been suggested that it is caused by a retinal toxicity produced with the sudden release of retinal neurotransmitters. Retinal cells from affected dogs have been found to have undergone apoptosis (Miller et al., 1998).

- Electroretinography reveals no retinal activity and is diagnostic for SARD. This is a very useful diagnostic test as the total absence of retinal activity eliminates other important differential diagnoses such as retrobulbar optic neuritis and central lesions which may present with similar clinical signs.
- Blood tests for routine haematology and biochemistry should be performed, and more specific tests for hyperadrenocorticism if indicated.
- There is no treatment and affected animals do not regain vision.
- Classic features of retinal degeneration occur with time, i.e. vascular attenuation, tapetal hyper-reflectivity and optic nerve atrophy.

Optic neuritis

Optic neuritis is usually idiopathic and immune mediated but can also be caused by infectious agents (fungal, viral or protozoal) or neoplasia (lymphosarcoma).

Dogs with optic neuritis present with acute visual impairment or blindness and dilated, unresponsive pupils. Optic neuritis can be unilateral or bilateral. Clinical features seen on fundoscopy include swelling and oedema of the optic disc manifested by blurred disc margins, apparent loss of the physiological cup, focal haemorrhages and distortion of the retinal vasculature as the vessels seem to 'climb' up onto the swollen papilla. Peripapillary lesions such as retinal oedema, retinitis and haemorrhages may also be present. These signs may be subtle and the diagnosis is often challenging from fundic signs alone. Retrobulbar optic neuritis is even more difficult to diagnose as the optic disc and surrounding retina appear normal on examination because it is the section of optic nerve posterior to the globe which is affected. As mentioned above, electroretinography is a very helpful diagnostic test and CT and/or MRI scanning techniques may also be indicated. Animals affected with optic neuritis may show other signs of neurological disease and again the more sophisticated imaging techniques in conjunction with cerebrospinal fluid analysis may be indicated.

Management

- Investigation for an underlying cause is indicated and specific treatment should be instigated as necessary.
- Intensive anti-inflammatory therapy is indicated to control the inflammation. Once any underlying causes, particularly infections, are controlled, immunosuppressive doses of systemic corticosteroids should be administered, prednisolone 1–2 mg/kg twice daily for 3–5 days, gradually reducing over several weeks in response to improvement and resolution of clinical signs. Azathioprine can be considered in refractory cases.
- The prognosis for vision is guarded. The amount of vision that returns depends on the amount of damage inflicted on the optic nerves, which in turn depends on the severity and duration of the inflammation as well as how quickly the inflammation responds to therapy. In some cases maintenance therapy is required to prevent recurrence, which is not uncommon.

RETINAL DETACHMENT

Retinal detachments (Fig. 3.46) are generally extensive by the time the patient presents with vision loss. The pupil is usually dilated in the affected eye(s) and the pupillary light reflex is slow, incomplete or virtually absent. The fundoscopic appearance will vary depending on the type and extent of the retinal detachment. Generally the tapetal reflection is reduced, and the neurosensory retina can be observed to be closer to the lens. The retinal vasculature may be visible through the pupil with a pen torch, without the need for an ophthalmoscope. Infundibular or 'morning glory' detachments appear as a grey, billowing 'curtain' posterior to the lens. Total detachment (with disinsertion at the ora ciliaris retina) creates an exceptionally reflective appearance as the tapetum is being viewed *directly* with the neurosensory retina lying ventrally.

There are a number of causes of retinal detachment in the dog including inflammatory, infectious, neoplastic, hypertensive, traumatic, inherited retinal dysplasias and in association with vitreal traction bands.

Management

- The prognosis for restoration of vision is generally poor as retinal degeneration at a cellular level begins within hours of the neurosensory retina becoming separated from the underlying retinal pigment epithelium. However, it is important to search for an underlying cause as some conditions, for example hypertension, will respond to medication.
- A thorough physical examination is indicated when no ocular cause for the detachment has been identified. Blood tests for routine haematology and biochemistry, urinalysis and blood pressure measurement should be performed.
- Specific medical therapy for systemic hypertension and management of concurrent or underlying conditions are indicated. There is little response to either medical or surgical intervention for large retinal detachments but it is important to control any underlying condition.
- Cage rest is helpful to prevent a partial retinal detachment from extending further and progressing to a total detachment.
- In some cases intensive systemic anti-inflammatory therapy may help to restore normal retinal anatomy; these have been called 'steroid-responsive retinal detachments'. In such cases complete retinal reattachment usually occurs within 4–39 days if no vitreal haemorrhage is present; if blood is present in the vitreous then the time taken for reattachment is much longer, 12–144 days.
- Retinal detachment surgery is practised by some veterinary ophthalmologists but is a complicated procedure and not widely available (Vainisi and Packo, 1995).

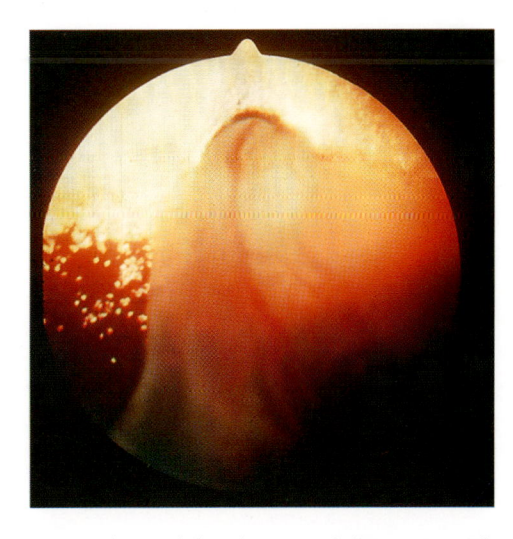

Fig. 3.46 Total retinal detachment and disinsertion. The retina hangs down in folds from the edge of the optic disc, which is obscured.

REFERENCES

Carpenter JL, Schmidt GM, Moore FM, Albert DM, Abrams KL, Elner VM (1989) Canine bilateral extraocular polymyositis. *Veterinary Pathology* **26**: 510–512.

Carter JD, Blevins WE (1970) Intraocular copper retention (chalcosis) in a dog: a case report. *Journal of the American Animal Hospital Association* **6**: 28–36.

Coleman ES (1998) Clostridial neurotoxins. *The Compendium on Continuing Education* **20**: 1089.

Collins BK, Moore CP (1999) Diseases and surgery of the canine anterior uvea. In Gelatt KN (ed.) *Veterinary Ophthalmology*, 3rd edn, pp. 755–795. Lippincott, Williams and Wilkins, Philadelphia.

Crispin SM (1993) Ocular manifestations of hyperlipoproteinaemia. *Journal of Small Animal Practice* **34**: 500–506.

Featherstone HJ, Sansom J (2000) Intestinal submucosa repair in two cases of feline ulcerative keratitis. *Veterinary Record* **146**: 136–138.

Gilger BC, Hamilton HL, Wilkie DA, van der Woerdt A, McLaughlin SA, Whitley RD (1995) Traumatic ocular proptoses in dogs and cats: 84 cases (1980–1993). *Journal of the American Veterinary Medical Association* **206**: 1186–1190.

Johnson BW, Brightman AH, Whitely HE (1988) Conjunctival mast cell tumour in two dogs. *Journal of the American Animal Hospital Association* **24**: 439–442.

Lane IF, Roberts SM, Lappin MR (1993) Ocular manifestations of vascular disease: hypertension, hyperviscosity and hyperlipidemia. *Journal of the American Animal Hospital Association* **29**: 28–36.

Mattson A, Roberts SM, Isherwood JME (1992) Clinical features suggesting hyperadrenocorticism associated with sudden acquired retinal degeneration syndrome in a dog. *Journal of the American Animal Hospital Association* **28**: 199–302.

Miller PE, Galbreath EJ, Kehren JC, Steinberg H, Dubielzig RR (1998) Photoreceptor cell death by apoptosis in dogs with sudden acquired retinal degeneration syndrome. *American Journal of Veterinary Research* **59**: 149–152.

Millichamp NJ, Spencer CP (1991) Orbital varix in a dog. *Journal of the American Animal Hospital Association* **27**: 56–60.

Roberts SM (1985) Assessment and management of the ophthalmic emergency. *The Compendium on Continuing Education* **7**: 739–752.

Rühli MB, Spiess BM (1995) Therapy of orbital cellulitis and abscesses in dogs and cats. *Tierärztl Prax* **23**: 398–401.

Samuelson DA (1999) Ophthalmic anatomy. In Gelatt KN (ed.) *Veterinary Ophthalmology*, 3rd edn, pp. 35–36. Lippincott, Williams and Wilkins Philadelphia.

Sansom J, Barnett KC (1997) Soft contact lenses in small animals. *Waltham Focus*, **7**: 21–23.

Schmidt GM, Dice PF, Koch SA (1975) Intraocular lead foreign bodies in four canine eyes. *Journal of Small Animal Practice* **16**: 33–39.

Simison WG (1993) Sialoadenitis associated with periorbital disease in a dog. *Journal of the American Veterinary Medical Association* **202**: 1983–1985.

Spiess BM, Wallin-Håkanson N (1999) Diseases of the canine orbit. In Gelatt KN (ed.) *Veterinary Ophthalmology*, 3rd edn, pp. 520–522. Lea and Febiger, Philadelphia.

Vainisi SJ, Packo KH (1995) Management of giant retinal tears in dogs. *Journal of the American Veterinary Medical Association* **206**: 491–495.

Watson TD, Barrie J (1993) Lipoprotein metabolism and hyperlipidaemia in the dog and cat: a review. *Journal of Small Animal Practice* **34**: 479–487.

Whitney JC (1970) A case of cranial myodegeneration (atrophic myositis) in a dog. *Journal of Small Animal Practice* **11**: 735–742.

4 GLOBE AND ORBIT

INTRODUCTION

The globe in the dog is large and almost spherical with a greater anteroposterior dimension than either a vertical or a transverse one. As with other predators, the eyes are located frontally with a wide field of binocular vision. The globe is divided horizontally, when viewed from behind, by the long posterior ciliary artery.

As might be expected, globe size varies among the breeds from approximately 20–25 mm in diameter, the cornea having a smaller curvature than the globe. There have been several attempts at globe measurement by various means over the years, but more recently Long (1992) carried out an interesting biometric study of the canine eye using B-mode ultrasonography. He used a direct corneal contact method with only topical anaesthesia on 364 purebred dogs representing 33 breeds. He reports a narrow range of axial length for each breed but no significant difference between male and female or right and left eyes. The breeds with the largest eyes were the larger dolichocephalic breeds (long, narrow skulls, e.g. Dobermann, Afghan and Greyhound), although others in this group (Irish Wolfhound, Deerhound, Rough Collie) were further down the list. The mesocephalic breeds (intermediate skull shape) revealed a considerable variation in axial globe length from the Giant Schnauzer to the German Shepherd Dog. Brachycephalic breeds (broad, short skulls) produced measurements much smaller than external eye appearance indicates, in particular the Bulldog and Pekingese. Classification of head type was not a reliable guide as to expected globe size, prominent eyes not necessarily being large and deep set eyes (enophthalmic) not necessarily being small. The results clearly showed that globe size was related more to breed than to skull type, eye appearance or body weight (see Table 4.1).

Globe development starts very early in embryogenesis, being one of the first parts of the central nervous system to form; subsequent development is rapid. The eye forms from neural and surface ectoderm, mesoderm and neural crest; there is no endoderm in its formation. The optic plate, the first recognisable ocular structure, develops into the primary optic vesicle from neural ectoderm which invaginates to form the optic cup. The lens placode develops from surface ectoderm and in turn also invaginates to form the lens vesicle. The globe develops from the optic cup and brief notes on the embryology of each part of the globe are to be found in subsequent chapters.

Table 4.1 Relationship between globe size and breed and body weight. (after Long, 1992)

Breed	Mean body weight (kg)	Mean axial length of globe (mm)
Dobermann	33.5	20.5
Rottweiler	50	20.5
Giant Schnauzer	31	20.3
Afghan	30	20
Greyhound	25.7	20
Labrador	33	19.7
Flat-coated Retriever	36	18.6
Golden Retriever	32.5	17.6
Basset	26	17.2
Irish Wolfhound	55	17
Chow	31.5	16.9
Bulldog	19.5	16.4
Weimaraner	45	16.1
German Shepherd Dog	33	15.3
Rough Collie	28	15.3
Cavalier King Charles Spaniel	9.6	14
English Cocker Spaniel	16	14
Cairn Terrier	5.4	13.1
Pekingese	3.7	13
Yorkshire Terrier	4.3	11.2
Shetland Sheepdog	6	10.2

Some conditions affecting the globe relate to the size of the globe and therefore must relate to the normal globe sizes which vary considerably from breed to breed (see above). Anophthalmos and microphthalmos are congenital conditions and buphthalmos may be defined as congenital glaucoma. Hydrophthalmos is an increase in globe size due to glaucoma, and phthisis bulbi is a decrease in globe size following severe trauma, infection or inflammation and including glaucoma. Conditions involving the orbit, enophthalmos and exophthalmos (or proptosis), and ultimate prolapse of the globe, are conditions relating to the position of the globe. Orbital disease is common in the dog but presents problems in accurate diagnosis of the primary cause, including the

GLOBE AND ORBIT

differential diagnosis of the conditions listed above (see following section on Diagnostic Imaging). Secondary signs of orbital disease may include: swelling of the eyelids and/or chemosis; lagophthalmos and exposure keratitis; pain on opening the mouth; epiphora or ocular discharge; fundus changes, including retinal detachment, haemorrhage and papilloedema. Orbital disease may also be influenced by the proximity of the masticatory muscles, the frontal and maxillary sinuses, the nasal chamber, the pharynx, the zygomatic salivary gland and the roots of the molar teeth.

Strabismus (see Figs 4.29 and 4.30), or squint, due to cranial nerve involvement, and ocular nystagmus are other clinical signs which may accompany certain diseases of the globe and orbit (see also Chapter 15).

The shape of the skull in the dog varies considerably with the breed, from the dolichocephalic (long-headed) to the brachycephalic (short-headed), and hence the orbit, in particular its depth but also its size and shape, also varies. The orbit of the dog is described as open or incomplete, on the temporal side, where it is completed by the orbital ligament stretching from the frontal to the zygomatic bones, thereby completing the lateral orbital rim. The contents of the orbit are enclosed within a cone-shaped fibrous periorbital membrane with its apex at the optic foramen (second cranial or optic nerve); other foramina for cranial nerves III, IV, V (ophthalmic) and VI and blood vessels are present. Tenon's capsule, or fascia bulbi, is a connective tissue sheath attached near the corneoscleral junction (limbus) and continuous with the fascia of the extraocular muscles. The contents of the orbit include the globe (eyeball), the extraocular muscles (4 rectus, 2 oblique, 1 retractor bulbi), lacrimal gland, zygomatic salivary gland, nerves, blood vessels and retrobulbar fat.

DIAGNOSTIC IMAGING OF GLOBE AND ORBIT
R DENNIS

Although most of the eye is usually readily examined directly there are occasions when this is not possible, for instance if severe eyelid swelling, corneal or lenticular opacity or intraocular haemorrhage are present. Other parts of the eye may be difficult to see, such as the areas behind the ciliary body. The retrobulbar space is completely surrounded by opaque soft tissues and so of course is not amenable to visual inspection. These limitations to the normal ocular examination can be overcome by using various forms of diagnostic imaging, namely radiography, ultrasound and the advanced cross-sectional techniques of computed tomography (CT) and magnetic resonance imaging (MRI). Each of these techniques has advantages and limitations, and they are often used together to provide complementary information (Dennis, 2000; Hendrix and Gelatt, 2000).

RADIOGRAPHY

Radiography is not likely to be helpful in patients where changes are confined to the globe, but should be used as part of the work-up of suspected orbital disease. The patient will usually require general anaesthesia or heavy sedation to allow accurate positioning and non-manual restraint. High-definition film/screen combinations should be used together with careful processing to produce optimum contrast and definition on the radiographs. A knowledge of normal radiographic anatomy and conformational variants is required, and this can be quite a challenge owing to the complex nature of the skull. It is recommended that a library of normal radiographs for different breeds is compiled, and anatomy textbooks, radiological atlases and bone specimens are also helpful.

A number of radiographic projections may be needed to demonstrate the area of the bony orbit, although the shape of the skull means that in each view some superimposition of other structures will occur. A straight lateral projection is often used although this means that the right and left sides are superimposed. Lateral oblique projections will separate the two sides although they can be hard to interpret, especially if they are not identically positioned. The dorsoventral (DV) or ventrodorsal (VD) radiograph is very helpful for comparing the two sides, but the patient must be positioned symmetrically. This projection will also allow assessment of the frontal sinuses which may be secondarily involved in orbital disease. The DV intraoral radiograph will show nasal disease, which may be extending to involve the orbit or nasolacrimal duct, and the rostrocaudal skyline view shows the frontal sinuses and the medial wall of the orbits.

Radiographs will only show areas of marked bony change or radiopaque foreign bodies, and when orbital disease is confined to the soft tissues or when bony involvement is minor, the radiographs will be normal. Radiography is therefore of most value when orbital neoplasia has extended into normally air-filled surrounding areas, namely the caudal nasal cavity or the frontal sinus, or conversely when a nasal or frontal tumour has eroded into the orbit. Radiographic signs include opacification of the caudal nasal cavity with loss of turbinate detail, loss of frontal sinus air lucency and evidence of local osteolysis or new bone production (Figs 4.1 and 4.2). Normal radiographs do not exclude the possibility of neoplasia that is still confined to the soft tissues of the orbit or that has entered the cranium. Radiopaque foreign bodies such as pieces of lead shot will be visible radiographically although it may not be possible to say whether they are within or outside the globe (Fig. 4.3). A normal radiographic variant not to be confused with disease is partial mineralisation of the orbital ligaments, which may be seen on the DV/VD projection.

Dacryocystorhinography is a radiographic contrast study which is used to outline the nasolacrimal ducts, although it can be rather difficult to perform and interpret. Following cannulation of the punctum of the lower eyelid, a small quantity of oily or water-soluble iodinated contrast medium is instilled slowly, taking care to avoid leakage onto the animal's skin. Lateral oblique radiographs are of most value, and may demonstrate blockage, rupture, irregularity or cyst formation associated with the duct.

DIAGNOSTIC IMAGING OF GLOBE AND ORBIT

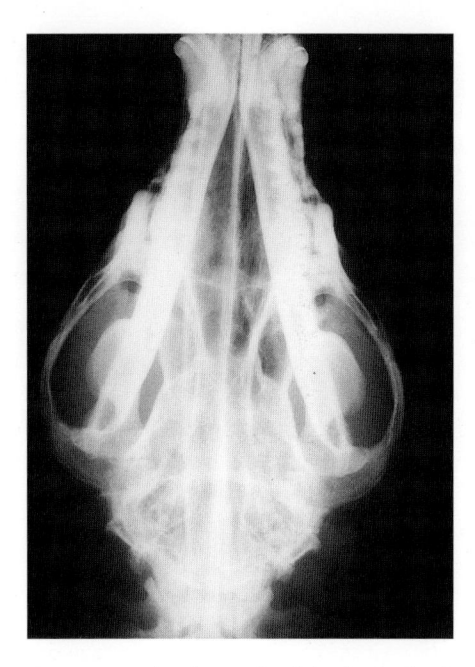

Fig. 4.1 Dorsoventral radiograph of the skull of a dog with orbital neoplasia, showing opacification of the right frontal sinus (on the left of the image) and increased soft tissue radiopacity in the caudal nasal cavity.

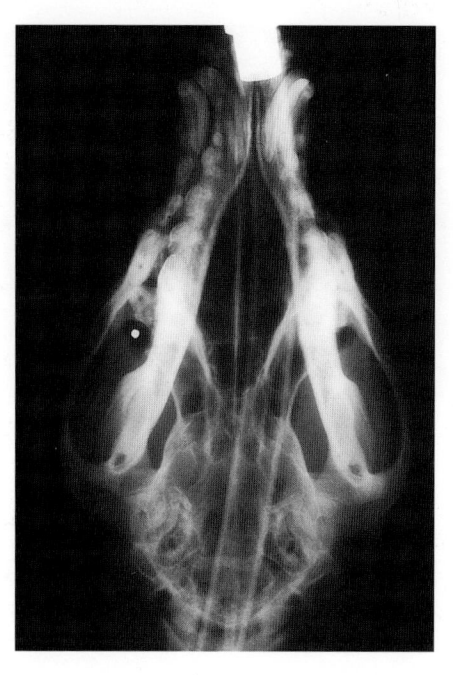

Fig. 4.3 Dorsoventral radiograph of a Labrador which had been accidentally shot. A metallic pellet is seen in the region of the orbit but it is not possible to say whether it is within or outside the globe.

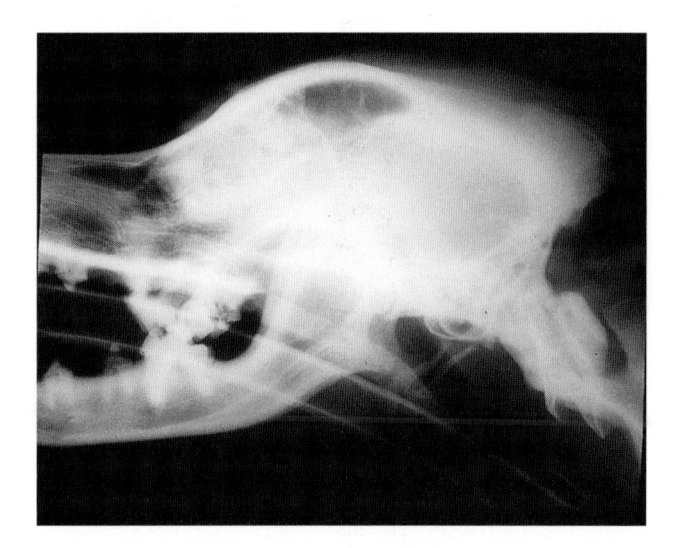

Fig. 4.2 Lateral radiograph of a dog with orbital neoplasia, showing opacification of the frontal sinus and granular sclerosis in the region of the orbit caused by new bone production.

Thoracic radiographs should be obtained in cases of known or suspected ocular or orbital neoplasia, since the presence of lung metastases will confirm a tentative diagnosis of neoplasia and may save the patient from invasive treatment, which is unlikely to be of long-term benefit. Right and left lateral recumbent radiographs with or without a DV or VD view should always be obtained since masses in the relatively poorly aerated dependent lung lobes may be overlooked.

ULTRASONOGRAPHY

Ultrasonographic examination is employed when the eye cannot be examined directly because of eyelid defects, periorbital swelling or opacity of parts of the eye which are normally translucent. Some ophthalmologists recommend routine ultrasonographic examination of eyes before cataract surgery to check for conditions such as retinal detachment which would prevent resumption of vision and would render cataract surgery inappropriate. Measurements of the globe can be made allowing confirmation of subjective assessments of changes in globe size. Ultrasound can also be used to investigate the retrobulbar space.

In general, higher frequency ultrasound transducers produce images with better definition but with a shallower depth of penetration into the tissues. For ocular and orbital ultrasonography, high frequency transducers are used since the depth of penetration required is small but fine detail is essential. Ideally a 10 or 12 MHz transducer is required although 7.5 MHz will produce acceptable images. If the front of the globe is to be examined, a stand-off should be used (a device of soft tissue equivalent built onto the front of the transducer so that the confusing 'transducer artefact' at the top of the image does not overlie structures of interest). If the area of interest is the retrobulbar space then a stand-off is not necessary.

Although the eye can be scanned through the lids, the image is poor because of interference by air trapped between the eyelid hairs, even if they are clipped. The preferred approach is using direct corneal contact, which conscious dogs and cats tolerate remarkably well following topical anaesthesia (Fig. 4.4).

GLOBE AND ORBIT

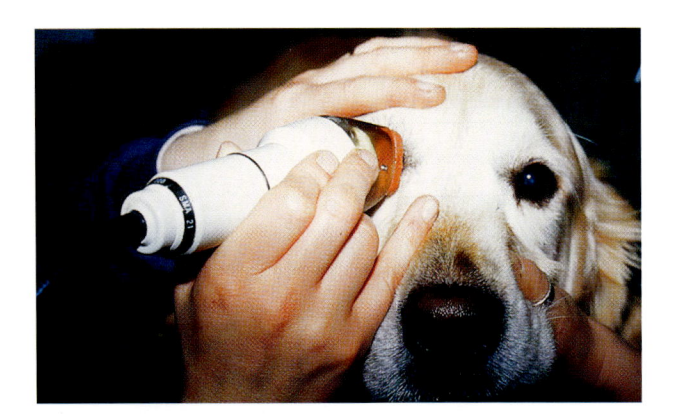

Fig. 4.4 Technique for ocular ultrasonography using the direct corneal contact method.

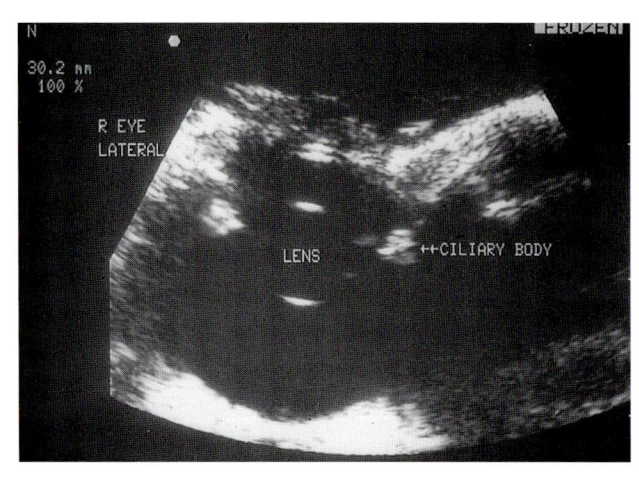

Fig. 4.5 Normal ocular ultrasonogram. The ciliary body and the centre of the lens are identified.

Sedation is rarely required and anaesthesia is contraindicated since the eyeball will retract and rotate downwards making it hard to image. An assistant is required to steady the patient's muzzle and perhaps to help hold the eyelids apart, depending on which eye is being scanned and whether the operator is right- or left-handed. Animals which are blind in the eye that is not being scanned may panic at first when the sighted eye is covered, but this can soon be overcome with sympathetic handling. Normal viscous ultrasound gel is used as a contact medium, scanning being performed through the gel rather than by pressing on the cornea.

Images are usually obtained first in the horizontal plane, sweeping up and down to cover the eye and orbit from top to bottom. The image can be zoomed to show the globe only, or expanded to cover the retrobulbar space. The eye can also be interrogated vertically, sweeping from side to side for completeness. Often the opposite eye can act as a control.

The normal globe is an anechoic or black sphere, the aqueous and vitreous humour and the lens producing no ultrasound echoes. Tissues which are more or less at right angles to the sound beam create echoes which return to the transducer, producing echogenic (bright) lines on the image. The front and back of the cornea and lens, the ciliary body and the back of the eye are seen in this way (Fig. 4.5). Interfaces which are angled relative to the ultrasound beam produce echoes which may not return to the transducer and these are poorly visualised; thus the normal lens capsule is not seen in its entirety and the sides of the globe are unclear. Behind the eye the retrobulbar fat and muscles appear hyperechoic (bright) and hypoechoic (dark) respectively, forming a cone shape towards the apex of the orbit. A dark band running vertically towards the transducer is often said to be the optic nerve, although in many cases this is probably acoustic shadowing from the head of the nerve. Medially, the concave frontal bone, which forms the medial wall of the orbit, can be seen as a curved, highly echoic line creating total acoustic shadowing distally.

Ultrasound can be used to detect intraocular masses, although it will give no suggestion as to histological type and cannot differentiate neoplastic masses from blood clots (Fig. 4.6). Free blood, areas of vitreal liquefaction and other debris can be seen as an unstructured increase in echogenicity, often swirling around with eye movements. Retinal detachments can easily be recognised, the complete detachment producing a 'bird's wing' appearance as it remains attached at the ora serrata and the optic nerve head (Fig. 4.7). Other linear echogenicities may be produced by vitreoretinal traction bands and by certain intraocular foreign bodies. Some foreign bodies may produce characteristic reverberations or acoustic shadowing (Fig. 4.8). Lens luxations can be identified easily, especially if the lens is cataractous (in which case it appears echogenic) or if it is surrounded by ocular haemorrhage (when it appears as an anechoic 'filling defect') (Fig. 4.9).

Behind the eye, ultrasound is especially rewarding for the diagnosis of focal masses and will usually differentiate between solid masses and fluid-filled lesions such as abscesses (Figs 4.10 and 4.11). However, it is often much harder to detect large and diffuse masses. Foreign bodies can sometimes be demonstrated, usually by virtue of acoustic shadowing or other artefacts created by their non-soft tissue composition (Martin *et al.*, 2000).

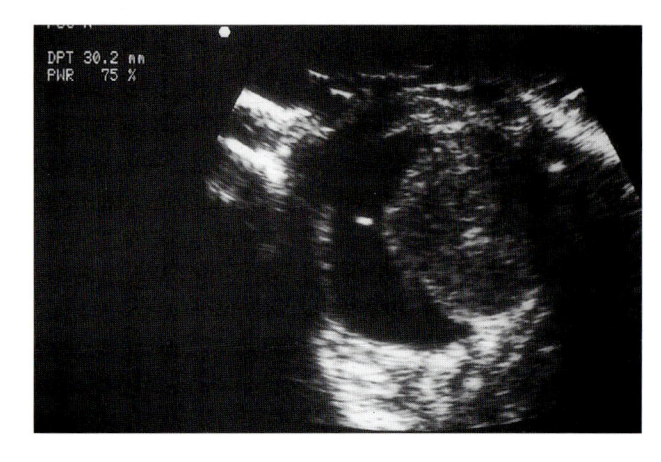

Fig. 4.6 Ultrasonogram of a large ocular melanoma. The lens is displaced to one side.

DIAGNOSTIC IMAGING OF GLOBE AND ORBIT

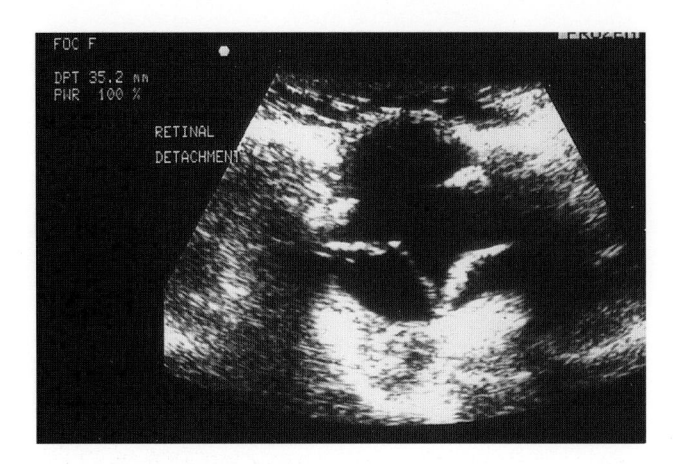

Fig. 4.7 Total retinal detachment producing the characteristic 'bird's wing appearance' on ultrasonography.

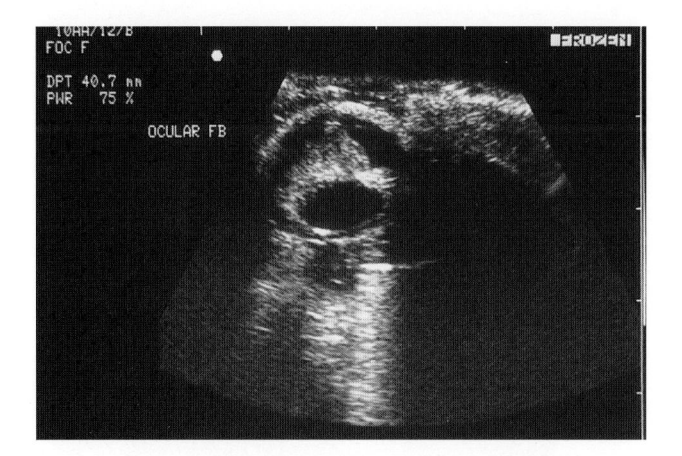

Fig. 4.8 Metallic pellet in the eye of a dog seen with ultrasonography (same patient as in Fig. 4.3). The pellet produces a short, linear, echogenic shadow with distal reverberations. Although the wall of the eye is not clearly seen, the position of the pellet suggests that it is intraocular. Haemorrhage is seen in the anterior segment.

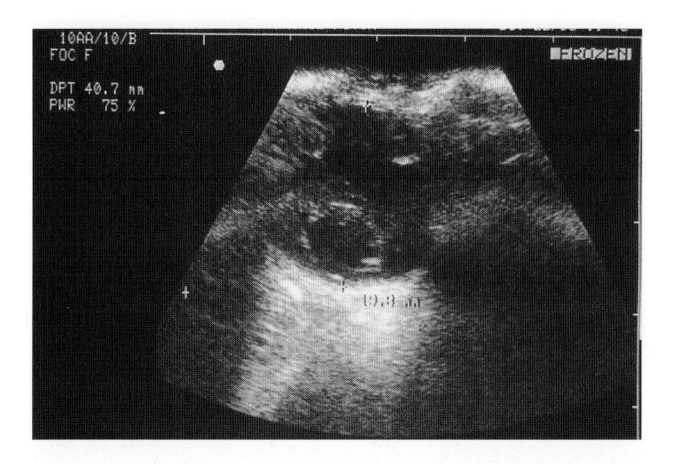

Fig. 4.9 Ultrasonographic appearance of caudal lens luxation in a terrier. The lens is seen as a dark, oval structure lying against the posterior wall of the eye. The ciliary bodies create two echogenic spots nearer the top of the image.

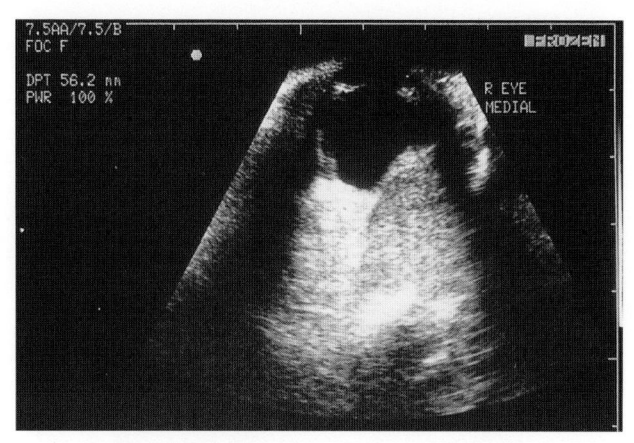

Fig. 4.10 Retrobulbar tumour seen with ultrasound. A hypoechoic mass displaces normal orbital tissues and indents the back of the eye.

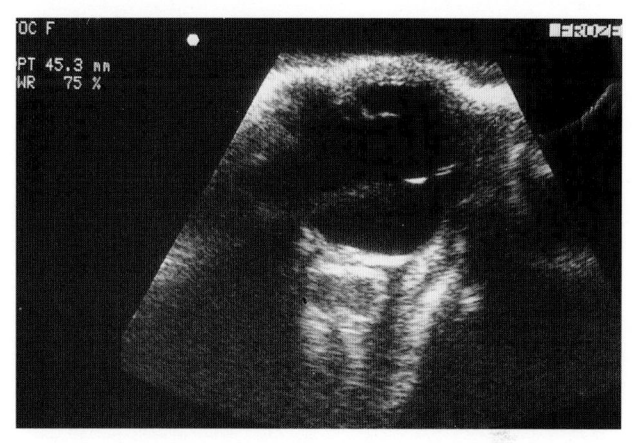

Fig. 4.11 Retrobulbar abscess on ultrasonography; a small, hypoechoic to anechoic lesion with echogenic walls.

MAGNETIC RESONANCE IMAGING AND COMPUTED TOMOGRAPHY

The advanced imaging techniques of MRI and CT both produce cross-sectional images which yield more three-dimensional information and far better tissue definition than do radiography and ultrasound. CT uses X-rays, producing cross-sectional radiographs of thin slices of the body which are computer-manipulated to increase differentiation compared with normal radiographs. Bone definition is excellent and CT is very sensitive for detecting early osteolysis or the presence of mineralisation. Soft tissue differentiation is superior to conventional radiography although much less than with MRI. One of the main drawbacks of CT is that primary images often can be obtained only in the transverse plane, and computer-reformatted images in other places are much poorer. CT requires chemical immobilisation of the patient but is relatively quick to perform. MR scanning uses an entirely different physical principle, working by a combination of magnetism and radio signals to map out the distribution of hydrogen nuclei (protons) in tissues. The images are

GLOBE AND ORBIT

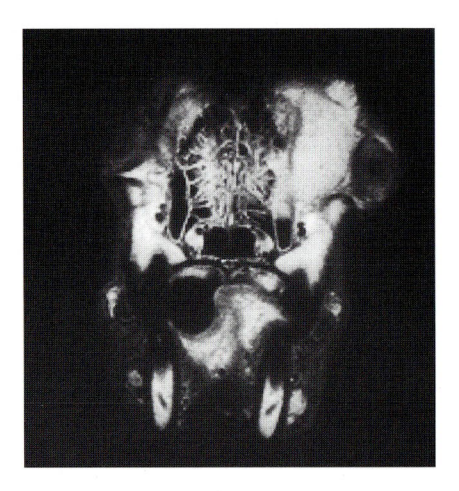

Fig. 4.12 MRI scan of an orbital chondrosarcoma. The mass displaces the eye laterally and erosion through the medial wall of the orbit into the maxillary recess is evident; this was not seen radiographically.

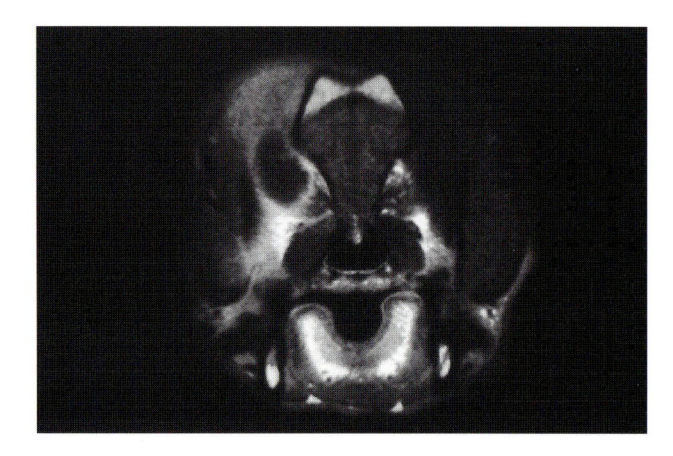

Fig. 4.13 Large retrobulbar abscess and cellulitis seen on an MRI scan. There is a well-defined hypointense area in the orbit with diffuse contrast enhancement of surrounding soft tissues indicating inflammation.

also thin cross-sectional slices but can be obtained in any plane with no loss of quality. Additionally, different types of scan can be performed to emphasise different tissues or to suppress the signal from orbital fat. Soft tissue resolution is vastly superior to CT, even allowing visualisation of the optic chiasm and optic nerves, although sensitivity for bone involvement is slightly lower. General anaesthesia is required and the studies take longer than with CT. With both techniques, contrast studies allow assessment of vascularity of tissues or damage to the blood–brain barrier and extension of disease into the brain.

Orbital neoplasia is seen as a mass lesion displacing normal orbital tissues; erosion into surrounding structures, which influences treatment and prognosis, can be clearly seen (Fig. 4.12). However, the histological nature of the tumour cannot be assessed without a biopsy or fine needle aspirate. Tumour extension into the cranium and sphenoid bones can be seen, as well as minor involvement of the orbital wall which is not evident radiographically. Abscesses can be clearly identified by their imaging features and diffuse inflammation may be differentiated from a focal mass using MRI (Fig. 4.13). Both modalities allow precise localisation of ocular and orbital foreign bodies permitting easier retrieval, although patients with metallic foreign bodies should not be imaged with MRI since the scanner's powerful magnetic field may cause ferrous materials to migrate (Fig. 4.14).

Postnatal growth of the globe

In an attempt to measure eyeball size and growth in the puppy, litters of Miniature Longhaired Dachshunds were studied and globes measured by B-mode ultrasound. Both right and left eyes were measured at regular intervals until 12 months of age. The measurements were the same for both right and left eyes and there was no difference between the sexes. Table 4.2 presents the results, in millimetres, averaged

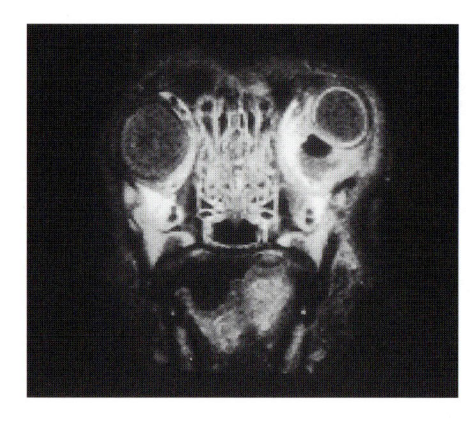

Fig. 4.14 Retrobulbar foreign body (a piece of plastic) and small abscess seen on MRI. The plastic appears as a signal void (black).

Table 4.2 Ultrasound globe measurements of postnatal Miniature Longhaired Dachshund puppies.

Age of puppy	Size of globe (mm)
2 weeks	10.1
3 weeks	11.2
4 weeks	11.8
5 weeks	12.1
7 weeks	13.3
10 weeks	14.7
12 weeks	15.1
14 weeks	15.9
18 weeks	16.7
6 months	16.9
8 months	17.7
10 months	17.8
12 months	17.9

CONGENITAL ANOMALIES

for the two readings taken for each eye of the three litters (eight puppies) studied.

CONGENITAL ANOMALIES

Anophthalmos complete absence of the globe, is extremely rare. Apparent anophthalmos (Fig. 4.15) usually proves to be severe microphthalmos with the presence of a small pigmented rudimentary cyst.

Microphthalmos (Figs 4.16–4.18), an abnormally small globe, is common in the dog. It may be unilateral or, more usually, bilateral and the two eyes may be similar or exhibit different degrees of severity. Microphthalmos is, by

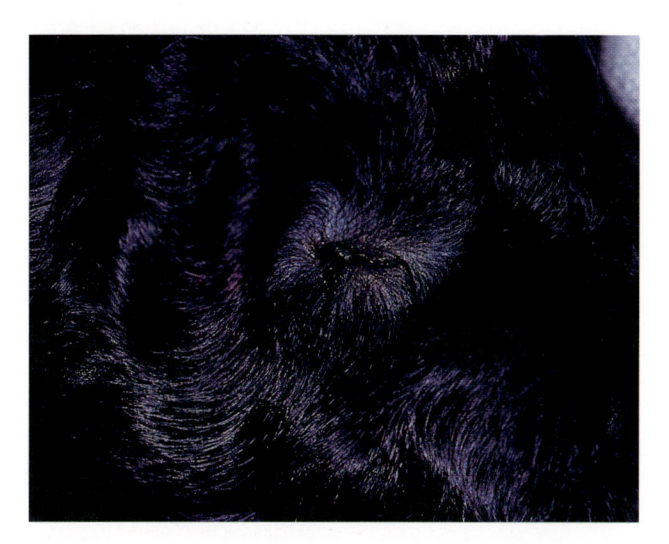

Fig. 4.15 Apparent anophthalmos in a Miniature Poodle puppy. Note small palpebral orifice and ocular discharge. This was not a case of true anophthalmos as a small pigmented cyst was found in the orbit on post-mortem examination.

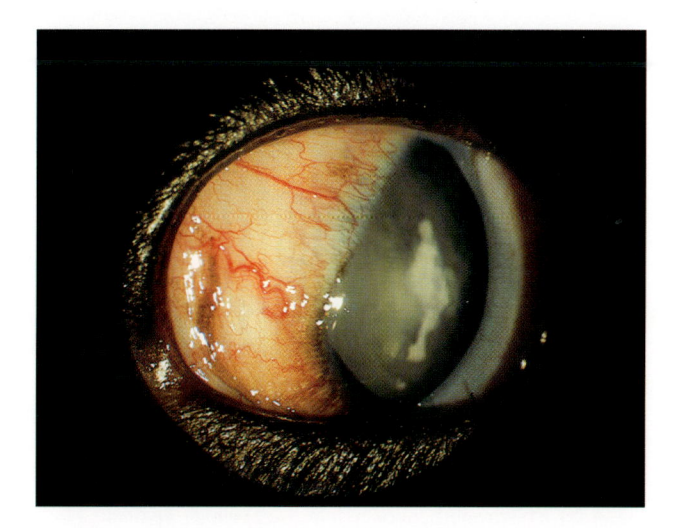

Fig. 4.16 Microphthalmos in an English Cocker Spaniel puppy. Note prominence of third eyelid, abnormal limbus and cataract, including dense white cataract on the anterior lens capsule.

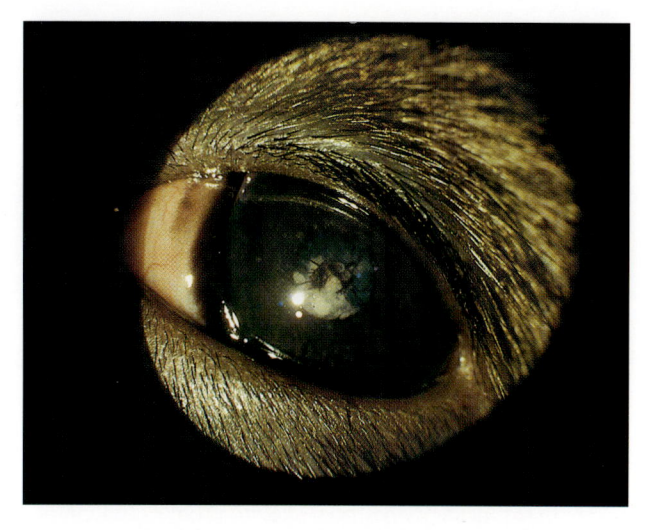

Fig. 4.17 Microphthalmos and multiocular defects in a German Shepherd Dog puppy. Note prominence of third eyelid, iris hypoplasia, pupillary membranes and cataract.

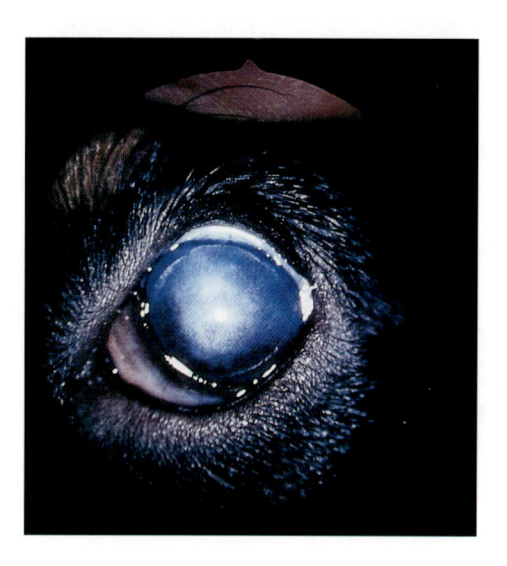

Fig. 4.18 Severe microphthalmos in a Dobermann puppy. Note prominence of third eyelid, exposure of sclera, corneal opacity and pigmentation.

definition, congenital and it may, or may not, be inherited – isolated cases do occur but cases also occur which exhibit a marked breed incidence and in some breeds inheritance has been proven.

Nanophthalmos is a term reserved for a small but otherwise normal globe but the common condition is microphthalmos accompanied by other ocular anomalies. In fact, cases of microphthalmia are usually, if not invariably, cases of multiple ocular defects (MOD). The commonest accompanying defect is cataract, often the presenting sign and frequently nuclear in position or pyramidal with a dense white anterior protuberance through the pupil. Vision is defective but total blindness is uncommon; these cataracts

GLOBE AND ORBIT

usually remain stationary, although just occasionally progression does occur depending upon their location within the lens. Anomalies of the uveal tract, particularly iris hypoplasia and persistent pupillary membranes, are other fairly frequent accompaniments to microphthalmos. In addition, irregular, usually posterior, corneal opacities, ciliary body anomalies, lens colobomata and retinal dysplasia are other abnormalities found not infrequently.

Mild degrees of microphthalmos together with cataract severe enough to cause defects in vision has been shown to be inherited in both the Miniature Schnauzer and Cavalier King Charles Spaniel (see Chapter 11). In several other breeds, notably the English Cocker Spaniel (Fig. 4.16), West Highland White Terrier and Old English Sheepdog, cataract and microphthalmos have been recorded and, although a strong breed incidence has been shown, proof of inheritance is lacking. In fact, the pattern of occurrence of cases in a kennel, and the fact that several or all in a litter are affected from clear parents, indicates a cause other than inheritance. Such cases are more accurately diagnosed as multiocular defects although cataract is frequently the presenting sign. Hereditary, and severe, microphthalmos, with other ocular defects, has been reported in the Dobermann in the UK (Lewis et al., 1986) (Fig. 4.18) and elsewhere (Peiffer and Fischer, 1983).

The microphthalmic eye tends to be sunken in the orbit and, as with other cases of enophthalmos, the nictitating membrane is prominent. In many cases with cataract, intermittent oscillatory bouts of ocular nystagmus are also present.

The microphthalmic eye should be distinguished from the phthitic eye, a non-congenital condition.

Buphthalmos (Fig. 4.19) is the term usually reserved for congenital glaucoma with globe enlargement. It is rare in the dog in comparison with hydrophthalmos, globe enlargement due to glaucoma occurring later in life, but in all other respects is similar to hydropthhalmos.

HYDROPHTHALMOS

Hydrophthalmos (Fig. 4.20) is globe enlargement due to glaucoma, an increase in intraocular pressure, although with hydrophthalmos the increase in intraocular pressure may remain or actually decrease owing to stretching of the globe. The globe enlargement leads to mild increased prominence, i.e. minimal proptosis, but the nictitating membrane is usually retracted and not more but less prominent. Retropulsion of the globe is accompanied by very little resistance. Buphthalmic and hydrophthalmic eyes are blind eyes due to pressure atrophy of the retina and, because of their size, must cause some pain due to pressure in the orbit; enucleation is the correct treatment. Corneal changes of oedema and vascularisation and fractures in Descemet's membrane are often accompanied by ocular discharge, and the appearance of the enlarged globe is another reason for enucleation. Hydrophthalmos must be distinguished from exophthalmos.

PHTHISIS BULBI

Phthisis (Fig. 4.21) is a shrunken globe which sinks into the orbit and is accompanied by prominence of the nictitating membrane and ocular discharge. The condition follows severe trauma, intraocular infection or inflammation and glaucoma. The eye is irreparably blind and enucleation is the answer.

ENOPHTHALMOS

Enophthalmos is defined as sinking, or recession, of the globe into the orbit and occurs for a variety of reasons:

- In marked dolichocephalic breeds, e.g. Flat-coated Retriever, Dobermann, Rough Collie, it is often accom-

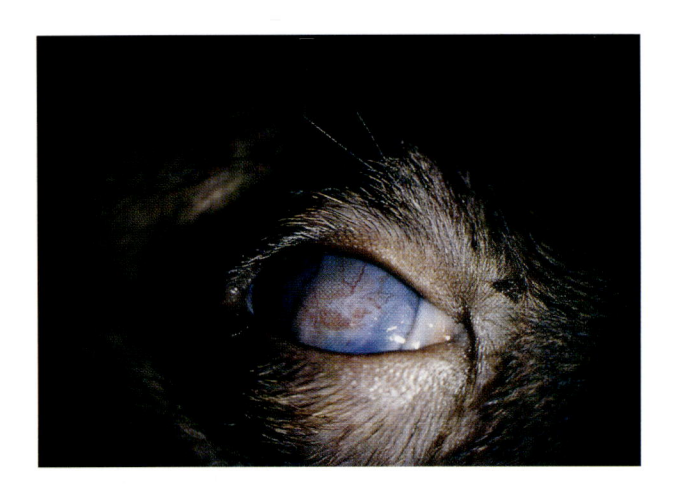

Fig. 4.19 Buphthalmos in a Greyhound puppy. Note corneal opacity and vascularisation. Another case of multiocular defects with other affected puppies in the litter.

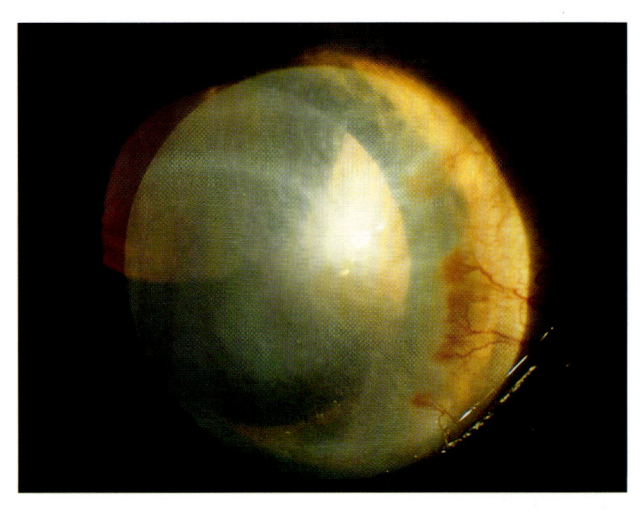

Fig. 4.20 Hydrophthalmos in a Welsh Springer Spaniel following primary glaucoma. Note diffuse corneal opacity with denser fractures in Descemet's membrane, superficial vascularisation and upward displacement of lens.

EXOPHTHALMOS OR PROPTOSIS

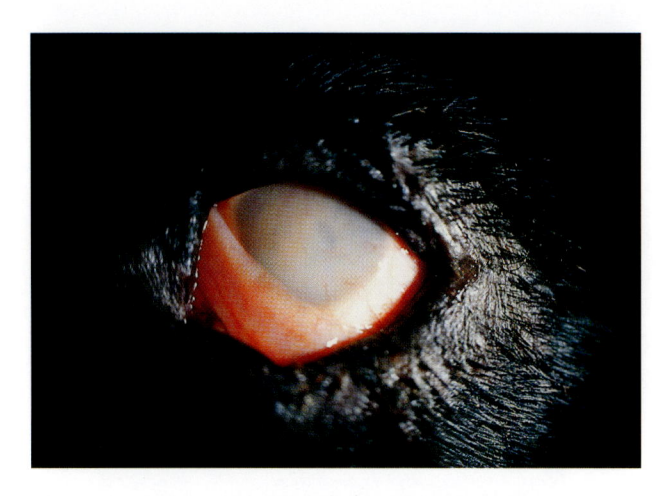

Fig. 4.21 Phthisis in an English Cocker Spaniel. Note enophthalmos and prominence of nictitating membrane, corneal opacity and discharge. The primary condition in this case was glaucoma.

panied by a grey mucoid ocular discharge present at the deep and pocket-like inner canthus.
- With small eyes, microphthalmos or phthisis, accompanied by mild prominence of the nictitating membrane (see Figs 4.18 and 4.21).
- In cases of severe anterior segment pain, e.g. corneal ulcer, foreign body, glaucoma with retraction of the globe due to the retractor oculi muscle of the dog and again accompanied by prominence of the nictitating membrane (see Fig. 6.1).
- As part of Horner's syndrome together with miosis, ptosis, globe retraction and again third eyelid prominence (see Fig. 6.2).
- Rarely due to tumours of the orbit (Fig. 4.22), depending upon the actual site of the tumour (exophthalmos and third eyelid prominence is a much more common sign with retrobulbar tumours).
- Possibly as a bilateral condition in cases of chronic illness with loss of orbital fat and with atrophy of the muscles of mastication.

Exophthalmos or proptosis

Exophthalmos (proptosis) is the prominence of a normal sized globe caused by some retrobulbar space-occupying lesion. It is, like enophthalmos, usually unilateral but is frequently accompanied by prominence of the nictitating membrane. It may vary in degree from a relatively subtle widening of the palpebral orifice (Fig. 4.23) in early or mild cases, to obvious prominence of the globe and third eyelid (Fig. 4.24). Proptosis is always more obvious when viewed from above and the two eyes are compared; perhaps the most useful clinical test is retropulsion of the globe which meets with an

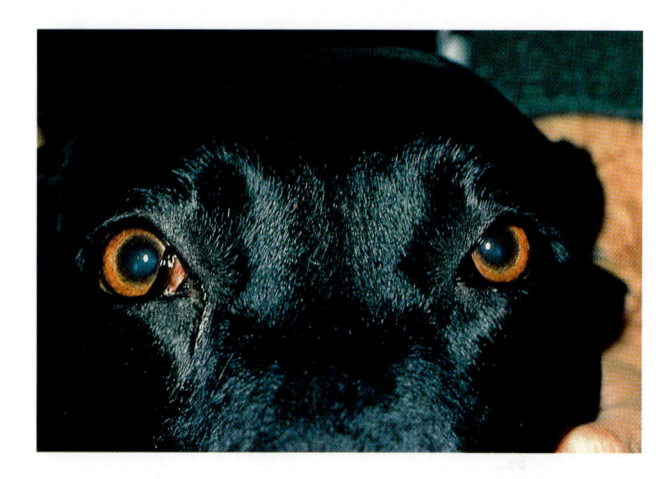

Fig. 4.23 Exophthalmos in a Labrador with retrobulbar tumour. Note wider palpebral orifice, prominence of the nictitating membrane and mild epiphora on the right side. Ophthalmoscopic examination also revealed partial retinal detachment.

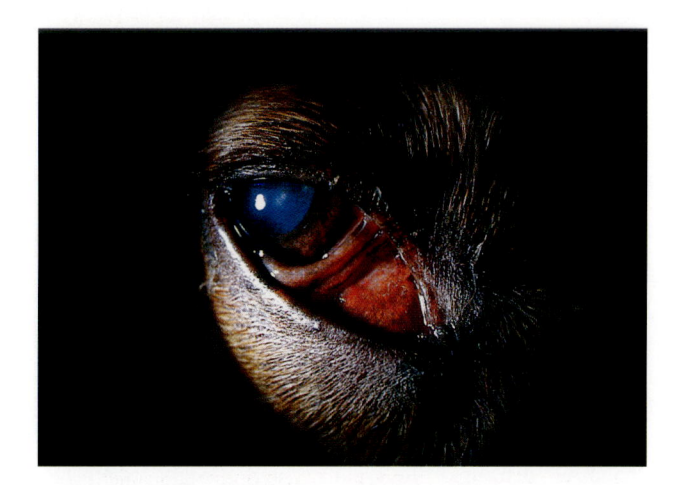

Fig. 4.22 Enophthalmos in a Standard Longhaired Dachshund. The mass at the medial canthus proved to be a nictitating gland carcinoma.

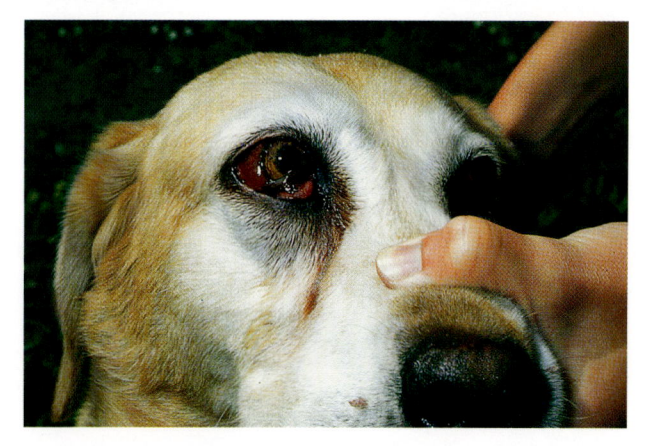

Fig. 4.24 Exophthalmos in a Labrador with retrobulbar tumour. Note prominence of both globe and nictitating membrane, chronic epiphora and chemosis.

GLOBE AND ORBIT

increased resistance. For example, hydrophthalmos may present with an enlarged palpebral orifice and some prominence of the globe (enlarged) but with no difference in retropulsion of the two eyes. Exophthalmos may be accompanied by ocular discharge (retrobulbar abscess) or simply epiphora (interference with normal tear drainage); pain on retropulsion may be present (abscess or cellulitis) or absent (neoplasia). Exophthalmos may also exhibit a change in the direction of the globe (strabismus) dependent upon both the size and location of the mass, together with limitation of globe movement.

Causes of exophthalmos are many and varied:

- Degrees of exophthalmos are exhibited in the brachycephalic breeds with their shallow orbits, e.g. Pekingese, Shih Tzu.
- Retrobulbar cellulitis (Figs 4.25 and 4.26), diffuse inflammation of orbital tissue, and retrobulbar abscess (Fig. 4.27) – these may be accompanied by difficulty in opening the mouth and pain also on retropulsion; heat around the orbit; swelling behind the last upper molar; pyrexia. Foreign bodies such as grass awn, slivers of wood and shotgun pellets are common causes.
- Orbital neoplasia – the tumour may be primary arising from any of the various orbital tissues; metastasis or part of multifocal neoplastic disease, e.g. lymphoma, extension from adjacent structures such as oral or nasal cavities and paranasal sinuses. The course of the exophthalmos is usually slow, progressive and painless and usually unilateral with prominence of the nictitating membrane. Fundus examination may reveal retinal detachment and/or papilloedema. Orbital tumours are frequently malignant with a wide variety of types.
- Eosinophilic myositis occurs mainly in the German Shepherd Dog and Weimaraner; it is bilateral with protrusion of the nictitating membranes and is often acute and painful.
- Retrobulbar haemorrhage resulting from trauma or possibly coagulation defect is rare.
- Other recorded causes of exophthalmos in the dog include craniomandibular osteopathy in the Scottish and West Highland White Terrier (not all cases); zygomatic mucocele; congenital orbital arteriovenous fistula.

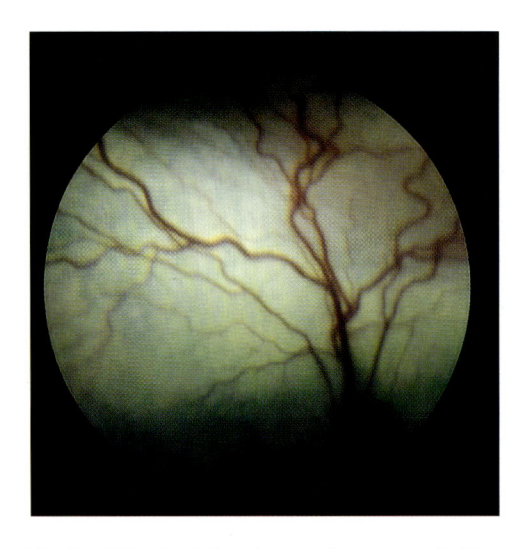

Fig. 4.26 Partial retinal detachment due to retrobulbar pressure in the same case as in Fig. 4.25. This dog made a complete recovery following removal of the foreign body and medical treatment.

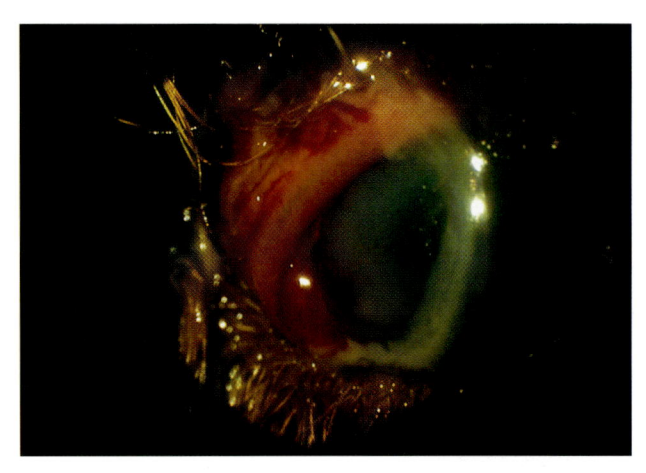

Fig. 4.27 Exophthalmos in a Lakeland Terrier with retrobulbar abscess. Note bloody ocular discharge.

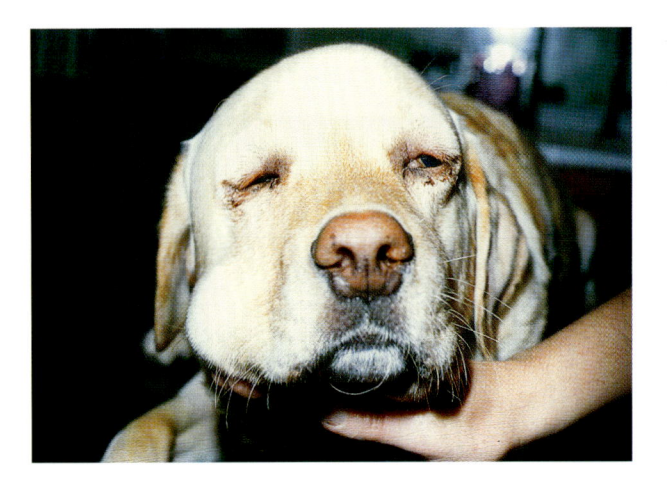

Fig. 4.25 Exophthalmos in a Labrador with retrobulbar cellulitis. Note prominence of both globe and nictitating membrane on the left side, partially obscured by gross swelling of the head. The cause was a foreign body (piece of stick) lodged in the orbit with entry via the oral cavity.

PROLAPSE OF THE GLOBE

Prolapse, sometimes referred to as proptosis, is dislocation of the globe in front of the eyelids which prevents its replacement in the orbit. It is particularly seen in the brachycephalic breeds (Fig. 4.28) because of their shallow orbits; it is traumatic in origin (traffic accidents or fight wounds and even

REFERENCES

excessive restraint) and is a dire emergency. Prolapse is often accompanied by optic nerve damage resulting in blindness occurring at the time of insult and appearing as optic atrophy ophthalmoscopically several weeks after the accident. The replaced eye often exhibits a divergent strabismus which may improve with time (Fig. 4.29). See also Chapter 3.

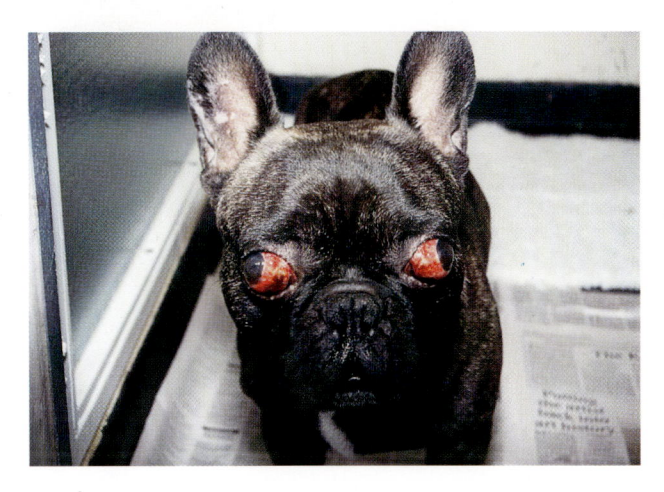

Fig. 4.28 Prolapse in a French Bulldog with bilateral prolapsed globes following a road traffic accident.

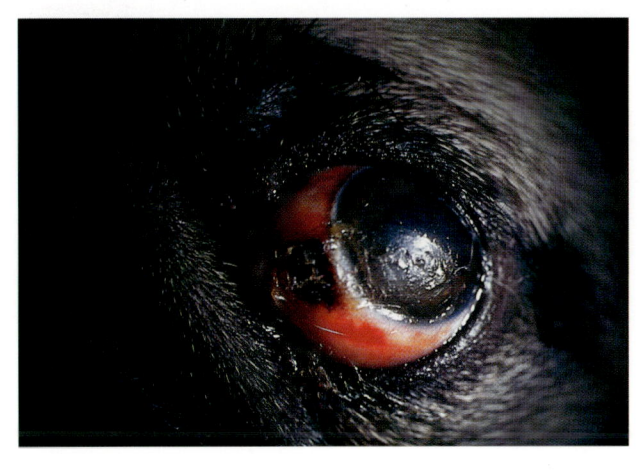

Fig. 4.29 Divergent strabismus in a Pug puppy following prolapse of the globe. Note retraction of the nictitating membrane and exposure keratitis.

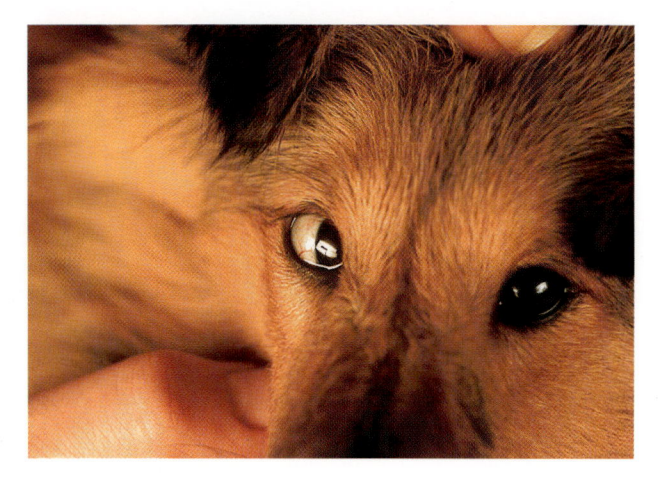

Fig. 4.30 Convergent strabismus in a Shetland Sheepdog puppy. Unilateral and congenital case.

References

Dennis R (2000) Use of magnetic resonance imaging for the investigation of orbital disease in small animals. *Journal of Small Animal Practice* **41**: 145–155.

Hendrix DVH, Gelatt KN (2000) Diagnosis, treatment and outcome of orbital neoplasia in dogs: A retrospective study of 44 cases. *Journal of Small Animal Practice* **41**: 105–108.

Lewis D, Kelly D, Sansom J (1986) Congenital microphthalmia and other developmental ocular anomalies in the Dobermann. *Journal of Small Animal Practice* **27**: 559–566.

Long RD (1992) Biometric study of the canine eye using B-mode ultrasonography: Globe size and breed differences. DVOphthal Dissertation, Royal College of Veterinary Surgeons.

Martin E, Perez J, Mozos E, Lopez R, Molleda JM (2000) Retrobulbar anaplastic astrocytoma in a dog: Clinicopathological and ultrasonographic features. *Journal of Small Animal Practice* **41**: 354–357.

Peiffer R, Fischer C (1983) Microphthalmia, retinal dysplasia and anterior segment dysgenesis in a litter of Doberman Pinschers. *Journal of American Veterinary Medical Association* **183**: 875–878.

5 UPPER AND LOWER EYELIDS

INTRODUCTION

The canine eyelids consist of an outer layer of thin skin with loose subcuticular tissue containing the orbicularis oculi muscle. The inner surface consists of the palpebral conjunctiva, below which is a poorly defined fibrous sheet known as the tarsus. The tarsus is continuous with the orbital septum and attaches to the periosteum at the bony orbital rim. The upper lid contains a row of cilia or eyelashes. Associated with the cilia are sebaceous and apocrine sweat glands. Modified sebaceous glands, known as meibomian glands, are within the tarsus and can frequently be seen on eversion of the lid margin. They look like a piano keyboard. Their ducts exit at the mucocutaneous junction in a furrow referred to as the 'grey-line'. The contents of these sebaceous glands have a very important function and contribute to the precorneal tear film. The eyelid margin is an extremely important anatomical structure and is responsible for protecting the cornea and maintaining the tear film. Interference with this margin can therefore have serious consequences for ocular health. The eyelid skin, because of its thin and loose nature, is predisposed to a number of disorders and the clinical presentation is frequently exaggerated. This is clearly demonstrated in hypersensitivity reactions when severe dermal oedema may occur. Focal mucinosis (Fig. 5.1) may produce exaggerated folding, the Shar Pei is a breed particularly prone to this problem (see Chapter 8). Disorders of collagen, seen in cutaneous asthenia, (Fig. 5.2) will also affect the lids. This congenital and inherited collagen defect results in hyperextensibility of the skin.

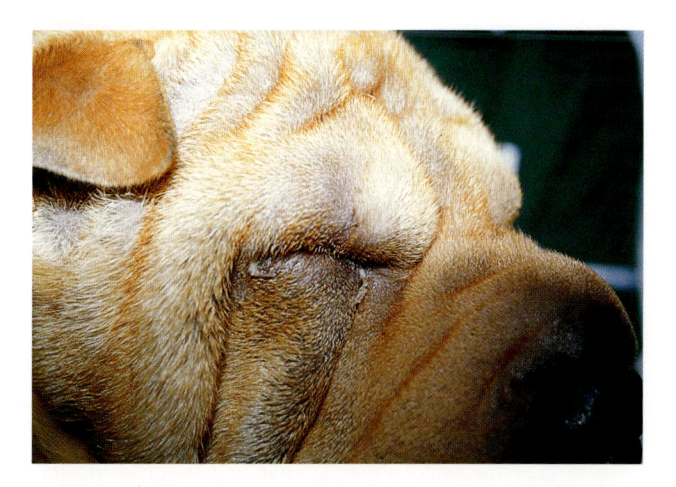

Fig. 5.1 Mucinosis and severe upper and lower lid entropion in a Shar Pei. The apparent lid swelling results from mucinosis, a connective tissue disorder in this breed and frequently confused with oedema.

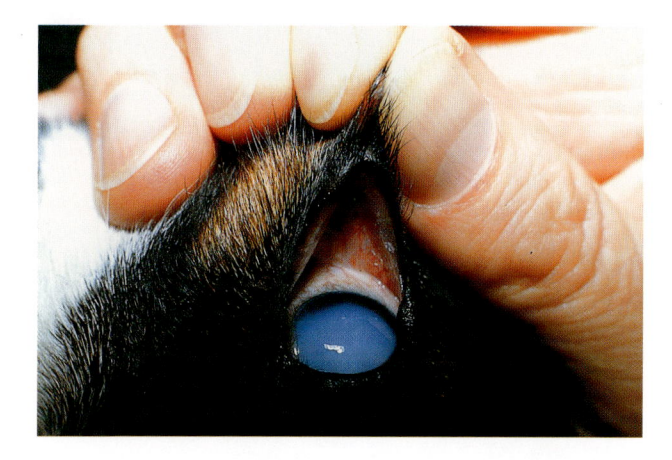

Fig. 5.2 Cutaneous asthenia (Ehlers–Danlos syndrome) in a 12-month-old crossbred bitch.

CONGENITAL ANOMALIES

DERMOID

Dermoids (Figs 5.3–5.6) are benign, congenital tumours known as choristomas. They are caused by displacement of embryonic tissue. Lids, cornea and conjunctiva are the areas mainly affected and a simple resection of the tissues involved with direct closure of the defect is corrective. They resemble skin and usually have a large number of hair follicles which can cause trichiasis and irritation. There seems to be a breed incidence in the Golden Retriever, German Shepherd Dog and St Bernard.

COLOBOMA

Colobomata (Figs 5.6 and 5.7) are congenital lid defects and may be partial or full thickness; they may present as partial notching to complete agenesis. Usually the lower lid towards the lateral canthus is affected. They are unusual, particularly in the dog, and may cause exposure keratitis and conjunctivitis. Where there is extensive absence of the eyelid margin a sliding skin flap may be required for surgical correction. They have been reported in the Staffordshire Bull Terrier in association with dermoids (Peiffer, 1989).

UPPER AND LOWER EYELIDS

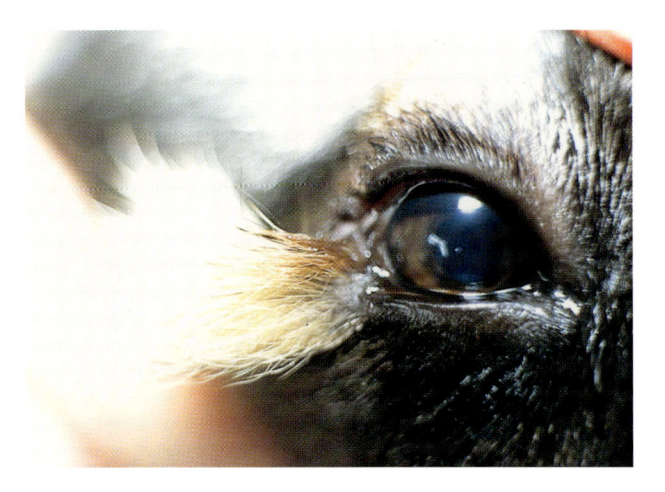

Fig. 5.3 Very hairy dermoid in a German Shepherd Dog puppy, bilateral condition in this case.

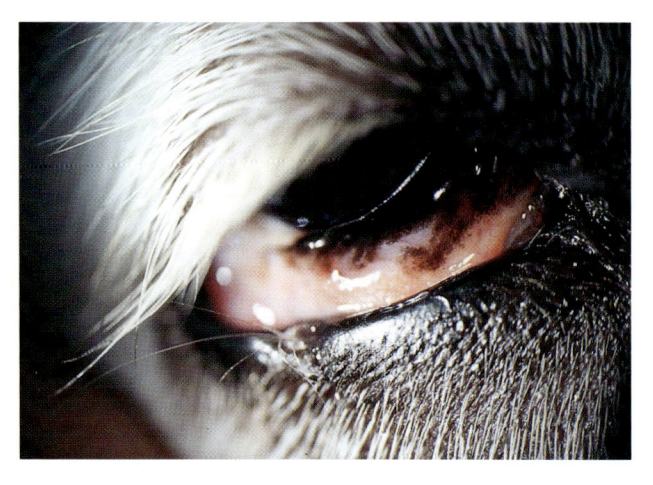

Fig. 5.6 Partial lid coloboma and small dermoid on the conjunctival surface in a Labrador Retriever puppy.

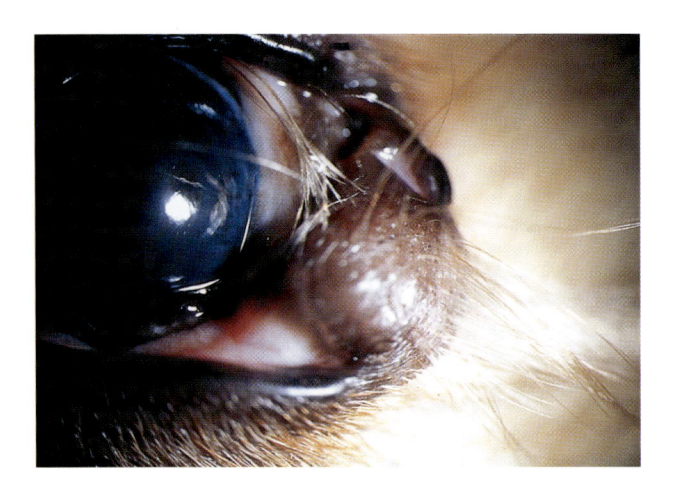

Fig. 5.4 Large dermoid involving the outer one-third of the lower lid including conjunctiva, with associated corneal oedema due to trichiasis in a Golden Retriever puppy.

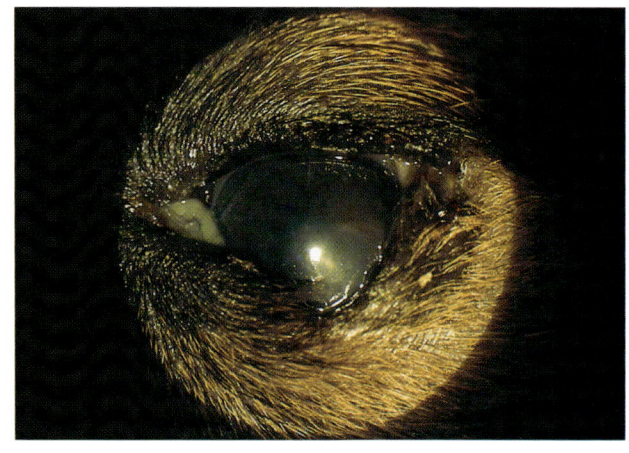

Fig. 5.7 Full-thickness eyelid coloboma in a Staffordshire Bull Terrier puppy.

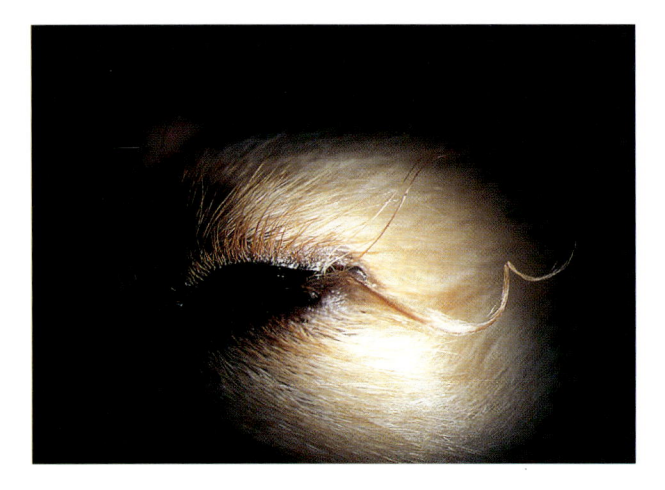

Fig. 5.5 The same case as in Fig. 5.4 showing the extremely long hairs growing from the dermoid.

Eyelid disorders

Ophthalmia neonatorum

Infection of the conjunctival sac in the neonate, usually with a coagulase positive *Staphylococcus*, causes a delayed opening of the lids (ankyloblepharon) (Fig. 5.8). The condition is extremely painful resulting in swollen lids and a profuse purulent discharge trapped within the conjunctival sac.

Treatment requires drainage and flushing of the conjunctival sac, best achieved by introducing a pair of blunt curved scissors into the small opening that exists at the medial canthus separating the upper and lower lids. Topical broad spectrum antibiotics, such as chloramphenicol or tetracycline, should be given. Complications of this condition are corneal ulceration, perforation and loss of the globe.

EYELID DISORDERS

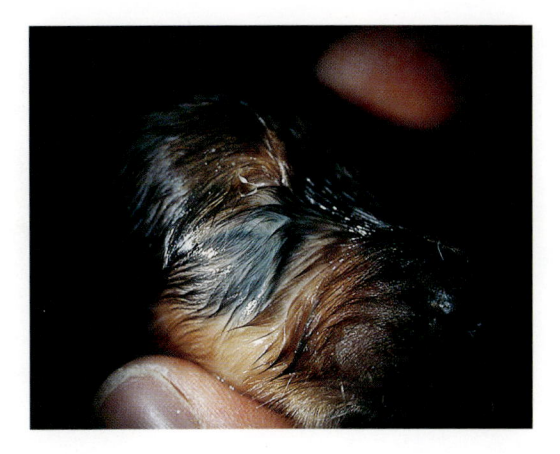

Fig. 5.8 Ophthalmia neonatorum in a Miniature Longhaired Dachshund puppy.

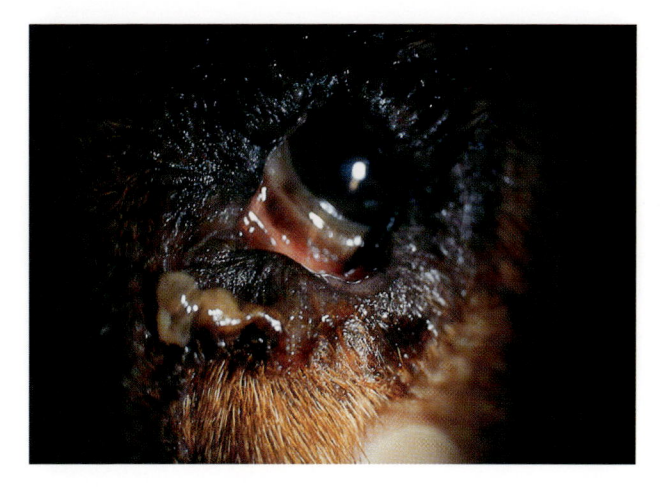

Fig. 5.10 Juvenile cellulitis in a 5-month-old female Cocker Spaniel. Swelling of the eyelids and muzzle occur with a serosanguineous to mucopurulent discharge.

BLEPHARITIS

Inflammation of the lid is usually a manifestation of a dermatological condition with secondary conjunctival involvement. A large number of dermatoses have a predilection for the periorbital area and may occur in isolation or in conjunction with lesions elsewhere. It is important when presented with a case of blepharitis that a thorough examination of the skin is carried out. Skin scrapings, hair plucks and a skin biopsy should be performed as part of a full diagnostic work-up.

Bacterial infection, usually with *Staphylococcus* sp., is a frequent occurrence. The lids may be affected by acute or chronic pyodermas (Fig. 5.9). In puppies, juvenile pyoderma (Fig. 5.10) invariably affects the periorbital region and is frequently complicated by a lymphadenitis. Chronic hair loss and scarring results, often with pigmentation. This is probably an immune-mediated disease for, although cocci can be isolated, it does not respond to antibiotics alone and corticosteroids are the treatment of choice. In addition to bacteria (Fig. 5.11), fungal and parasitic agents may be implicated in

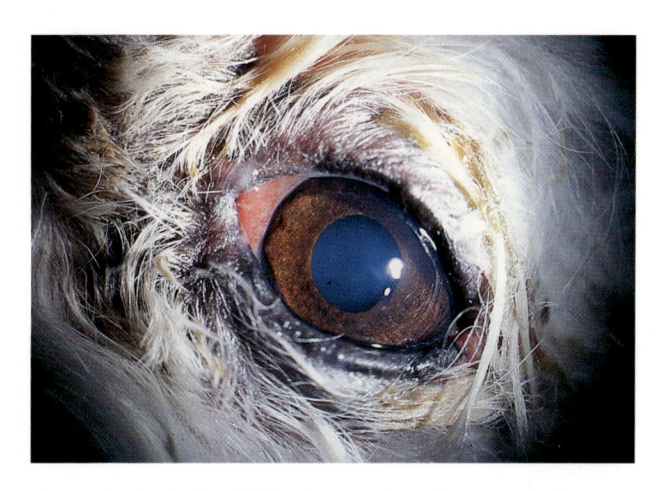

Fig. 5.11 Periorbital folliculitis resulting from a mixed bacterial infection (coagulase positive *Staphylococcus* sp. and beta-haemolytic *Streptococcus* sp.) in a female neutered 8-year-old Maltese Terrier. Note the inflammation of the skin, mild depigmentation of the lid margins, particularly towards the medial canthus, and a secondary conjunctivitis.

periorbital inflammation. The eyelids are a predilection site for *Demodex canis* infection (Fig. 5.12) in young dogs; the lesions are pruritic and accompanied by hair loss and inflammation. The clinical signs may be localised or generalised. Diagnosis is confirmed by a skin scraping. *Sarcoptes scabiei* (Fig. 5.13) may also affect this site but the condition is usually generalised and accompanied by severe pruritus.

Fungal infections, particularly with the sylvatic (wild animal) ringworm show a predilection for the facial hair including the lids (Fig. 5.14). The terrier breeds are predisposed.

MEIBOMIANITIS

Inflammation of the meibomian glands (Fig. 5.15) may be acute or chronic and accompany a blepharitis or conjunctivitis. Chronic inflammation of the meibomian gland results

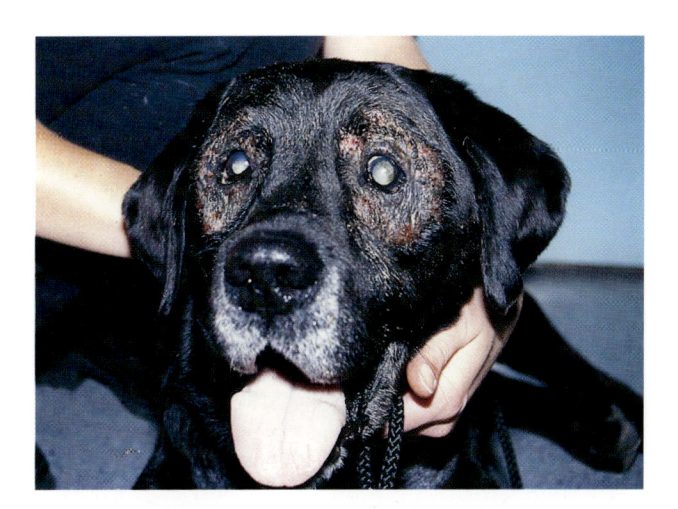

Fig. 5.9 Chronic deep periorbital pyoderma, bilaterally symmetrical, in an old Labrador with chronic renal disease.

UPPER AND LOWER EYELIDS

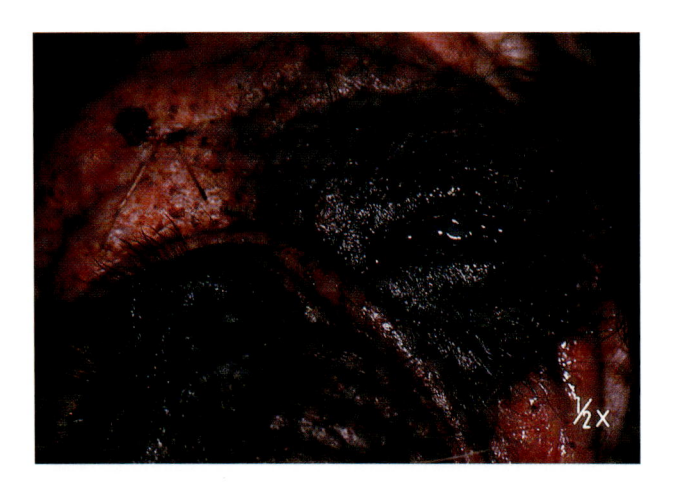

Fig. 5.12 Adult-onset demodicosis in a 13-year-old Pekingese. (Courtesy of SC Shaw.)

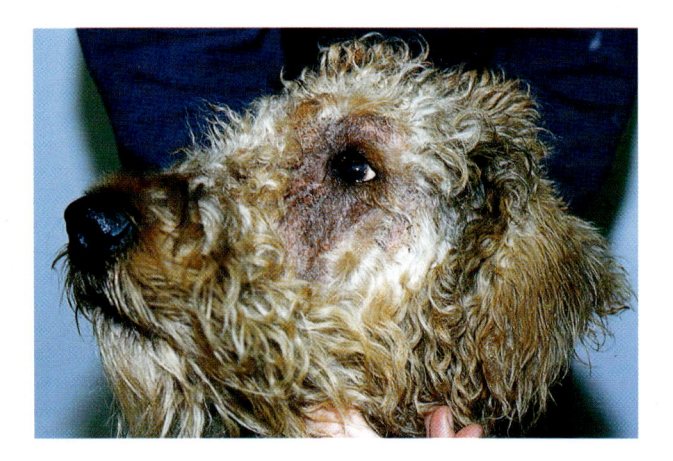

Fig. 5.13 Sarcoptic mange affecting the periorbital area of an 18-month-old Airedale. (Courtesy of JD Littlewood.)

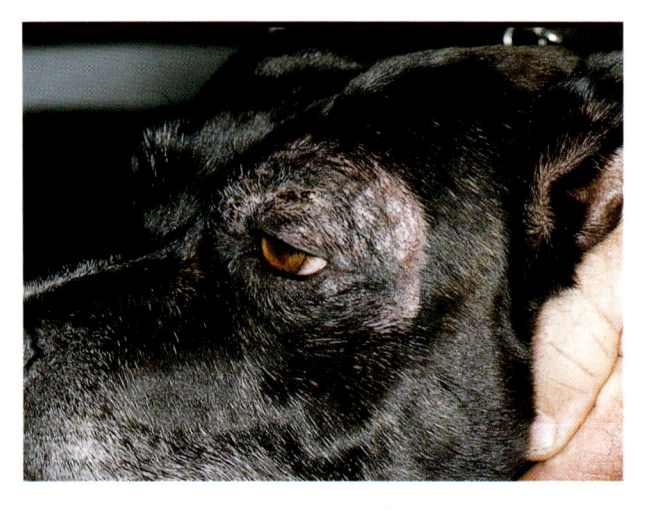

Fig. 5.14 Periorbital infection with *Trichophyton erinacei* in a 6-year-old male Staffordshire Bull Terrier. (Courtesy of JD Littlewood.)

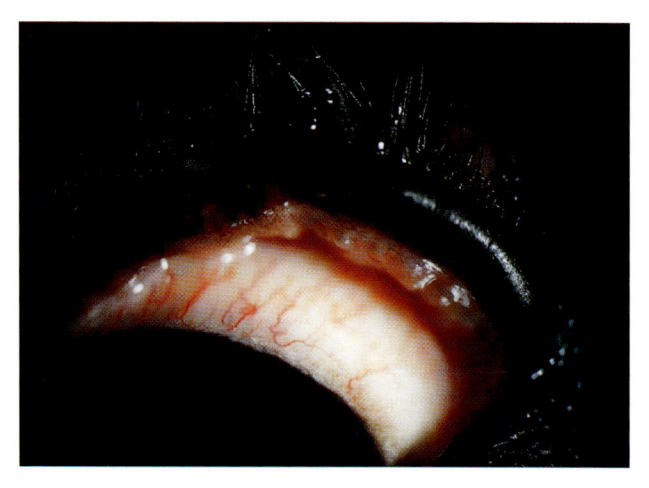

Fig. 5.15 Meibomitis, acute inflammation and abscessation of the meibomian glands in a Cairn Terrier.

in a pyogranuloma or chalazion (Figs 5.16 and 5.17). This may occur as an isolated lid lesion or may involve multiple glands (Fig. 5.18) and different lids. The condition may be seen in association with cutaneous sterile pyogranulomatous syndrome (Panich *et al.*, 1991), or in isolation. Where a single lesion occurs, a biopsy or wedge resection may be indicated to reach a diagnosis. The causative agent in many cases remains obscure. Treatment with systemic antibiotics can provide an excellent result (Fig. 5.19) (Sansom *et al.*, 2000) and in some cases anti-inflammatory drugs are required.

HYPERSENSITIVITY REACTIONS

Acute lid inflammation as a result of degranulation of mast cells and basophils can occur for a variety of reasons. These may have an immunological basis, as in atopic dermatitis. However, tick bites (Fig. 5.20) or bee stings will provoke a similar reaction, as will certain drugs (Fig. 5.21) and chemicals. Infection with *Staphylococcus* sp. may also provoke a hypersensitivity response. Food intolerance may manifest as severe lid oedema (Paterson, 1998).

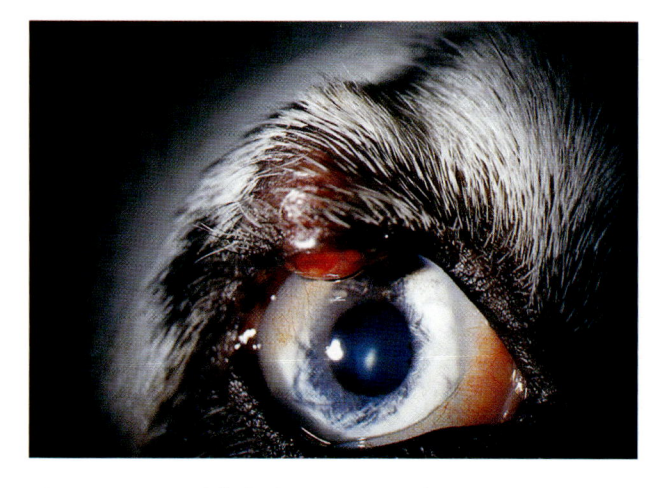

Fig. 5.16 Large full-thickness pyogranulomatous lesion affecting the right upper lid of a 1-year-old Dalmatian bitch.

EYELID DISORDERS

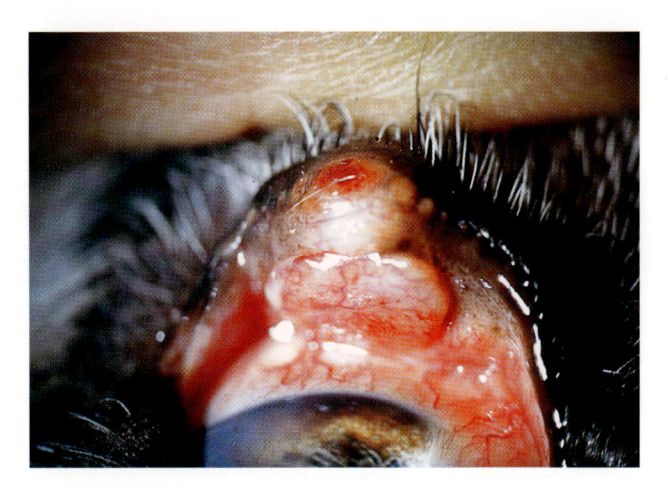

Fig. 5.17 Eversion of the right upper lid to demonstrate the soft tissue appearance of the pyogranulomatous lesion (same dog as in Fig. 5.16).

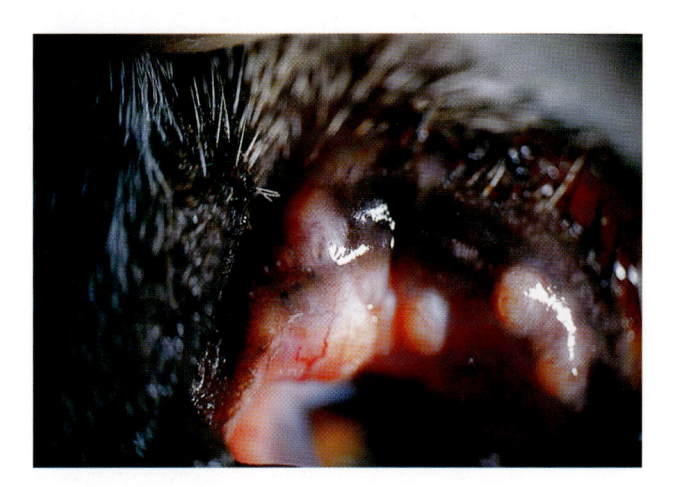

Fig. 5.18 Dalmatian, 11-year-old male, with multiple pyogranulomatous lesions of the left upper lid.

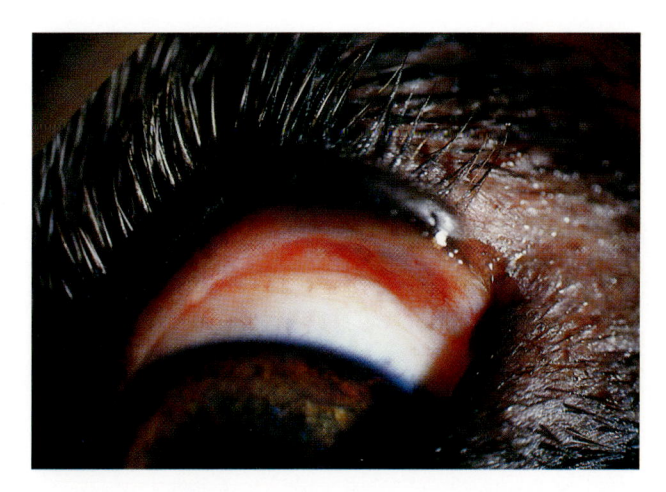

Fig. 5.19 Complete resolution of the lesions following 6 weeks of antibiotic treatment (same dog as in Fig. 5.18).

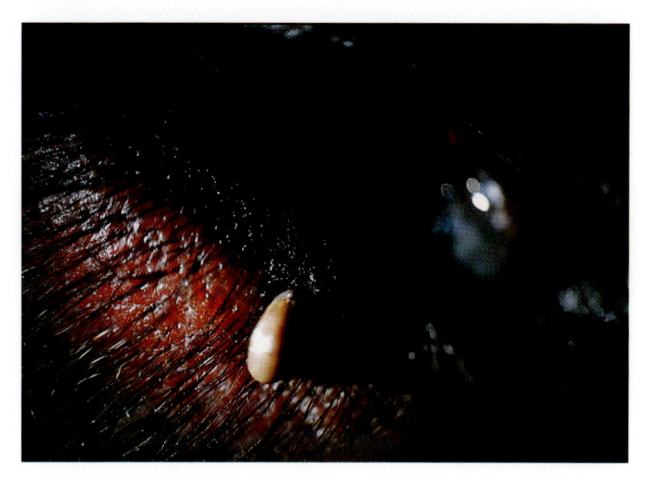

Fig. 5.20 Localised blepharitis in a Border Collie as a result of tick infestation.

Adverse reactions are not uncommon as a result of topical drug application and the aminoglycoside antibiotics (Fig. 5.21) are frequently implicated. Lid swelling, inflammation, ulceration and discharge may be accompanied by self-inflicted trauma and blepharospasm when the treatment is applied. Withdrawal of treatment results in resolution of the problem.

ATOPIC DISEASE

Atopic dermatitis (Fig. 5.22) may be accompanied by conjunctivitis and inflammation of the periorbital area. An age-related incidence is apparent and it is usually young dogs (under 2 years of age) that manifest this problem. There is also a breed incidence in the Labrador, West Highland White Terrier and English Setter. Atopy is an inherited disease (Shaw, 2000). The dog frequently suffers from facial irritation and excessive grooming and careful examination may

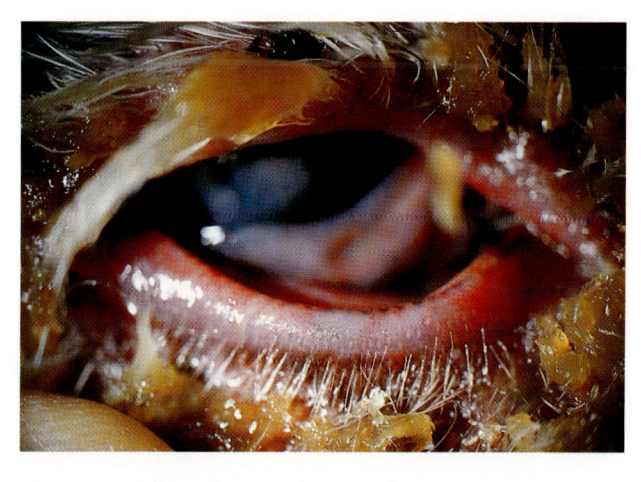

Fig. 5.21 Contact hypersensitivity reaction to gentamycin in a West Highland White Terrier with keratoconjunctivitis sicca. Note the complete depigmentation on the eyelid margins with severe inflammation and swelling of the lids accompanied by a secondary discharge.

UPPER AND LOWER EYELIDS

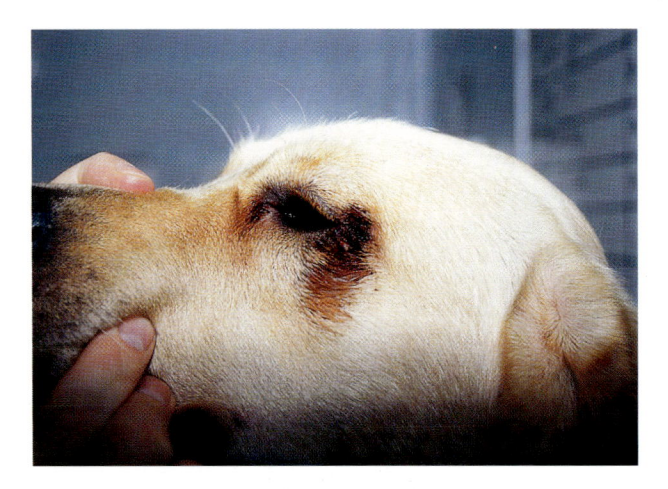

Fig. 5.22 Atopic dermatitis in a young Labrador. Note the marked periorbital tear staining as a result of dermatitis and conjunctivitis.

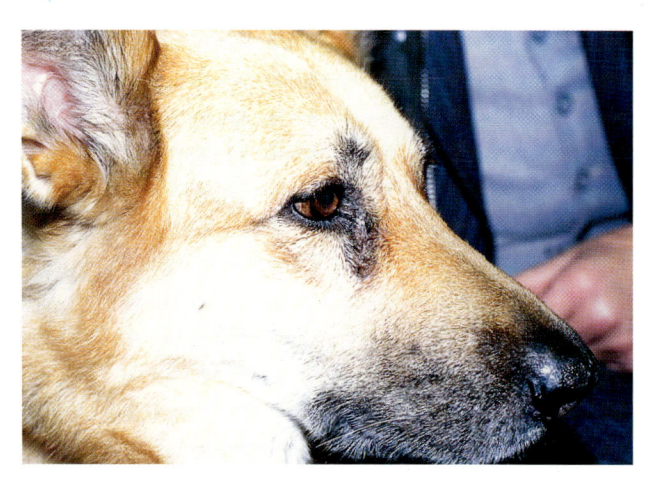

Fig. 5.24 Mucocutaneous pyoderma, the nose and medial canthus are affected in a 7-year-old German Shepherd Dog. (Courtesy of JD Littlewood.)

AUTOIMMUNE DISEASE

Autoimmune disease that affects the skin may involve the periorbital area and the lids as they represent a mucocutaneous junction (Fig. 5.25). Pemphigus foliaceus is more common than pemphigus vulgaris but does not usually affect the mucocutaneous junctions. Although pemphigus vulgaris is rare it usually causes erosion and ulceration of the oral cavity and the lids may be similarly affected. Discoid lupus may manifest as facial lesions involving the periorbital area but the lesions usually involve the nose.

The lids may also become involved in immune-mediated connective tissue disorders such as systemic lupus erythematosus. Diagnosis relies on a skin biopsy and laboratory tests.

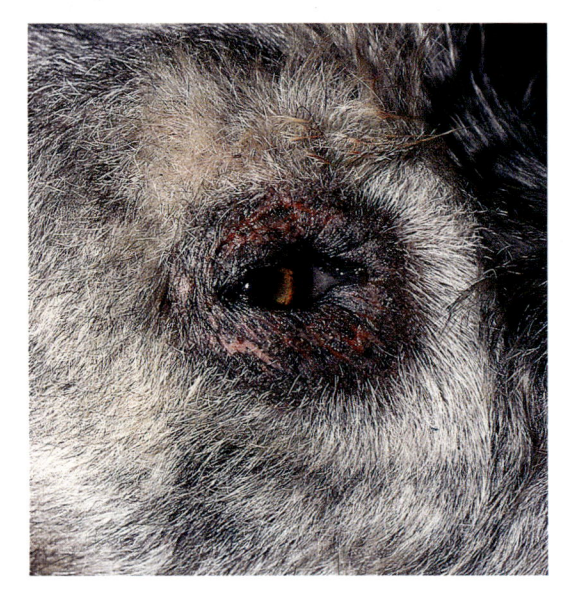

Fig. 5.23 Chronic thickening of the periorbital skin in a Lurcher suffering from atopic dermatitis. The skin shows evidence of lichenification, hyperpigmentation with alopecia and self-excoriation. (Courtesy of JD Littlewood.)

reveal minor lesions elsewhere in the early stages of the disease. Secondary bacterial infection may occur. Irreversible hypertrophy and keratosis of the skin occur with the passage of time (Fig. 5.23). An intradermal skin test or a blood sample for IgE may identify the allergen.

MUCOCUTANEOUS PYODERMA

Mucocutaneous pyoderma affects the mucocutaneous junctions and may involve the lids (Fig. 5.24). Aetiology is unknown but there is a breed predisposition in the German Shepherd Dog. The lesions respond to topical and systemic antibiotics.

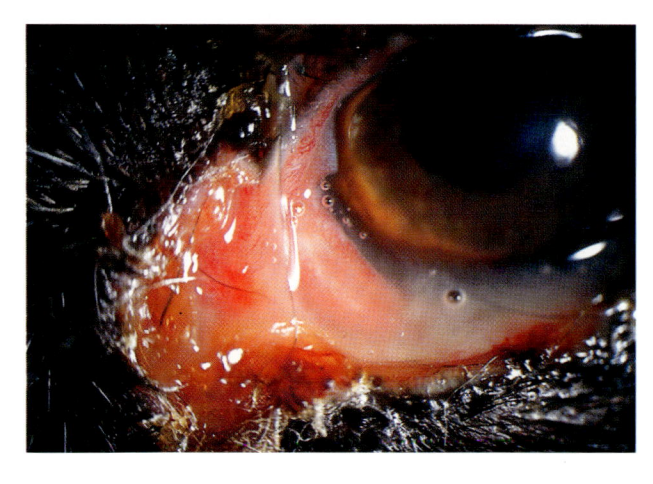

Fig. 5.25 Loss of upper and lower lid margins as a result of chronic ulcerative lesions in a Bearded Collie. Although no diagnosis was reached, the histopathology demonstrated pyogranulomatous inflammation and the condition responded to azathioprin, suggesting immune-mediated disease.

LID ANOMALIES

VITILIGO

Vitiligo is an autoimmune reaction against melanocytes, resulting in depigmention of the skin and hair. It is a benign autoimmune disease that can occur anywhere on the body, but it shows a predilection for the face, particularly the periorbital region. There is a breed predisposition in the German Shepherd Dog, Rottweiler and Dobermann. The differential diagnosis would include epitheliotropic lymphoma, discoid lupus erythematosus and uveal dermatologic syndrome or Harada's disease (see Chapter 12).

ZINC DERMATOSES

Zinc dermatoses (Fig. 5.26) may manifest as a periocular problem with crusting and scaling of the periorbital area. The diagnosis is confirmed by a skin biopsy. It can be a genetic problem in the Alaskan Malamute and Siberian Husky, requiring lifelong supplementation. In young growing puppies a zinc deficient diet may require only temporary supplementation.

LID ANOMALIES

ANKYLOBLEPHARON

Ankyloblepharon is the congenital fusion of the upper and lower lids at the lid margin; it usually occurs in association with bacterial infection (see Fig. 5.8). It is, of course, normal in the first few days of life (see Chapter 2).

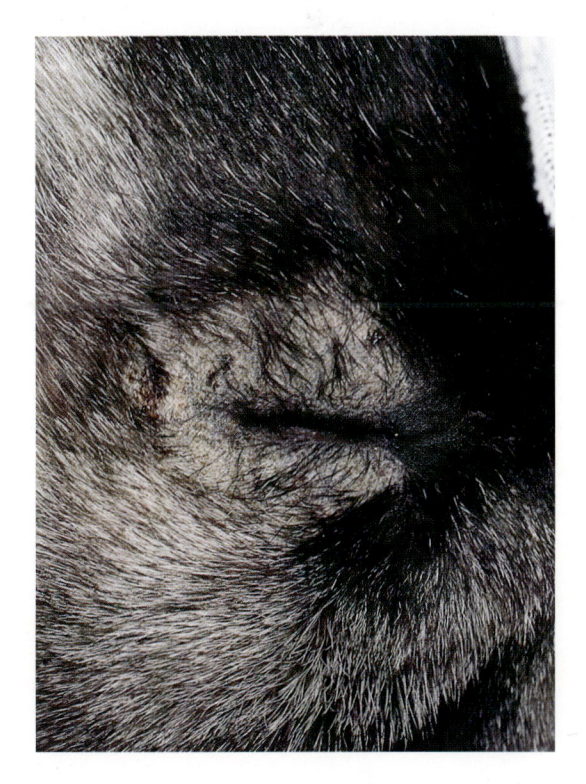

Fig. 5.26 Zinc responsive dermatosis in a 4-year-old female Akita. There is periorbital crusting and scaling with facial involvement. (Courtesy of JD Littlewood.)

PALPEBRAL FISSURE

The size and shape of the palpebral fissure will vary from breed to breed. A macropalpebral fissure is seen in the giant breeds, frequently in the form of a 'diamond eye' (see Fig. 5.29), resulting in medial and lateral lid entropion and a central ectropion. Assessment of the size, shape and laxity of the palpebral fissure is very important in the evaluation of eyelid conformation.

A micropalpebral fissure, which is a congenitally small or narrowed palpebral fissure, may be seen in breeds such as the Chow and the collies (Rough, Smooth and Shetland Sheepdog). Microphthalmia, with multiocular defects, may accompany a micropalpebral fissure. A small fissure may result in entropion, as also may too long a lower eyelid.

ENTROPION

Entropion is a deviation or inturning of the lid margin towards the globe, resulting in hairs at the lid margin coming into contact with the cornea (Figs 5.27–5.29 and see Fig. 5.1). In very mild cases this may manifest as a wetness over the affected area with depigmentation of the lid margin in chronic cases. In more severe cases there is blepharospasm, conjunctivitis and ulcerative keratitis. The diagnosis is made on very careful examination of the lid and by manual retraction to expose the in-turned lid margin. Sedation and general anaesthesia are contraindicated as part of the examination as they will alter the lid conformation.

The condition is hereditary in a large number of breeds and the presentation and age incidence is usually breed-specific with a particular area of lid being affected. It is unusual to have upper lid entropion (Fig. 5.27); usually the outer two-thirds of the lower lid, sometimes with canthal involvement, is affected, e.g. Golden Retriever, Labrador Retriever. In some breeds all four lids may be affected, e.g. Shar Pei and Chow. Entropion due to other causes, such as trauma and senility, is far less common and secondary entropion as a result of ocular pathology is extremely rare.

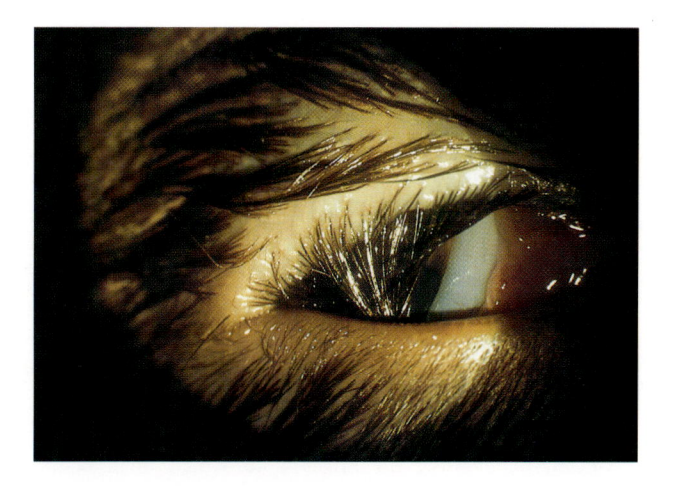

Fig. 5.27 Upper lid entropion in an 8-week-old English Springer Spaniel puppy.

UPPER AND LOWER EYELIDS

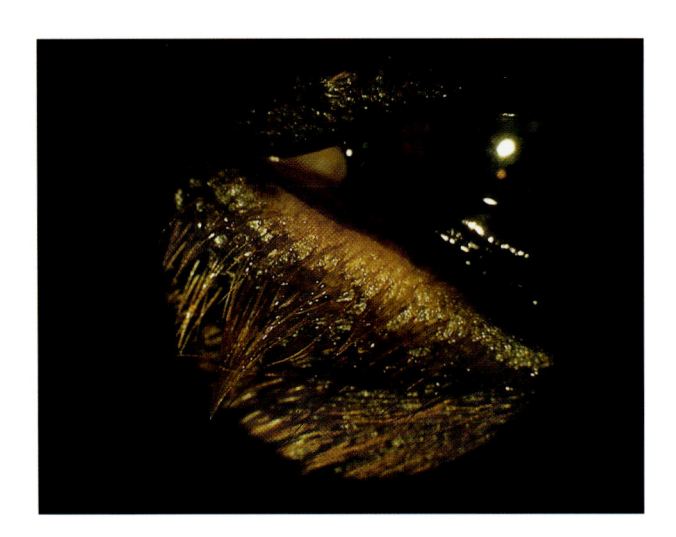

Fig. 5.28 Severe entropion in a Golden Retriever, the lid has been everted to demonstrate the chronic lid depigmentation over the affected area.

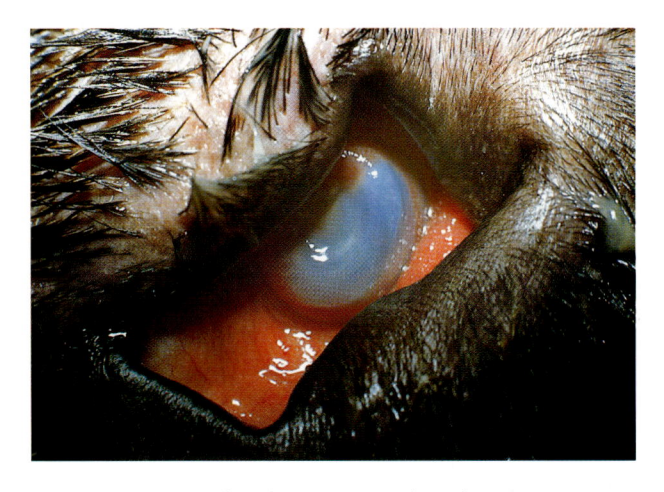

Fig. 5.29 Diamond eye in a St Bernard resulting in severe lower lid ectropion and medial canthal entropion of the lower lid, lateral and medial entropion of the upper lid, secondary stromal ulceration, total corneal oedema and associated vascular fringe and chronic conjunctivitis.

However, a senile upper lid entropion, often accompanied by a lower lid ectropion, classically occurs in the Cocker Spaniel with heavy ear flaps and prominent nuchal crest.

There are a large number of surgical techniques described for correcting entropion. They are often unnecessarily complicated and may not give superior results. The most effective and simple treatment for entropion is the Hotz–Celsus technique in which an ellipse of skin is removed close to the lid margin and corresponding to the affected area. Where entropion occurs because of an abnormally long palpebral fissure, assessed by everting the affected lid which then extends beyond the lateral canthus, a simple wedge resection will correct the deformity by shortening the lid.

ECTROPION

Ectropion is the converse of entropion but is much more rare and involves only the lower lids. The lids become everted exposing conjunctival tissue. There is also a breed incidence to this lid defect.

Surgical correction is carried out by a full-thickness wedge resection over the affected area or by removal of a wedge of tissue near the lateral canthus which results in a tightening of the lower lid. Complicated lid splitting procedures do not give superior results and frequently result in severe and irreversible complications.

DIAMOND EYE

Macropalpebral fissures may result in a central ectropion of the lower lid and medial and lateral canthal entropion in conjunction with an upper lid entropion (Fig. 5.29). More than one surgical procedure may be necessary for correction. However, a generous wedge resection of the lower lid to correct the severe ectropion and shorten the lid is usually adequate. For the upper lid, a wedge resection performed in combination with the Hotz–Celsus technique will shorten and evert the lid margin.

DISTICHIASIS

The upper lids normally have between two and four rows of eyelashes but there are none on the lower lids. Distichiasis (Fig. 5.30) is a condition where extra lashes arise from, or adjacent to, the meibomian gland orifices. There is a predisposition to this condition in a large number of breeds and it is probably the most common hereditary defect in the dog. It may be asymptomatic and, for this reason, a careful history and examination should be conducted when presented with a history of ocular irritation or epiphora. In many cases it is not the distichia which is the cause of the problem but ectopic cilia. If the extra lashes come into contact with the cornea or conjunctiva, then chronic conjunctivitis, mild

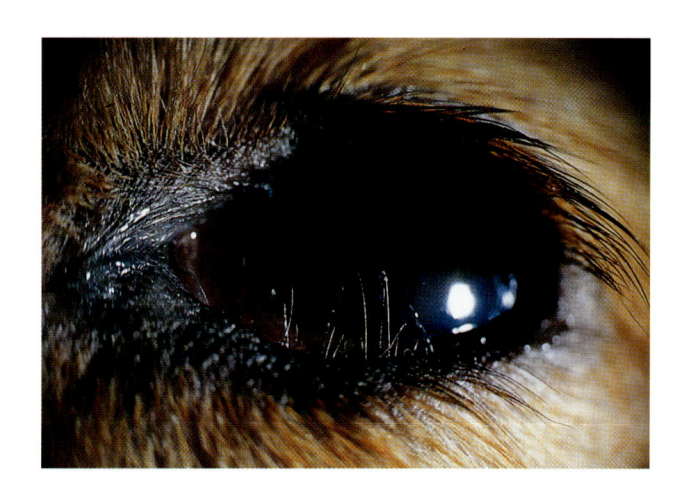

Fig. 5.30 Distichiasis of the lower lid in a Miniature Longhaired Dachshund. Note that the lashes are easily visualised when tangentially illuminated.

LID ANOMALIES

blepharospasm and, only occasionally, corneal ulceration result. Puppies may present with severe problems but the situation may improve as the animal grows. It has been diagnosed as early as 3 weeks of age in a Miniature Longhaired Dachshund, a breed frequently affected like the American Cocker Spaniel, Miniature Poodle and others.

Focal illumination, magnification and the use of local anaesthesia to remove the distichia by epilation will determine whether they are the cause of the problem. For more permanent results, lid electrolysis or cryotherapy are probably the most helpful techniques. These procedures often have to be repeated as it is usually impossible to remove all the distichia successfully at the first attempt. Surgical techniques, such as lid splitting, should be avoided as they can result in loss of lid margins and severe permanent scarring.

Ectopic cilia

Ectopic cilia emerge from the palpebral conjunctiva (Fig. 5.31) and usually impinge directly on to the cornea. They may arise singly or in clumps and usually cause severe discomfort as evidenced by blepharospasm, tearing and the development of a corneal erosion. Diagnosis may be difficult, particularly when the hairs are pale or poorly pigmented. Careful examination, under good magnification, is essential. Occasionally ectopic cilia arise on the back of the third eyelid. A localised excision around the hair and follicle resolves the condition.

There is a breed incidence for ectopic cilia. It is a common condition in the Flat-coated Retriever and Boxer and is often accompanied by degrees of distichiasis.

In some cases, groups of unerupted cilia (Fig. 5.32) can be seen subconjunctivally at the level of the meibomian gland. They are best left untreated unless they erupt.

Trichiasis

Normal facial hair coming into contact with the ocular surfaces will result in chronic conjunctivitis, keratitis and epiphora (Figs 5.33–5.35). This is a common condition in

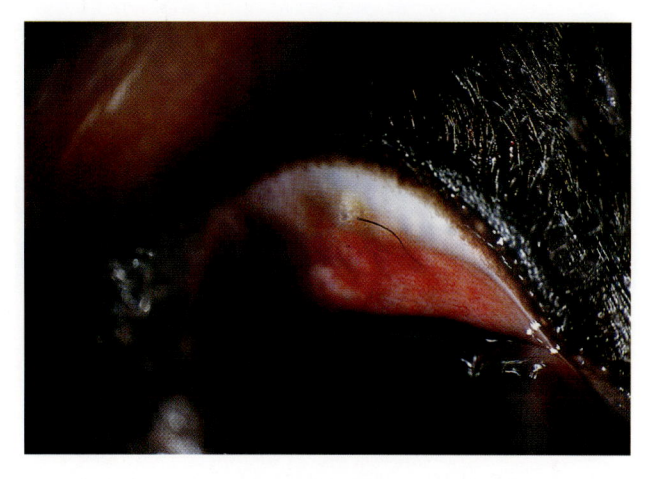

Fig. 5.32 An ectopic cilium emerging from the palpebral conjunctiva at the level of the meibomian glands in a 6-year-old male Miniature Poodle.

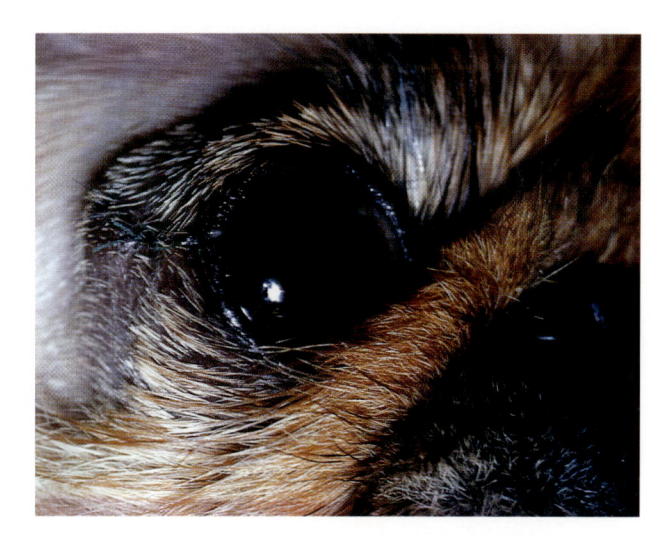

Fig. 5.33 Trichiasis due to nasal folds in a Pekingese.

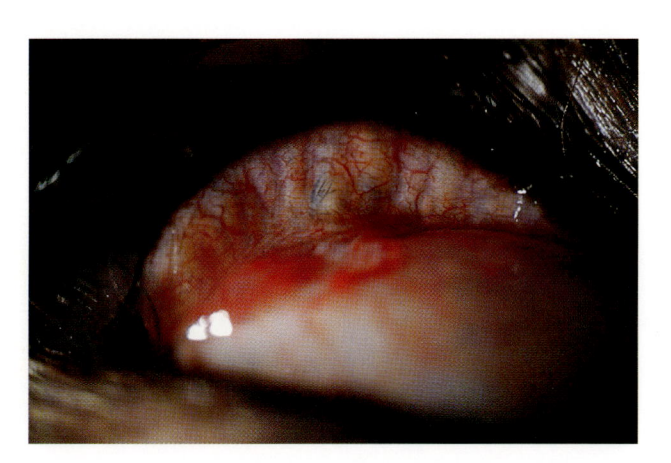

Fig. 5.31 A clump of non-erupted ectopic cilia below the palpebral conjunctiva at the level of the meibomian glands in the upper lid of a 7-year-old male Shih Tzu.

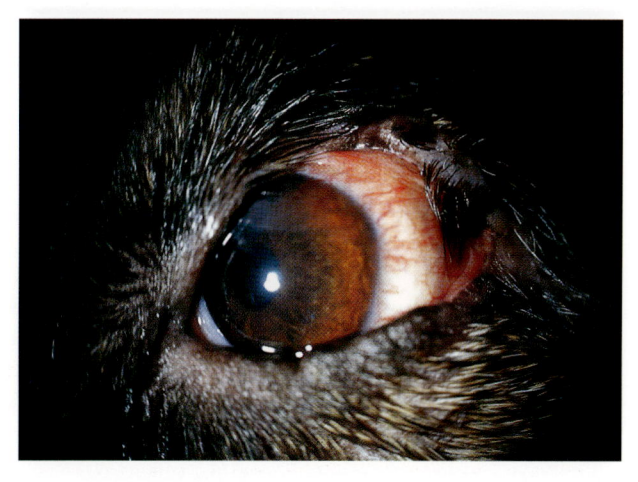

Fig. 5.34 Trichiasis due to a traumatic lateral lid defect resulting in exposure of the cornea and sclera and an inadequate blink reflex in a Jack Russell Terrier.

UPPER AND LOWER EYELIDS

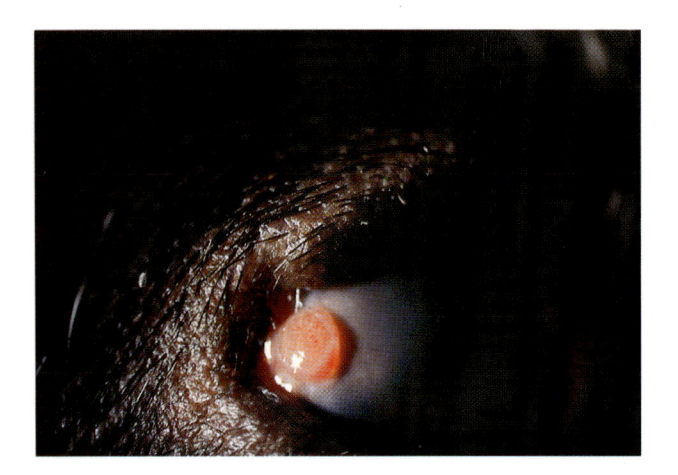

Fig. 5.35 Trichiasis and lateral canthal entropion in a Pointer resulting in a corneal granuloma.

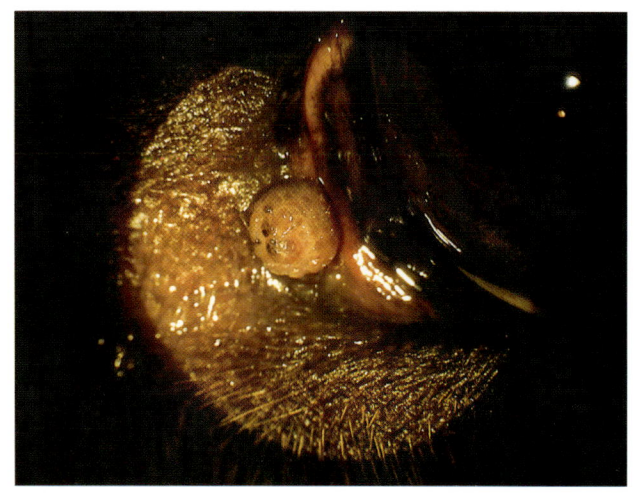

Fig. 5.36 Viral papilloma in a 1-year-old Golden Retriever.

breeds such as the Pekingese and Pug because of their nasal folds. In the Cocker Spaniel it may occur with senility where the upper eyelid skin droops onto the corneal surface. Surgical excision of the responsible skin folds or the Stades technique is usually corrective.

Neoplasia

Papillomas, adenomas, adenocarcinomas and melanomas are the most common tumours involving the eyelids of the dog. Basal cell carcinoma and squamous cell carcinoma occur rarely. The upper eyelid tends to be more frequently affected than the lower eyelid. When tumours present at the eyelid margin they may cause a secondary conjunctivitis, keratitis and corneal ulceration; early removal by wedge resection (V-plasty) is recommended before one-third of lid involvement occurs, as this might require a more complicated surgical procedure.

Papilloma

Papillomas (Fig. 5.36) are elevated cauliflower-like neoplasms that arise from the epithelium with minimal involvement of the underlying tissue. They may have a viral aetiology and typically develop in the young (under 1 year of age) or old (7–8 years of age) dog. They may arise on the eyelid, at the mucocutanous junction, or from the palpebral or bulbar conjunctiva. Papillomas arising from conjunctiva have a distinctive, but different, appearance from the cutaneous papilloma (see Figs 8.13 and 8.14). They assume a characteristic frond-like appearance (Sansom *et al.*, 1996). The diagnosis of papilloma is usually made on their very characteristic wart-like appearance. However, the differential diagnosis is to squamous cell carcinoma which may have a similar papillary appearance. In contrast to squamous cell carcinoma, which invades the deeper tissues, the papilloma is superficial and grows rapidly. Squamous cell carcinoma is usually slow growing and is an unusual tumour in the dog.

Papillomas may resolve spontaneously in young dogs. Where there is involvement of the eyelid margin, with the likelihood of damage to the cornea, a wedge resection is the treatment of choice. Care should be taken when removing these tumours as seeding with virus particles is a possibility (Bonney *et al.*, 1986).

Adenoma/adenocarcinoma

Tumours arising from sebaceous glands (Fig. 5.37), and the meibomian gland can be regarded as a modified sebaceous gland, are the most commonly reported tumours affecting the canine eyelids (Krehbiel and Langham, 1975; Roberts *et al.*, 1986). The adenocarcinomas, although malignant, rarely metastasise. These tumours may assume a pedunculated form at the mucocutaneous junction or they may extend into the substance of the lid. Epitheliomas (Figs 5.38 and 5.39), which are less well differentiated but more aggressive sebaceous gland tumours, appear to have a greater tendency to recur. Like all tumours they should be removed in their entirety and this will involve some resection of eyelid tissue.

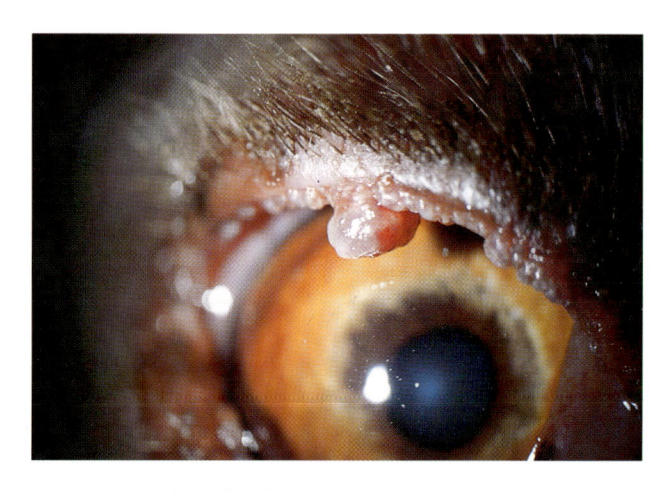

Fig. 5.37 Pedunculated upper lid adenoma with adjacent meibomian glandular hyperplasia in a 7-year-old female Weimaraner.

NEOPLASIA

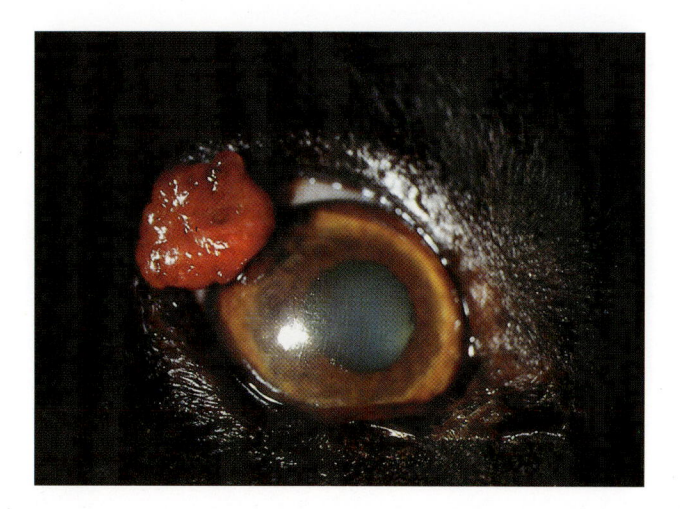

Fig. 5.38 Sebaceous gland epithelioma, well demarcated and extending from the upper lid margin in an 11-year-old male neutered Labrador. A mass had been removed at this site a year previously.

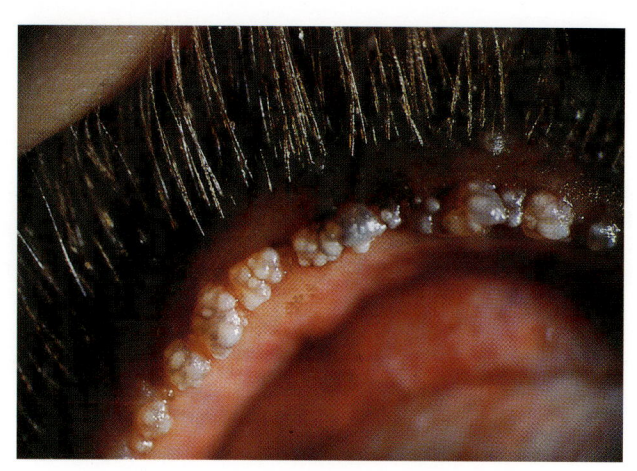

Fig. 5.40 Meibomian gland hyperplasia in a 7-year-old female Weimaraner. The aetiology of this condition was obscure but the dog also had multiple skin haemangiomas and mast cell tumours.

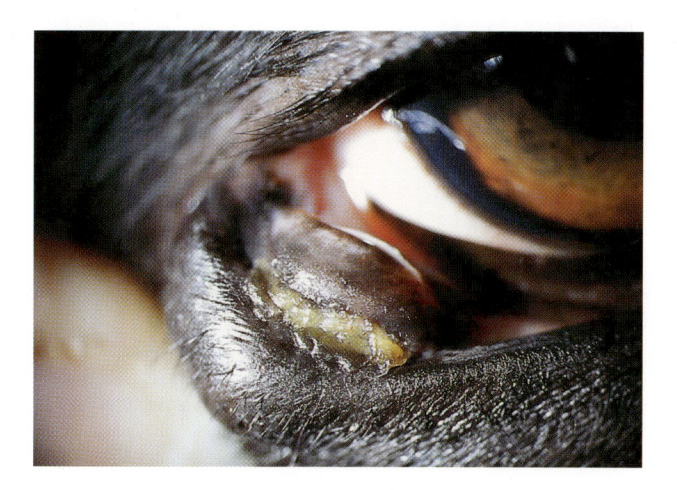

Fig. 5.39 Sebaceous gland epithelioma affecting the lower lid of a 3-year-old male entire crossbred. This diffuse lesion was accompanied by lipogranulomatous inflammation due to ductal rupture. A small mass had previously been excised at the site 2 years previously and, in spite of its size, the lesion was subsequently successfully removed by a wedge resection.

Meibomian gland hyperplasia (Fig. 5.40) is rare. It has been observed affecting all four lids and was confirmed on histopathology (J. Sansom, personal communication).

HISTIOCYTOMA

Histiocytomas usually present as rapidly growing solitary pink masses affecting the eyelid skin (Fig. 5.41). They tend to be broad based and are described as button tumours because of their appearance. In young dogs they will regress spontaneously over weeks or months and no treatment is indicated. Their presence is confirmed with a needle aspirate. When they occur in the older dog surgical excision may be necessary, although spontaneous regression may also occur (Fig. 5.41(b)).

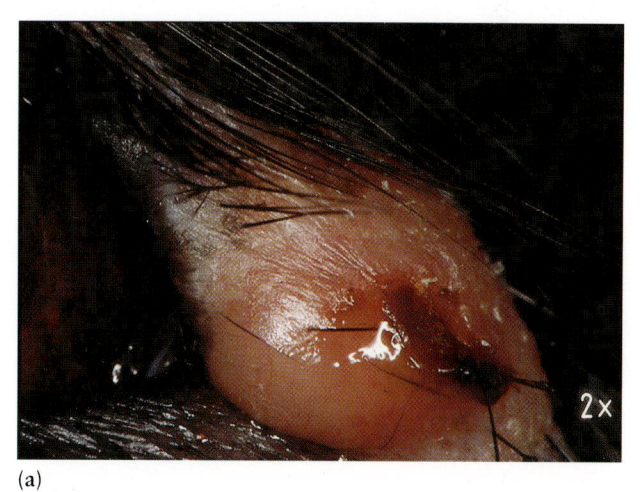

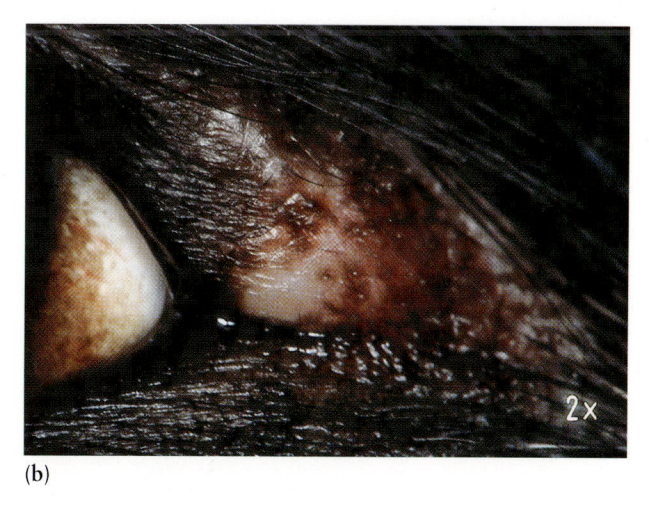

(a)

(b)

Fig. 5.41 (a) Histiocytoma in a 7-year-old Flat-coated Retriever. Spontaneously resolved over a 3-week period. (b) The same dog 20 days later.

MELANOMA

Eyelid melanomas (Fig. 5.42) are pigmented masses arising at the eyelid margin. They all behave in a benign manner but on the basis of their cell morphology will be classified as benign or malignant. They frequently present as nodular growths at the eyelid margin.

MAST CELL TUMOUR

Mast cell tumours arise in the dermis and usually affect the posterior parts of the body although they may develop in the periorbital area (Fig. 5.43). They cause swelling and pruritus; this may be intermittent. A diagnosis is based on a needle aspirate. Excision is the treatment of choice; a wide 2 cm margin is essential to prevent recurrence and frequently necessitates a reconstructive blepharoplasty. The prognosis depends on the level of differentiation of the neoplastic cells. Local recurrence and metastases do occur.

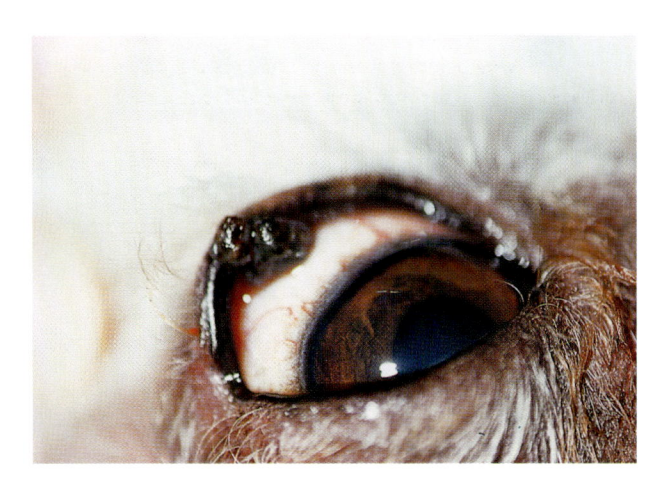

Fig. 5.42 Upper eyelid melanoma.

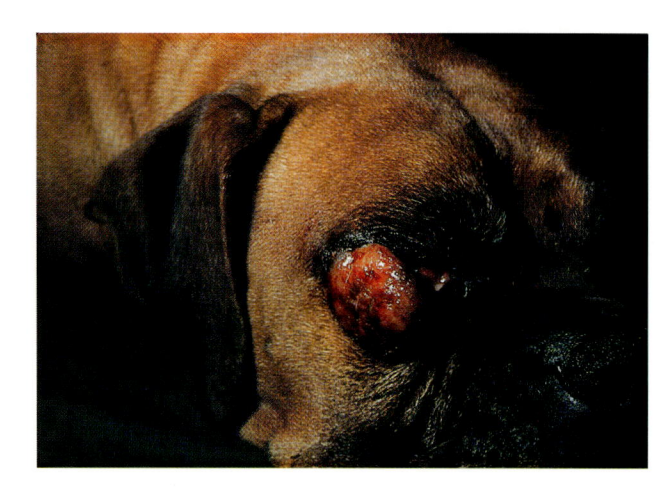

Fig. 5.43 Mast cell tumour in a 9-year-old Boxer.

REFERENCES

Bonney CH, Koch SA, Dice PF, Confer AW (1986) Papillomatosis of conjunctiva and adnexa in dogs. *Journal of the American Veterinary Medical Association* **176**(1): 48–51.

Krehbiel JD, Langham RF (1975) Eyelid neoplasms of dogs. *American Journal of Veterinary Research* **36**: 115–119.

Panich R, Scott DW, Miller WH (1991) Canine cutaneous sterile pyogranuloma/granuloma syndrome: a retrospective analysis of twenty-nine cases. *Journal of American Animal Hospital Association* **27**: 519–528.

Paterson S (1998) *Skin Diseases of the Dog*. Blackwell Science, Oxford.

Peiffer RL (1989) *Small Animal Ophthalmology. A Problem Orientated Approach*, p. 146. WB Saunders, London.

Roberts SM, Severin GA, Lavach JD (1986) Prevalence and treatment of palpebral neoplasms in the dog – 200 cases (1975–1983). *Journal of the American Veterinary Medical Association* **189**: 1355–1359.

Sansom J, Barnett KC, Blunden AS, Smith KC, Turner S, Waters L (1996) Canine conjunctival papilloma: a review of five cases. *Journal of Small Animal Practice* **37**: 84–86.

Sansom J, Heinrich C, Featherstone H (2000) Pyogranulomatos blepharitis in two dogs. *Journal of Small Animal Practice* **41**: 80–83.

Shaw SC (2000) The immune response in canine atopy: hypersensitivity to house dust mites (*Dermatophagoides* spp). PhD Thesis, Open University.

6 THIRD EYELID

INTRODUCTION

The third eyelid (nictitating membrane, membrana nictitans or haw) is situated at the medial canthus, or nasal angle, of the palpebral aperture. Under normal circumstances only the free border is visible and as this is usually pigmented and black it is hardly noticeable.

The third eyelid is covered on both sides by palpebral conjunctiva, the conjunctiva being continuous with that lining the upper and lower lids (palpebral) and the globe (bulbar) and extending into the fornices. It is, therefore, involved with forms of conjunctivitis (see Chapter 8). The free border of the third eyelid extends to partly or completely encircle the globe behind the limbus and may appear as a pigmented shallow flap. The third eyelid retains its shape and form due to the presence of a T-shaped cartilaginous plate, the horizontal part of the 'T' being parallel to the free border, the shaft of the 'T' being perpendicular to the free border. The surface of the third eyelid is covered with stratified squamous epithelium with a stroma of fibrous connective tissue containing much glandular and lymphoid tissue and rich in elastic tissue.

The nictitans gland (seromucous) is pink, is situated at the base of the shaft of the cartilage and is surrounded by fat. This gland is not Harder's gland and at one time was incorrectly called the Harderian gland.

In the dog, but not the cat, the membrana nictitans does not contain any muscle tissue for movement across the globe. Movement is entirely passive and is dependent upon action of the retractor oculi muscle and displacement of ocular fat with consequent protrusion of the third eyelid across the cornea in a lateral and upward direction.

Functions are important and include protection and contribution to the aqueous portion of the precorneal tear film, the nictitans gland being classed as an accessory lacrimal gland. Because of these functions it should be preserved whenever possible and only removed when affected by malignant neoplasia, rare in the dog.

DISORDERS OF THE THIRD EYELID (Barnett, 1978)

PROMINENCE OR PROTRUSION

Bilateral prominence of the nictitating membrane is seen in a number of the larger breeds, in particular the Bloodhound and St Bernard, and may be classed as normal in such breeds. Unilateral prominence can be the concern for an owner whose dog has one unpigmented third eyelid, in comparison with the pigmented one, but examination will reveal no abnormality. In chocolate or brown-coated dogs, the edge of the third eyelid is pale brown or pink and again may appear more prominent.

Ocular pain of whatever cause, e.g. corneal ulcer, foreign body or glaucoma, will lead to active retraction of the globe and consequent prominence of the third eyelid (Fig. 6.1). Similarly, enophthalmos as part of Horner's syndrome (see Chapter 15), together with miosis and ptosis, to an owner is often the most obvious, and therefore presenting, sign (Fig. 6.2). Such cases are almost invariably unilateral. Idiopathic Horner's syndrome is remarkably common in the Golden Retriever in the United Kingdom (Boydell, 1995). Cases have been seen in dogs of all ages, including young animals under 12 months of age; in Golden Retrievers of two generations; and in crossbred Golden Retrievers. These cases of Horner's syndrome occur in either eye and are temporary, the clinical signs no longer being apparent, but repeated episodes do occur.

In addition to enophthalmos, prominence of the third eyelid may occur with microphthalmos due to sinking of the small eye in the orbit (see Figs 4.16–4.18).

Exophthalmos, together with prominence of the third eyelid (see Figs 4.23–4.25), due to a retrobulbar space occupying lesion, e.g. tumour or abscess, is again almost invariably unilateral. Prominence of the third eyelid in such cases

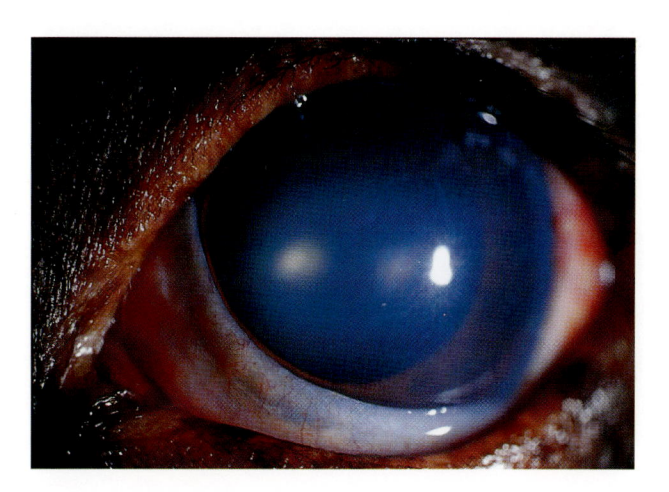

Fig. 6.1 Prominence of the third eyelid associated with pain (acute glaucoma).

THIRD EYELID

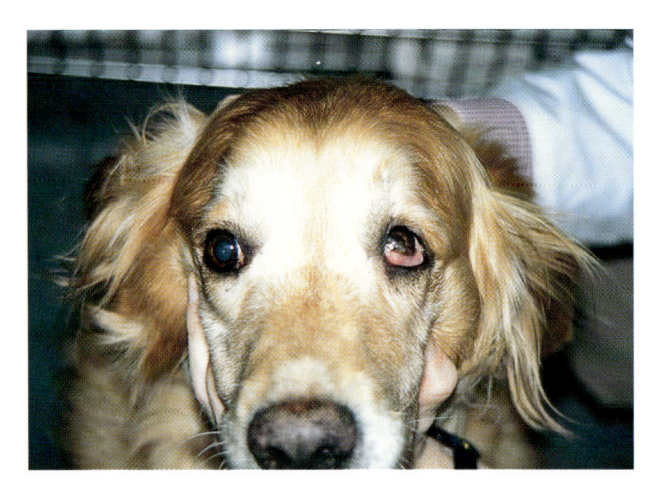

Fig. 6.2 Prominence of the third eyelid in Horner's syndrome in a 7-year-old Golden Retriever. Note the miosis and mild ptosis. (Courtesy of L Garosi.)

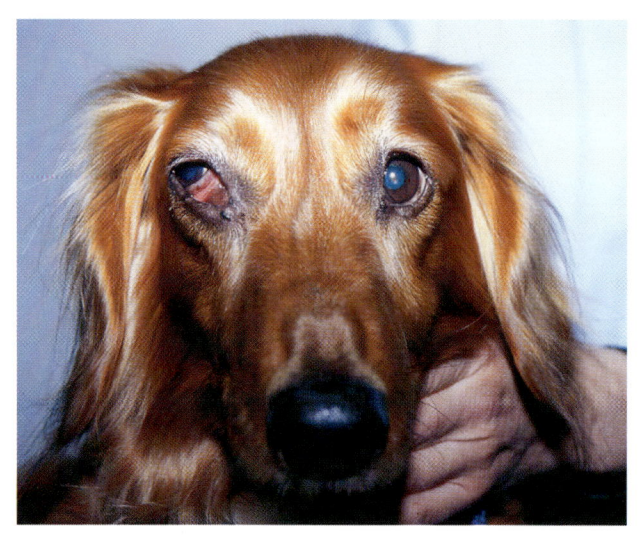

Fig. 6.4 Neoplasia of the nictitans gland, carcinoma, in a 9-year-old male Standard Longhaired Dachshund.

is dependent upon the actual site of the lesion and, therefore, does not always accompany the exophthalmos.

Neoplasia of the third eyelid or the nictitans gland, both rare in the dog, should also be considered in this category of prominence (Figs 6.3 and 6.4). Conjunctival cysts in young dogs often involve the base of the third eyelid leading to prominence (see Fig. 8.10 and Chapter 8).

Prominence of the third eyelid may also accompany tetanus (Fig. 6.5) and rabies.

TRAUMA AND FOREIGN BODIES

Trauma, particularly of the free border, is a common injury mainly following dog and cat fights and may become secondarily infected leading to ocular discharge. Small flaps may be successfully trimmed under local anaesthesia but more extensive wounds should be carefully sutured, preferably with 6/0 or 8/0 absorbable material.

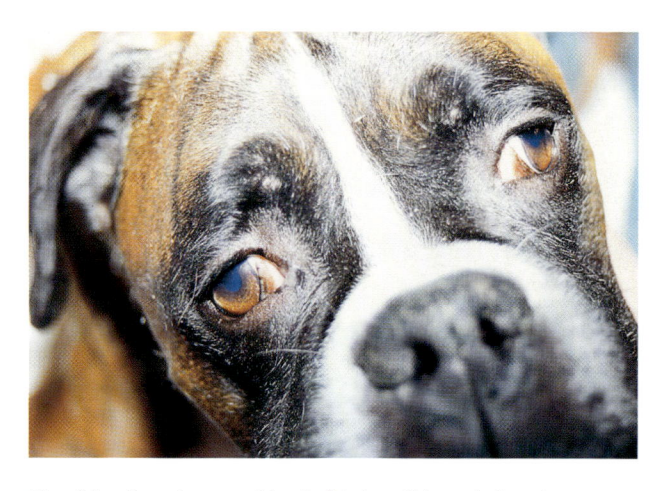

Fig. 6.5 Prominence of both third eyelids and rigor in a case of tetanus in an adult Boxer.

The pocket behind the third eyelid and in front of the globe is a favourite site for foreign bodies, in particular grass awns (Fig. 6.6).

INFLAMMATION

Both surfaces of the third eyelid are covered by conjunctiva and may be involved in cases of general conjunctivitis (Figs 6.7 and 6.8 and see Chapter 8).

Follicular conjunctivitis, in particular, affects both aspects of the nictitating membrane but especially the bulbar surface. It will be accompanied by lacrimation and/or mucoid discharge.

Canine nictitans plasmacytic conjunctivitis, plasma cell infiltration or plasmoma, may affect several breeds but especially the German Shepherd Dog and Belgian Shepherd Dog and collie types. The condition is a chronic, immune mediated, essentially bilateral but not always symmetrical,

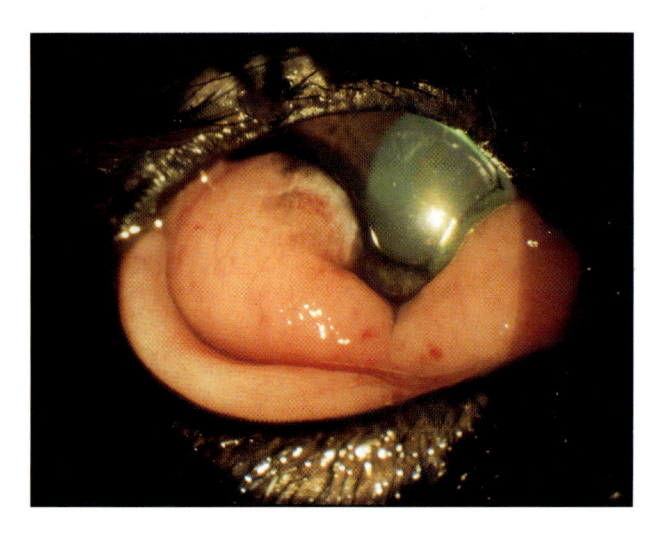

Fig. 6.3 Neoplasia of the nictitating membrane, lymphoma, in an 8-year-old male Scottish Terrier.

DISORDERS OF THE THIRD EYELID

occasionally unilateral, specific form of conjunctivitis affecting the nictitating membrane (Figs 6.9 and 6.10). It affects both sexes, usually in middle to old age (i.e. 6–10 years old) and commonly accompanies pannus (see Chapter 9).

Diagnosis is on the appearance of raised, pin-head, non-pigmented lesions near the free border of the anterior surface of the nictitating membrane, leading to an increase in size, thickening, depigmentation and inflammation of the exposed surface often with a mucopurulent discharge and conjunctival hyperaemia. Confirmation by biopsy reveals an infiltrate of plasma cells, lymphocytes and other inflammatory cells. Treatment with 0.2% cyclosporin in oil is best (Read, 1995) but topical corticosteroids can also be successful. However, recurrence following cessation of treatment does occur.

Inflamed third eyelids should never be removed.

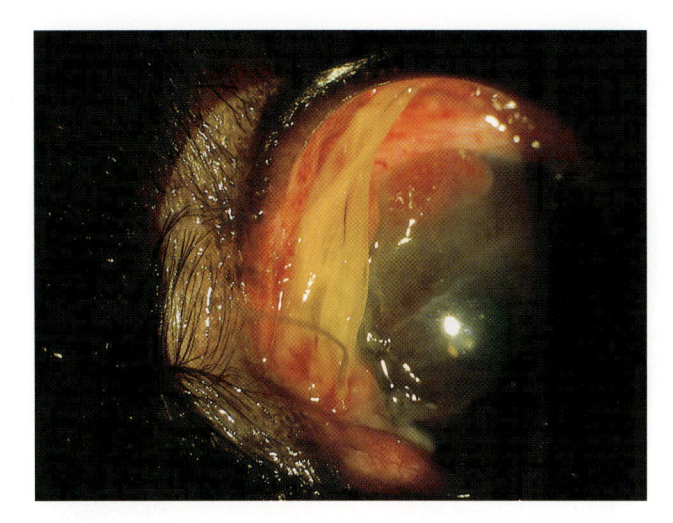

Fig. 6.6 Foreign body (grass awn) behind the third eyelid. Note the associated keratitis.

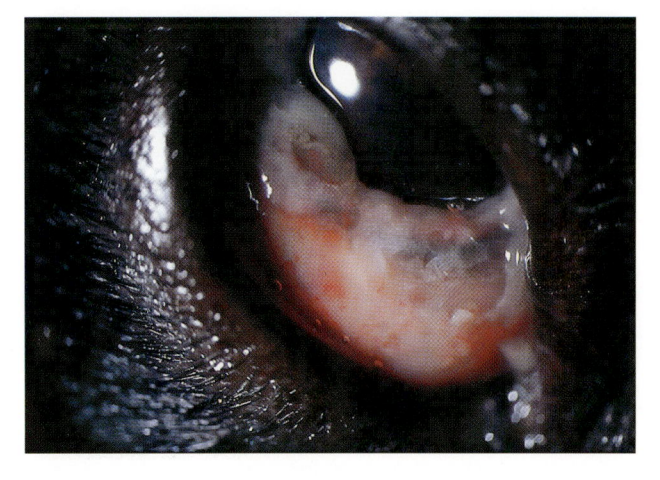

Fig. 6.7 Ligneous conjunctivitis in an adult Dobermann bitch. Similar lesions were also present in the mouth.

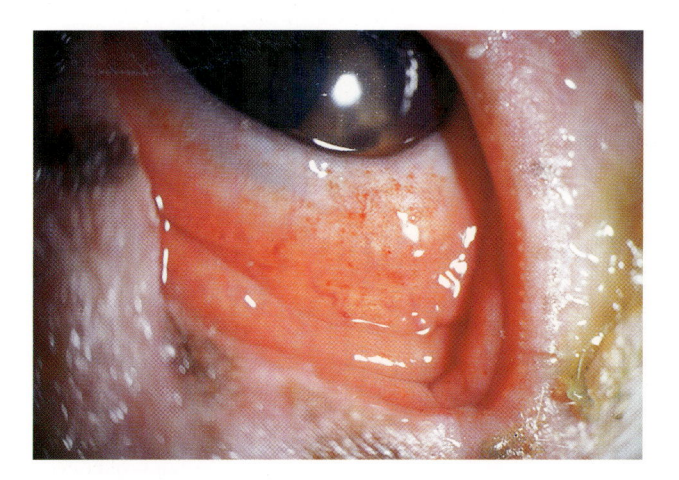

Fig. 6.8 Atopic conjunctivitis in a 5-year-old Clumber Spaniel bitch. Note the petechial haemorrhages.

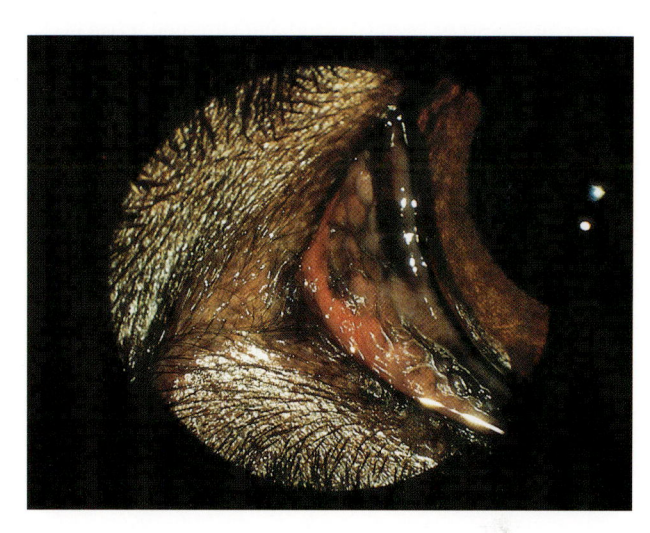

Fig. 6.9 Plasma cell infiltration, early case, in a 5-year-old German Shepherd Dog. Note the thickened nictitating membrane with inflammation and few non-pigmented spots.

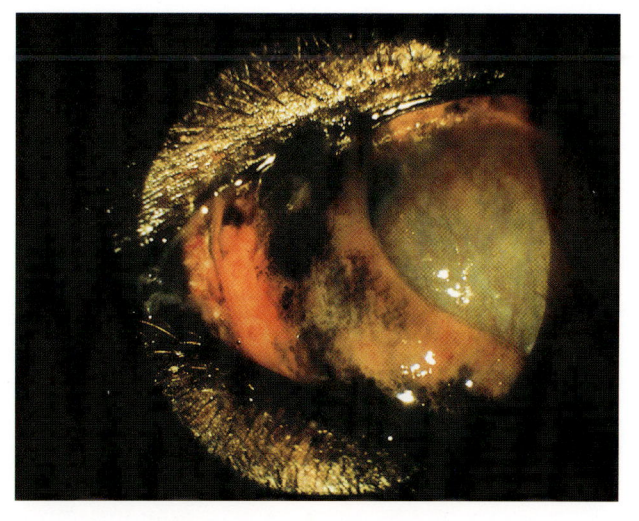

Fig. 6.10 Plasma cell infiltration, advanced case, in an 8-year-old German Shepherd Dog. Note discharge, large areas of depigmentation and associated pannus.

DISORDERS OF THE NICTITANS GLAND

Hyperplasia

Chronic hyperplasia of the nictitans gland can be the cause of excessive tear production and the prominent brown tear streak seen most frequently in young adults with white coats, classically the Toy Poodle. Following the elimination of obvious causes of epiphora and lacrimation, diagnosis is made by retropulsion of the globe producing prominence of the nictitating membrane and the appearance of a pink lump at its base, i.e. visible swelling of the gland through the anterior surface of the nictitating membrane. The Schirmer tear test in most cases is raised but often not excessively, usually 20–25. Treatment is the submucous resection of the enlarged gland with replacement, but no suturing, of the overlying conjunctiva. It should always be remembered that the nictitans gland is an accessory lacrimal gland and although it has been stated that excision of this gland may predispose to keratoconjunctivitis sicca, in our experience this has never occurred in suitable cases. Hodgman (1960) described the chemical cauterisation of the membrana nictitans with phenol, in cases of tear overflow, which afforded temporary relief, but a more permanent result is obtained by excision of the gland. Read *et al.* (1996) reported a histological study of nictitans glands removed from dogs with idiopathic tear overflow which revealed evidence of nictitans gland hyperplasia.

Prolapse of the nictitans gland

Prolapse of the nictitans gland or 'cherry eye' is a condition of young dogs, often small puppies, particularly in brachycephalic breeds especially the Bulldog (Fig. 6.11) but also the Beagle. One or both eyes may be involved, the latter simultaneously or not. The appearance is of a red lump at the medial canthus together with ocular discharge (Fig. 6.12). The actual cause is not known. Treatment used to consist of surgical removal of the prolapsed gland but, where possible, this gland should be retained; several procedures have been described for the surgical repositioning and anchoring of the nictitans gland. Manipulation of the gland with replacement is rarely permanently successful.

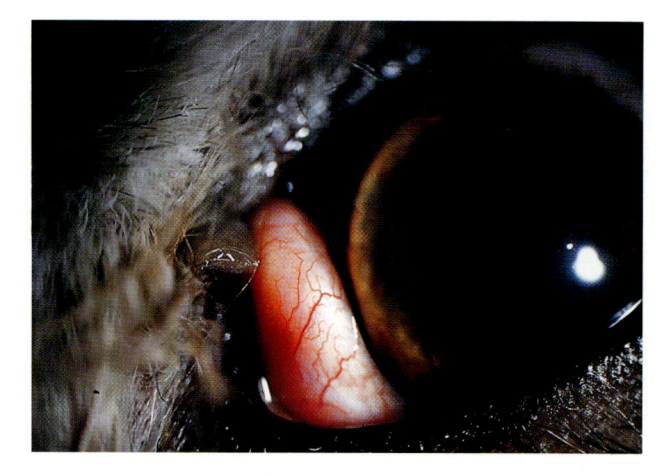

Fig. 6.12 Prolapsed nictitans gland in a 1-year-old Lhasa Apso. Note the similarity in appearance to Fig. 6.14.

DEFORMITY OF THE CARTILAGE OR BENT CARTILAGE

Deformity of the shaft of the cartilage, leading to 'scrolling' of the edge of the third eyelid occurs usually bilaterally and mainly in young adult dogs. This deformity leads to eversion (Fig. 6.13), or rarely inversion (Fig. 6.14), of the free border with a scroll-like and unsightly appearance at the inner canthus. It may lead to chronic or repeated bouts of conjunctivitis and even keratitis and ulceration. It is almost exclusively seen in the large breeds, the German Shepherd Dog, Great Dane and St Bernard being typical examples. It has been suggested to be an inherited defect (Martin and Leach, 1970). Treatment is the careful submucous dissection of the deformed cartilage under general anaesthesia, followed by conjunctival suturing with a fine absorbable material. If too much cartilage is removed prolapse of the nictitans gland may follow.

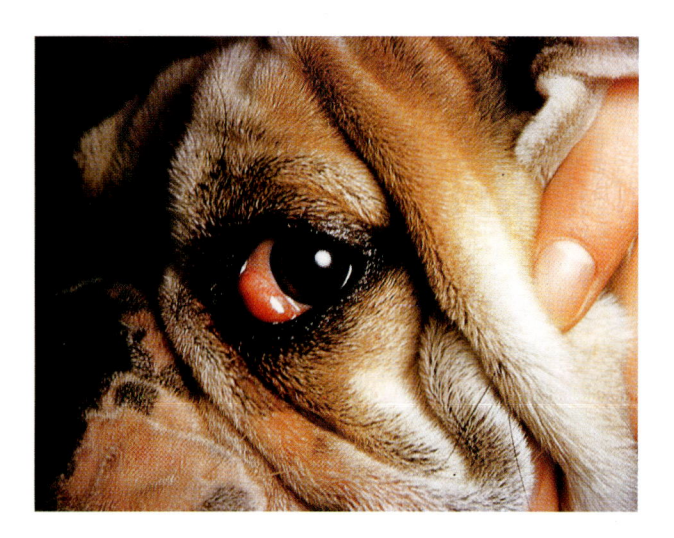

Fig. 6.11 Prolapsed nictitans gland in a young Bulldog.

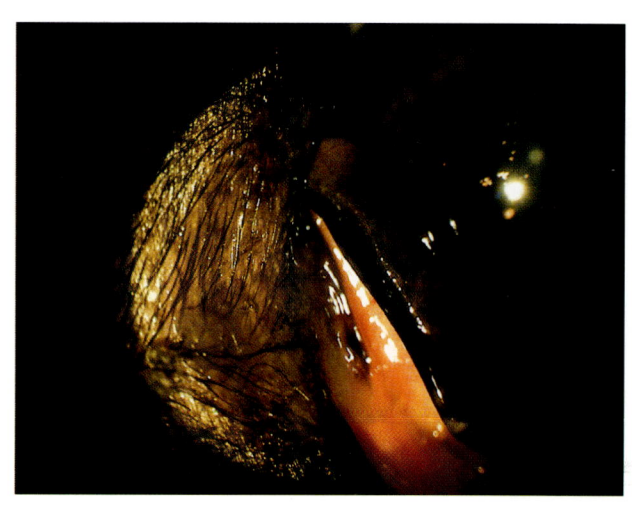

Fig. 6.13 Deformity of the cartilage, eversion, in a 16-month-old Bouvier bitch.

DISORDERS OF THE THIRD EYELID

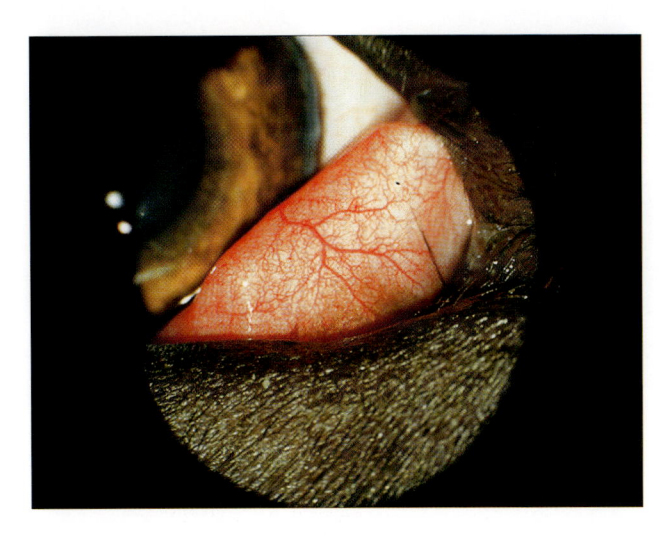

Fig. 6.14 Deformity of the cartilage, inversion, in a young adult Great Dane.

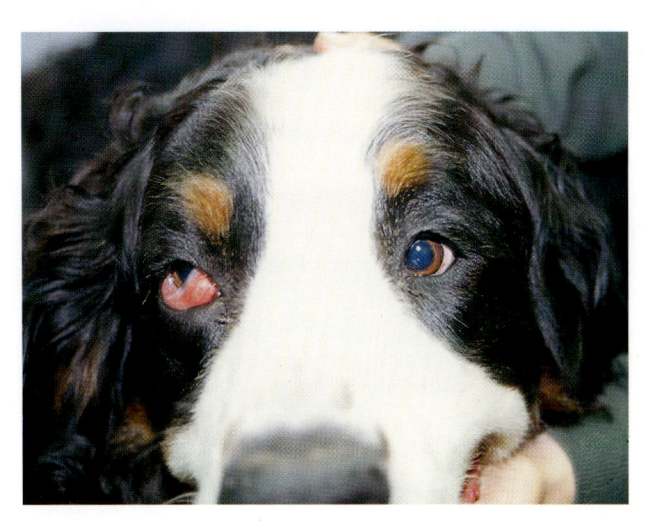

Fig. 6.16 Histiocytosis in a 4-year-old male Bernese Mountain Dog. Note the prominence and swelling of the nictitating membrane.

NEOPLASIA

The following neoplasms have been recorded but are uncommon in the dog: adenoma, adenocarcinoma, squamous cell carcinoma, melanoma, mastocytoma, papilloma, haemangioma, lymphosarcoma and angiokeratoma (Fig. 6.15). Adenocarcinomas, melanomas and papillomas are the most common.

Systemic histiocytosis particularly affects young adult and often male Bernese Mountain Dogs; several cases have been reported in the United Kingdom. Systemic histiocytosis is one of a number of histiocyte proliferative disorders with a predilection for the head, and in particular the ocular structures, together with multinodular skin lesions. The ocular signs may be the presenting sign and, in addition to prominence and swelling of the nictitating membrane (Figs 6.16 and 6.17), include episcleral masses, exophthalmos, uveitis and conjunctival and corneal lesions including chemosis and corneal oedema (Fig. 6.18) (Brearley *et al.*, 1994; Paterson *et al.*, 1995).

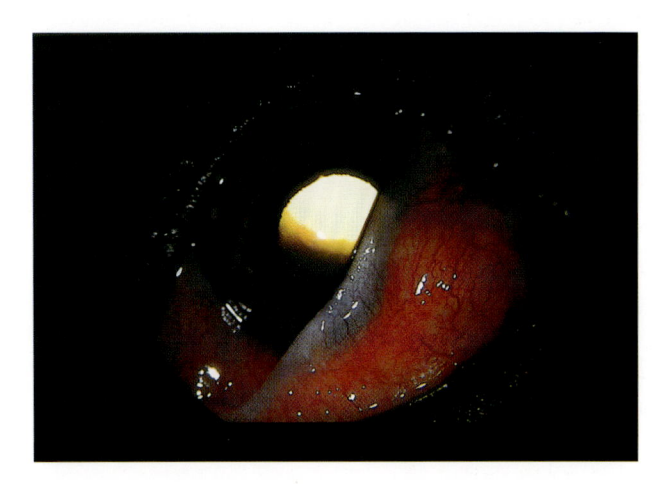

Fig. 6.17 Histiocytosis in the same dog as in Fig. 6.16.

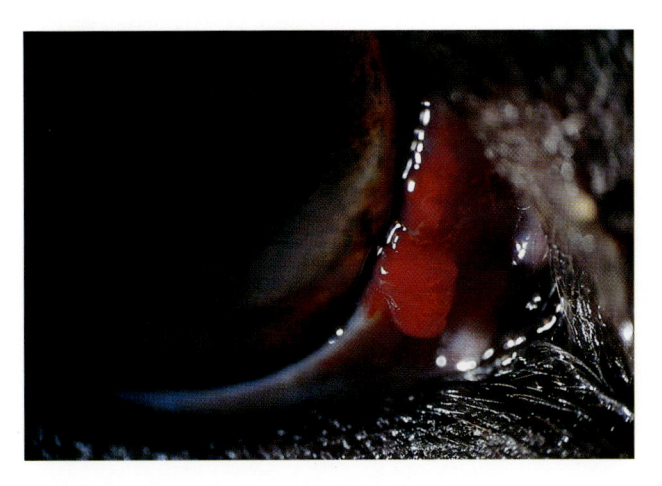

Fig. 6.15 Neoplasia of the nictitating membrane, angiokeratoma, in a 9-year-old male Beagle.

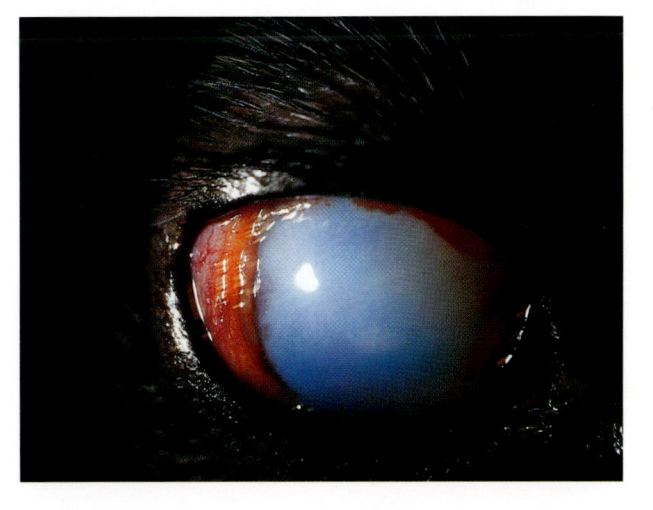

Fig. 6.18 Histiocytosis in a 5-year-old female Retriever/Border Collie cross. Note the corneal oedema and episcleral masses in addition to mild prominence of the nictitating membrane.

References

Barnett KC (1978) Diseases of the nictitating membrane of the dog. *Journal of Small Animal Practice* **18**: 101–108.

Boydell P (1995) Idiopathic Horner's syndrome in the golden retriever. *Journal of Small Animal Practice* **36**: 382–384.

Brearley MJ, Dunn KA, Smith KC, Blunden AS (1994) Systemic histiocytosis in a Bernese Mountain Dog. *Journal of Small Animal Practice* **35**: 271–274.

Hodgman SFJ (1960) Cauterization of the membrana nictitans. In Jones BV (ed.) *Advances in Small Animal Practice Volume II*, pp. 115–116. Oxford Press, Oxford.

Martin CL, Leach R (1970) Everted membrana nictitans in German Shorthaired Pointers. *Journal of the American Veterinary Medical Association* **157**: 1229–1232.

Paterson S, Boydell P, Pike R (1995) Systemic histiocytosis in the Bernese mountain dog. *Journal of Small Animal Practice* **36**: 233–236.

Read RA (1995) Treatment of canine nictitans plasmacytic conjunctivitis with 0.2% cyclosporin ointment. *Journal of Small Animal Practice* **36**: 50–56.

Read RA, Dunn KA, Smith KC, Barnett KC (1996) A histological study of nictitans glands from dogs with tear overflow of unknown cause. *Veterinary and Comparative Ophthalmology* **6**(3): 195–204.

7 LACRIMAL SYSTEM

INTRODUCTION

The canine lacrimal system comprises two separate tear-secreting glands, the lacrimal gland located superiotemporal to the globe and just below the supraorbital process of the frontal bone, and the nictitans gland situated at the base of the third eyelid. Both glands contribute to the lacrimal component of the tear film which is responsible for corneal and conjunctival wetting. Blinking is effective in maintaining wetness of the ocular surface and contributes significantly to the tear drainage mechanisms. Tears are driven down the nasolacrimal system through two small puncta. Both puncta are located at the medial canthus on the upper and lower lid. They can be found by everting the lid margin at the point where it terminates. Small horizontal elliptical openings can be seen on the palpebral conjunctiva (Fig. 7.1). Drainage occurs through the puncta into the canaliculi which meet to form a nasolacrimal sac which is very poorly developed in the dog. The nasolacrimal duct extends from this juncture to a distal opening in the nasal vestibule passing through the lacrimal and maxillary bones. The length of the nasolacrimal duct will vary with head conformation and therefore the breed of dog. In the brachycephalic breeds it is short and drainage may occur into the oropharynx rather than down the nose.

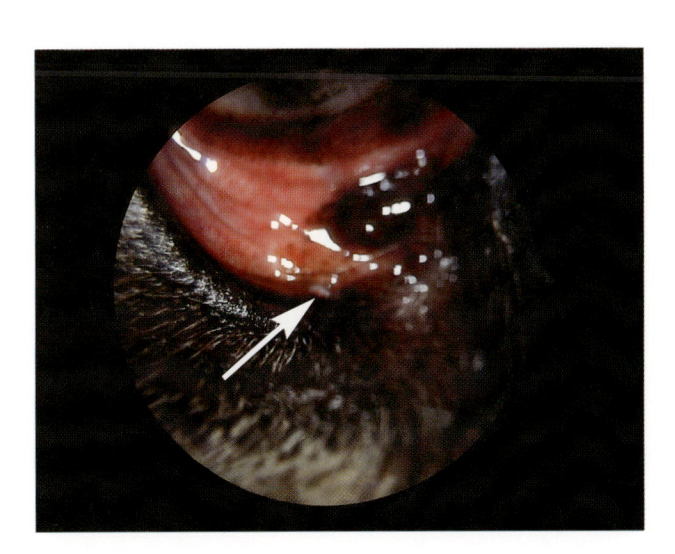

Fig. 7.1 Normal lower punctum located on the palpebral conjunctiva at the medial canthus in a 2-year-old Golden Retriever.

CONGENITAL ANOMALIES

ABSENCE OF THE PUNCTA

Imperforate punctum is congenital absence of the punctum; the lower opening is most commonly affected (Fig. 7.2) and, since it is responsible for the bulk of the lacrimal drainage epiphora (tear overflow), is the presenting sign (Fig. 7.3). It may present as a unilateral or bilateral problem. In some cases imperforate punctum occurs in one eye and micropunctum in

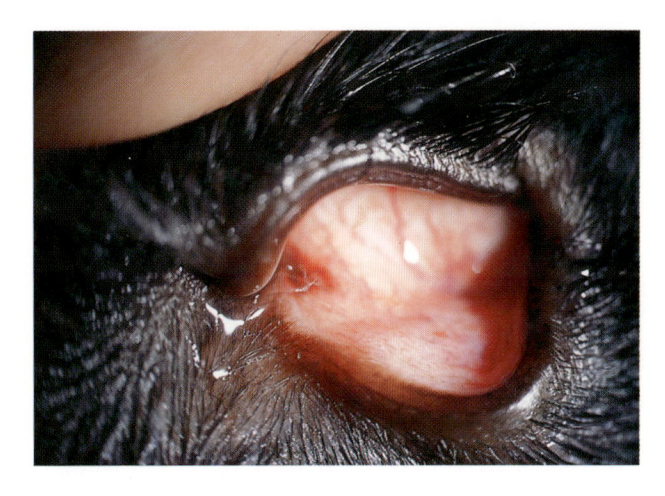

Fig. 7.2 Imperforate punctum.

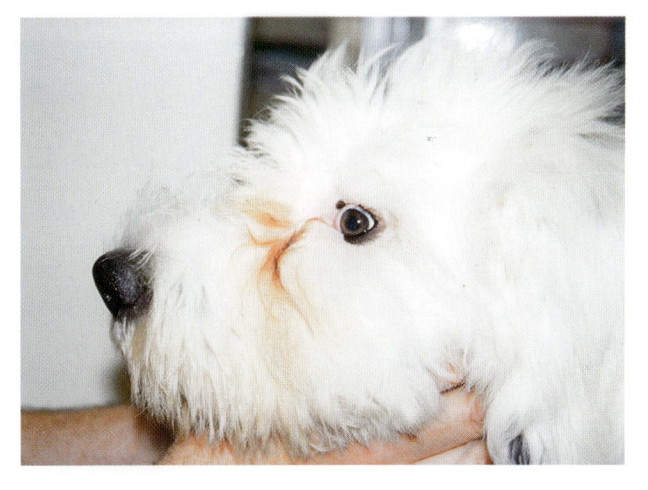

Fig. 7.3 Discoloration of the facial hair at the medial canthus (tear streak) associated with epiphora due to an imperforate punctum in an Old English Sheepdog puppy.

LACRIMAL SYSTEM

the other. In the dog the canaliculus is usually present and surgical correction with a three snip procedure, which removes the overlying conjunctiva, resolves the problem permanently. The placement of indwelling sylastic tubing is not necessary but it is important that surgery is performed with good magnification and accuracy. The initial incision must be made in the appropriate position. A small depression can often be seen at the appropriate site. Usually the imperforate punctum can be located by flushing from the upper punctum, a ballooning of the conjunctiva will then occur over the area of imperforation. If the incision is not made over the canaliculus, haemorrhage and postoperative scarring may result in permanent occlusion of the duct.

On rare occasions the upper puncta and/or canaliculi are absent. In these cases it is usually possible to manage the tear overflow by using medical treatment with barrier creams when appropriate. Conjunctivorhinostomy, the creation of a permanent fistula into the nasal cavity, is not usually considered.

There is a breed incidence for imperforate puncta in the American and English Cocker Spaniel and the Labrador and Golden Retriever.

MICROPUNCTUM

A small punctal opening may occur, often in conjunction with imperforate puncta. The diagnosis is based not only on the small size but also on its circular configuration (Fig. 7.4). The normal aperture assumes an elliptical shape. Enlargement of the puncta by dilatation with a dilator, or a three snip procedure to remove a triangle of conjunctiva over the canaliculus, rectifies the situation.

DISEASES OF THE LACRIMAL SYSTEM

OBSTRUCTION OF THE PUNCTA

The puncta may become obstructed by conjunctival and lid inflammation in cases of chronic conjunctivitis, blepharitis and neoplasia. Foreign bodies, particularly plant material

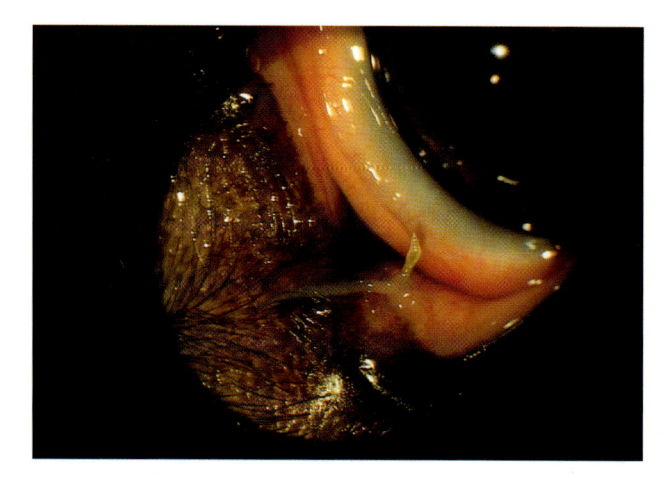

Fig. 7.5 Grass awn obstructing the lower punctum.

(Fig. 7.5), may enter the nasolacrimal system resulting in a dacryocystitis. Trauma to this area may result in cicatrisation of the punctal opening and canaliculus.

Careful examination of the area under local or general anaesthesia is necessary to arrive at a diagnosis. The patency of the nasolacrimal system can be assessed by monitoring the passage of fluorescein dye from the conjunctival sac to the nasal punctum or into the oropharynx. This test is often unhelpful as it may give a false negative result – the appearance of stain signifies patency of the duct but no stain does not necessarily imply a blocked duct. The placement of a nasolacrimal cannula into the upper puncta and gentle flushing of the system is the best method of establishing whether the system is patent or not and should always be used in cases where stain does not appear at the nose following fluorescein in the conjunctival sac. Cannulation and flushing via the upper (Fig. 7.6) and lower puncta can be performed in the conscious dog under local anaesthesia. Cannulation of the nasal punctum is more difficult and requires general anaesthesia. When there is erosion or rupture of the duct,

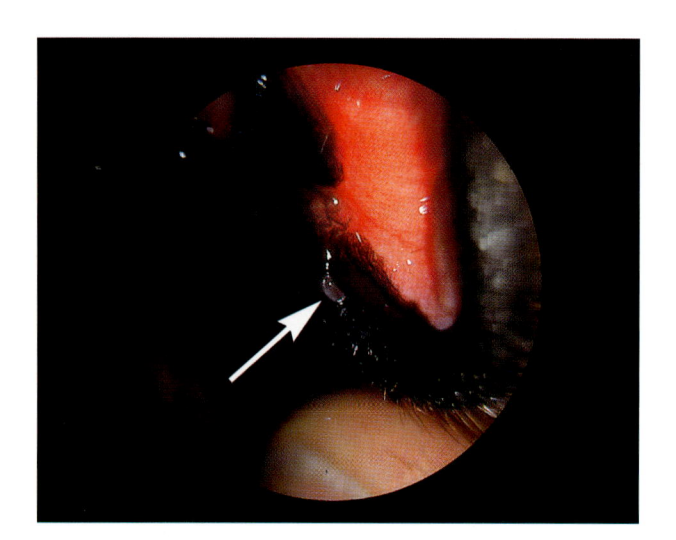

Fig. 7.4 Micropunctum.

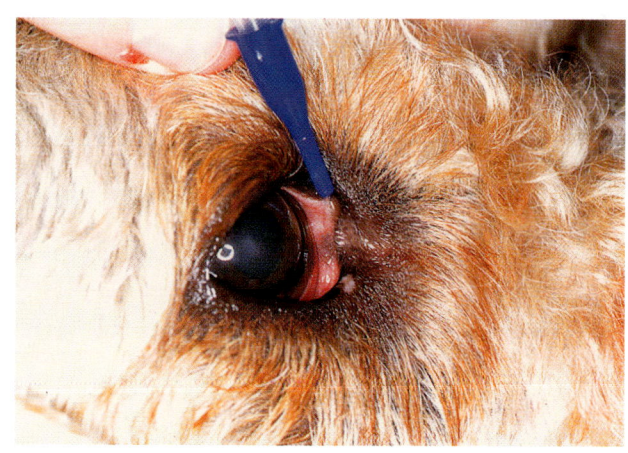

Fig. 7.6 Cannulation of the upper puncta using a plastic nasolacrimal cannula. This procedure is performed using local anaesthesia only.

DISEASES OF THE LACRIMAL SYSTEM

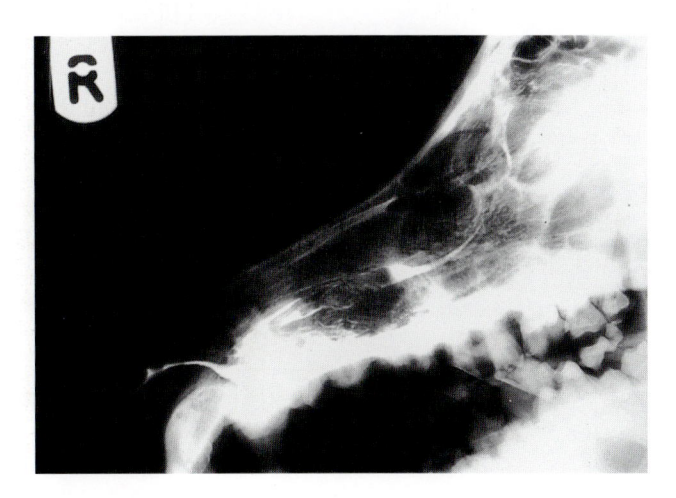

Fig. 7.7 Dacryocystorhinogram in a 3½-year-old German Shepherd Dog. Contrast studies of the nasolacrimal system demonstrate the proximal outline of the left nasolacrimal duct which becomes dilated followed by filling defects. A second injection of contrast material passed into the distal duct exiting at the left nostril. The dog presented with dacryocystitis of 18 months' duration; there was a good response to repeated nasolacrimal flushing and broad spectrum antibiotic cover over a 6-week period.

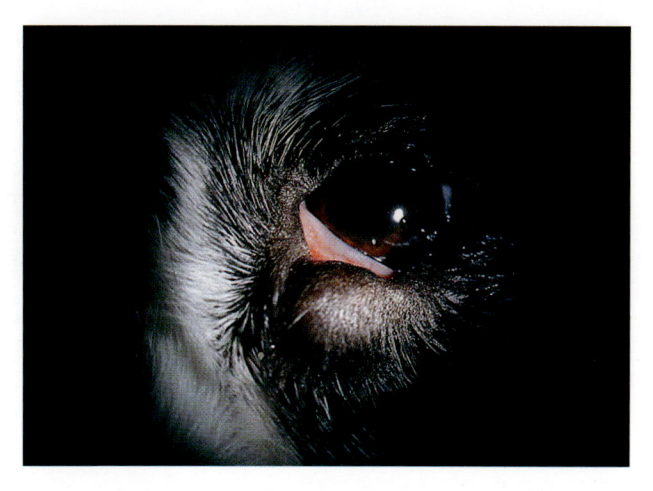

Fig. 7.8 Infection and cystic dilatation of the lower canaliculi in a 1-year-old English Springer Spaniel.

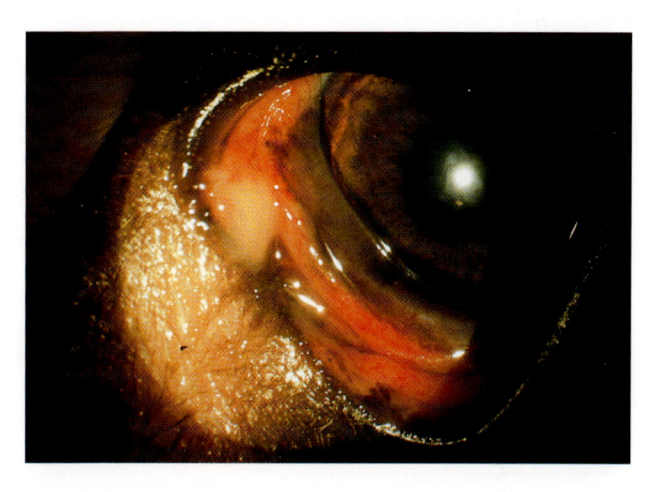

Fig. 7.9 Dacryocystitis with pus exuding from the upper punctum.

haemorrhage and discomfort will occur on flushing. In such cases the procedures should be performed under general anaesthesia to avoid further soft tissue damage.

Plain and contrast radiography (dacryocystorhinography) may be helpful (Gelatt et al., 1972) but may merely tend to confirm rupture or blockage of the duct when this has occurred. Cystic dilatation of the nasolacrimal duct is not common, but when present it can be demonstrated very clearly with the use of contrast materials (Fig. 7.7). In cases where duct obstruction or infection is secondary to dental or nasal disease or neoplasia, radiography is of diagnostic value. Magnetic resonance imaging has also been reported as a useful diagnostic tool.

DACRYOCYSTITIS

Infection or inflammation of the nasolacrimal sac and nasolacrimal duct (dacryocystitis) (Fig. 7.8) is not uncommon. Infection may be primary or secondary to obstruction of the nasolacrimal duct or canaliculi, usually following foreign body penetration. Acute infection will respond to repeated nasolacrimal duct flushing and antibiotic treatment. With chronic infection it is necessary to establish an aetiology; it may be secondary to an obstruction resulting from trauma to this area, or dental or nasal disease. In addition, space-occupying lesions will prevent drainage. The presentation is as for chronic conjunctivitis but careful examination of the puncta and the gentle application of pressure over the canaliculus will reveal pus exuding from the punctum (Fig. 7.9). Culture and sensitivity tests should be performed followed by appropriate systemic antibiotic treatment. Gentle and repeated flushing of the duct until patency is established is essential if treatment is to be successful. Topical antibiotics will be helpful only when drainage can occur. Systemic treatment may be necessary for several weeks and repeated flushing is usually carried out at fortnightly intervals until the infection has cleared. In some cases it may not be possible to establish complete patency because of narrowing or obliteration of the nasolacrimal duct.

Where cystic dilatation of the nasolacrimal duct occurs in association with chronic infection, rhinotomy and drainage of the cyst into the nasal cavity can be considered (van der Woerdt et al., 1997).

TRAUMA

Trauma may result in damage to the nasolacrimal puncta (Fig. 7.11). The canaliculus should be identified where possible and cannulated, and a nasolacrimal catheter sutured in place until healing is complete. It may be necessary to leave in situ for 3–4 weeks.

LACRIMAL SYSTEM

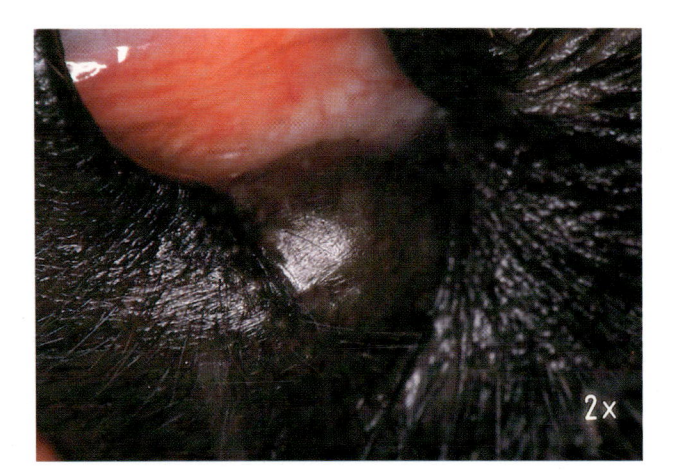

Fig. 7.10 Inclusion cyst (contained hair) at the medial canthus of a 6-year-old Cavalier King Charles Spaniel; acute onset 3 weeks previously, possible traumatic origin.

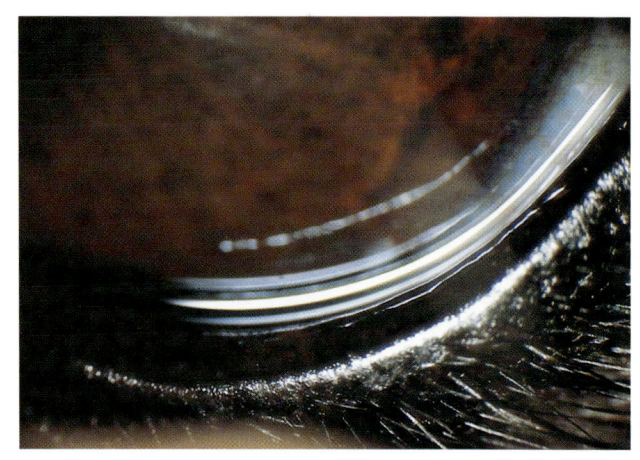

Fig. 7.12 Normal tear film covering the cornea and forming a meniscus.

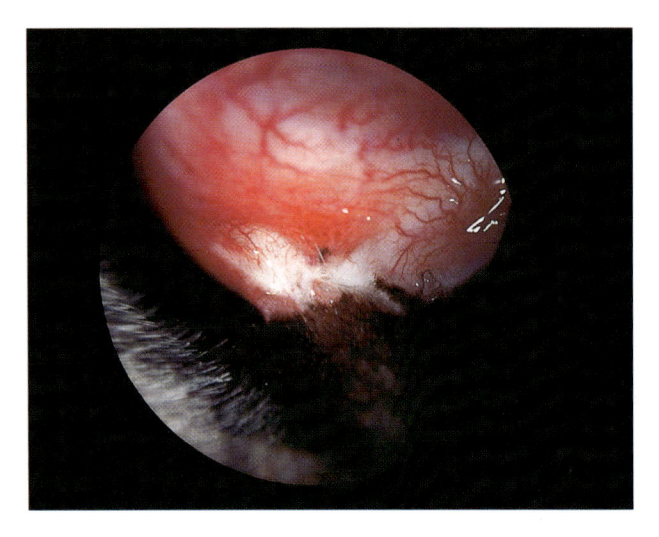

Fig. 7.11 Permanent occlusion of the lower punctum with scar tissue resulting from trauma.

KERATOCONJUNCTIVITIS SICCA

Dry eye is due to a deficiency or excessive evaporation of the tear film; a combination of these two features may be seen in some cases, particularly the brachycephalic breeds. The tear film is no longer regarded as a clear-cut three-layered structure and there is probably an intermingling of the mucous, aqueous and lipid components. The tear film will adhere to the conjunctiva and cornea, the latter due to the presence of a glycocalyx. A deficiency in any of these components may cause a dry eye, although it is the reduction in the aqueous component of the tear film that can be measured. The function of the tear film is to cover and protect the cornea and conjunctival sac, in addition to a lubricating and optical function. Three-quarters of the tears will lie in the tear meniscus or reservoir and this can be visualised between the lid margin and the corneal surface (Fig. 7.12). Changes in the conjunctival or corneal surface, lid conformation and the blink reflex will affect the stability of the tear film. The lipid layer is secreted from the meibomian glands and meibomianitis may lead to tear film instability. Likewise, quantitative or qualitative changes in aqueous secretion from the lacrimal and nictitans gland or mucus secretion from the goblet cells may manifest as a dry eye.

The diagnosis is based on the clinical presentation and quantitative assessment of the tear film using the Schirmer tear test (see Fig. 1.7). A reading of 10 mm of wetting per minute is borderline and usually diagnostic when values are less than this. The normal values are usually in excess of 15 mm of wetting per minute. It may be necessary to repeat the Schirmer tear test reading on more than one occasion in order to establish an average value and confirm the diagnosis. It is obviously imperative that there has been no interference, cleaning or medication of the eye prior to performing the Schirmer tear test. The severity of the clinical presentation may not correlate well with the Schirmer tear test value.

There is a breed incidence of dry eye. It is usually seen in small dogs and is very common in the United Kingdom in the West Highland White Terrier. The Spaniel breeds, the Yorkshire Terrier and the Dachshund (Miniature and Standard) are frequently affected. In addition to a genetic predisposition there is an age incidence (middle age) and a sex incidence, being more common in the female (Barnett and Joseph, 1987). This has been disputed (Kaswan *et al.*, 1991) suggesting that neutered animals are predisposed to develop dry eye.

Keratoconjunctivitis sicca is a common cause of chronic conjunctivitis in the dog. Inflammation and destruction of the tear-secreting lacrimal and nictitans glands will result in a reduction or absence of tear secretion. It can occur as an acute presentation particularly if the condition has an infectious aetiology, as with distemper virus. However, most cases are chronic due to immune-mediated destruction of the lacrimal gland. Rarely in the dog is a dry eye associated with a dry mouth (xerostomia) or with immune-mediated

DISEASES OF THE LACRIMAL SYSTEM

connective tissue disorders. However, dry eye and dry mouth, known as Sjögren's syndrome in man, has been reported in the dog (Quimby *et al.*, 1979) It is therefore important to check that there is adequate salivary secretion to the mouth before considering a parotid duct transposition.

In acute cases the eye is painful with severe blepharospasm, profuse discharge with severe conjunctival hyperaemia (Figs 7.13 and 7.14). In more chronic cases the eye is uncomfortable with conjunctival hyperaemia and hypertrophy (Fig. 7.15). A pigmentary and vascular keratitis develops in conjunction with irregularities of the corneal surface. The upper half of the cornea is primarily affected (Fig. 7.16). The discharge is profuse, muco to mucopurulent and adherent to the cornea (Figs 7.17 and 7.18). The latter can be

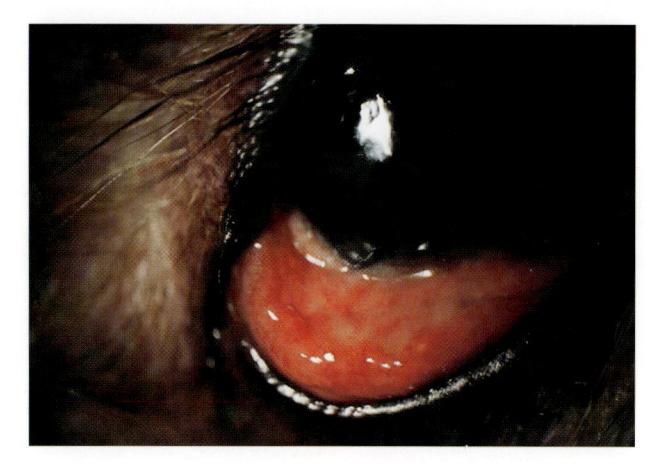

Fig. 7.15 Conjunctival hyperaemia and hypertrophy resulting in folding of the conjunctiva following 18 months of keratoconjunctivitis sicca.

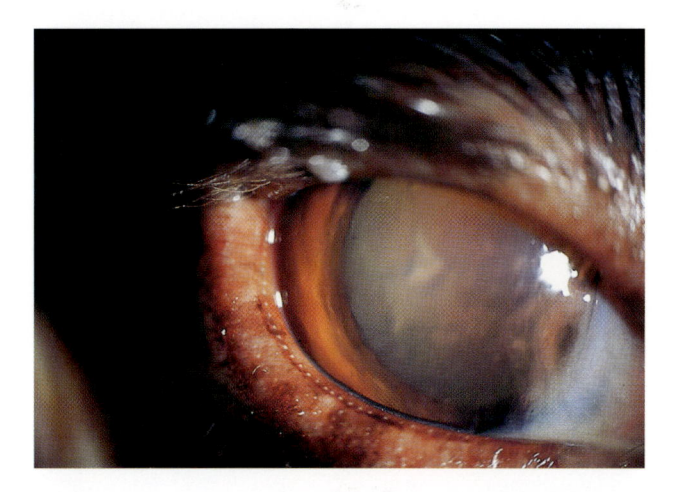

Fig. 7.13 Acute keratoconjunctivitis sicca in an 8-year-old male English Springer Spaniel. There was severe corneal dryness (Schirmer tear test 0), marked conjunctival inflammation and severe ocular discomfort, in association with a secondary staphylococcal conjunctivitis. This unilateral problem responded dramatically to a 10-day course of systemic steroids in conjunction with antibiotic cover and topical lubricants. (The pupil is dilated following the application of a mydriatic.)

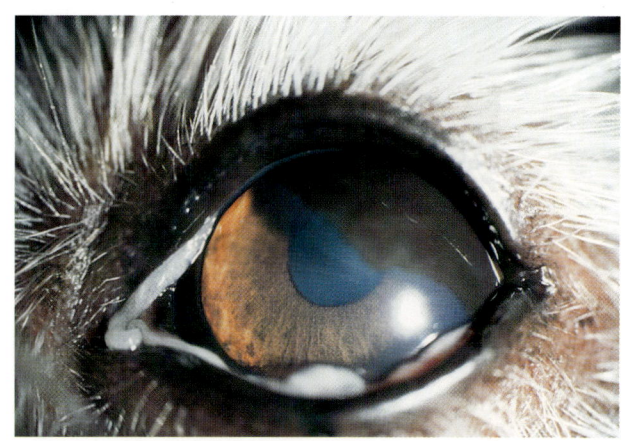

Fig. 7.16 Bilateral keratoconjunctivitis sicca of 15 months' duration in a 4-year-old female neutered West Highland White Terrier. Left eye with a pigmentary keratitis affecting the dorsotemporal cornea with a very obvious mucus thread.

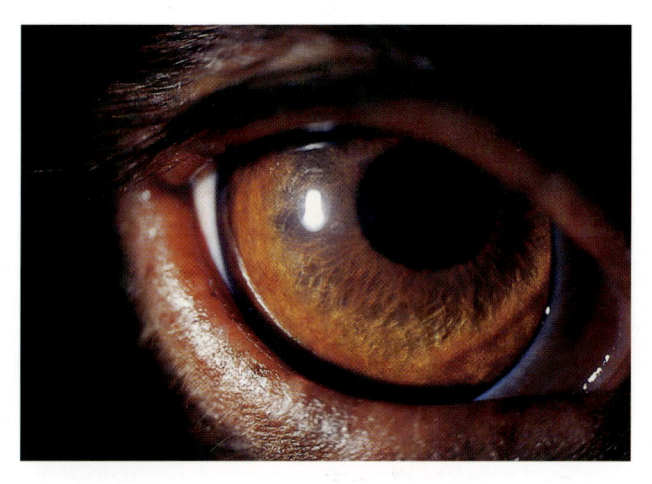

Fig. 7.14 The same eye as in Fig. 7.13 after 10 days' treatment, Schirmer tear test 8 mm of wetting.

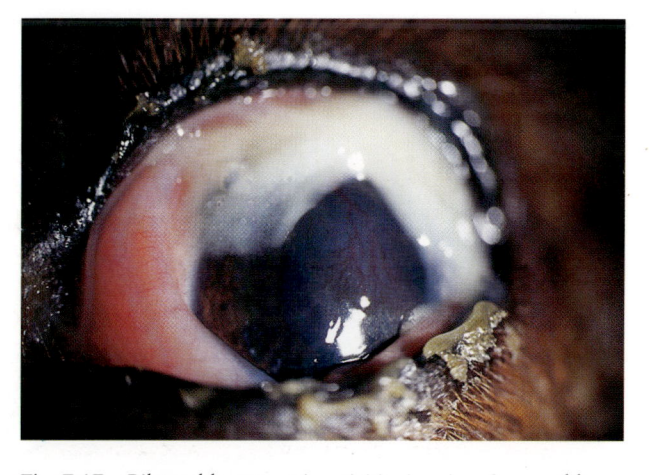

Fig. 7.17 Bilateral keratoconjunctivitis sicca in a 2-year-old female entire Cavalier King Charles Spaniel. Profuse discharge adherent to the cornea with a mild vascular keratitis. Littermate was similarly affected at the same age.

LACRIMAL SYSTEM

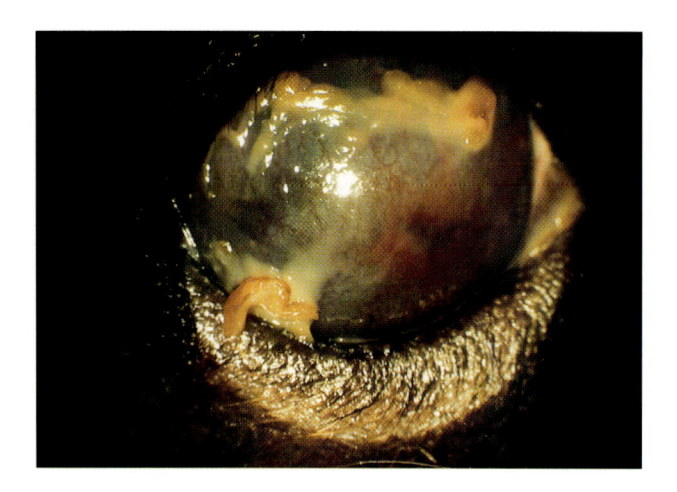

Fig. 7.18 Severe keratoconjunctivitis sicca in a 4-year-old Lhasa Apso bitch with a Schirmer tear test reading of zero. Purulent discharge is adherent to the cornea, there is marked corneal vascularisation associated with patchy pigmentation and corneal oedema.

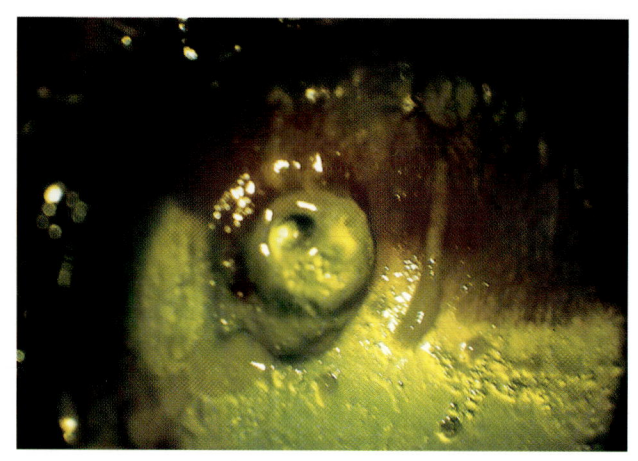

Fig. 7.20 A descemetocoele associated with keratoconjunctivitis sicca in a West Highland White Terrier. There is deep corneal vascularisation to the oedematous edge of the descemetocoele.

regarded as pathognomonic for a tear film deficiency. In extreme cases the discharge may dry on the surface of the cornea, producing a crust (Fig. 7.19). Ulceration may occur with keratoconjunctivitis sicca and this is typically a descemetocoele (Fig. 7.20). The condition is particularly severe in exophthalmic breeds such as the Pug and the Pekingese, where poor lid closure will exacerbate the problem (Fig. 7.21).

Keratoconjunctivitis sicca may be congenital with a bilateral or unilateral presentation. In the United Kingdom there is a breed incidence of congenital keratoconjunctivitis sicca in association with dermatological disease in the Cavalier King Charles Spaniel. Here the condition is frequently bilateral in association with an abnormally curly coat. Certain drugs are lacrimotoxic in the dog and these include the

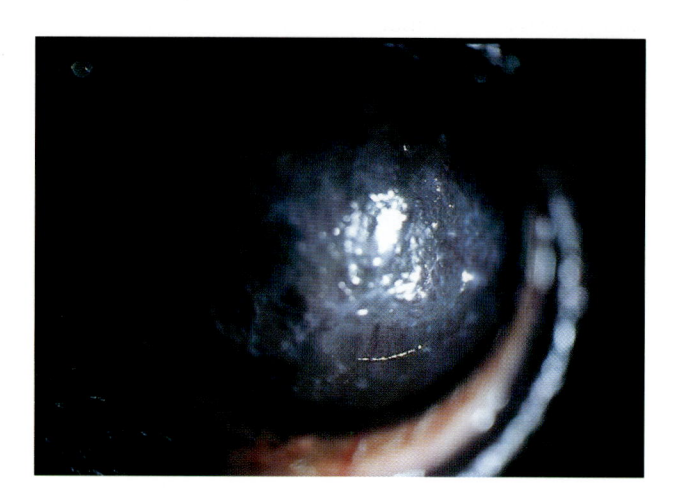

Fig. 7.21 A severe pigmentary keratitis in a $2\frac{1}{2}$-year-old Pug as a result of dry eye. Schirmer tear test 4 mm of wetting. The corneal surface is irregular with loss of corneal transparency and the corneal reflection. The presence of dense pigmentation obscures any intraocular detail.

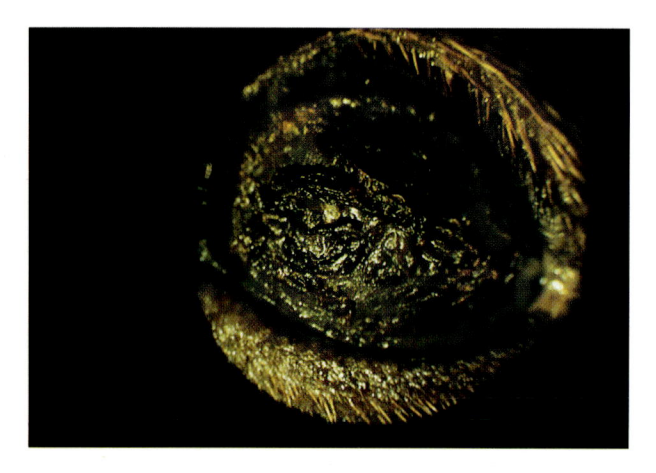

Fig. 7.19 Extreme dryness resulting in irreversible corneal changes in a 4-year-old Jack Russell Terrier bitch. The pigmentation and crusting obscure any corneal or intraocular detail.

sulphonamides (Sansom *et al.*, 1985), 5-aminosalicylic acid (Barnett and Joseph, 1987), and phenazopyridine (Slatter, 1973). Overzealous use of atropine may also produce a dry eye. General anaesthesia will reduce lacrimal secretion and this is particularly pertinent in subclinical borderline cases as clinical signs of dry eye may be precipitated. Facial trauma and middle ear disease may cause a unilateral or bilateral neurogenic dry eye. Neurogenic dry eye is a result of damage to parasympathetic fibres that originate in the nucleus of the facial nerve. These fibres also supply the lateral nasal gland which is responsible for producing a serous secretion to the nasal mucosa. A dry discharge will accumulate at the affected nostril (Fig. 7.22) and is frequently misinterpreted as a failure of lacrimal secretion to the respective nostril, rather than a loss of secretion from the nasal gland. When a dry

DISEASES OF THE LACRIMAL SYSTEM

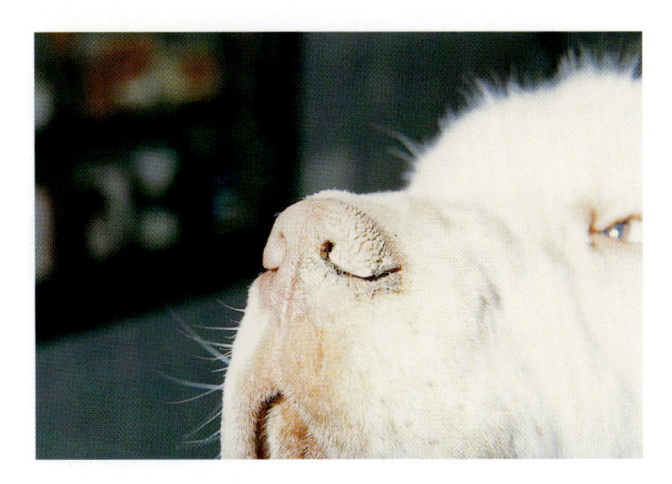

Fig. 7.22 Unilateral keratoconjunctivitis sicca in a Clumber Spaniel associated with a dry nose, indicative of a neurogenic aetiology.

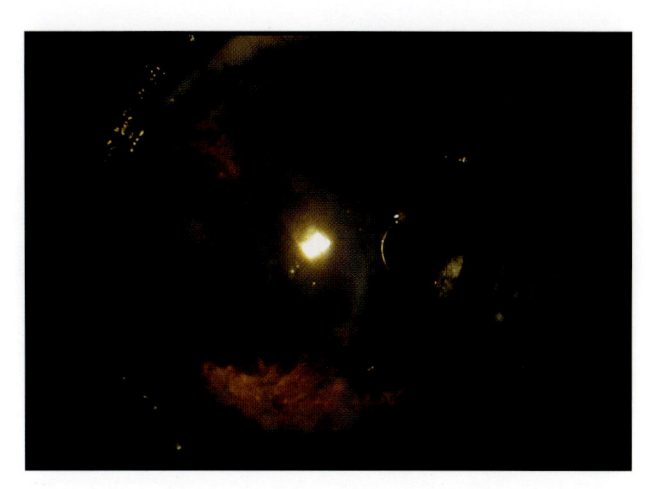

Fig. 7.24 Severe corneal pigmentation in a 4-year-old Pekingese as a result of keratoconjunctivitis sicca. Schirmer tear test reading 14 mm of wetting in response to cyclosporine treatment.

nose occurs in association with a dry eye it is likely that the preganglionic parasympathetic fibres proximal to the pterygopalatine ganglion have been damaged and a diagnosis of neurogenic keratoconjunctivitis sicca can be made. The lesion may be localised to the petrous temporal bone. Loss of corneal sensation (cranial nerve V) will also lead to a dry eye (neuroparalytic). Destruction of the lacrimal gland may also result from infection or neoplasia (Fig. 7.23). Systemic disease such as hypothyroidism, diabetes mellitus and Cushing's disease have been associated with decreased tear secretion.

The treatment of choice is topical cyclosporine ophthalmic ointment (Figs 7.24 and 7.25) as it is lacrimogenic (Sansom *et al.*, 1995). It is usually effective within 2 weeks of twice daily topical application although some dogs may take longer to respond. In many cases it is necessary, in the first

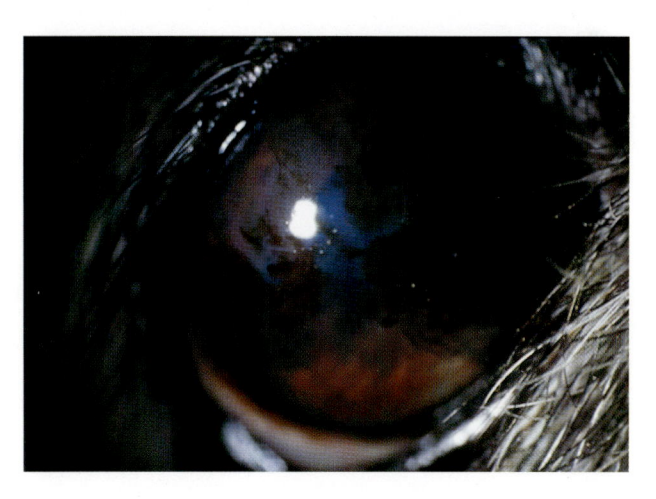

Fig. 7.25 The same eye as in Fig. 7.24 showing clearing of the cornea after 2 years of treatment.

instance, to provide additional ocular lubrication with false tear preparations until tear secretion returns. If there is no improvement after 6 weeks on cyclosporine treatment then it should be discontinued. Long-term monitoring is essential as in some cases there will be a deterioration of tear secretion with time despite an initially good response (Sansom and Smitherman, 1994). Many cases will need adjunctive treatment in the form of ocular anti-inflammatories, antibiotics and false tears. There is no entirely satisfactory false tear product, but sodium hyaluronate, which is a visco-elastic, may prove to have superior properties to other false tear preparations. Ointments act as long-term lubricants and are particularly good for overnight use. It should be remembered that topical treatment will contribute to tear film instability and overzealous treatment can be unhelpful. For those cases that fail to respond to medical treatment a parotid duct transposition procedure is indicated.

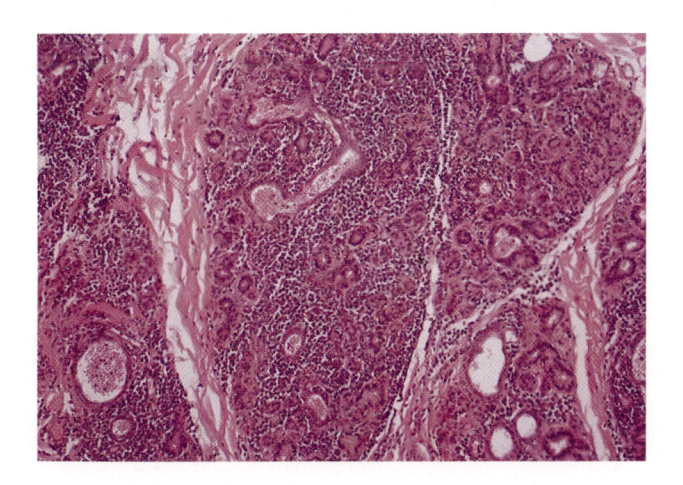

Fig. 7.23 Lymphosarcomatous infiltration of the lacrimal gland in an 8-year-old male Corgi that presented with unilateral keratoconjunctivitis sicca and facial paresis before the onset of a generalised lymphadenopathy and multicentric lymphosarcoma 10 months later.

References

Barnett KC, Joseph EC (1987) Keratoconjunctivitis in the dog following 5-aminosalicylic acid administration. *Human Toxicology* 6: 377–383.

Gelatt KN, Cure TH, Guffy MM, Jessen CL (1972) Dacryocystorhinography in the dog and cat. *Journal of Small Animal Practice* 13: 381–397.

Kaswan RL, Salisbury MA, Lothrop CD Jnr (1991) Interaction of age and gender on the occurrence of canine keratoconjunctivitis sicca. *Veterinary and Comparative Ophthalmology* 1: 93–97.

Quimby FW, Schwartz RS, Poskitt T, Lewis RM (1979) A disorder of dogs resembling Sjögren's syndrome. *Clinical Immunology and Immunopathology* 12: 471–479.

Sansom J, Smitherman P (1994) Cyclosporine veterinary applications in ophthalmic disease. Meeting of the ESVO/ECVO September 14, Dresden, Germany, Schering Plough Animal Health Proceedings, pp. 41–43.

Sansom J, Barnett KC, Long RD (1985) Keratoconjunctivitis sicca in the dog associated with the administration of salicylazosulphapyridine. *Veterinary Record* 116: 391–393.

Sansom J, Barnett KC, Neumann W *et al.* (1995) Treatment of keratoconjunctivitis sicca in dogs with cyclosporine ophthalmic ointment: a European clinical field trial. *The Veterinary Record* 137: 504–507.

Slatter DH (1973) Keratoconjunctivitis sicca in the dog produced by oral phenazopyridine hydrochloride. *Journal of Small Animal Practice* 14: 749–771.

van der Woerdt A, Wilkie DA, Gilger BC, Smeak DD, Kerpsack SJ (1997) Surgical treatment of dacryocystitis caused by cystic dilatation of the nasolacrimal system in three dogs. *Journal of the American Veterinary Medical Association* 211: 445–447.

8 Conjunctiva and sclera

Conjunctiva

Introduction

The conjunctiva is a thin, translucent, highly vascular, mucous membrane that lines the lids (palpebral conjunctiva) and is reflected on to the sclera at the fornices (cul de sac) where it forms the bulbar conjunctiva. The palpebral and bulbar conjunctiva cover their respective surfaces of the third eyelid. Closure of the lids forms the conjunctival sac. The conjunctival epithelium is continuous with the corneal epithelium at the limbus and with the skin at the mucocutaneous junction of the lid margin. The substantia propria contains the conjunctival associated lymphoid tissue (CALT), found predominantly at the dorsal and ventral conjunctival fornices and on the bulbar aspect of the third eyelid where the excretory ducts of the nictitans gland occur. Below this adenoid layer is a more fibrous layer that blends with the subconjunctival tissue.

The conjunctiva has a secretory function with large numbers of goblet cells, mainly in the fornices, producing mucus that contributes to the tear film. Mucus collects in the dorsal and ventral conjunctival fornix to form a mucous thread. Under disease conditions such as keratoconjunctivitis sicca, or where the fornices are deep as in the Standard Poodle, the mucous thread will become more obvious. The lacrimal gland has excretory ducts which empty into the temporal conjunctival fornix. Drainage of these secretions occurs through the lacrimal puncta and canaliculi, allowing the conjunctival sac direct access to the nasal cavity.

The sensory nerve supply to the conjunctiva is from the trigeminal nerve and is responsible for reflex tear secretion and blinking.

The conjunctival vessels are branching, freely moveable and bright red in appearance. These superficial vessels form arcades at the limbus and are responsible for superficial corneal vascularisation. It is important to differentiate the conjunctival from the deeper ciliary vessels as ciliary hyperaemia is an indicator of intraocular disease.

In addition to the third eyelid a small modified skin nodule at the medial canthus, which may contain hairs, forms the caruncle. In some animals the conjunctiva of the third eyelid may continue over the bulbar surface in an encircling manner.

Congenital disorders

Symblepharon

Conjunctival adhesions in the dog are uncommon and rarely occur as a result of a congenital malformation (Fig. 8.1).

Mucinosis

This condition results in an apparent swelling of the conjunctiva and lids. It occurs in certain breeds, like the Shar Pei, where it is idiopathic. It should not be confused with conjunctival oedema. It has also been reported in association with hypothyroidism, acromegaly, dermatomyositis and systemic lupus (Fig. 8.2).

Dermoids

See Chapters 5 and 9.

Conjunctivitis

Infectious conjunctivitis

Bacteria are found normally in the conjunctival sac and studies have been undertaken to ascertain the normal conjunctival flora (Urban *et al.*, 1972). *Staphylococci* are most frequently isolated, followed by *Streptococcus* species, diphtheroids, *Neisseria* and *Pseudomonas* species. The organisms isolated from the conjunctival sacs of dogs vary with geographical location, season and breed. The latter is no surprise

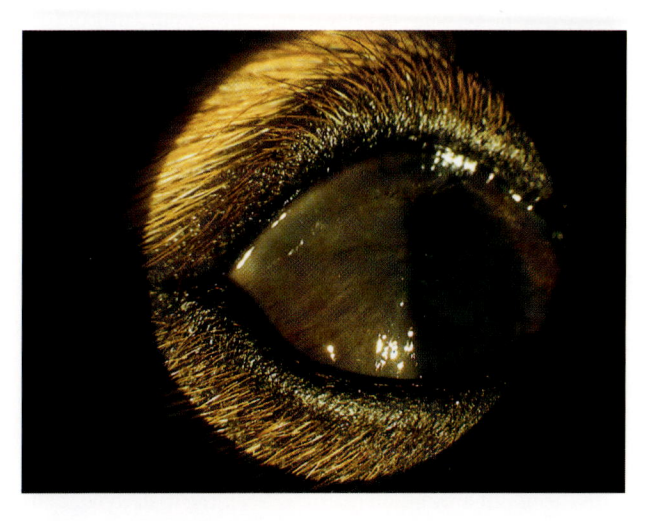

Fig. 8.1 Congenital conjunctival adhesions in a 15-week-old male Cavalier King Charles Spaniel.

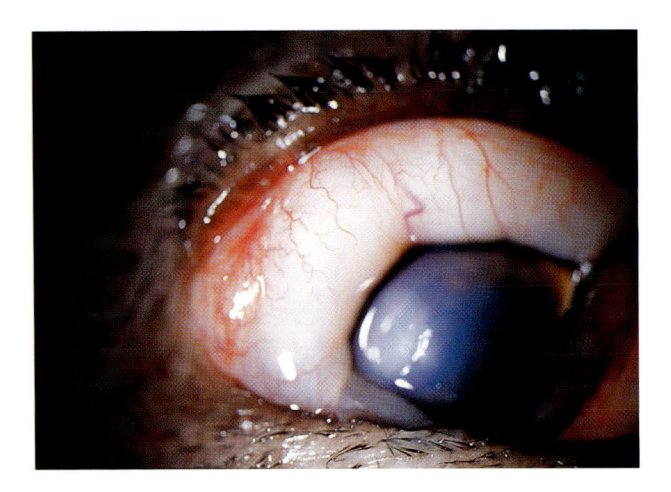

Fig. 8.2   Idiopathic mucinosis in a Shar Pei.

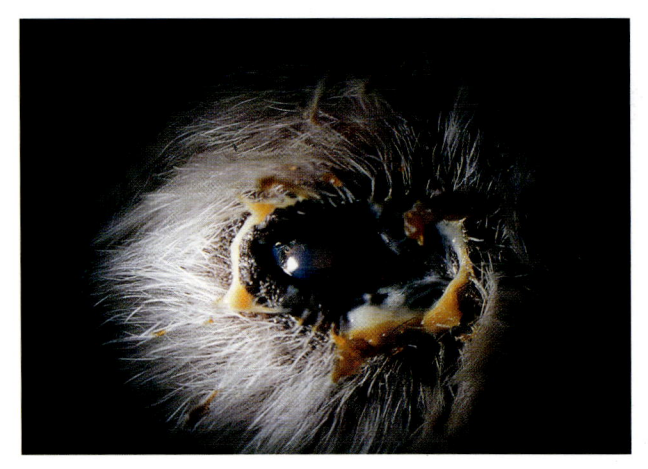

Fig. 8.3   Purulent conjunctivitis in a 14-year-old male West Highland White Terrier.

when one considers the frequency of bacterial conjunctivitis in certain breeds, particularly the Cocker Spaniel, from which greater number of organisms, particularly *Staphylococci* and *Streptococci* (Urban *et al.*, 1972), were isolated. Breed-related ocular disorders such as trichiasis, lagophthalmos, dry eye, entropion and ectropion will compromise the local ocular defence mechanisms, upsetting the normal conjunctival flora and predisposing to either excessive proliferation of these organisms or the introduction of pathogens.

Contact lenses provide a focus for infectious agents such as bacteria or fungi to colonise and they should not be placed in eyes where pre-existing infection is suspected.

The primary causes of infectious conjunctivitis in the United Kingdom are usually bacterial, occasionally viral (distemper and adenovirus) but parasites and fungal agents are not recognised. Viral infections are usually associated with systemic disease, often upper respiratory tract infections, and tend to be self-limiting.

Bacterial conjunctivitis may be unilateral or bilateral. The conjunctiva (bulbar and palpebral) is acutely inflamed in association with chemosis, which is usually mild, hyperaemia and a discharge. The discharge may be serous, mucoid or mucopurulent, but neutrophils usually predominate whatever the cause (Fig. 8.3). Opportunist infections are not uncommon; gram-positive organisms predominate in the conjunctival sac, particularly staphylococcus species. Mixed infections do occur but anaerobic infections are uncommon. In the neonate (ophthalmia neonatorum – see Chapter 5) *Staphylococcus* is usually the causative agent.

Treatment with a topical broad-spectrum antibiotic should address most cases of bacterial conjunctivitis and there should be a rapid improvement within 48 hours.

When bacterial infection is chronic or recurring the diagnosis should be reviewed. Referral may be considered. A thorough ocular examination should be repeated. If the initial treatment was inappropriate, and this may happen with the use of anti-inflammatories, then the underlying condition may have been masked. Stopping all treatment will allow for a complete reassessment of the situation and will eliminate those ongoing cases of conjunctivitis that result from an allergic reaction due to the overuse of topical antibiotic preparations (see Fig. 5.21). The latter is not uncommon, particularly the aminoglycosides, antibiotics which can cause severe irritation, discomfort and inflammation. On withdrawal of treatment the conjunctiva and lids return rapidly to normal. Cytology and bacteriology should be carried out in chronic cases of conjunctivitis. Recurring infection may be secondary to ocular or systemic pathology. The conjunctival sac is more prone to secondary infection in the presence of tear film abnormalities, autoimmune disease, lid abnormalities and the presence of skin disease. Persistent and severe infections are frequently associated with foreign body penetrations of the conjunctival sac (fornices or canthus), or behind the third eyelid. A thorough investigation under general anaesthesia is warranted in such cases as the foreign body can be well hidden or can even have penetrated the conjunctival sac resulting in a discharging sinus. A common cause of recurring conjunctivitis is qualitative or quantitative changes in the tear film. It should be remembered that the tear film not only covers the cornea but also the conjunctiva and is responsible for flushing bacteria and debris from the conjunctival sac into the nasolacrimal system. Conjunctivitis in these cases may be acute and accompanied by severe discomfort and ulceration or may be chronic and accompanied by a keratitis. The discharge characteristically sticks to the cornea or forms a large thread in the conjunctival fornices, because of the inadequate tear film (see keratoconjunctivitis sicca – Chapter 7).

Allergic eye disease

It is likely there are a number of allergic eye diseases in the dog and atopy, as described below, may be only one of the possible aetiological factors. The conjunctivitis may be acute and seasonal or persistent, depending on the allergen involved. Pollens, drugs, food and animal dander are all capable of inducing an allergic conjunctival reaction. (Figs 8.4 and 8.5).

CONJUNCTIVA

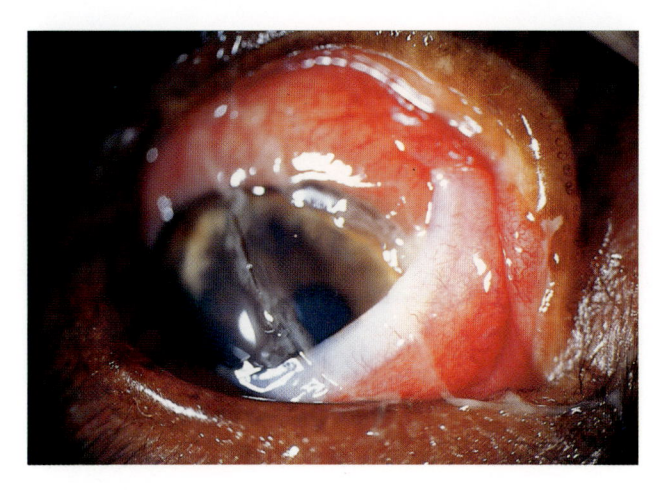

Fig. 8.4 Acute allergic conjunctivitis in a 7-year-old female Clumber Spaniel; there is severe conjunctival hyperaemia and chemosis and a mucoid discharge.

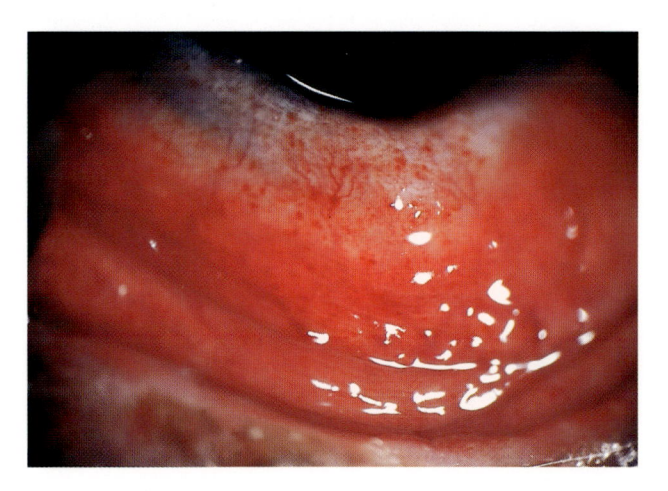

Fig. 8.5 Acute allergic conjunctivitis (in the same case as in Fig. 8.4) demonstrating petechiae on nictitating membrane.

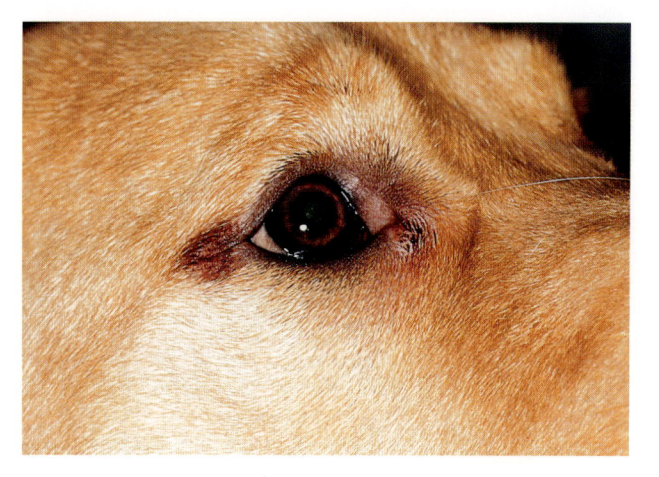

Fig. 8.6 Mild periorbital dermatitis and conjunctivitis associated with atopic skin disease in a Labrador Retriever.

Atopic conjunctivitis

The signs of atopic conjunctivitis are not well defined and in making a definitive diagnosis a number of factors need to be considered. Atopic dermatitis, presenting as alopecia, erythema, saliva staining, pyoderma or *Malassezia* dermatitis, may be present. Initially the conjunctiva, invariably the palpebral conjunctiva, become bilaterally inflamed with an increase in lacrimation. The discharge may become mucopurulent to purulent with the development of a secondary opportunist infection. Follicle formation is common. The condition is frequently irritant but not painful, a distinction that is sometimes difficult to make in animals. There may be self-inflicted trauma and an accompanying periorbital blepharitis (Fig. 8.6). Facial pruritus is a feature of these cases. The condition in the United Kingdom has a breed and age incidence in the young Golden Retriever and Labrador Retriever and their crosses. The mean age is 29 months. In many cases the skin disease may be mild and not immediately apparent, especially to the ophthalmologist. A definitive diagnosis will depend on the presence of atopic dermatitis. A conjunctival biopsy or scrape may be helpful if eosinophils and/or mast cells are present. It is obviously important to rule out other causes of conjunctival inflammation and lacrimation, such as entropion, which may also be present in these breeds.

Treatment involves control of the underlying inflammatory conjunctival disease. The efficacy of topical antihistamines and mast cell inhibitors has not been studied adequately in the dog. In the absence of a secondary infection topical corticosteroids are beneficial. A change of environment is sometimes helpful.

Follicular conjunctivitis

Follicle formation almost always involves the palpebral conjunctiva and the conjunctival fornices with predilection sites at the medial canthus, involving both the follicular and bulbar aspect of the third eyelid. It appears to be a non-specific response to a variety of causes. It is commonly seen in association with chronic irritation in cases of entropion and distichiasis. It is often severe in cases of atopic conjunctivitis. It can be particularly severe in young dogs. The aetiology remains obscure in many cases.

The follicular appearance of the conjunctival sac is diagnostic and treatment is symptomatic, usually in the form of topical anti-inflammatories. The condition occurs frequently in those breeds with deep fornices such as the Great Dane, Standard Poodle (Fig. 8.7) and Doberman Pinscher. This condition, also known as medial canthal pocket syndrome, results in poor tear drainage and an accumulation of debris in the conjunctival fornix. Irrigation may be helpful in these particular cases (Hendrix, 1999).

Ligneous conjunctivitis

This unusual form of chronic membranous conjunctivitis has been reported in the Doberman Pinscher, with a sex incidence in the female. It is thought to be a manifestation of a

CONJUNCTIVA AND SCLERA

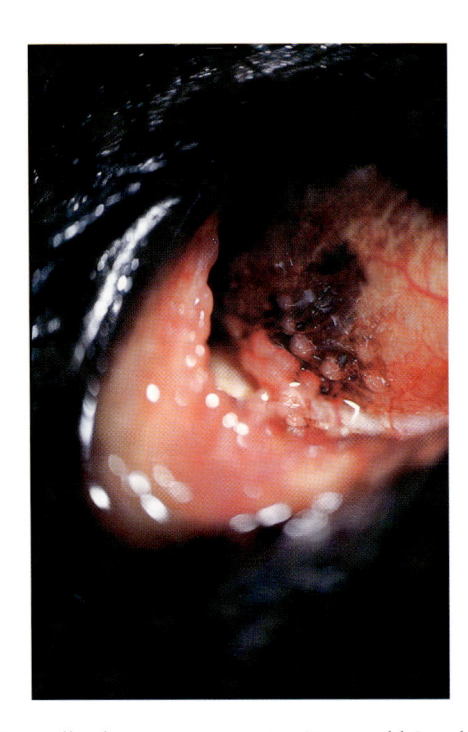

Fig. 8.7 Follicular conjunctivitis in a 5-year-old Standard Poodle. There is follicle formation affecting the palpebral conjunctiva and fornix of the upper lid in association with conjunctival hyperaemia as a chronic allergic response to cat dander.

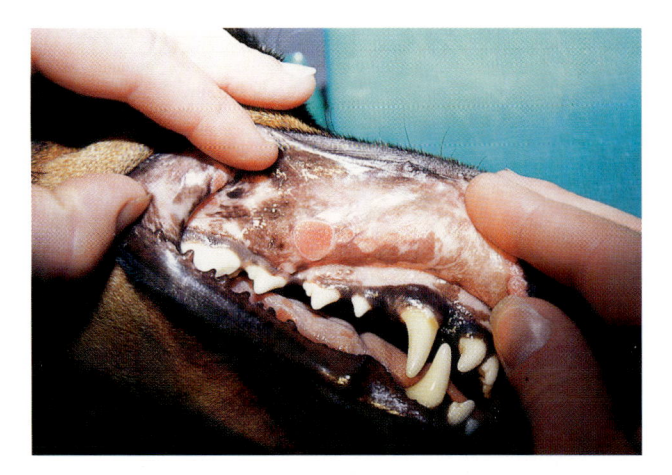

Fig. 8.9 Oral ulceration with ligneous conjunctivitis (same case as in Fig. 8.8).

Pyogranulomatous blepharitis

See Chapter 5.

Conjunctival trauma and foreign bodies

See Chapter 3.

Conjunctival cysts

Conjunctival epithelial cysts may arise in the conjunctival sac or involve the third eyelid, particularly the base (Fig. 8.10); they may have a lucent 'blue' appearance (Fig. 8.11). Cystic dilatations of the lacrimal duct may also involve the conjunctival sac at the medial canthus (Fig. 8.12). In these cases an aspirate usually consists of mucus and blood.

The treatment of choice for inclusion cysts is total surgical removal.

NEOPLASIA

Neoplasia of the conjunctival sac is an uncommon condition although a variety of tumours have been reported. It is the interpalpebral corneoscleral junction that is most commonly

multisystemic disorder. The palpebral conjunctiva assumes a grey ulcerated appearance with a tendency to bleed and is covered by an amorphous membrane (Fig. 8.8). The oral mucosa (Fig. 8.9), respiratory and urinary tract may be affected in a similar fashion. Azathioprine may be helpful in the treatment of this condition (Ramsey et al., 1996).

Plasmacytic conjunctivitis

See Chapter 6.

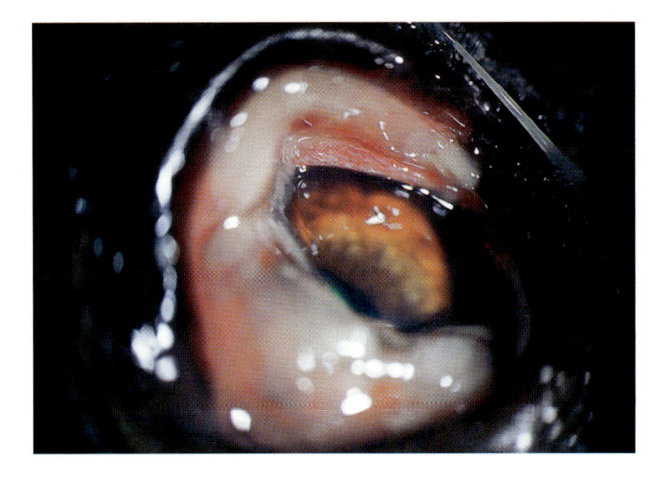

Fig. 8.8 Ligneous conjunctivitis in a 5-year-old female Dobermann. The conjunctiva and third eyelid have a grey appearance and are covered by a thick opaque membrane.

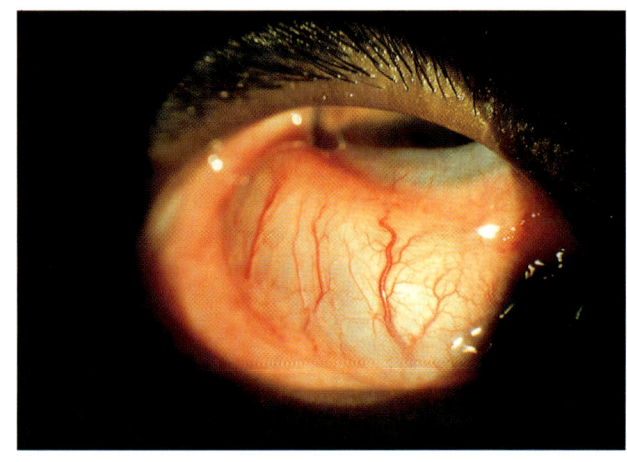

Fig. 8.10 Conjunctival cyst affecting the third eyelid of an English Springer Spaniel.

CONJUNCTIVA

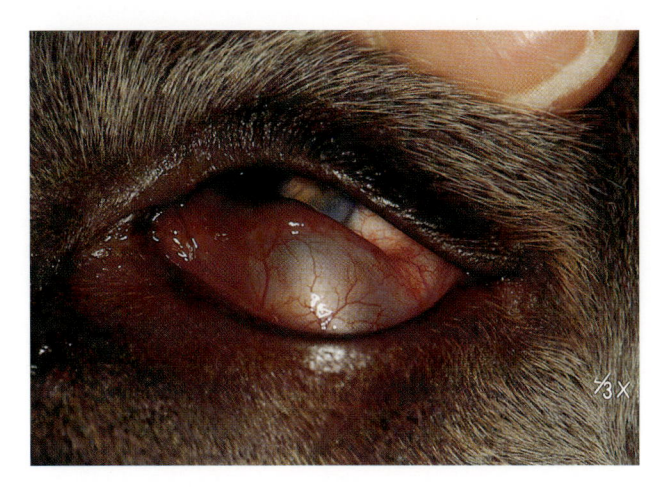

Fig. 8.11 Third eyelid cyst present for 2 months and causing protrusion of the third eyelid in a 5-month-old male Weimaraner. The cyst extended to the base of the nictitating membrane.

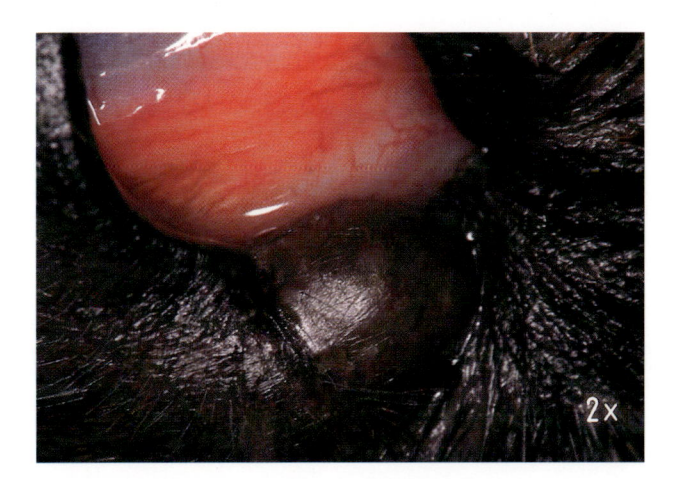

Fig. 8.12 Pigmented inclusion cyst at the medial canthus of a male 6-year-old Cavalier King Charles Spaniel.

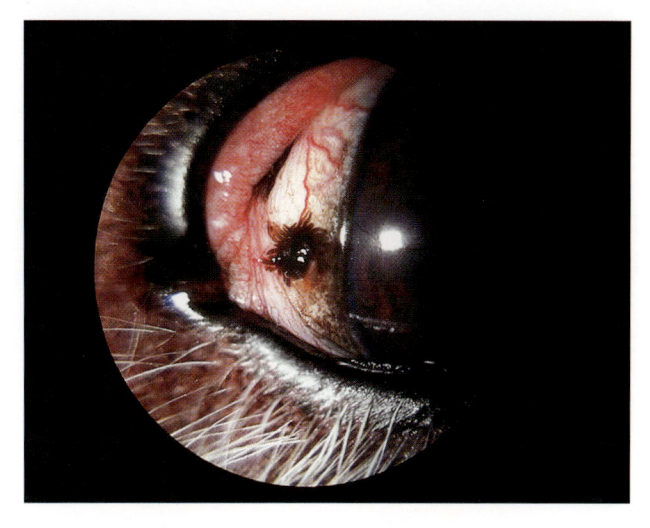

Fig. 8.13 Pigmented papilloma on the bulbar conjunctiva of a $4\frac{1}{2}$-year-old female West Highland White Terrier.

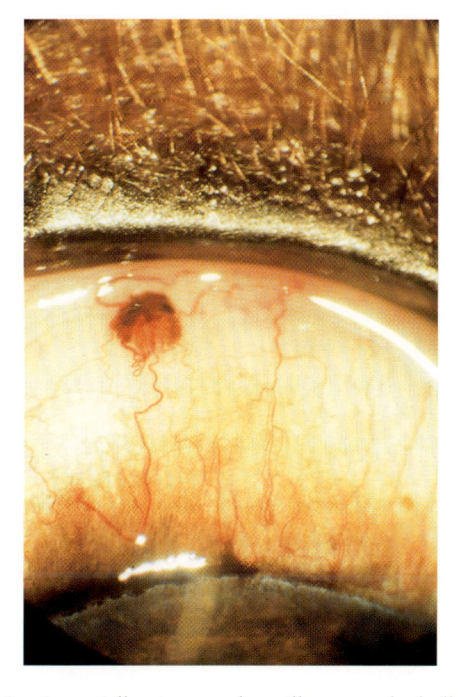

Fig. 8.14 A partially pigmented papilloma on the bulbar conjunctiva of a 9-year-old female Airedale.

affected by neoplasia or chronic inflammatory lesions. Most develop at the temporal limbus which is the area most exposed to irritants and ultraviolet light (Hargis et al., 1978)

Papillomas

These are benign and may have a very characteristic frond-like appearance on the bulbar conjunctiva (Fig. 8.13) (Sansom et al., 1996). They may show variable degrees of pigmentation (Fig. 8.14). Appearances on other surfaces can be variable, assuming irregular cauliflower-like masses (Fig. 8.15). They should be differentiated from other more aggressive tumours such as squamous cell carcinomas and conjunctival melanomas.

Vascular tumours

Haemangiomas and haemangiosarcomas affect the bulbar conjunctiva particularly in the temporolimbal area or involve the third eyelid. Telangiectasis (angiokeratoma) may also occur (see Fig. 6.15). Excision is the treatment of choice.

Melanomas

Melanomas may be recurring and do have a tendency to metastasise. They have been reported on the palbebral conjunctiva of the third eyelid and upper eyelids. There may be a predilection in the older bitch with a possible incidence in the Weimaraner. The material excised should be submitted for histopathology and if the margins are not free of tumour tissue then follow-up with cryosurgery has been reported to give good results (Collins et al., 1993).

CONJUNCTIVA AND SCLERA

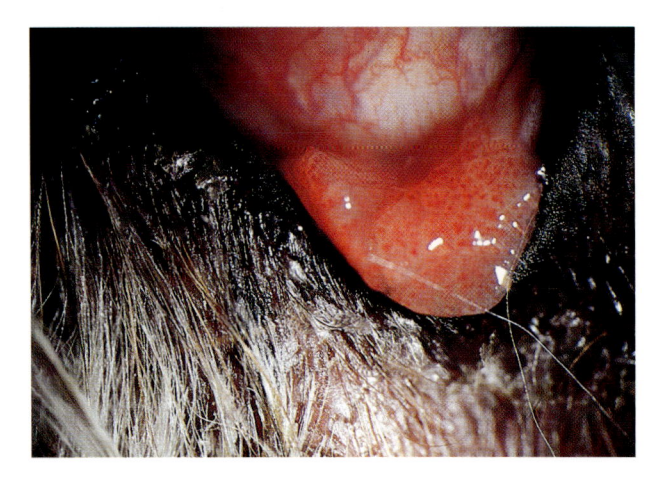

Fig. 8.15 Large non-pigmented papilloma arising from the palpebral conjunctiva of the lower lid of a 12-year-old male Lhasa Apso.

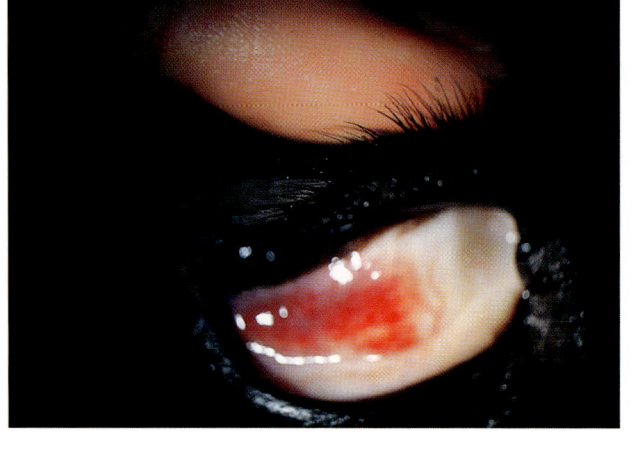

Fig. 8.17 Conjunctival haemorrhage and pallor as result of thrombocytopenia in a $3\frac{1}{2}$-year-old female Labrador Retriever.

Squamous cell carcinoma

These arise in the perilimbal area as elevated caruncular-like and ulcerated tumours. In contrast to other species they are very uncommon in the dog.

MANIFESTATIONS OF SYSTEMIC DISEASE

The conjunctiva may reflect underlying blood dyscrasias in the following ways. Anaemia will produce pallor of the conjunctival surfaces (Fig. 8.16) and coagulopathies may result in either petechial or echymotic haemorrhages (Fig. 8.17). In coumarin poisoning there may be massive subconjunctival haemorrhage and chemosis. Congestion of the conjunctival blood vessels may occur in hyperviscosity syndromes such as multiple myeloma or with polycythemia. Where there is severe jaundice the conjunctiva will become involved (Fig. 8.18) along with other mucous membranes and the skin.

In systemic inflammatory disorders, such as histiocytosis, there may be conjunctival involvement along with ocular and skin lesions (see Figs 6.16–6.18). In diffuse neoplastic conditions, classically lymphosarcoma, there may be infiltration of the conjunctiva and chemosis (see Fig. 8.16). A general clinical examination will help confirm the diagnosis. In idiopathic granulomatous diseases, where there is a breed incidence in the Border Collie, eyelids, conjunctiva, sclera and skin may be affected by multiple sterile granuloma (Collins *et al.*, 1992) (Figs 8.19–8.21).

Chemosis will occur because of the loose arrangement of the conjunctival and subconjunctival tissue. It is not a common presentation but when it does occur it is very dramatic and it may be the presenting sign for a number of different conditions. It will occur as an acute severe reaction to insect bites or food intolerance, in association with lid swelling. Contusive injuries will cause subconjunctival haemorrhage and severe swelling. It is a feature of polymyositis for which there is a breed incidence in the Golden Retriever. It should not be confused with mucinosis.

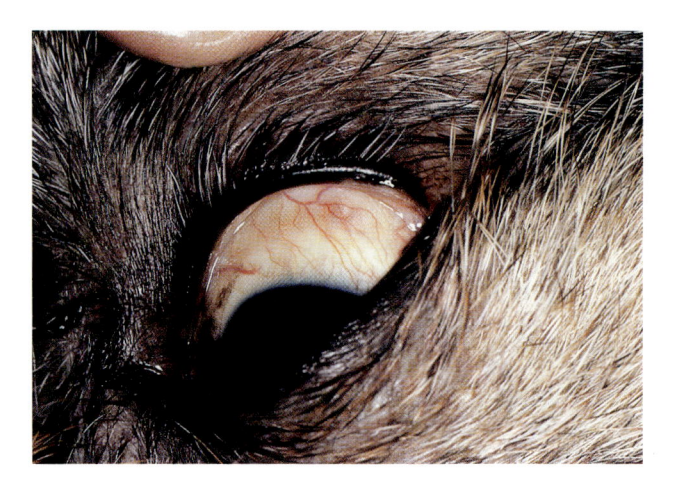

Fig. 8.18 Jaundice causing discoloration of the bulbar and palpebral conjunctiva. (Courtesy of JD Littlewood.)

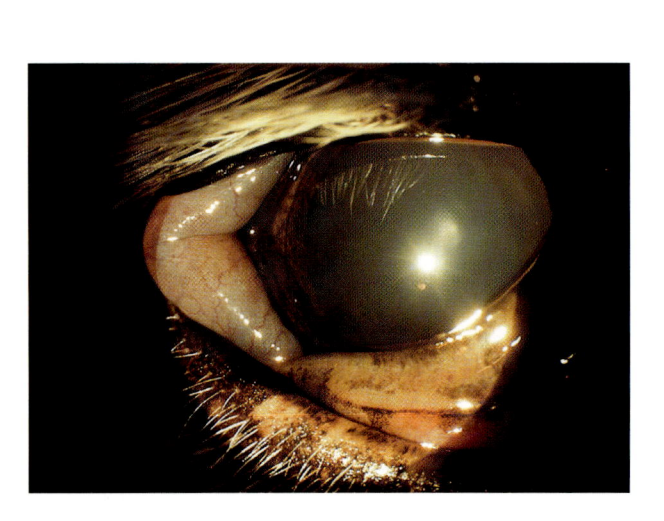

Fig. 8.16 Conjunctival chemosis and pallor associated with leukaemia.

SCLERA

Sclera

Introduction

The sclera is the fibrous connective tissue tunic that forms the outermost layer of the globe. It can be divided into episclera, stroma and lamina fusca. At the transitional zone, the limbus, the collagen assumes a uniform layer of parallel lamellae rendering the cornea transparent.

The episclera is a loose fibrous and elastic tissue that lies directly under the conjunctiva and is closely apposed to the underlying sclera. This fibrovascular layer extends from the limbus to the insertion of the extraocular muscles. It contains nerve fibres and the deeper layers contain blood vessels.

The scleral stroma consists of intermingling collagen fibres with fibroblasts and melanocytes.

The internal lamina fusca blends with the suprachoroid.

Congenital disorders

Scleral thinning, or ectasia, is an unusual condition and is usually associated with collie eye anomaly in the form of a coloboma affecting the posterior segment. Inherited collagen diseases are rare in the dog but Ehlers–Danlos syndrome may result in scleral thinning (blue sclera).

Inflammatory disorders

The sclera and episclera are prone to inflammatory disease. A clear distinction between episcleritis and scleritis is not always apparent either on clinical presentation or on the basis of histopathology. Histologically these inflammatory conditions can be described as proliferative or non-proliferative.

The aetiology of these conditions is not known. There may be a variety of precipitating factors and the possibility of underlying systemic disease, either of an infectious or immunological nature, should be considered in every case.

Episcleritis

The terminology for the various presentations of this inflammatory condition is extremely confusing and the disease processes involved in the different morphological appearances may be similar. Episcleritis may present as a diffuse or nodular lesion.

Nodular episcleritis

Nodular episcleritis (Figs 8.22–8.24) is a sessile granulomatous inflammatory condition, acute in onset, affecting both eyes but not involving the nictitating membrane. It is described as synonymous with non-necrotising scleritis.

Nodular granulomatous episclerokeratitis

Nodular granulomatous episclerokeratitis (Fig. 8.25) is the most common form of episcleral inflammation, presenting as multiple fleshy proliferations at the limbus with third eyelid

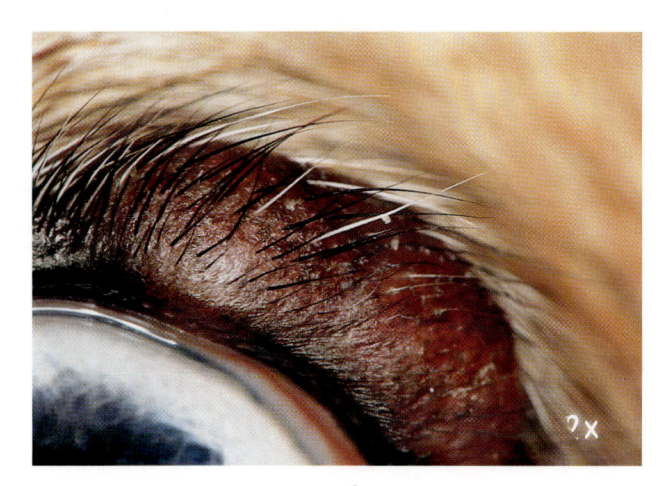

Fig. 8.19 Eyelid involvement as a result of sterile granulomata in a 7-year-old female Border Collie.

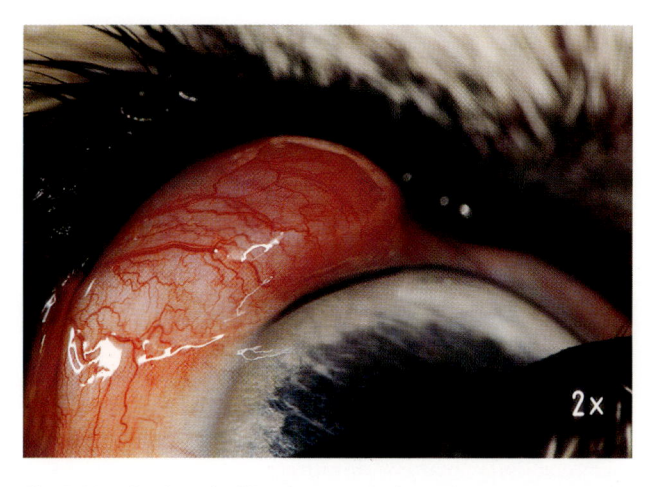

Fig. 8.20 Conjunctival involvement in the same case as Fig. 8.19.

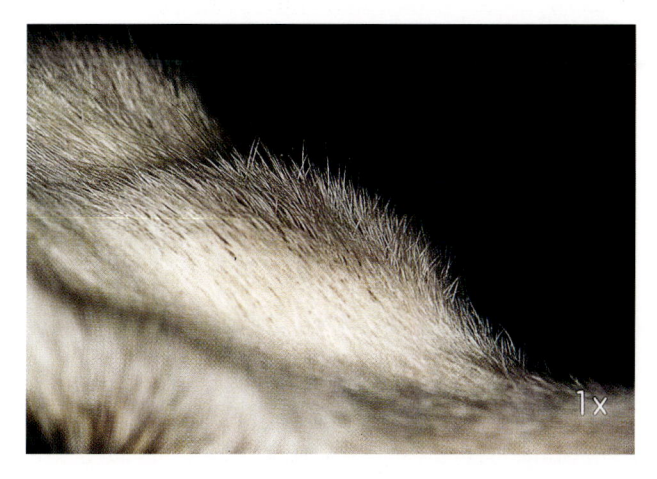

Fig. 8.21 Skin involvement in the same case as Fig. 8.19.

The conjunctiva will also become secondarily inflamed in association with local ocular disorders such as episcleritis, uveitis, keratitis and blepharitis.

CONJUNCTIVA AND SCLERA

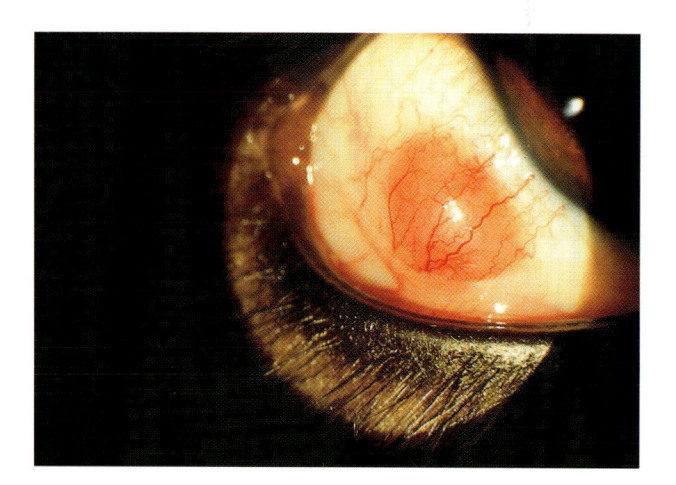

Fig. 8.22 Nodular episcleritis in a 4-year-old male Bearded Collie.

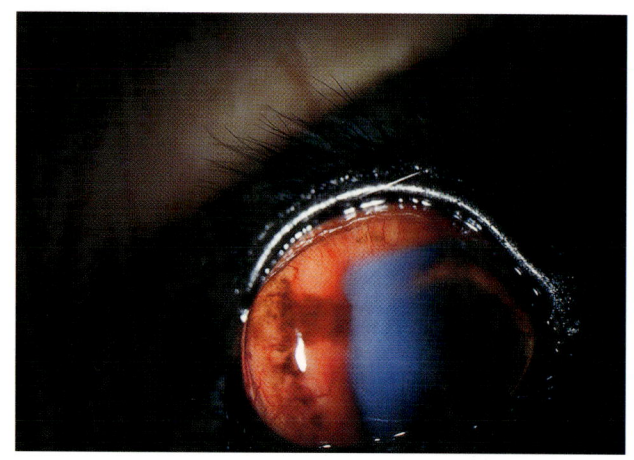

Fig. 8.25 Nodular granulomatous episclerokeratitis in a 9-year-old Border Collie.

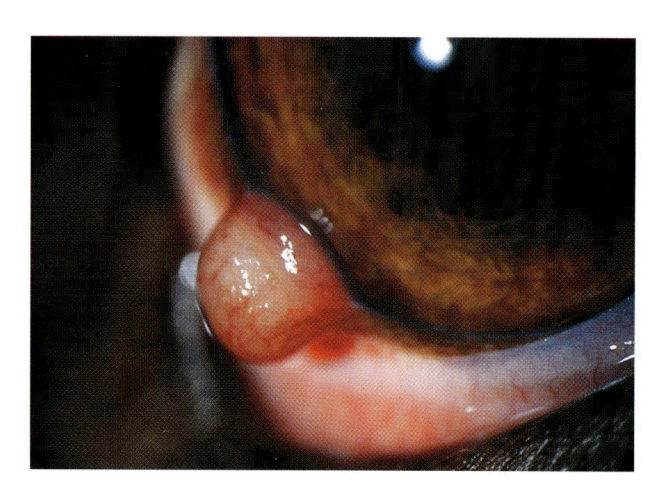

Fig. 8.23 Nodular episcleritis in a 5½-year-old Welsh Springer Spaniel.

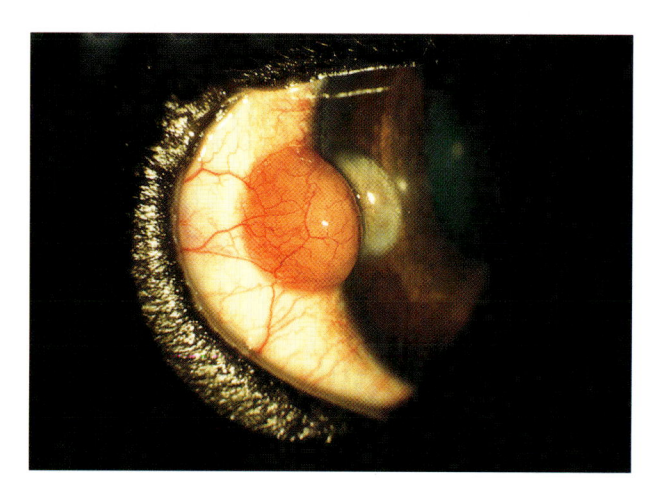

Fig. 8.24 Nodular episcleritis with secondary corneal lipidosis in a 3-year-old female Boxer.

involvement. In some cases there may be additional involvement of the iris, lid and mucocutaneous junctions (Dugan et al., 1993). The condition is often bilateral. There is a breed predisposition in the Rough Collie and Shetland Sheepdog (Paulsen et al., 1987). The histopathology is consistent with a chronic granulomatous inflammatory response, with histiocytes, lymphocytes, plasma cells and neutrophils; fibroblasts are not a feature of this condition.

Scleritis

Inflammation of the sclera in the dog is usually non-necrotising and there is no breakdown of the underlying collagen, as in man. Scleritis is usually a proliferative granulomatous inflammatory disorder that may present as a sectorial inflammatory lesion or with diffuse scleral involvement. The inflammation may be anterior or posterior with secondary effects on the cornea and choroid respectively.

Regional proliferative scleritis

Here a region of scleral tissue becomes infiltrated and thickened just posterior to the limbus, frequently with secondary corneal involvement, but does not extend to involve the posterior segment. Histopathology will demonstrate a granulomatous inflammatory response.

Generalised proliferative scleritis

Where there is diffuse scleral inflammation of a proliferative nature this will present with 360° scleral oedema and vascular engorgement. In severe cases there may be proptosis. The condition is painful and there may be photophobia and lacrimation. The uveal tracts may become involved and present as an anterior uveitis and choroiditis, later manifesting as areas of abnormal pigmentation in the tapetal fundus (Fig. 8.26). Retinal detachment and hyalitis may also occur.

In the United Kingdom there appears to be a breed incidence in the Cavalier King Charles Spaniel, sometimes at a very young age (under 12 months). The granulomatous

SCLERA

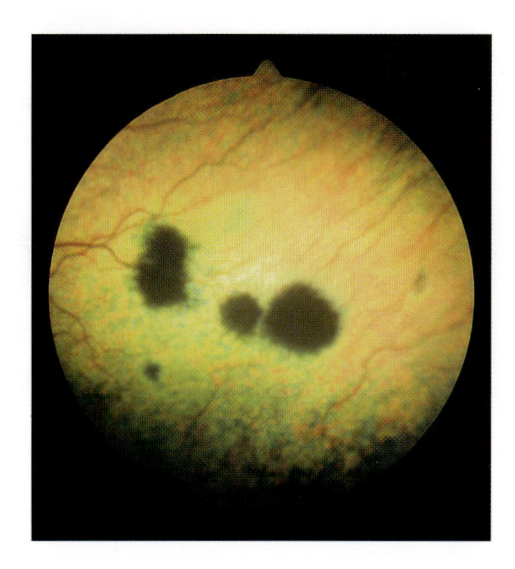

Fig. 8.26 Post-inflammatory pigmented tapetal lesion following scleritis in a 6-year-old female Golden Retriever. This dog also showed optic atrophy in this eye.

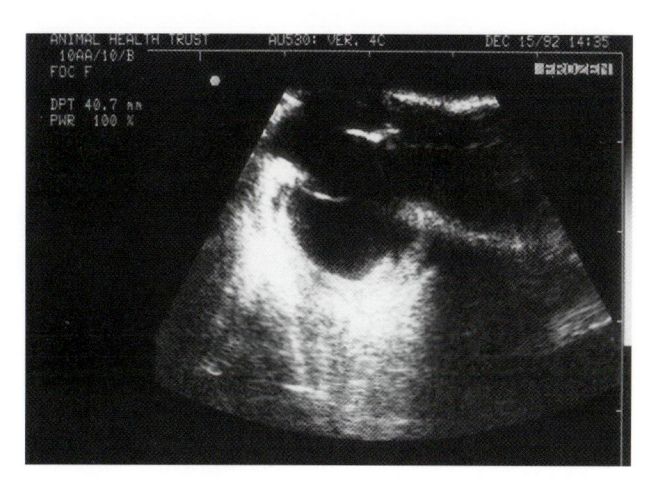

Fig. 8.28 Ocular ultrasound demonstrating posterior segment inflammation with thickening of the choroid and scleral tunic.

inflammatory response is aggressive and may present either as a diffuse or sectorial inflammation of the episclera, sclera and overlying conjunctiva (Fig. 8.27). The condition can be very painful and palpation of the globe is frequently resented. There may be unilateral or bilateral involvement and the posterior segment may be affected (Fig. 8.28).

The treatment of choice for scleritis and episcleritis is topical and systemic anti-inflammatories in the form of corticosteroids. Initially topical application should be frequent (six times daily) and given to effect over 4–6 weeks depending on the response. In many cases these conditions are recurring. In the absence of a response to corticosteroids, immunosuppressive agents such as azathioprine should be given, but blood biochemistry and routine haematology should be carried out to ascertain there are no serious side effects from this treatment.

NEOPLASIA

Limbal melanoma

These tumours (Figs 8.29–8.31) arise on the scleral side of the limbus, presenting as raised pigmented masses that progress in a circumferential fashion to involve large areas of sclera and cornea. They should be differentiated from conjunctival and ciliary body melanomas. There appears to be a breed incidence in the German Shepherd Dog and Golden Retriever. In young dogs (2–4 years) tumours are reported as more aggressive than in the older animal (8–11 years). Resection and a course of strontium-90 can give extremely good results. Cryosurgery, photoablation and excision are other possible approaches. The prognosis is good if treated at an early stage.

Squamous cell carcinoma

Squamous cell carcinoma (Fig. 8.32) may arise from the cornea but may also involve the limbus. They appear as raised multilobular masses. Surgical excision in the form of a keratectomy with follow-up treatment as for limbal melanomas is indicated.

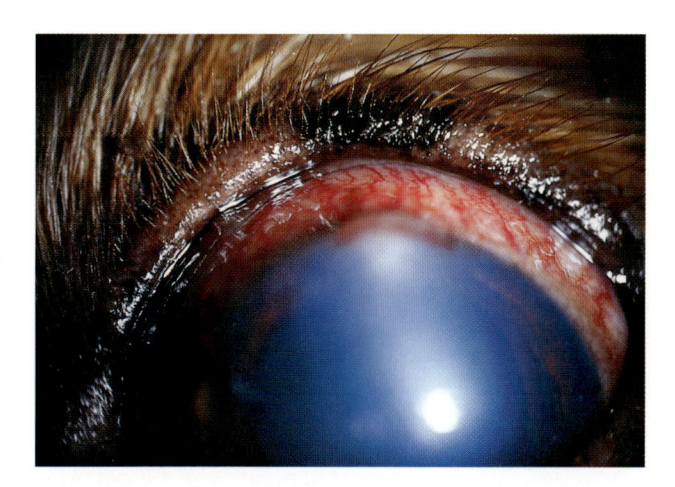

Fig. 8.27 Diffuse episcleritis/scleritis in a 9-year-old female Cavalier King Charles Spaniel.

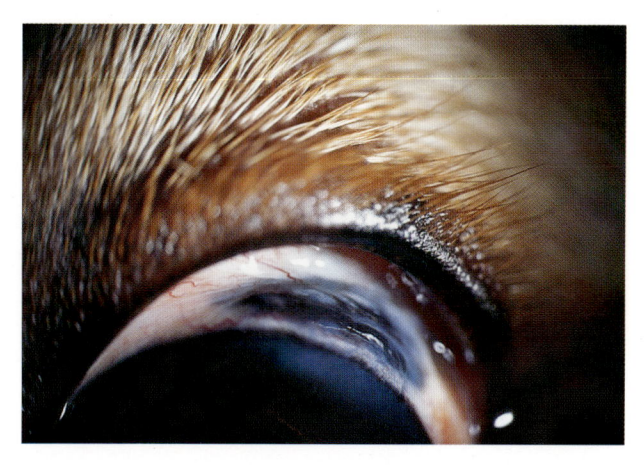

Fig. 8.29 Limbal melanoma in a 3-year-old male Labrador.

CONJUNCTIVA AND SCLERA

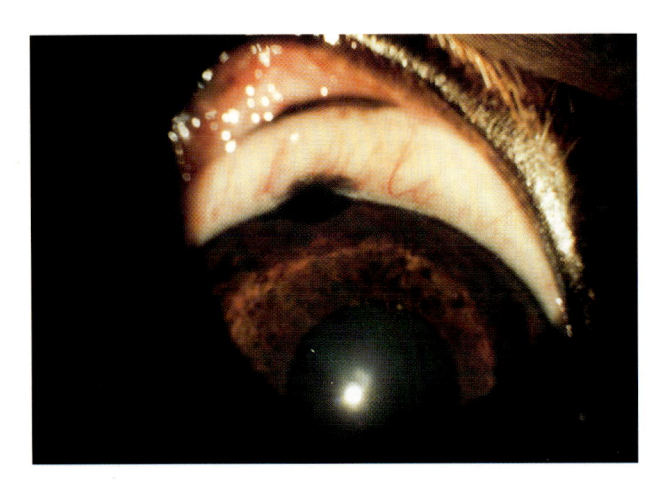

Fig. 8.30 Small limbal melanoma in a 6-year-old female Golden Retriever.

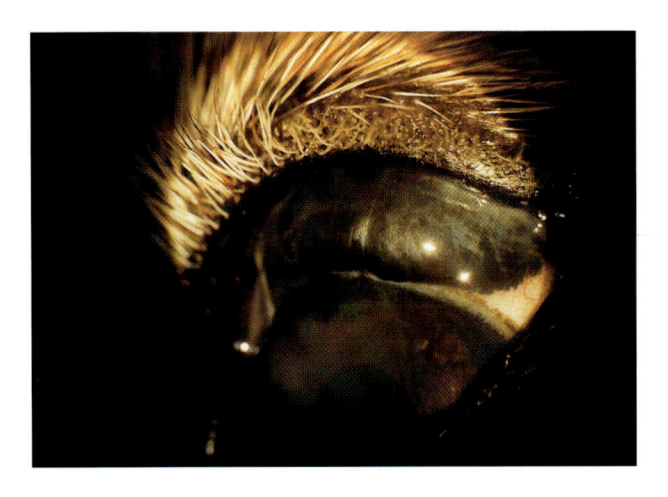

Fig. 8.31 Large limbal melanoma with corneal extension but absence of intraocular involvement and no pupillary distortion. Compare with Figs 12.63–12.69 (uveal melanomas).

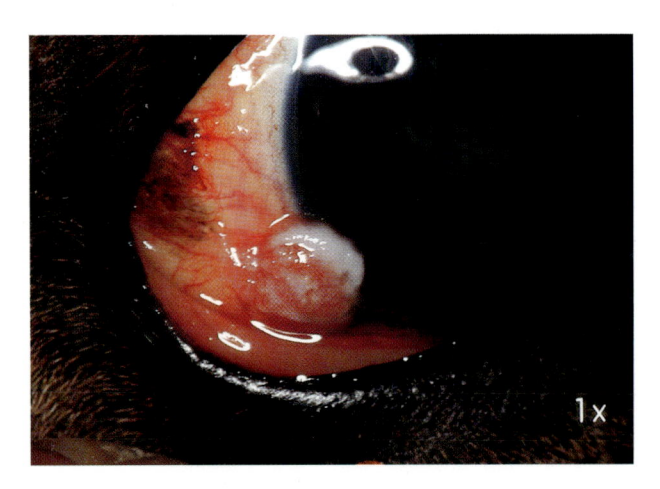

Fig. 8.32 Squamous cell carcinoma at the limbus.

References

Collins BK, MacEwan EG, Dubielzig RR, Swanson JF (1992) Idiopathic granulomatous disease with ocular adnexal and cutaneous involvement in a dog. *Journal of the American Veterinary Medical Associataion* **201**: 313–316.

Collins BK, Collier LL, Miller MA, Linton LL (1993) Biologic behaviour and histologic characteristics of canine conjunctival melanoma. *Progress in Veterinary and Comparative Ophthalmology* **3**(4): 135–140.

Dugan SJ, Ketring KL, Severin GA, Render JA (1993) Variant nodular granulomatous episclerokeratitis in four dogs. *Journal of The American Animal Hospital Association* **29**: 403–409.

Hendrix DVH (1999) Diseases of the canine conjunctiva. In Gelatt KN (ed.) *Veterinary Ophthalmology*, 3rd edn, p. 624. Lippincott, Williams and Wilkins, Philadelphia.

Hargis AM, Lee AC, Thomassen RW (1978) Tumour and tumour-like lesions of perilimbal conjunctiva in laboratory dogs. *Journal of the American Veterinary Medical Association* **173**(9): 1185–1190.

Paulsen ME, Lavach JD, Snyder SP, Severin JA, Eichenbaum JD (1987) Nodular granulomatous episclerokeratitis in dogs: 19 cases (1973–1985). *Journal of the American Veterinary Medical Association* **190**(12): 1581–1587.

Ramsey DT, Ketring KL, Glaze MV, Render JA (1996) Ligneous conjunctivitis in four Doberman Pinschers. *Journal of the American Animal Hospital Association* **32**: 439–447.

Sansom J, Barnett KC, Blunden AS, Smith KC, Turner S, Waters L (1996) Canine conjunctival papilloma: a review of five cases. *Journal of Small Animal Practice* **37**: 84–86.

Urban M, Wyman M, Rheins M, Marraro RV (1972) Conjunctival flora of clinically normal dogs. *Journal of the American Veterinary Medical Association* **161**(2): 201–206.

9 Cornea

Introduction

The canine cornea is almost circular, slightly smaller vertically than horizontally, with a diameter of 12.5–17 mm and with obvious variation between the breeds. The cornea is derived from surface ectoderm and neural crest mesenchyme.

The cornea occupies the anterior fifth of the fibrous tunic of the eye filling most of the palpebral aperture. It is approximately 0.5 mm thick and is slightly thicker peripherally. Except for a fine arcade at the limbus there is complete absence of blood vessels and lymphatic vessels but a rich supply of non-myelinated sensory nerves (ophthalmic branch of cranial V), particularly superficially. The cornea is covered by the preocular tear film with its lipid aqueous and mucin components.

Histologically the canine cornea can be divided into four parts:

- The epithelium is non-keratinised, stratified squamous epithelium on a basement membrane with a single layer of columnar basal cells firmly attached to the basal membrane by hemidesmosomes; two to four layers of wing cells; a few layers of squamous cells. The corneal epithelium is pigmented only at the limbus and not in all dogs.
- Bowman's layer is poorly defined in the dog.
- The stroma (substantia propria) amounts to 90% of the thickness of the whole cornea, consisting of collagen fibrils organised in parallel bundles running across the cornea, keratocytes and ground substance.
- Descemet's membrane is an acellular, homogeneous, collagen and elastic structure.
- The mesothelium (endothelium) is a single layer of flattened cells between Descemet's membrane and the aqueous of the anterior chamber.

Nutrition is from the aqueous and perilimbal vessels and the active pump mechanism, which regulates the fluid content of the cornea keeping it transparent, is mainly dependent upon the integrity of the endothelium.

The classification of corneal disease is difficult and variable and certain conditions may appear under more than one heading, for example corneal oedema and corneal opacities and dystrophies. In addition, much information on the canine cornea is still required for a full understanding of this structure and its diseases. The classification in this chapter has been devised to try and aid the clinician as much as possible in diagnoses.

Congenital diseases

Changes in size and contour

Changes in corneal size and contour usually arise as a result of a congenital anomaly. Abnormal corneal size, in the form of either a small or large cornea, in an otherwise normal globe is extremely rare. Microcornea is more frequently associated with microphthalmos and multiocular anomalies (Fig. 9.1) for which there is a breed predisposition in the Old English Sheepdog, St Bernard, Australian Shepherd Dog, Cocker Spaniel and Rough Collie. Severe perforating trauma whilst the globe is still developing, particularly during the first 3 months of life, may affect subsequent development resulting in an abnormally small globe.

Megalocornea is usually associated with congenital glaucoma (buphthalmos), a very uncommon problem in this species.

Changes in corneal contour may result due to thinning of the central cornea and/or localised defects in Descemet's membrane, which result in focal oedema predisposing to a conical or globular distortion (keratoconus (Fig. 9.2), keratoglobus).

Congenital opacities

Congenital opacity of the posterior cornea, in the form of a diffuse central area (Fig. 9.3) or multiple small spots, occurs in association with persistent pupillary membranes, the corneal opacity often being the presenting sign (see also Chapter 12).

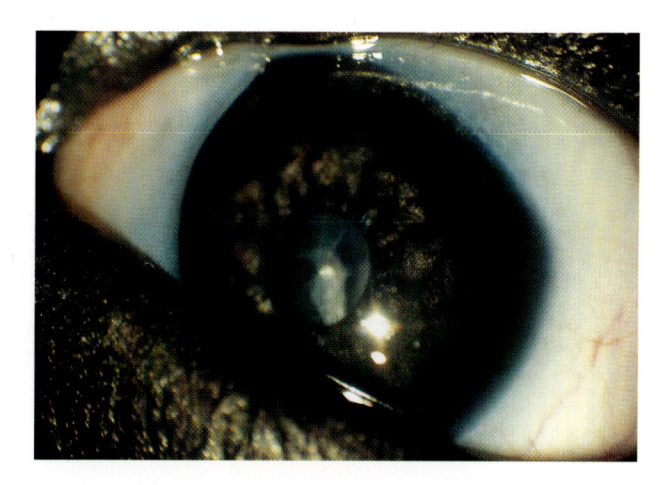

Fig. 9.1 Microcornea in microphthalmic eye in an Old English Sheepdog. Note also cataract and persistent pupillary membranes.

CORNEA

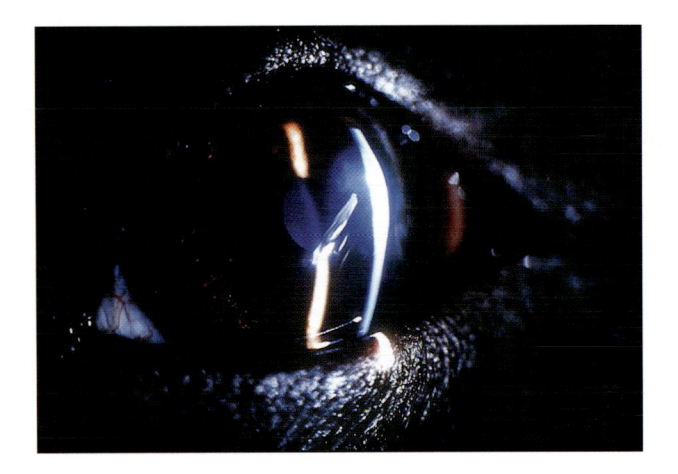

Fig. 9.2 Congenital keratoconus in a Dachshund puppy. The slit beam demonstrates corneal distortion and increased thickness, due to oedema, of the central area.

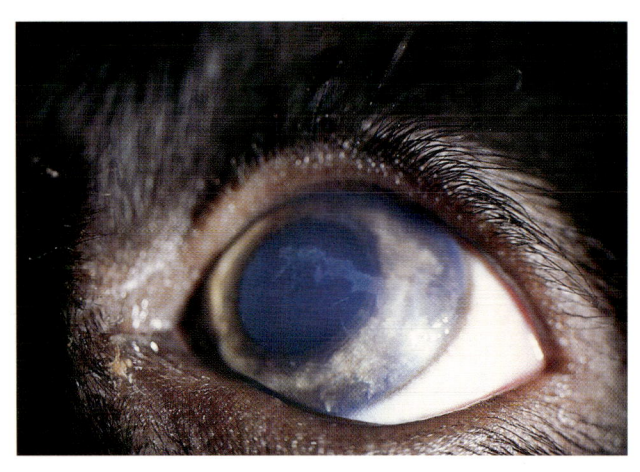

Fig. 9.4 Irregular subepithelial transient corneal opacity in a 6-week-old Border Collie.

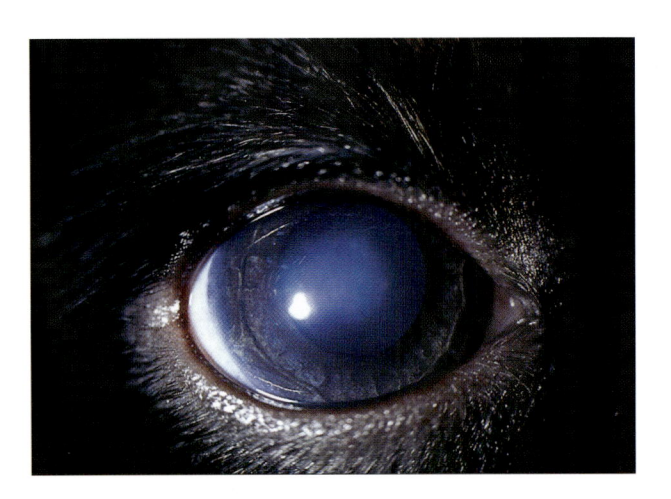

Fig. 9.3 Diffuse central corneal opacity associated with persistent pupillary membranes in a Miniature Longhaired Dachshund puppy.

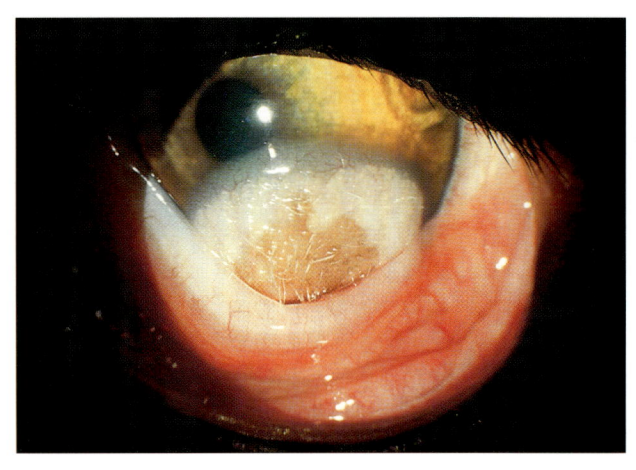

Fig. 9.5 Unpigmented dermoid with white hair in a Pointer.

INFANTILE DYSTROPHY

A superficial and transient opacity (Fig 9.4) is often present in puppies around 6 weeks of age. This subepithelial opacity is not significant and requires no treatment. It has been described as an infantile dystrophy (Wyman, 1986).

DERMOIDS

Dermoids (Figs 9.5–9.8) that involve the cornea are located at the limbus. They are slow growing and may be asymptomatic if hairless. However, the presence of hair follicles causes secondary corneal irritation. They may be pigmented or not. The treatment of choice is keratectomy, usually performed around 12 weeks of age. Breed predisposition has been described, in particular the German Shepherd Dog and St Bernard (see also Chapter 5).

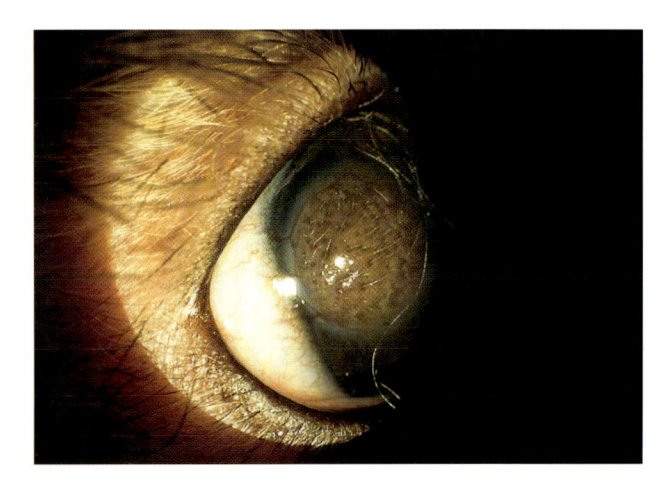

Fig. 9.6 Hairy pigmented corneal dermoid localised to the corneal side of the lateral limbus – common site – in a German Shepherd Dog.

CORNEAL OPACITIES

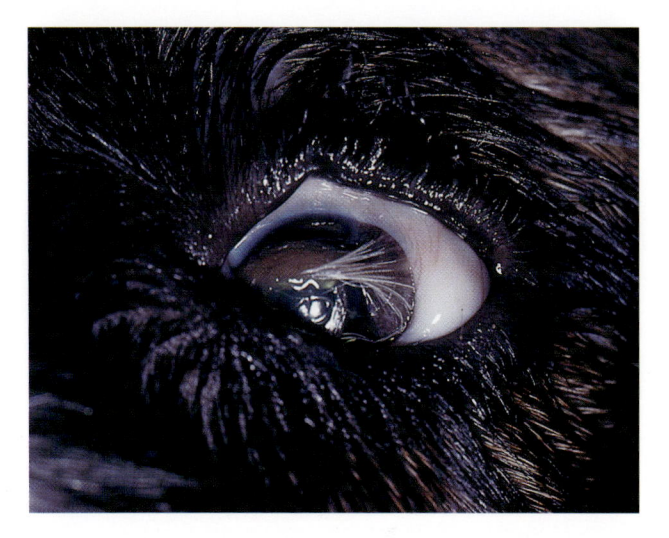

Fig. 9.7 Dermoid arising from the limbus in a St Bernard.

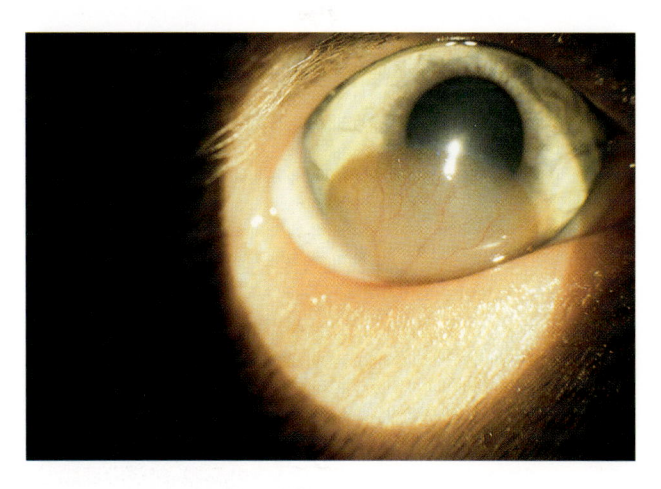

Fig. 9.8 An atypical hairless dermoid in a Weimaraner.

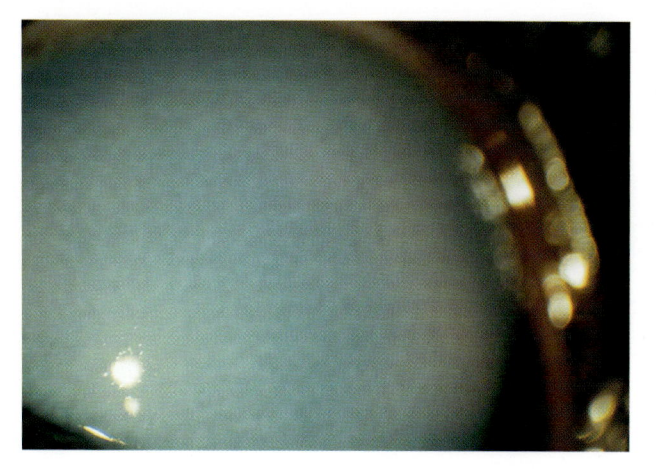

Fig. 9.9 Typical mottled or ground glass appearance of corneal oedema.

Corneal opacities

Corneal oedema

Corneal oedema is a common condition, presenting as a diffuse or focal opacity and due to a variety of causes. Focal oedema has no effect on vision; diffuse oedema causes some visual impairment. Corneal oedema is most frequently due to endothelial dysfunction as a result of endothelial cell degeneration or death, less often it is due to loss of corneal epithelium. Predisposing factors to the loss of endothelial cells are age, intraocular surgery, intraocular inflammation and the mechanical effect of a dislocated lens or intraocular mass pressing on the endothelium. Changes in intraocular pressure either alone or in combination with endothelial dysfunction will result in aqueous entering the corneal stroma. Mild stromal oedema will also be seen in association with corneal inflammation (vascular keratitis). In mild cases the cornea assumes a hazy or steamy appearance. In severe cases the corneal stroma has a dense blue appearance described as 'ground glass' or 'blue eye' (Fig. 9.9). The diagnosis of corneal oedema relies on its characteristic appearance and can be confirmed by the gentle application of pressure to the eye which spreads the oedema if it is focal or increases the density if it is diffuse. This test allows differentiation from other corneal opacities, such as scars, dystrophies, degenerations, etc.

Frequently corneal oedema is a manifestation of more serious intraocular problems such as lens luxation (Figs 9.10 and 9.11), uveitis (see Fig. 12.4), glaucoma (see Fig. 10.9) or neoplasia (Fig. 9.12). (See also interstitial keratitis.) Tears or ruptures in Descemet's membrane are characteristically seen in hydrophthalmos (see Fig. 4.20). They are described as striae and present as linear streaks resembling 'ice cracks' across the cornea.

In severe cases fluid accumulates to form cysts or bullae, resulting in a bullous keratopathy (Fig. 9.13). Whilst oedema alone is not a painful condition bullous keratopathy causes discomfort and pain as the bullae rupture. The presence of corneal ulcers and erosions in conjunction with corneal

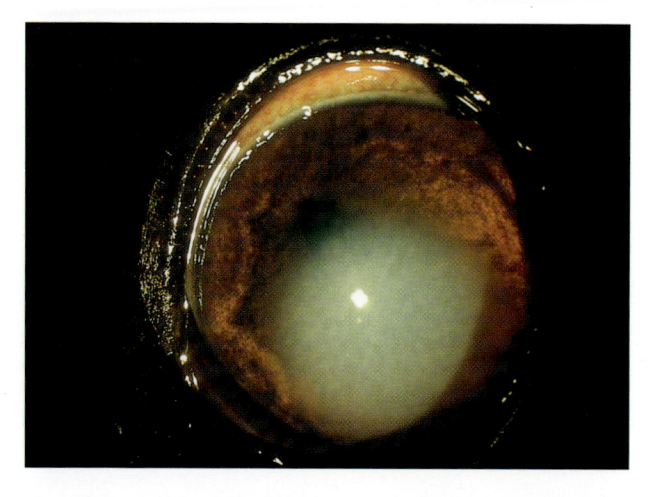

Fig. 9.10 Subcentral localised corneal oedema secondary to endothelial damage due to anterior lens luxation in a Tibetan Terrier.

CORNEA

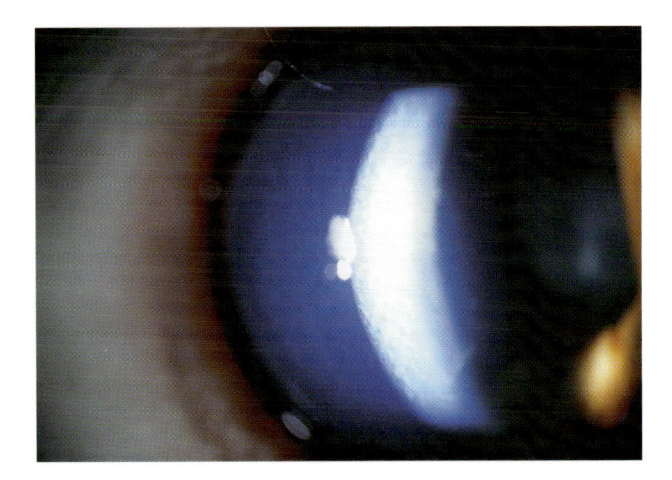

Fig. 9.11 Slit-lamp photograph to demonstrate increased thickness of the corneal stroma in a Jack Russell Terrier with lens luxation.

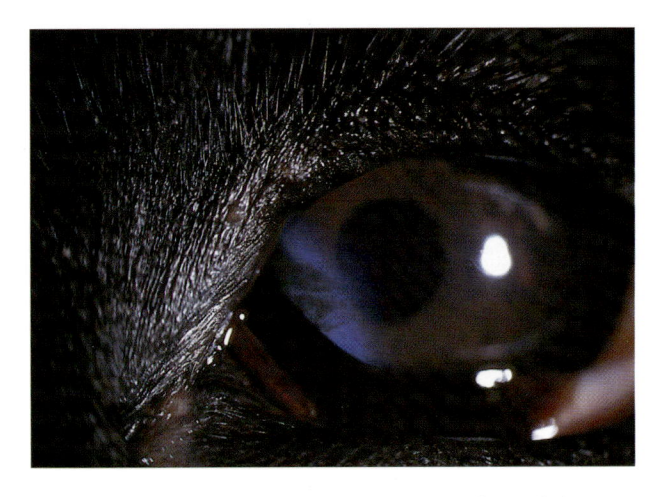

Fig. 9.12 Mild oedema and pigmentation at the medial canthus due to an intraocular iris melanoma (not visible) in a Labrador Retriever. Note pupil distortion.

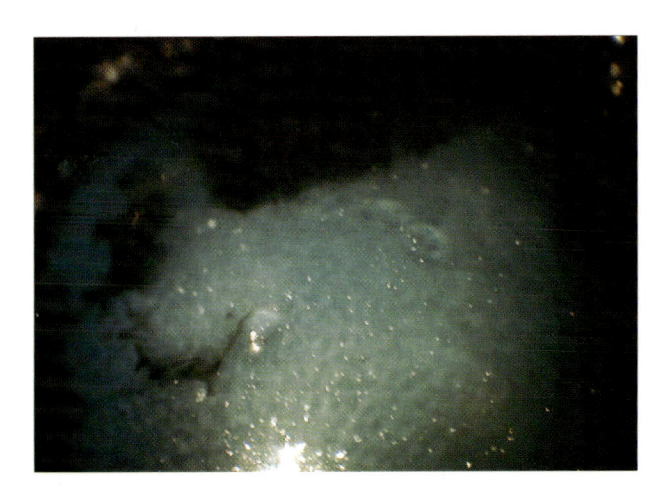

Fig. 9.13 Bullous keratopathy with secondary pigmentation.

oedema means that healing is extremely slow. Treatment for oedema alone, secondary to an endothelial dystrophy or degeneration, can only be symptomatic. Soft contact lenses and ocular lubricants are the treatment of choice. In severe cases thermokeratoplasty may be indicated.

CORNEAL DYSTROPHIES

Corneal dystrophies are primary inherited conditions that may affect the corneal epithelium, stroma or endothelium. They are not associated with inflammatory corneal disease. The mode of inheritance for most of these conditions in the dog is not known but there is an obvious breed predisposition.

Epithelial basement membrane dystrophy/recurrent epithelial erosions (Fig. 9.14)

Uncomplicated and recurring superficial ulceration where there is a breed predisposition particularly in the Boxer and Pembroke Corgi may represent an epithelial dystrophy due to structural abnormalities in the corneal epithelium and basement membrane. (See also corneal ulceration.) The diagnosis is based on the very characteristic appearance and breed predisposition.

Lipid dystrophies (also termed corneal lipidosis) (Figs 9.15–9.17)

The lesions are usually bilateral, not necessarily symmetrical and have a shiny metallic scintillating appearance. The opacities represent intracellular and extracellular lipids in the form of cholesterol crystals and esters and are usually deposited in the anterior corneal stroma in central or subcentral positions, unassociated with ocular inflammation. Crystalline cholesterol deposition is thought to occur due to an accumulation of lipid within the fibroblast. Subsequent death and necrosis of this keratocyte results in the lipid dystrophy. This very characteristic appearance, sometimes described as looking like glass fibres or sugar crystals, can be

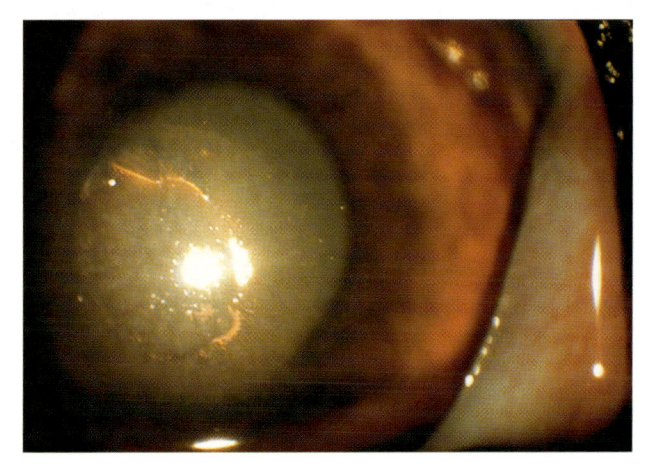

Fig. 9.14 Recurrent epithelial erosion in a Bearded Collie. Note the large epithelial defect with a ragged undermined edge, mild stromal oedema and break in the corneal reflection.

CORNEAL OPACITIES

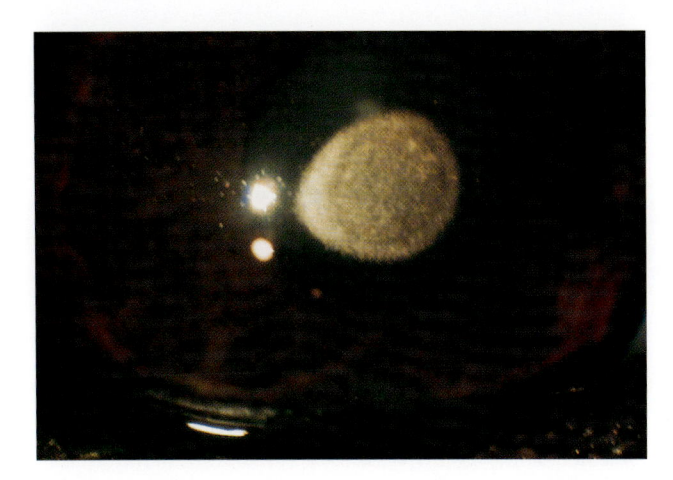

Fig. 9.15 Lipid dystrophy in a 4-year-old Cavalier King Charles Spaniel.

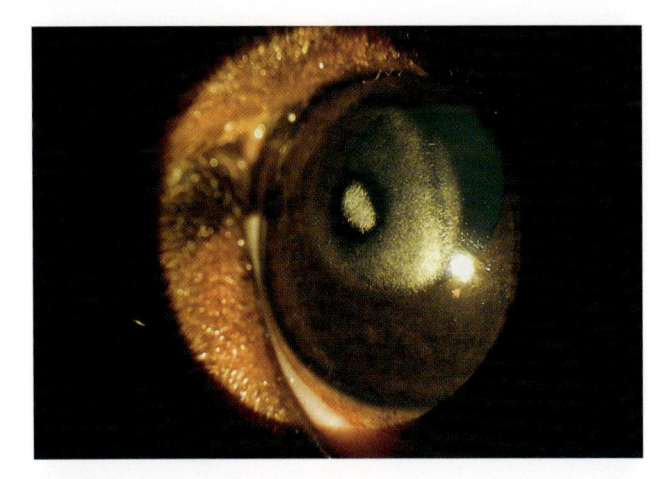

Fig. 9.16 Lipid dystrophy in a 3-year-old Cavalier King Charles Spaniel.

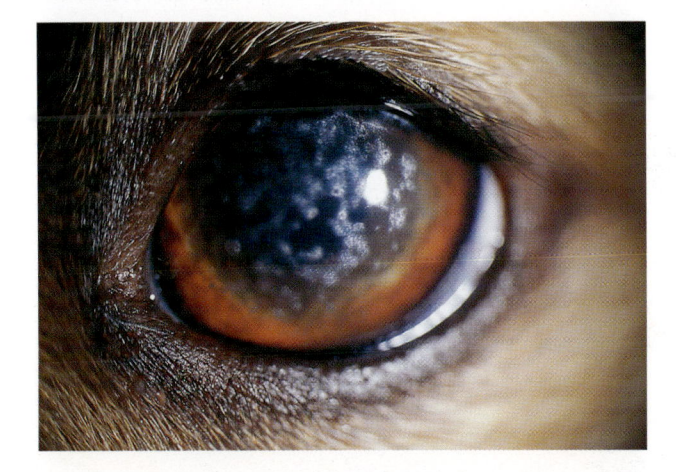

Fig. 9.17 Corneal lipidosis in an 18-month-old Shetland Sheepdog.

years) with a sex incidence in the female (Crispin and Barnett, 1983).

Differentiating between inherited dystrophies and local degenerative conditions is not always easy. However, the lipid dystrophies do not cause epithelial disruption or discomfort and they are not associated with pre-existing ocular pathology. No treatment is usually indicated. Topical corticostreroids and local factors such as distichiasis may exacerbate the problem. Where the condition is progressive a lipid and lipoprotein analysis should be carried out, but it is unlikely to be helpful.

The main breed incidence of this corneal dystrophy is in the Rough Collie, Cavalier King Charles Spaniel, Bichon Frise and Shetland Sheepdog, and the cholesterol and lipid deposits are subepithelial. Depending on the breed they may present as multiple circular rings, as in the Shetland Sheepdog, or as a paracentral lesion as in the Cavalier King Charles Spaniel. In the Siberian Husky the clinical presentation is variable, the deposits may occur at various levels and up to five clinical patterns for this condition have been described.

Endothelial dystrophy

Endothelial dystrophy (Figs 9.18 and 9.19) is a bilaterally progressive condition resulting in total corneal oedema. The eyes are classically quiet and visual in the early stages of the disease. Only in advances cases, where keratoconus and/or a secondary bullous keratopathy develop, are there signs of ocular inflammation and discomfort. Treatment is as for corneal oedema. There is a breed incidence in the Boston Terrier, Chihuahua and Dachshund in the United States and in the English Springer Spaniel in the UK. The age of presentation is variable but usually in the older dog.

In the American Cocker Spaniel endothelial cell dysfunction presents as multiple opacities in contrast to diffuse oedema. It has been described as a posterior polymorphic dystrophy and is thought to be inherited in a dominant fashion.

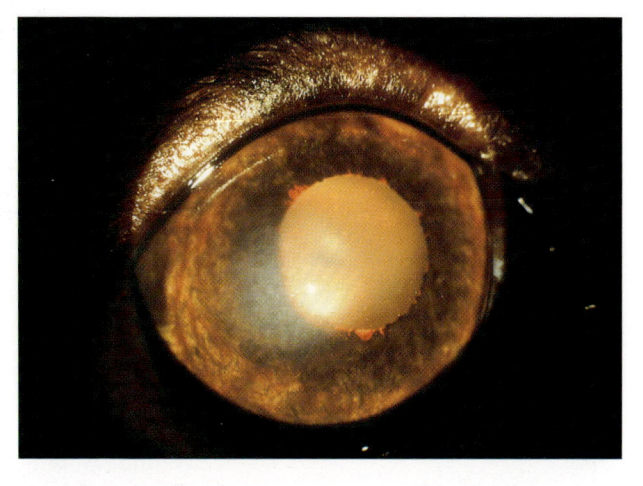

Fig. 9.18 Endothelial dystrophy. Mild corneal oedema in an 11-year-old female English Springer Spaniel (right eye).

seen with good illumination and magnification. The deposits may increase in size with time and in the bitch may vary with hormonal status. The condition affects the young adult (2–4

CORNEA

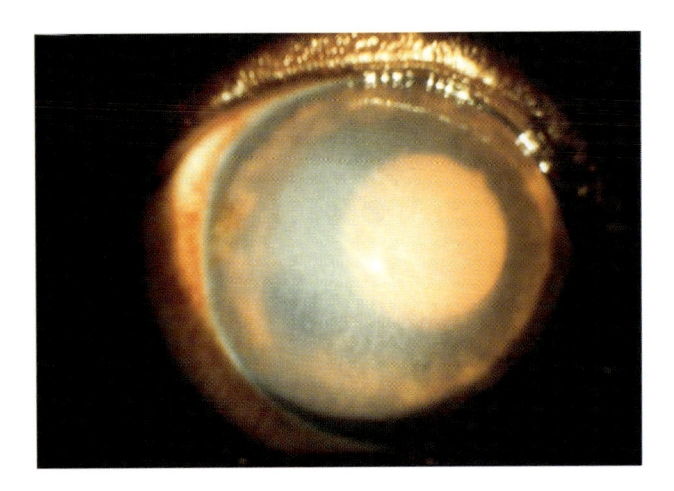

Fig. 9.19 Same dog as in Fig. 9.18 (left eye). Note typical difference in severity between the two eyes.

Corneal pathology, particularly corneal vascularisation, changes in corneal temperature, ocular hypotension, low-grade trauma (distichiasis or trichiasis) and plasma hyperlipoproteinaemia may be contributing factors to the stromal deposition of lipid within one or both corneas. Corneal vascularisation is always present in lipid keratopathy and it is likely that such vessels are the source of lipid for direct stromal deposition.

Treatment of such cases is difficult unless an underlying cause can be determined. A lipid and biochemical profile should be performed to ascertain whether there are underlying systemic abnormalities. The presence of other ocular abnormalities should be identified. A keratectomy may be indicated if the lesion is causing discomfort or interfering with vision; the latter is unlikely.

ARCUS LIPOIDES

Infiltration of the peripheral cornea with lipid material, known as arcus lipoides (Figs 9.21 and 9.22), has been

OTHER CORNEAL OPACITIES

A variety of deposits may develop within the corneal stroma. Lipid deposits may be seen in association with other corneal or ocular diseases such as chronic superficial keratitis and keratoconjunctivitis sicca.

Keratopathies may result in calcium deposits, which have a dense chalky white appearance. They may be associated with corneal ulceration.

Fibrous tissue in the form a scar will form irregular opacities within the cornea at any depth depending on the aetiology.

Cellular infiltrates occur with keratitis and these may present as localised opaque deposits or more diffuse lesions if there is stromal involvement.

The term lipid keratopathy is reserved for an aetiology that is inflammatory or unknown (Fig. 9.20). This is in contrast to the corneal dystrophies that occur as primary inherited conditions.

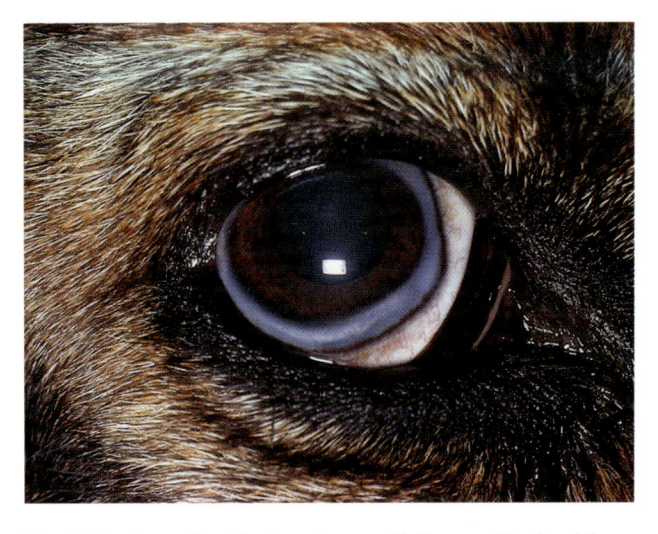

Fig. 9.21 Arcus lipoides in a 4-year-old German Shepherd Dog.

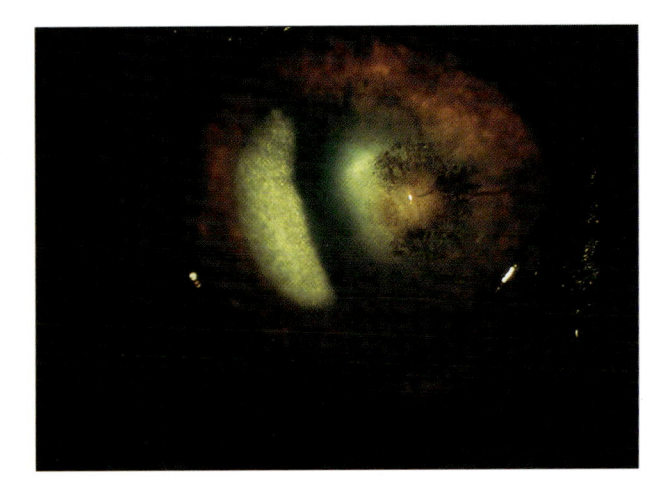

Fig. 9.20 Lipid keratopathy in association with a pigmentary and vascular keratitis in a Boxer.

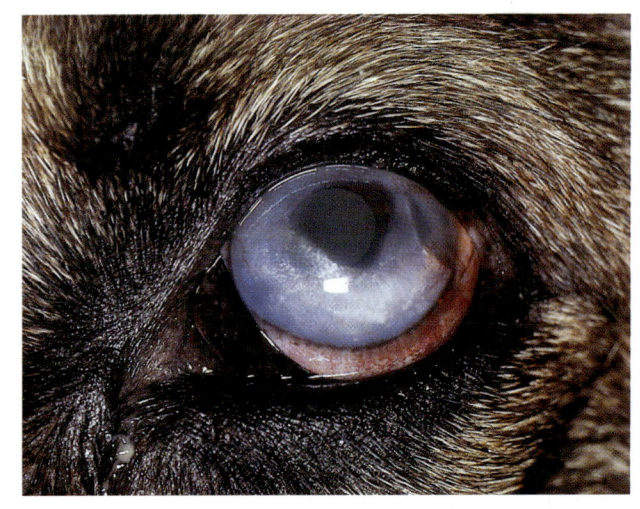

Fig. 9.22 Arcus lipoides in a 6-year-old German Shepherd Dog.

CORNEAL PIGMENTATION

reported secondary to hyperlipoproteinaemia in hyperthyroidism in the Alsatian breed (Crispin and Barnett, 1978). This is always a bilateral condition and associated with hyperlipoproteinaemia. It is suggested that the increased permeability of blood vessels at the limbus allows large-sized lipoproteins to enter the cornea to form an arcus. There may be some vascularisation of the opacities. The lesions tend not to regress even when the underlying condition is treated successfully.

CORNEAL DEGENERATIONS

Corneal degenerations may be fatty, hyaline or calcareous in nature and associated with inflammation, vascularisation and ulceration. They may occur secondary to systemic or ocular disease.

Lipid and calcareous degeneration (Figs 9.23–9.25) has been reported in the Golden Retriever where it probably represents a corneal dystrophy. The corneal opacities occupy a paraxial or peripheral position well inside the limbus. As with arcus lipoides there is clear cornea between the lesion and the limbus. Calcium and lipid deposition within the cornea result in vascularised, sausage-shaped opacities with secondary epithelial disruption. The latter results in discomfort and blepharospasm and may require surgery.

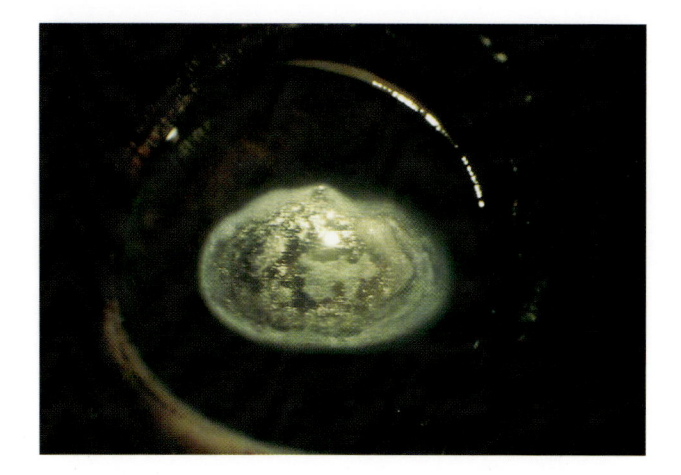

Fig. 9.25 Corneal degeneration/dystrophy in a Golden Retriever. This lesion is more central than in Figs 9.23 or 9.24, but note the obvious epithelial involvement with break-up of the corneal reflection.

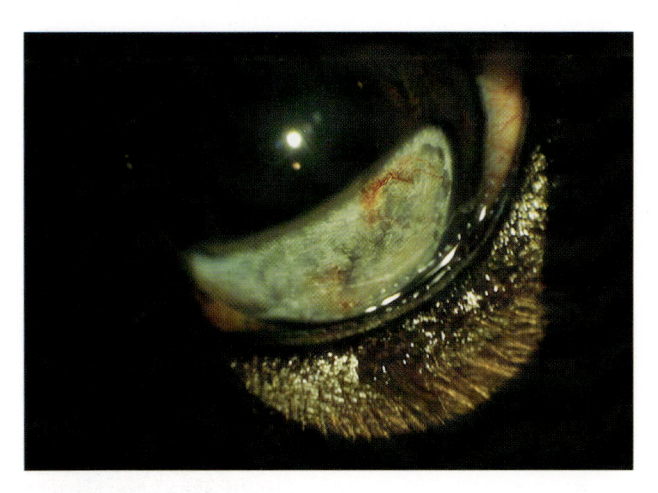

Fig. 9.23 Corneal degeneration/dystrophy in a 3-year-old Golden Retriever bitch. Note the obvious vascularisation of this lesion.

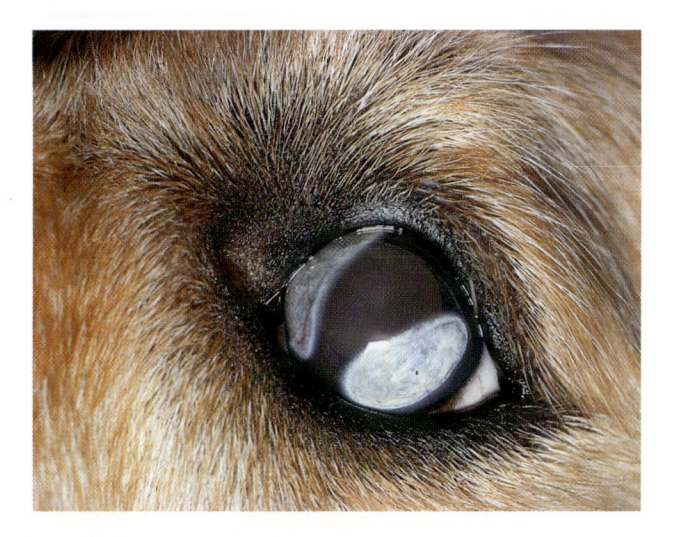

Fig. 9.24 Corneal degeneration/dystrophy in a Golden Retriever. There are two large opaque vascularised lesions inside the limbus.

CORNEAL PIGMENTATION

Pigment deposition in the cornea (Figs 9.26 and 9.27) may be secondary to a variety of diseases; it is usually post-inflammatory and associated with vascularisation of the cornea. Superficial pigmentation is common in the brachycephalic breeds particularly at the medial canthus. In many cases it is associated with an active keratitis but in others it appears to occur in the absence of inflammation and at a

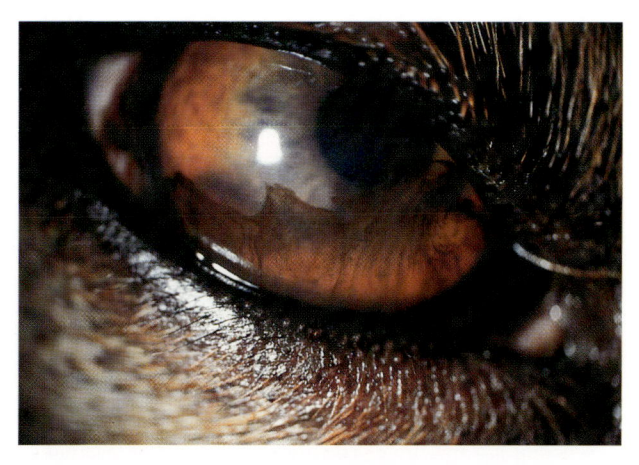

Fig. 9.26 Pigmentation of the ventral superficial corneal quadrant in a 12-year-old crossbred dog. This case had been treated for chronic superficial keratitis over a 6-week period.

CORNEA

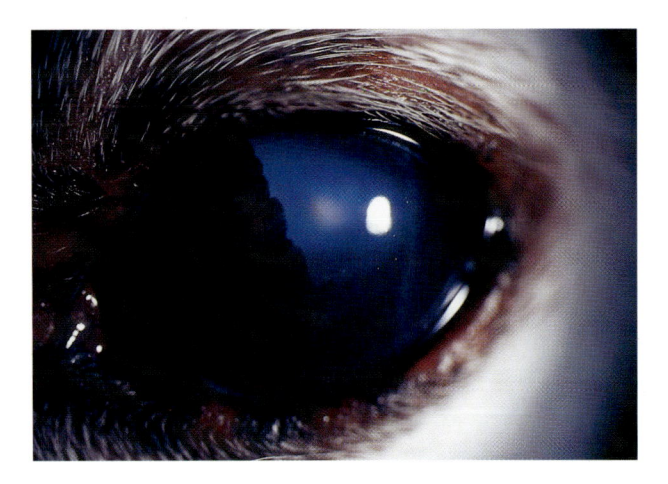

Fig. 9.27 Pigmentation of the corneal endothelium in a 13-year-old Whippet.

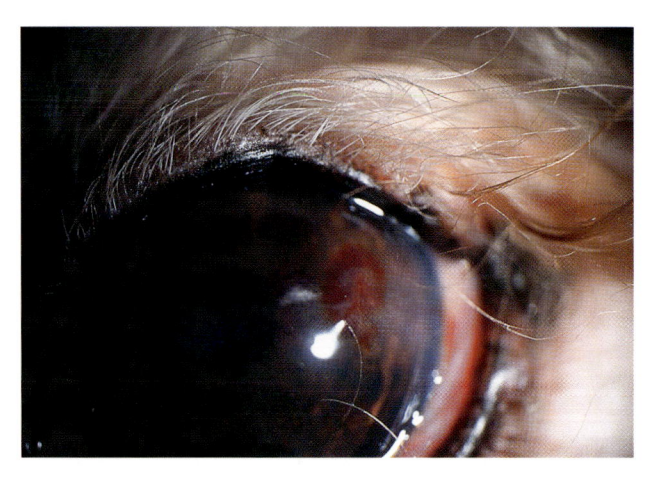

Fig. 9.28 Corneal haemorrhage and vascularisation in a 12-year-old Bichon Frise. Note the small area of lipid keratopathy medial to the haemorrhage.

very young age. It is also a feature of chronic superficial keratitis (pannus) seen in the German Shepherd Dog and related breeds, where again it may occur independently of vascularisation and is not necessarily progressive but the distribution of the pigment may change and sometimes even disappear with the passage of time.

Endothelial pigmentation is a benign condition that occurs in the older dog; it does not appear to be associated with corneal disease. The pigmentation extends from the limbus onto the corneal endothelium and progresses in a benign fashion.

Pigment deposition on the corneal endothelium will also occur as a result of contact with uveal tissue either in the form of synechiae or as a result of congenital deposition with persistent pupillary membranes.

HAEMATOGENOUS PIGMENTATION

Blood staining of the cornea occurs with severe hyphaema, the cornea assuming a dark brown appearance precluding intraocular examination.

Haemorrhage into the cornea (Fig. 9.28) is an unusual condition but it may occur secondary to rupture of corneal blood vessels or as an extension from conjunctival haemorrhage.

CORNEAL ULCERATION

Corneal ulceration is an extremely common condition with a breed predisposition often related to facial conformation.

SUPERFICIAL ULCERATION

Superficial corneal ulceration, also known as an erosion, is usually an uncomplicated single lesion that will heal rapidly within 7 days unless infected. It has a well defined edge in the absence of stromal involvement; mild oedema is present in some cases. The presenting clinical signs are of discomfort and blepharospasm associated with increased lacrimation and mild conjunctival inflammation. A thorough clinical examination should be carried out to try and ascertain the aetiology. It may result from ectopic cilia, entropion, foreign bodies, abnormalities of the lid margin and space-occupying lesions. Removal of the inciting cause results in rapid healing usually by first intention but where the lesion is chronic, vascularisation will have already occurred. Visible ingrowth of vessels from the limbus will occur after 3–5 days but may take 2–3 weeks to reach the central cornea.

RECURRENT EPITHELIAL EROSIONS (see also epithelial basement membrane dystrophy)

These indolent ulcers present as superficial ulcers but have a very characteristic lip of undermined necrotic epithelium (see Fig. 9.14). They may affect one or both eyes and are frequently recurring in those breeds susceptible to this condition. Healing is always slow but usually not complicated by secondary infection unless the cornea is further compromised. Inappropriate medical treatment in the form of local anaesthetics, corticosteroids or epitheliotoxic antibiotics (aminoglycosides) will further delay healing. Treatment has traditionally been by debridement or phenol cautery under topical anaesthesia. A superficial keratectomy is claimed to give superior healing rates (Stanley et al., 1998). These lesions are always slow to heal and may take weeks if not months. Overzealous treatment, sometimes due to too frequent debridement (Fig. 9.29), will damage normal epithelium and stroma resulting in severe stromal ulceration or corneal melts. Keratotomies should not be performed in the presence of a secondary infection as this procedure may have the effect of dispersing infection throughout the cornea.

Healing is frequently by second intention and occasionally excessive granulation tissue may result at the site (Fig. 9.30). The vascularisation will usually regress slowly of its own accord over several weeks. Topical steroid treatment should not be used to control this unless a granuloma results.

CORNEAL ULCERATION

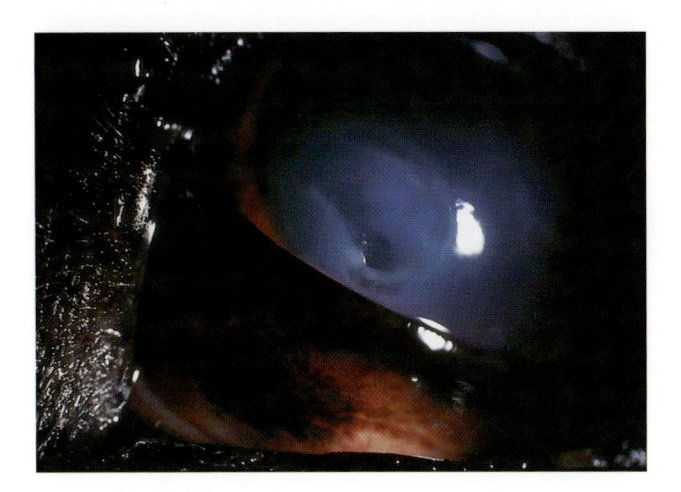

Fig. 9.29 Stromal ulceration in an 8-year-old Boxer. This result was secondary to aggressive and repeated debridement over a short period of time for what originally was a case of recurrent epithelial erosion. Bacterial culture was negative.

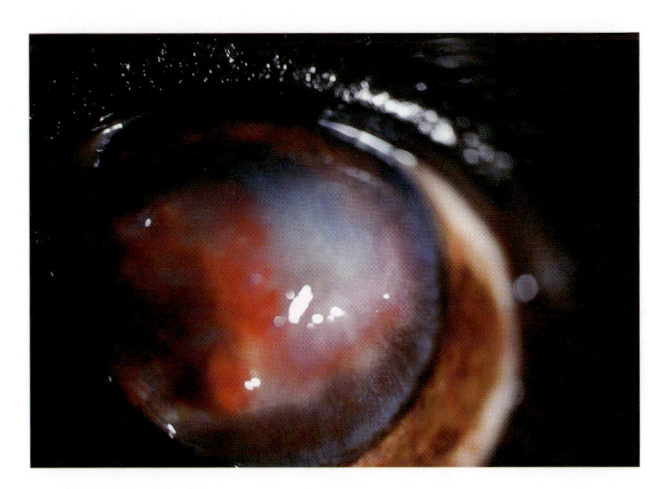

Fig. 9.30 The same eye as in Fig. 9.29, 4 weeks later following the placement of a conjunctival flap which resulted in excessive granulation tissue and migration of pigment from the ventral limbus.

Stromal ulceration

Stromal ulcers may be sterile or infected. They are commonly seen in the brachycephalic breeds where the aetiology is probably multifactorial as a result of exposure, trichiasis, tear-film abnormalities and secondary infection. The ulceration is usually central. The affected cornea is oedematous and there may be cellular infiltration and stromal breakdown. The diagnosis of stromal ulceration is based on the loss of normal corneal contour and clarity over the affected site. The ulcers will stain positively with fluorescein although this should not be necessary to make the diagnosis. This is a painful condition and will present with blepharospasm, lacrimation and conjunctival injection. With bacterial ulcerative keratitis a secondary uveitis and hypopyon are frequently present, in addition to the purulent discharge (Fig. 9.31). These ulcers are often rapidly progressive resulting in a descemetocoele.

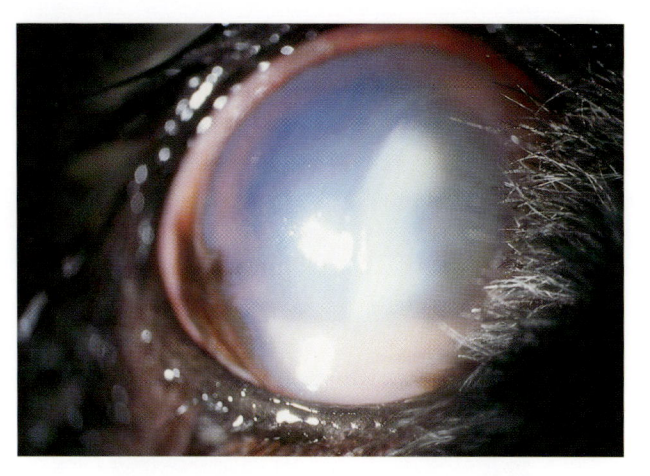

Fig. 9.31 Stromal ulcer with secondary uveitis and hypopyon in a Pekingese. The pupil is dilated following the use of topical atropine as a mydriatic.

Corneas with deep ulceration should be handled very carefully and samples taken for cytology and culture. A careful ocular examination should be performed to check for predisposing causes. A Schirmer tear test should be carried out in both eyes as dry eye can be a precipitating factor, but in the presence of corneal ulceration the reading is frequently elevated and may give a false positive. The contralateral eye is an aid to the diagnosis of underlying keratoconjunctivitis sicca as the reading may be borderline or reduced if the condition is bilateral, which it frequently is. Hospitalisation and intensive treatment with a broad-spectrum antibiotic, mydriatics and systemic analgesia is the required regimen. Additional protection in the form of a flap, preferably conjunctival, and partial lid closure, may be necessary if there is poor response to medical treatment.

Collagenase associated or melting ulcers

Rapid dissolution of the corneal stroma or melting, due to excessive production of enzymes such as proteases and collagenases, will result in a corneal melt (Figs 9.32 and 9.33). These ulcers are complicated ulcers, probably multifactorial in aetiology, but *Pseudomonas* infection should be regarded as a possible aetiology. Certain strains of *Pseudomonas* have the ability to produce large quantities of proteases which degrade the corneal stroma or secrete exotoxins that cause stromal cell death. Acid and alkaline burns and fungal infection (rarely seen in the United Kingdom) can produce the same effect. The cornea becomes oedematous, assuming a soft gelatinous appearance. Where there is collagen breakdown the corneal stroma disintegrates. In some cases a secondary bullous keratopathy may develop.

This condition should be regarded as an ocular emergency (see Chapter 3) and cases hospitalised for appropriate and vigorous therapy. Many will respond to a broad spectrum antibiotic (e.g. polymixin and gramicidin or the fluroquinolones), in addition to an anti-collagenase such as autologus serum, and systemic analgesia. It is important to obtain

CORNEA

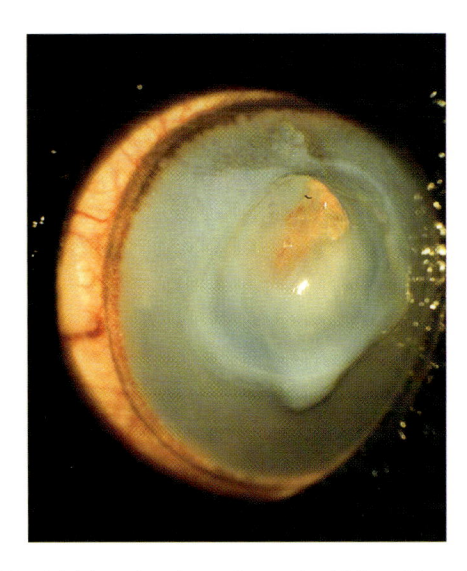

Fig. 9.32 Melting ulcer in an 8-month-old Pug. Note the total corneal oedema and dense central opacity as a result of degradation of the corneal stroma.

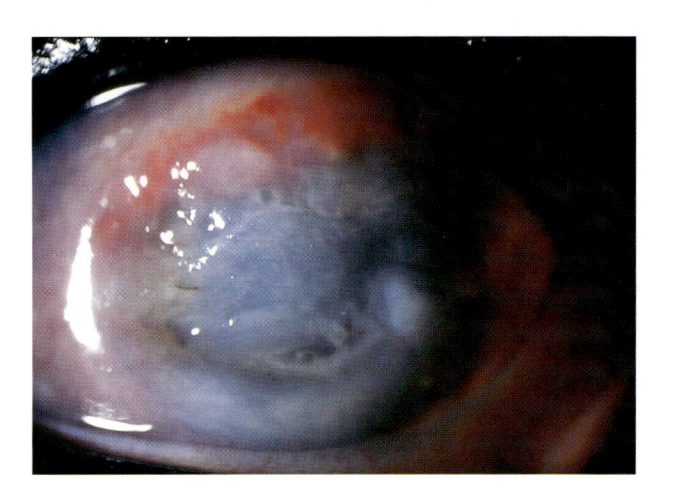

Fig. 9.33 Melting ulcer healing by second intention in a 10-year-old Border Collie. Note the large central defect and a secondary bullous keratopathy. This cornea healed uneventfully by second intention and cleared completely over a 3-month period.

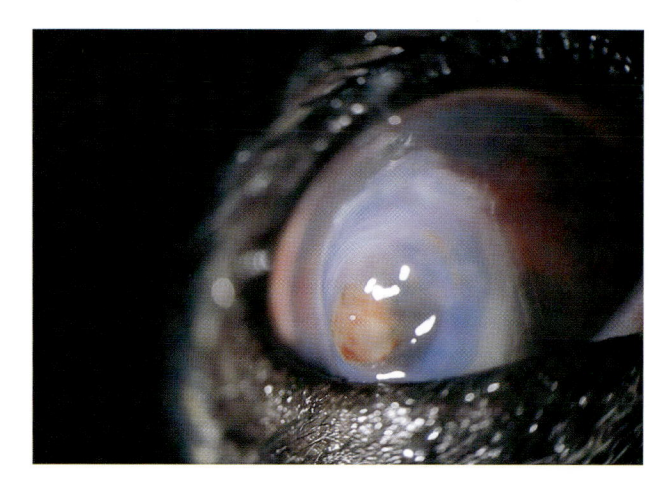

Fig. 9.34 Ruptured descemetocoele as a result of excessive debridement and keratectomy for a superficial ulcer in a Boston Terrier. Note the aqueous plug at the centre of the descemetocoele.

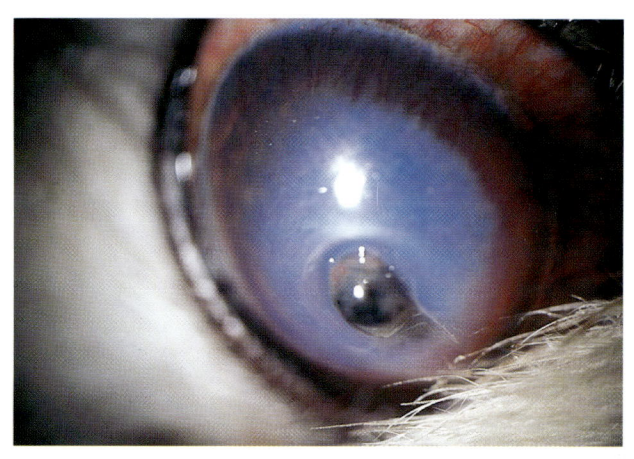

Fig. 9.35 Ruptured descemetocoele with incarcerated iris in a 2-year-old Pekingese. Note trichiasis of nasal fold.

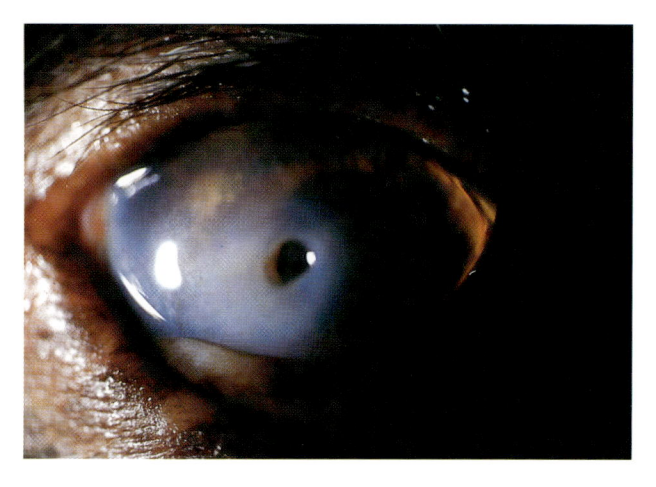

Fig. 9.36 Descemetocoele in a 10-year-old Labrador cross. Note the clear bulging base of the descemetocoele surrounded by cloudy cornea (oedema and fibrosis).

patient cooperation and making sure that the eye is comfortable is one way of achieving this. Frequent topical treatment is impractical if the patient is uncooperative and secondary self-inflicted trauma will result. Protective collars are frequently advocated but rarely necessary if pain is adequately controlled. In the event of impending perforation an extensive conjunctival flap is necessary. Healing will be slow by second intention but the results can be extremely satisfactory.

DESCEMETOCOELE

These deep ulcers (Figs 9.34–9.36) extend down to Descemet's membrane, which is transparent and characteristically does not stain with fluoroscein. Bulging and

KERATITIS

perforation of Descemet's membrane may occur. Perforation will result in loss of the anterior chamber and in severe cases haemorrhage into the anterior chamber with iris prolapse. Large defects will incarcerate iris and may be covered by exudate. These cases require surgical intervention. Very small perforations will seal with an aqueous plug and will heal by second intention from iridal or corneal vascularisation. Surgical intervention in the form of a conjunctival flap is the treatment of choice in most cases and is essential where the defect is large and vision is to be preserved. Descemetocoeles are usually regarded as an emergency (see Chapter 3) because of imminent perforation, but where the defect is small this may not occur. They can persist for many months and may eventually heal by second intention. However, in some cases healing will not occur and the defect persists.

KERATITIS

Corneal inflammation, or keratitis, is characterised by the presence of corneal blood vessels and the presence of leukocytes. Keratitis can be classified on the basis of whether it is ulcerative or non-ulcerative. The level at which the lesion occurs within the corneal stroma defines it as superficial or deep. The depth and position of the lesion is frequently an aid to diagnosis. For example chronic superficial keratitis almost invariably affects the ventral temporal quadrant of the cornea, whereas keratoconjunctivitis sicca usually starts at the dorsal limbus (keratoconjunctivitis sicca is not regarded by some as a true keratitis). Keratitis as a result of exposure due to an inadequate blink reflex, or of neurogenic aetiology, will affect the central cornea. Where corneal inflammation is due to mechanical irritation, in cases of entropion or canthal trichiasis, the result of space-occupying lid lesions or ectopic cilia, then the affected area will correspond to the inciting cause.

SUPERFICIAL DIFFUSE KERATITIS

The common causes of diffuse superficial keratitis in the dog are chronic degenerative conditions such as pannus and keratoconjunctivitis sicca. These conditions are characterised by the development of superficial vascularisation, corneal oedema and cellular infiltration, along with pigment migration. The latter will only occur if pigment is present at the limbus.

PANNUS OR SUPERFICIAL CHRONIC KERATITIS

Pannus (Figs 9.37–9.40) is a common condition in the adult German Shepherd Dog and Belgian Shepherd Dog and to a lesser extent the Dachshund, Greyhound, Lurcher, Border Collie and others. Both corneas are usually affected in a similar fashion. The lesion initially presents in the lower temporal quadrant of the cornea, later to involve the inferonasal quadrant. In the early stages there is mild inflammation, increased vascularisation at the limbus and a lymphocytic plasmacytic infiltrate of the superficial corneal

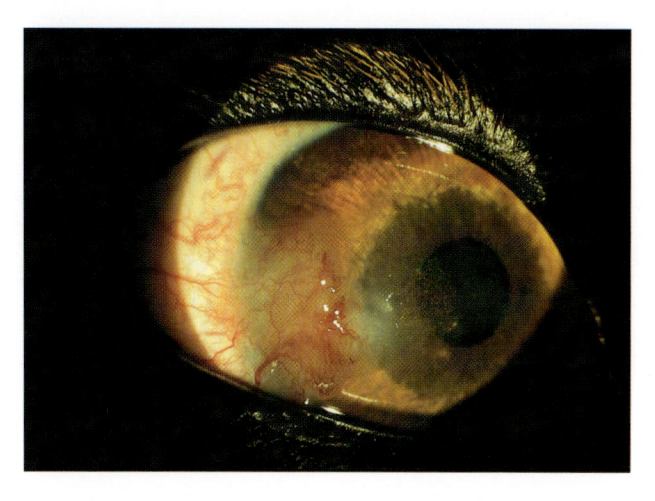

Fig. 9.37 Pannus in a German Shepherd Dog. Superficial vascularisation, infiltration and oedema at the inferotemporal corneal quadrant in an early case.

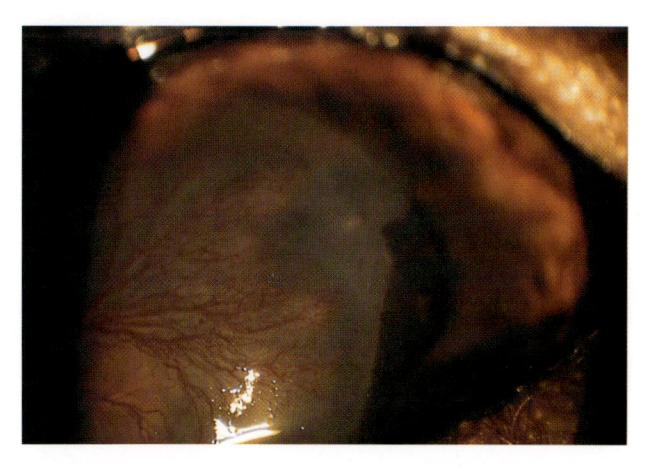

Fig. 9.38 Pannus in a German Shepherd Dog. Note the superficial keratitis with break-up of the corneal reflection and the pigmentation.

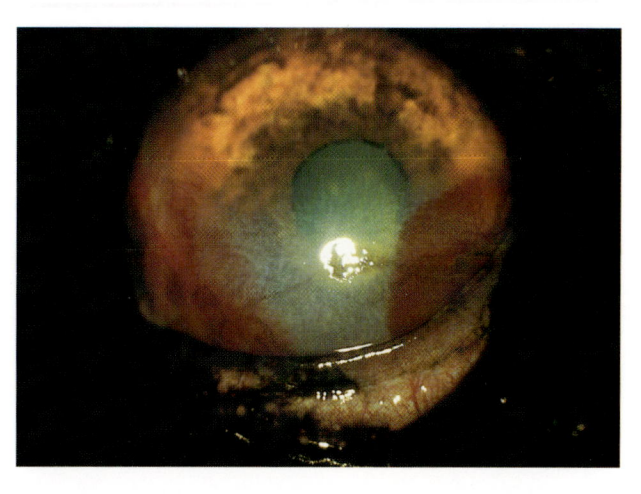

Fig. 9.39 Pannus and plasma cell infiltration of the third eyelid in a German Shepherd Dog. The inferotemporal and nasal quadrants are affected in this case.

CORNEA

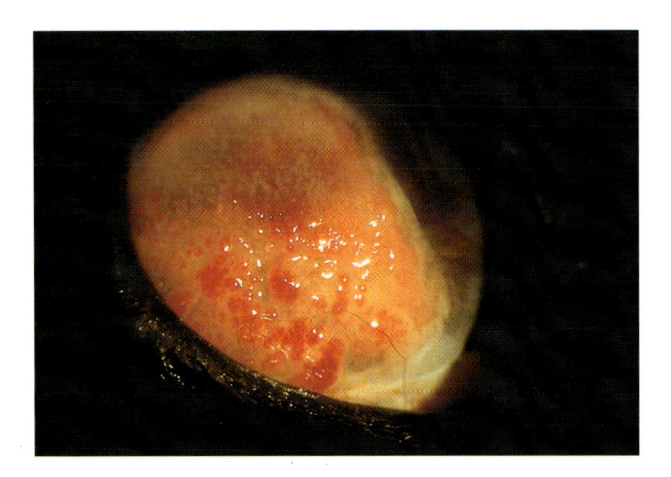

Fig. 9.40 Advanced and severe case of pannus in a 4-year-old German Shepherd Dog. Note the development of excessive granulation tissue over most of the cornea.

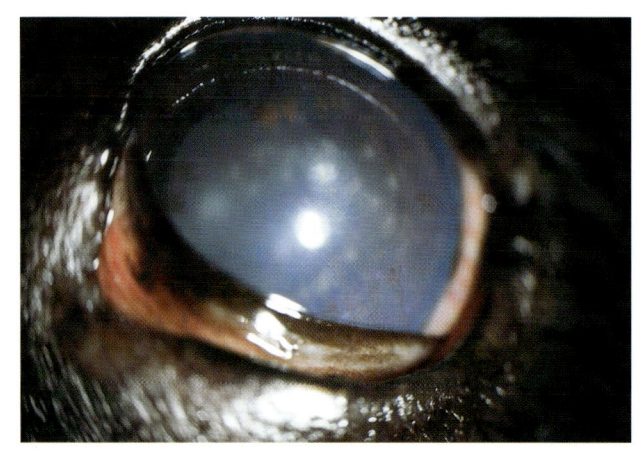

Fig. 9.41 Superficial punctate keratitis. Multiple small corneal opacities are associated with diffuse oedema and vascularisation.

stroma. The corneal lesion is similar to the discoid lupus lesion of the skin that also affects the German Shepherd Dog breed. The vascularisation progresses across the cornea with secondary oedema, cellular infiltration, sometimes lipidosis and often pigmentation. There may be the formation of exuberant granulation tissue and secondary epithelial ulceration. Blindness will result if the condition is not treated adequately.

This condition is often seen in association with plasma cell infiltration of the third eyelid (see Chapter 6), and less commonly with ulceration of the lid margins at the canthus.

The treatment of choice is frequent application (six times daily) of topical steroids (prednisolone acetate or dexamethasone alcohol) initially over a 6-week period. The frequency of the topical application can be tailed off over this period as the condition improves. A low maintenance dose is necessary in some cases. Cyclosporine can also be used in the treatment of this condition. Sunlight and other environments high in ultraviolet light will exacerbate pannus. A superficial keratectomy may be indicated in advanced cases. Pannus always tends to recur and treatment will need to be repeated, often on many occasions.

SUPERFICIAL PUNCTATE KERATITIS

This condition presents as multiple small corneal opacities involving the corneal epithelium (Fig. 9.41). Ulceration and vascularisation may occur to the corneal defects. The condition is steroid and cyclosporine responsive but frequently recurring. It has been suggested that it may have a viral aetiology as it is similar to herpetic infection in other species. In the Shetland Sheepdog it may represent a dystrophic lesion presenting as circular or irregular opacities in the central cornea resembling lipid deposition. It is most common in the Miniature Longhaired Dachshund.

KERATOCONJUNCTIVITIS SICCA

See Chapter 7.

INTERSTITIAL KERATITIS

The common causes of interstitial keratitis (Fig. 9.42) are infectious (bacterial, viral or fungal). In the United Kingdom, bacterial and infectious canine hepatitis virus are the common causes of deep or interstitial keratitis. In contrast to superficial keratitis, deep keratitis presents with extensive and dense corneal oedema. This may be accompanied by a circumferential vascular fringe or large deep vessels emerging below the limbus. Where there is deep stromal involvement a secondary uveitis is likely to be present.

Ocular lesions result from natural infection of infectious canine hepatitis or in the past following vaccination with attenuated canine adenovirus type I. The ocular lesions usually develop between 7 and 21 days after exposure. Mild transient (several hours) uveitis and photophobia may be followed by corneal opacification. The corneal changes consist of oedema, cellular infiltration and degeneration of the corneal endothelium (Curtis, 1973). The oedema usually starts at the limbus and extends towards the central cornea. It will clear in the same manner and this can be rapid, so

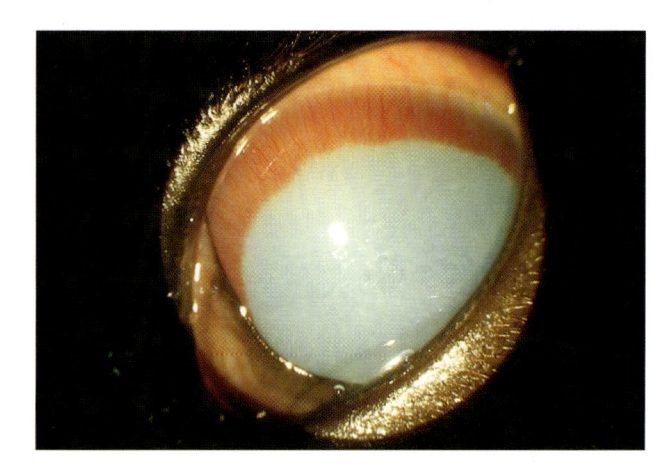

Fig. 9.42 Interstitial keratitis or 'blue eye' resulting from infectious canine adenovirus infection in an Airedale puppy.

cases may present with just a central corneal opacity. However, in some cases the oedema may take months to clear and is dependent on endothelial regeneration. These changes result from virus localising in tissues in the anterior segment, particularly the corneal endothelium, resulting in a type III hypersensitivity reaction. Secondary glaucoma and hydrophthalmos can follow if the condition fails to resolve. In the UK a high incidence of post-vaccination reactions were seen in the Afghan Hound. The diffuse and sudden onset of the corneal oedema seen in this form of interstitial keratitis has been referred to as 'blue eye'.

CORNEAL ABSCESS

Corneal abscess (Fig. 9.43) is an uncommon condition and results from an accumulation of inflammatory cells within the corneal stroma. The lesion is usually focal and yellow in appearance. It may be associated with the placement of sutures. The treatment of choice is a superficial keratectomy.

CORNEAL CYSTS

Cyst formation within the cornea (Fig. 9.44) is a most unusual condition, the aetiology is unknown and a keratectomy is the treatment of choice. The cyst may be superficial or deep and have a translucent 'blister-like' appearance.

CORNEAL INJURIES

See Chapter 3 for a discussion of corneal injuries caused by trauma, foreign bodies and burns (see also Fig. 9.45).

NEOPLASIA

Tumours of the cornea are extremely rare and most are due to secondary extension from limbal or scleral neoplasms

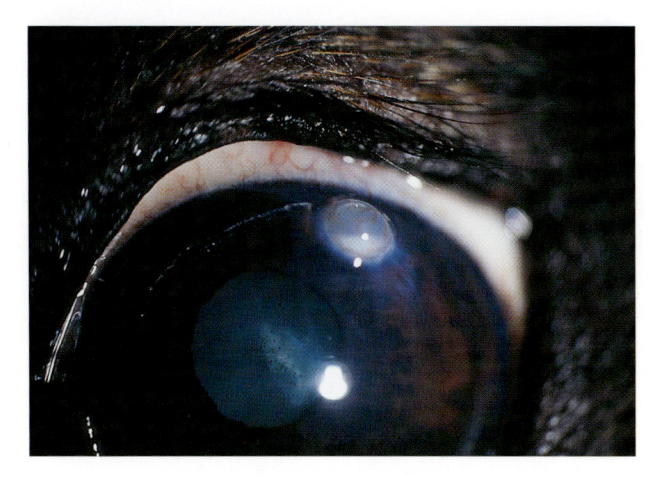

Fig. 9.44 Corneal cyst in a 9-year-old Boxer.

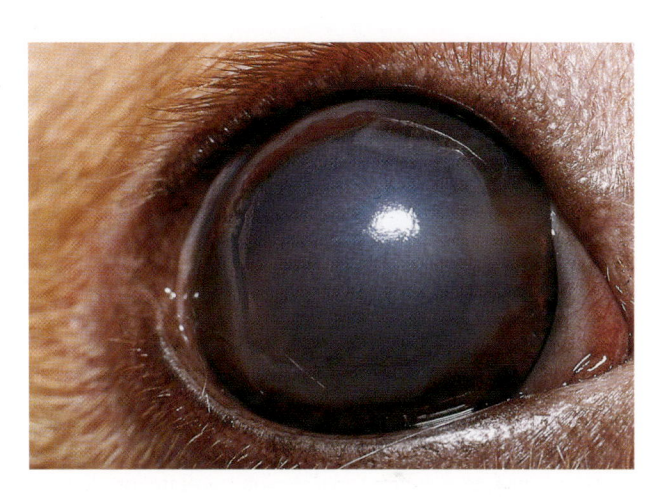

Fig. 9.45 Corneal burn due to washing-up liquid.

(see Chapter 8). Squamous cell carcinomas, fibrosarcomas, haemangiosarcomas and viral papillomas have been reported as primary corneal neoplasms.

REFERENCES

Crispin SM, Barnett KC (1978) Arcus lipoides corneae secondary to hypothyroidism in the Alsatian. *Journal of Small Animal Practice* **19**: 127–142.

Crispin SM, Barnett KC (1983) Dystrophy, degeneration and infiltration of the canine cornea. *Journal of Small Animal Practice* **24**: 63–83.

Curtis R (1973) Clinical and immunopathological aspects of ocular lesions attributable to canine adenovirus. A dissertation submitted to the University of Cambridge for the degree of Doctor of Philosophy.

Stanley RG, Hardman C, Johnson BW (1998) Results of grid keratotomy, superficial keratectomy and debridement for the management of persistent corneal erosions in 92 dogs. *Veterinary Ophthalmology* **1**: 233–238.

Wyman M (1986) *Manual of Small Animal Ophthalmology*, p. 158. Churchill Livingstone, New York.

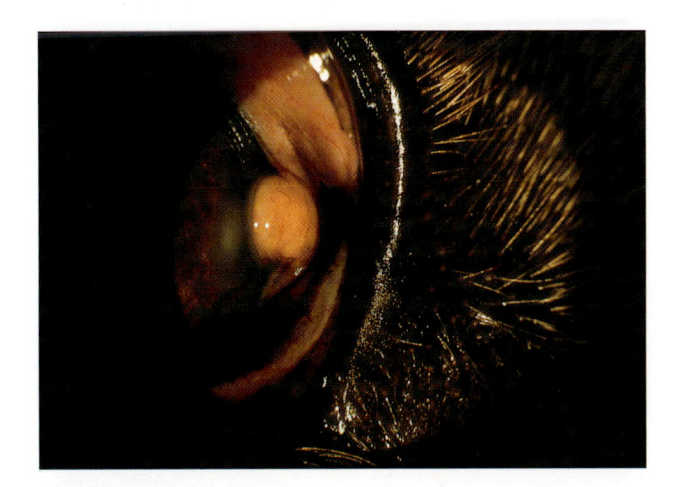

Fig. 9.43 Corneal abscess in a 10-month-old Golden Retriever.

10 GLAUCOMA

INTRODUCTION

Glaucoma is the term used to describe a group of conditions that lead to an increase in intraocular pressure, which eventually damages the retinal ganglion cells and their axons, resulting in vision loss and blindness. The optic nerve head is the structure most susceptible to increases in intraocular pressure and irreversible damage can result within short time spans of ocular hypertension. No single hypothesis has been proposed that adequately explains all changes seen in this complex disease, but it is likely that damage to the optic nerve fibres is due either to pressure-induced vascular disease of the optic nerve or to direct mechanical pressure disturbance of the normal axoplasmic flow (Brooks et al., 1999). Immediate diagnosis and intervention by the veterinary practitioner are required if sight is to be saved, and referral to a veterinary ophthalmologist should be considered. If undiagnosed or inadequately treated, glaucoma will almost inevitably lead to loss of sight and probably the globe.

The intraocular pressure is dependent on the equilibrium of aqueous humour production and drainage. An increase in intraocular pressure above the normal range is the result of a decrease in aqueous humour drainage, as glaucoma due to overproduction of aqueous humour has not been reported in the dog.

The aqueous humour is an optically clear fluid which not only assists in maintaining ocular turgidity but also acts as a nutrient supply and waste disposal system for intraocular structures. Avascular structures such as lens, cornea, trabecular meshwork and vitreous are especially dependent on the aqueous humour for their metabolism. Aqueous humour is formed by the processes of the ciliary body and the vast majority is produced by active secretion from the bilayered ciliary epithelium. Passive secretion in the form of diffusion, osmosis and ultrafiltration is responsible for only a small part of aqueous humour formation (see Chapter 12).

Following thermal convection currents, the aqueous humour passes from the posterior chamber through the pupil into the anterior chamber and there enters the ciliary cleft via the openings between the pectinate ligaments. The ciliary cleft is situated at the iris base within the iridocorneal angle and is filled with the fine trabecular meshwork. The trabecular meshwork is covered with an endothelial layer through which the majority of the aqueous humour leaves the anterior chamber by active vacuolation into scleral collecting vessels. This route of drainage is termed the conventional route and in the dog is responsible for approximately 85% of the total aqueous humour outflow. Glucosaminoglycans (GAGs) and other glycoproteins in the extracellular matrix of the trabecular meshwork are thought to be the major site of aqueous humour outflow resistance, and changes in the GAG composition have been related to increased outflow resistance in Beagles with primary glaucoma (Gum et al., 1993). A small amount of aqueous humour leaves the anterior chamber through a different route from the ciliary cleft via the ciliary body into the suprachoroidal space. This outflow pathway is also termed the unconventional or uveoscleral route and, together with aqueous humour drainage via iris and vitreous, is responsible for approximately 15% of all outflow.

Assessment of the intraocular pressure by indentation (Fig. 10.2) or applanation (Fig. 10.3) tonometry is the only reliable way to diagnose glaucoma (see Chapter 1). Mean intraocular pressures in the dog range from 11 to 29 mmHg and readings may vary depending on the type of tonometer used (Gelatt and MacKay, 1998). Gonioscopy is the visual inspection of the ciliary cleft opening and allows assessment of the pectinate ligaments and the width of the entrance to the ciliary cleft (Bedford, 1973, 1977). A contact lens is required to alter the refractive index of the cornea and both the Koeppe lens and the Lovac–Barkan lens have become established in canine ophthalmology (Fig. 10.3). The gonioscopy lens is applied to the corneal surface after the application of a topical anaesthetic (proxymetacaine hydrochloride) and the

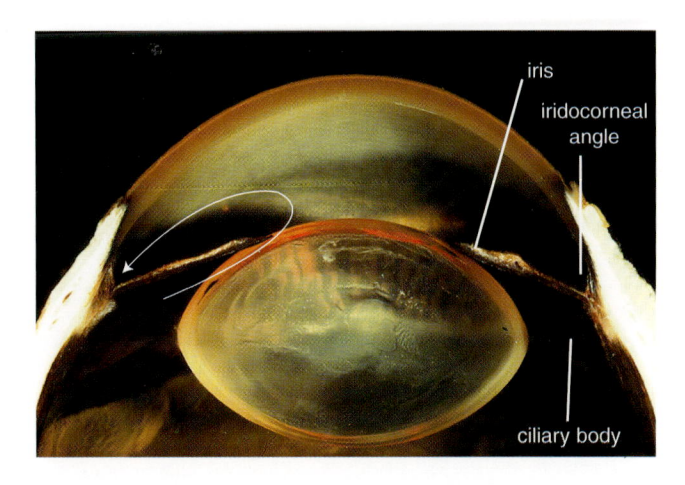

Fig. 10.1 Post-mortem photograph depicting flow of aqueous humour and ciliary body and posterior chamber through pupil into anterior chamber and iridocorneal angle. (Courtesy of JRB Mould.)

GLAUCOMA

iridocorneal angle is inspected with the help of either a slit-lamp biomicroscope, hand-held ophthalmoscope or retinal camera. Gonioscopy is a procedure that requires some expertise and is usually carried out by veterinary ophthalmologists. It is used in screening programmes for glaucoma and for assessment of the contralateral iridocorneal angle in classifying the type of glaucoma presented in clinical cases.

In the normal dog a wide entrance into the ciliary cleft is spanned by fine, more or less branching pectinate ligaments (Fig. 10.5). Varying degrees of dysplasia of the iridocorneal angle have been described for a number of breeds (see below) and partial (Fig. 10.6) or total (Fig. 10.7) closure of the iridocorneal angle can be seen. The iris base can be seen displaced forwards by intumescent diabetic cataracts, ciliary body neoplasia and other conditions, resulting in a narrowed or closed angle, and inflammatory debris may be found in cases of uveitis. Uveal cysts are a rare finding in the iridocorneal angle (Fig. 10.8).

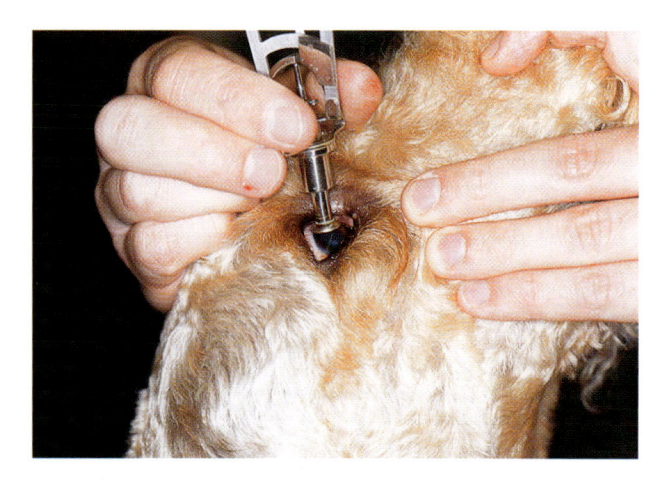

Fig. 10.2 Indentation tonometry with the Schiotz tonometer. This instrument can give reliable intraocular pressure estimations if used correctly and it is important that whilst the cornea is in a horizontal position care is taken to avoid pressure on the jugular veins.

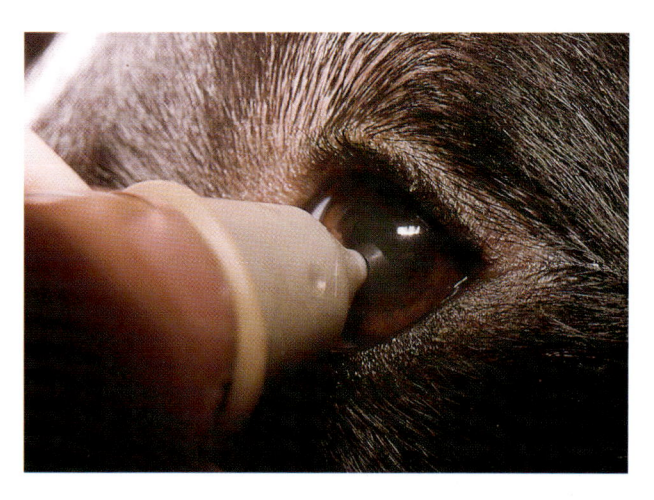

Fig. 10.3 Applanation tonometry with the TonoPen tonometer.

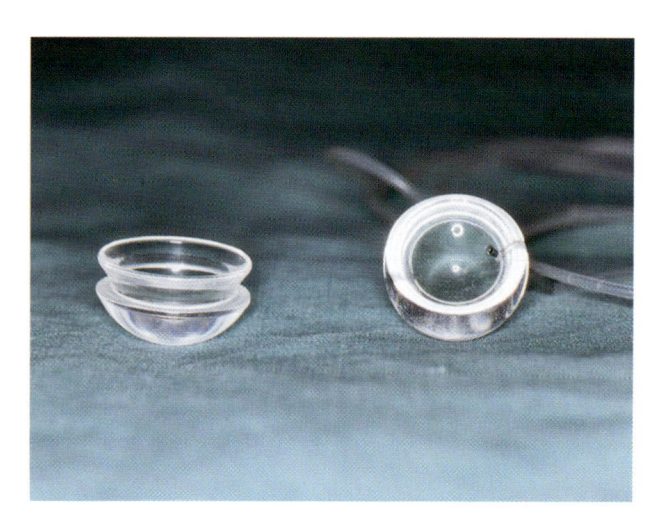

Fig. 10.4 Koeppe and Barkan gonioscopy lenses.

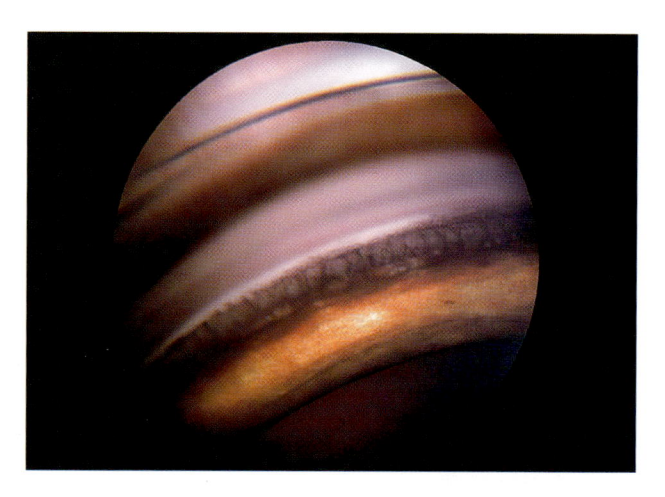

Fig. 10.5 Gonioscopic view of the normal iridocorneal angle. Note the fine branching pectinate ligaments and the wide spaces giving access to the ciliary cleft.

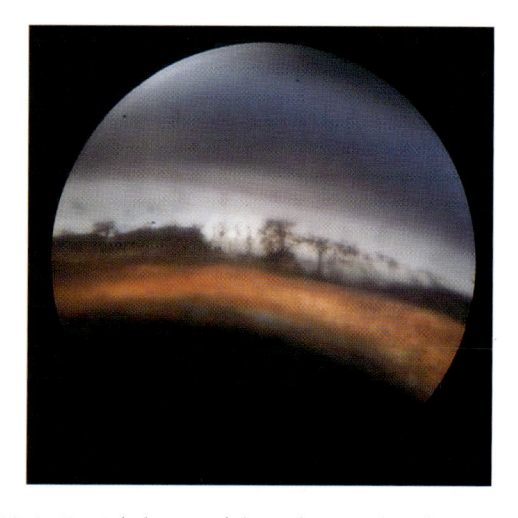

Fig. 10.6 Partial closure of the iridocorneal angle in a Welsh Springer Spaniel (goniophotograph).

CLINICAL SIGNS

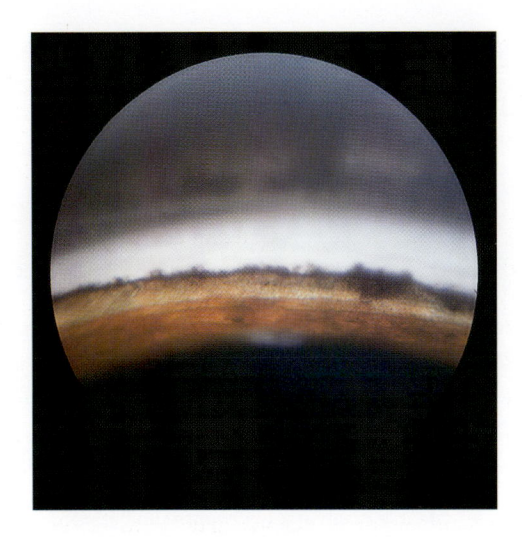

Fig. 10.7 Total closure of the iridocorneal angle in a Walsh Springer Spaniel (goniophotograph).

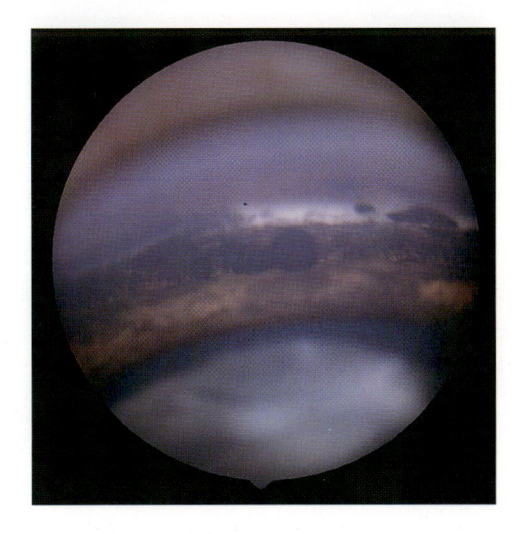

Fig. 10.8 Uveal cysts in the iridocorneal angle.

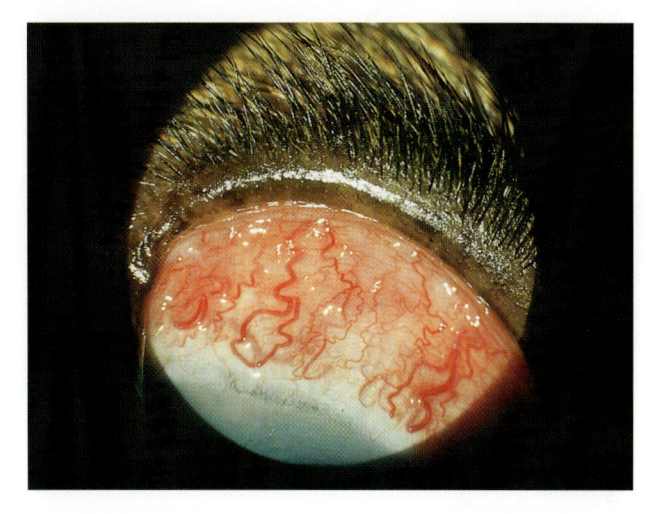

Fig. 10.9 Acute-onset glaucoma with corneal oedema and episcleral congestion.

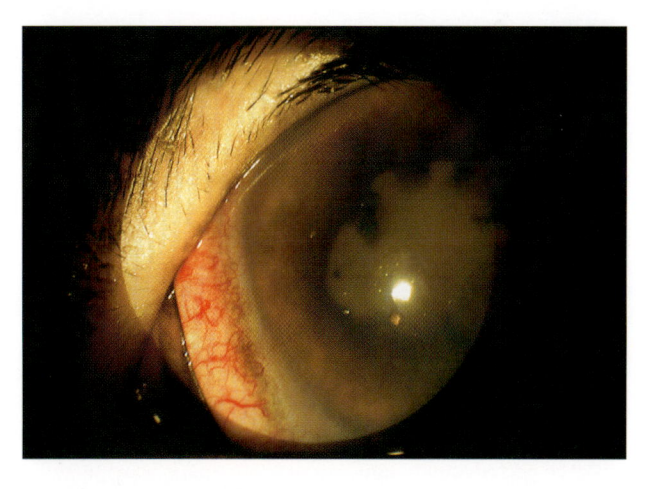

Fig. 10.10 Extensive posterior synechiae as the result of chronic uveitis in a Japanese Akita.

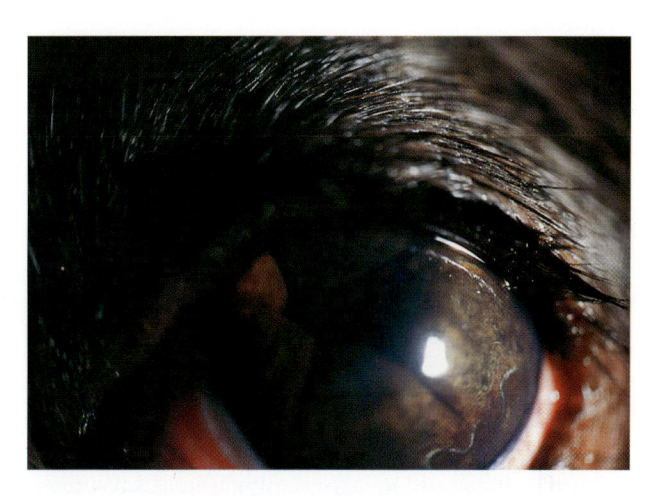

Fig. 10.11 Iris bombé formation as the result of total posterior synechiae.

Clinical signs

Clinical signs of glaucoma may be unspecific and vary according to whether the condition is acute or chronic. Pain, sometimes severe, with epiphora, blepharospasm and third eyelid prominence (see Fig. 6.1), is one of the most obvious features of acute onset glaucoma and is often accompanied by episcleral congestion, corneal oedema and a widely dilated pupil (Fig. 10.9). Pupil size is, however, not a reliable diagnostic feature as an episode of increased intraocular pressure and pupillary dilation may be followed by a sudden drop in intraocular pressure, anterior chamber flare and a more or less miotic pupil. Miotic pupils with extensive posterior synechiae can also be seen in glaucoma induced by uveitis (Fig. 10.10) and iris bombé formation (Fig. 10.11). Chronically affected and hydrophthalmic eyes are often apparently pain free (Fig. 10.12). Subluxated or luxated

101

GLAUCOMA

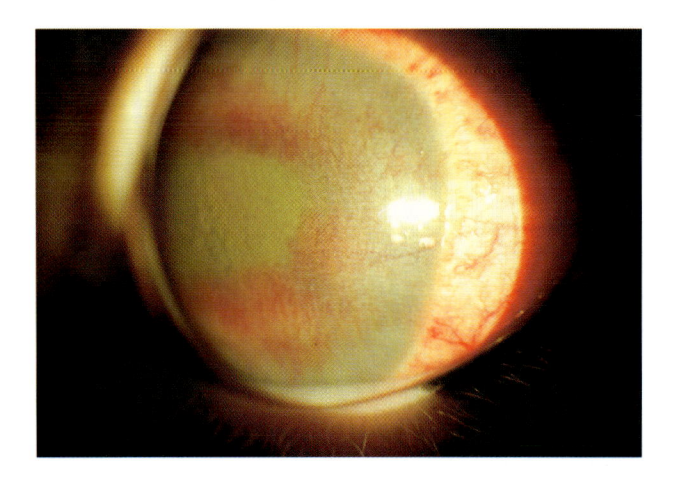

Fig. 10.12 Chronically glaucomatous globe.

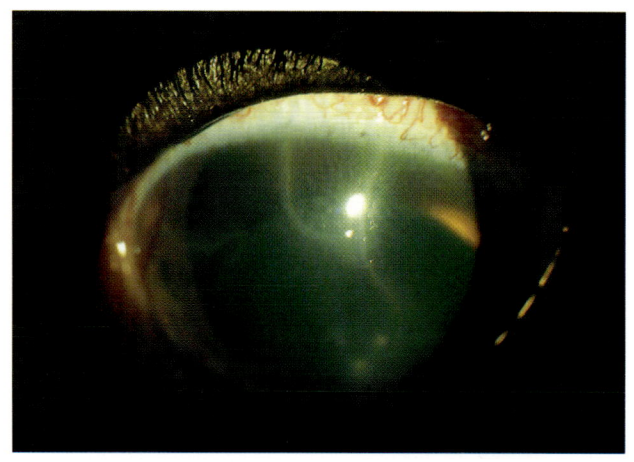

Fig. 10.14 Haab's striae in a hydrophthalmic globe.

lenses are common in these cases and are usually the result of zonular breakdown during globe enlargement (Fig. 10.13). Ruptures in Descemet's membrane result in linear corneal oedema, which is visible to the examiner as Haab's striae (Figs 10.14 and 4.20) and fundus examination reveals varying degrees of optic nerve atrophy and attenuation of the retinal vessels. The combined effect of nerve fibre loss and excavation of the scleral lamina cribrosa is clinically seen as optic disc cupping (Fig. 10.15) and may be more obvious on post-mortem examination (Fig. 10.16). Retinal necrosis can occur within 24 hours of an initial glaucoma attack and bands of hyperreflective tapetum radiating from the optic disc to the periphery are early signs of retinal atrophy in glaucoma (Fig. 10.17). These hyperreflective bands are described as watershed lesions and are due to pressure-induced circulation deficits in the choroidal vasculature. With time, the changes affect the whole retina and generalised hyperreflectivity and vascular attenuation are seen.

The degree of vision loss does not necessarily correlate simply with the duration of the disease but also with the

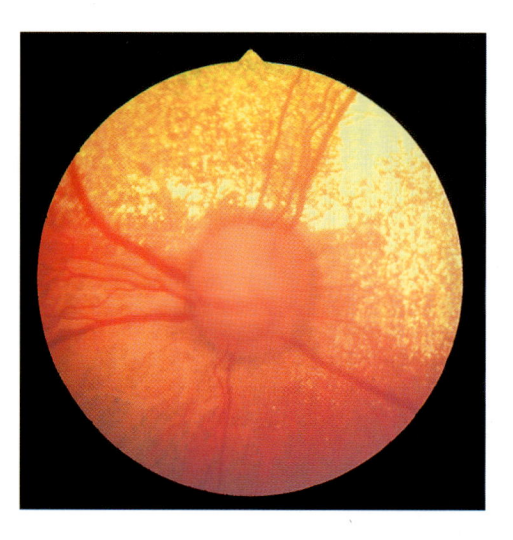

Fig. 10.15 Optic disc cupping as the result of sustained ocular hypertension. (Courtesy of JRB Mould.)

severity of the rise in intraocular pressure. Whereas some hydrophthalmic eyes with extensive optic cupping may retain sight, others are blind after an initial dramatic rise in intraocular pressure that has only been sustained for a relatively short time span. Hydrophthalmic eyes are prone to the development of corneal ulceration due to lagophthalmos (see Fig. 10.13). Phthisis bulbi can be the end result in chronic glaucoma and is usually due to pressure atrophy of the ciliary body processes (Fig. 10.18).

CLASSIFICATION

There are a number of classifications dividing glaucoma into different groups according to their aetiology. The most commonly used classification divides between congenital, primary and secondary glaucoma. Congenital glaucoma is rare in the dog and is usually related to the presence of anterior segment dysgenesis. Due to the much lower scleral rigidity in the neonate, globe enlargement is often rapid (see

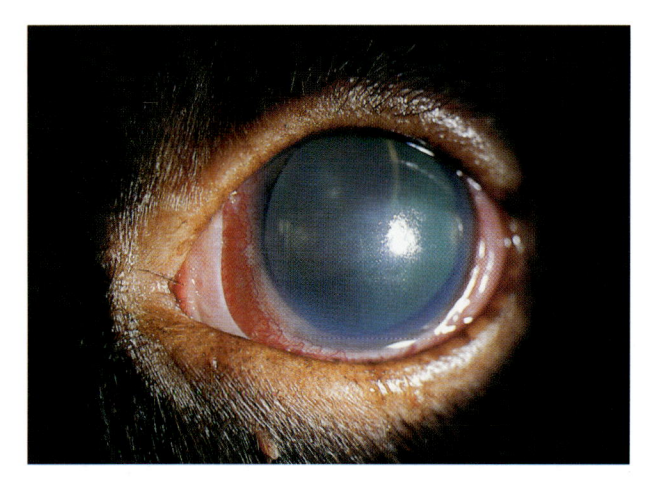

Fig. 10.13 Subluxated lens secondary to hydrophthalmos in chronic glaucoma. Note the broken specular reflection indicating corneal epithelial irregularities.

CLASSIFICATION

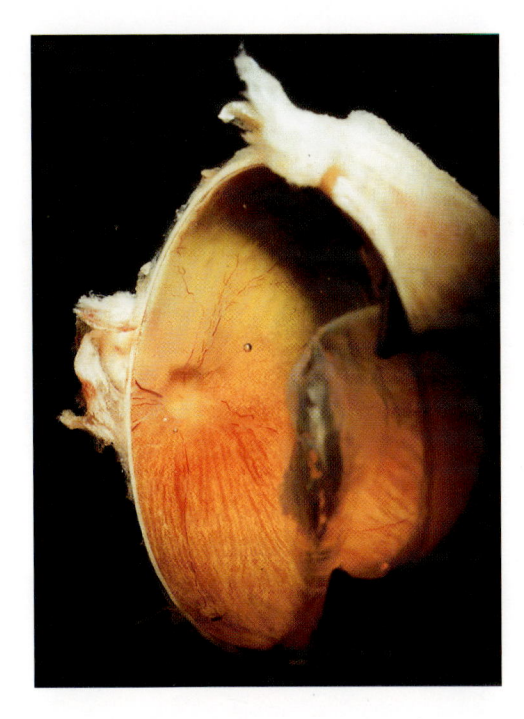

Fig. 10.16 Optic disc cupping on post-mortem examination, same dog as in Fig. 10.15. (Courtesy of JRB Mould.)

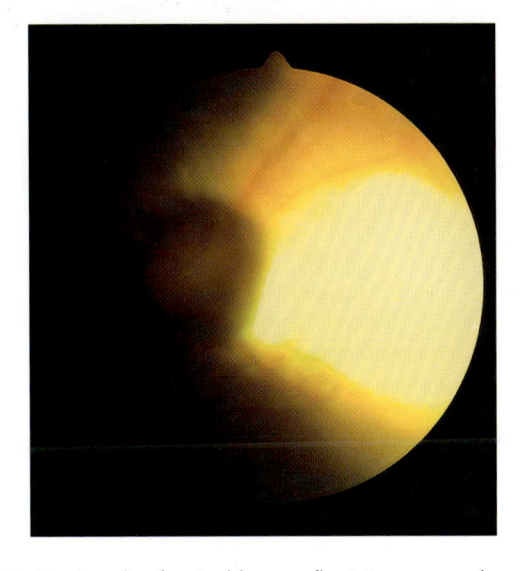

Fig. 10.17 Bands of retinal hyperreflectivity seen as the result of intraocular pressure effects on choroidal vasculature.

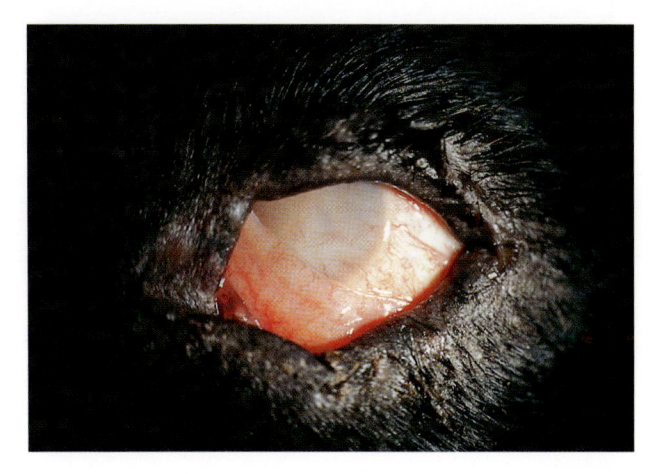

Fig. 10.18 Phthisis bulbi as the end-stage result of chronic glaucoma.

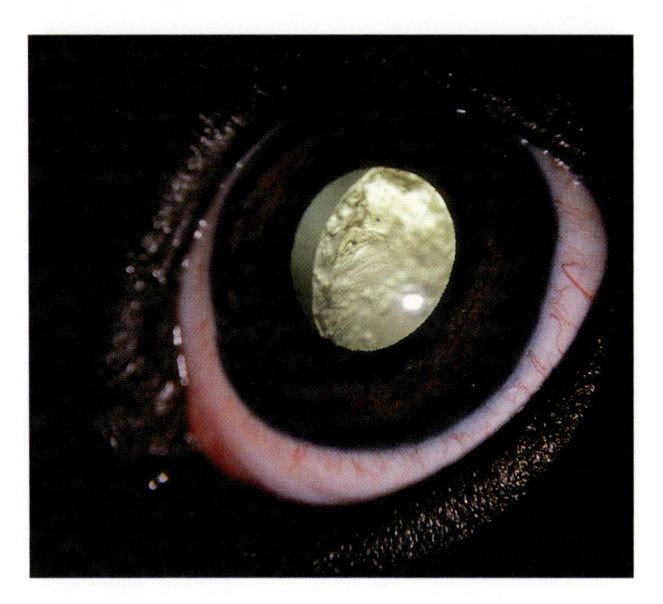

Fig. 10.19 Congenital glaucoma with microphakia and cataract formation in a 16-week-old Boxer puppy.

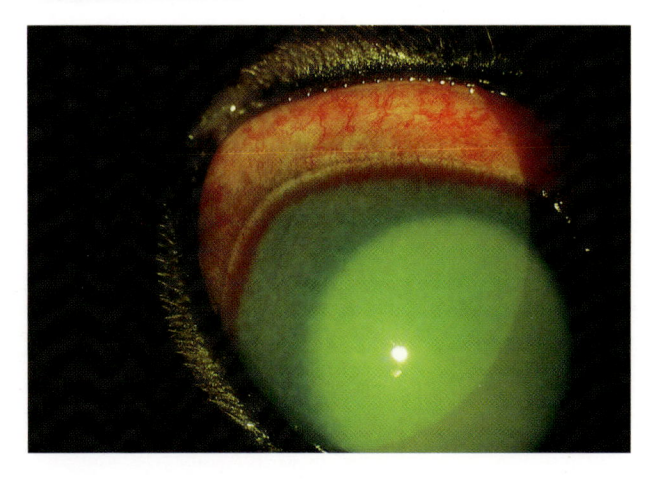

Fig. 10.20 Closed-angle primary glaucoma in a Welsh Springer Spaniel. Note dilated pupil, corneal oedema and fine vascular fringe and episcleral congestion.

Fig. 4.19). The elasticity of the young globe can have a protective effect on the retina and the optic nerve head and even dramatically enlarged globes often retain sight. Additional ocular abnormalities may be seen (Fig. 10.19).

PRIMARY

Primary glaucoma is not related to the presence of antecedent or concurrent ocular disease and is subdivided into open-angle glaucoma and glaucoma due to goniodysgenesis (Fig. 10.20). Open-angle glaucoma is rare in the dog although it is the most common form of glaucoma in man. Cases of canine open-angle glaucoma are only sporadically seen in the UK but the condition is thought to be inherited in the Norwegian Elkhound. Open-angle glaucoma has been extensively researched in a strain of laboratory Beagles in the USA (Peiffer and Gelatt, 1980).

Goniodysgenesis is the most common cause of primary glaucoma in dogs in the UK and has been shown to be inherited in a number of breeds in the UK, including the American Cocker Spaniel, Basset Hound, English Cocker Spaniel, Welsh Springer Spaniel, Siberian Husky, Great Dane and Flat-coated Retriever. Dogs affected with goniodysgenesis have abnormalities in the appearance of their iridocorneal angle with irregular-shaped or imperforated pectinate ligaments (see Fig. 10.6). In severe cases of goniodysgenesis the pectinate ligament forms a complete sheath across the iridocorneal angle and aqueous humour drainage is limited to small areas where flow holes are present (see Fig. 10.7). Although usually both eyes are affected, the abnormalities are not necessarily symmetrical. In breeds shown to be affected with goniodysgenesis, studies have shown that individuals with severe degrees of pectinate ligament dysplasia are more susceptible to develop glaucoma than other individuals of the same breed (Read *et al.*, 1998; Wood *et al.*, 1998).

SECONDARY

Secondary glaucoma is the most common form of glaucoma seen in the dog (Smith *et al.*, 1993). It is the result of antecedent or concurrent ocular disease which results in the obstruction of flow of aqueous humour from the posterior chamber to the scleral venous plexus whilst aqueous humour production is maintained. The obstruction may occur at the pupillary opening or at the level of the iridocorneal angle and in some globes flow of aqueous humour is impaired in both places. Many causes of secondary glaucoma in the dog are known and include primary lens luxation, uveitis, neoplasia, intumescent cataract, pre-iridal fibrovascular membrane formation, abnormal pigment deposition and vitreal prolapse and herniation.

Primary lens luxation is a common cause of secondary glaucoma in the terrier breeds (see Chapter 11) and has also been described in the Border Collie and the Shar Pei (Lazarus *et al.*, 1998). It is often the luxation of the lens into the anterior chamber which drags vitreous through the pupil and into the filtration angle because of the aqueous flow, so impeding the normal aqueous humour flow and leading to a very sudden rise in intraocular pressure. However, increases in intraocular pressure are also seen before the lens luxates fully as the chronic lens instability and lentodonesis can compromise the ciliary cleft and can be accompanied by vitreal degeneration and prolapse into the anterior chamber through areas of ruptured zonular fibres (Figs 10.21 and 10.22). Vitreous in the anterior chamber can block flow of aqueous humour through the pupillary aperture or by obstructing the iridocorneal angle. Slit-lamp examination can reveal lentodonesis and strands of vitreous in the anterior chamber can be highlighted with the slit beam (Fig. 10.23). It is not always possible to determine whether the lens luxation is secondary or primary and examination of the fellow eye, including gonioscopy, can give valuable information in these cases. Another helpful finding is the position of a subluxated lens – whereas subluxated lenses in primary lens luxation have a tendency to displace more ventrally it is often seen that subluxated lenses in hydrophthalmic eyes are positioned in the dorsal part of the pupillary opening (see Fig. 10.13) or in the centre of the pupil with a penumbra. Further information of assistance in diagnosis are the age and breed of the dog.

Glaucoma as the result of lens pathology can also be seen in lens-induced uveitis with hypermature cataracts and pre-iridal fibrovascular membrane formation (Peiffer *et al.*, 1990) or as the result of a traumatic or spontaneous rupture of the lens capsule resulting in a phacoclastic uveitis (Figs 10.24 and 10.25). Intumescent cataracts, especially those of sudden onset as in diabetic patients, can obstruct the ciliary cleft as the swollen lens pushes onto the iris base and causes

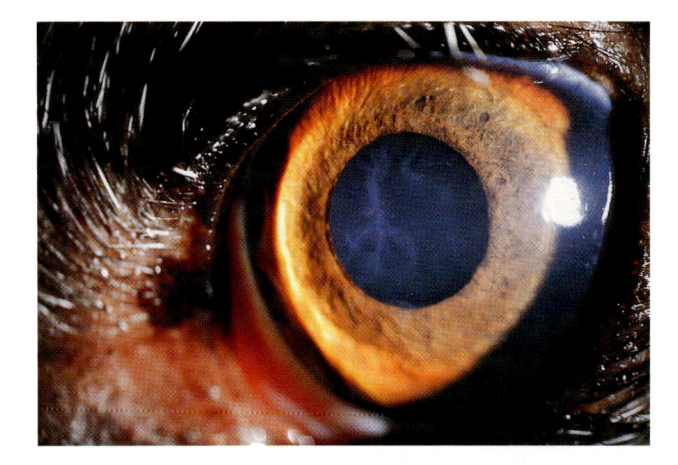

Fig. 10.21 Vitreal strands in the anterior chamber.

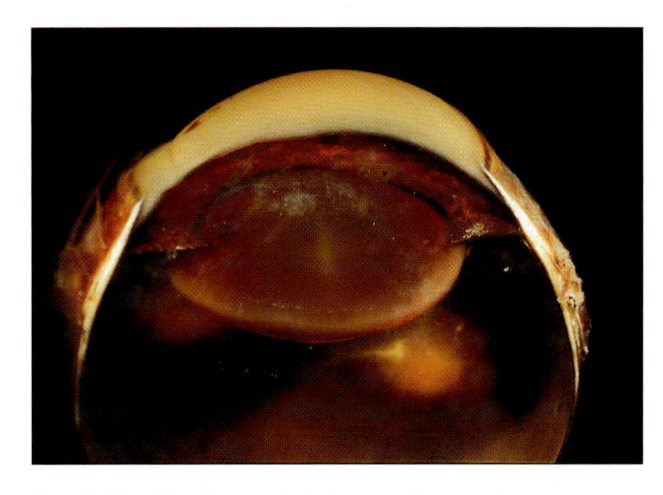

Fig. 10.22 Vitreal strands in the anterior chamber on post-mortem examination. (Courtesy of JRB Mould.)

CLASSIFICATION

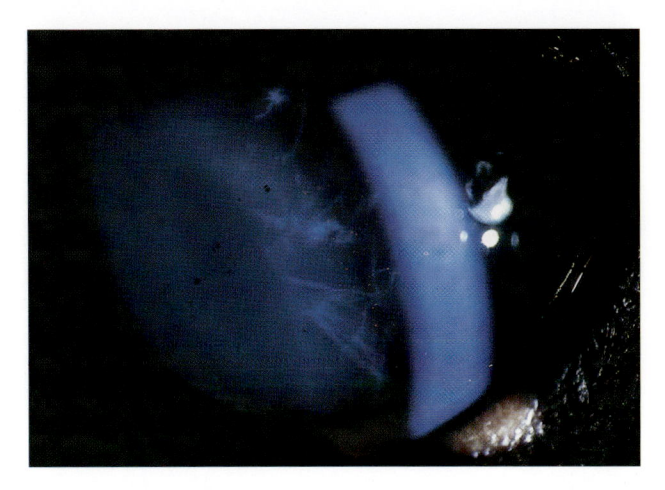

Fig. 10.23 Herniated vitreous in the anterior chamber visible through the Tyndall phenomenon on examination with the slit-lamp biomicroscope, same dog as in Fig. 10.21.

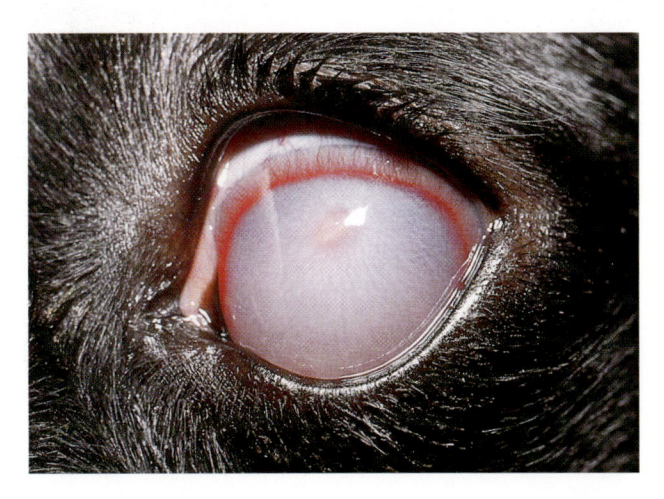

Fig. 10.24 Phacoclastic uveitis with glaucoma as the result of an anterior lens capsule rupture following a cat scratch injury. Note the site of corneal perforation and the peripheral corneal vascularisation.

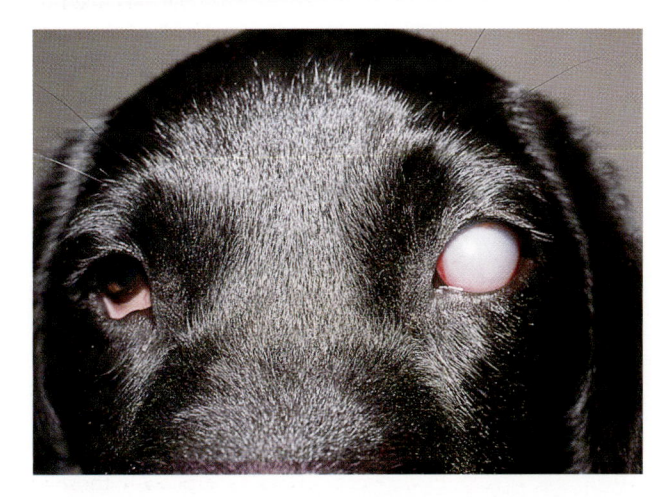

Fig. 10.25 Same dog as in Fig. 10.24 showing the degree of hydrophthalmos.

acute-onset glaucoma. Slit-lamp examination in this case will reveal an extremely shallow anterior chamber and peripheral anterior synechiae.

Uveitis may result in secondary glaucoma through a number of mechanisms including obstruction of the ciliary cleft with pre-iridal fibrovascular membranes, inflammatory cells, haemorrhage, fibrin and formation of peripheral anterior or posterior synechiae (see Fig. 10.10). Iris bombé formation is the result of impediment of the aqueous humour flow from the posterior chamber through the pupil by extensive posterior synechia formation. As a result, aqueous accumulates in the posterior chamber, leading to forward billowing of the iris with eventual total obstruction of the ciliary cleft (see Fig. 10.11). Only immediate and aggressive treatment with anti-inflammatories and pharmacological agents to mobilise the pupil may be able to prevent the onset of glaucoma. A severe and sudden-onset form of uveitis-induced glaucoma in association with ciliary body cyst formation has been reported in the Golden Retriever (Fig. 10.26) (Deehr and Dubielzig, 1998).

Acute-onset glaucoma is not uncommonly the presenting sign of ocular neoplasia and can be the result of occlusion of the iridocorneal angle by forward displacement of the iris, obliteration of the ciliary cleft by invasion or by the formation of pre-iridal fibrovascular membranes (Peiffer et al., 1990). Uveal melanomas, lymphoma and ciliary body tumours are common primary intraocular neoplasms, but metastatic spread of distant primary lesions must also be considered. Ocular ultrasound examination is mandatory in cases of unexplained intraocular pressure elevations if examination of intraocular detail is not possible due to the presence of corneal oedema.

Ocular melanosis is a rare condition that has been described in the Cairn Terrier (Petersen-Jones, 1991). Similar to pigmentary glaucoma in man, melanin is found to accumulate in the anterior segment of affected dogs and eventually also leads to occlusion of the aqueous humour outflow pathways. Pigmentation has also been reported in the retina

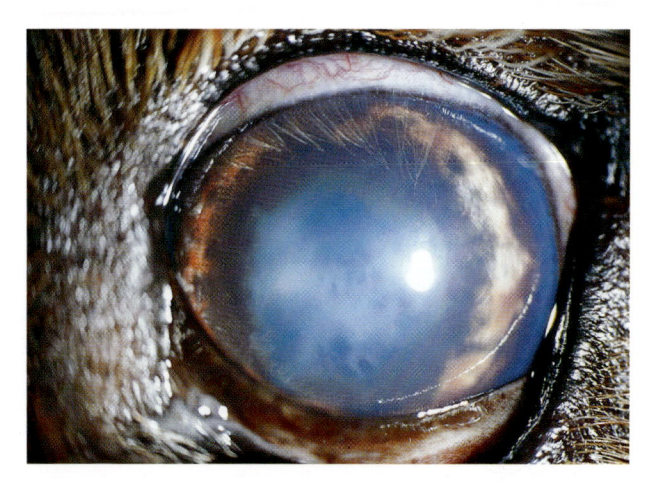

Fig. 10.26 Glaucoma and uveitis in a 6-year-old Golden Retriever. Ocular histopathology did not reveal the presence of ciliary body cysts in this case.

GLAUCOMA

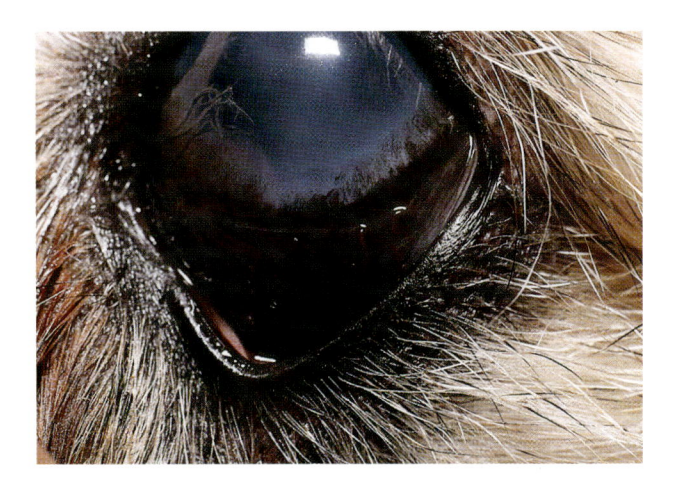

Fig. 10.27 Ocular melanosis in a Cairn Terrier. Note accumulation of pigment in the ventral sclera and corneal oedema. (Courtesy of PW Renwick.)

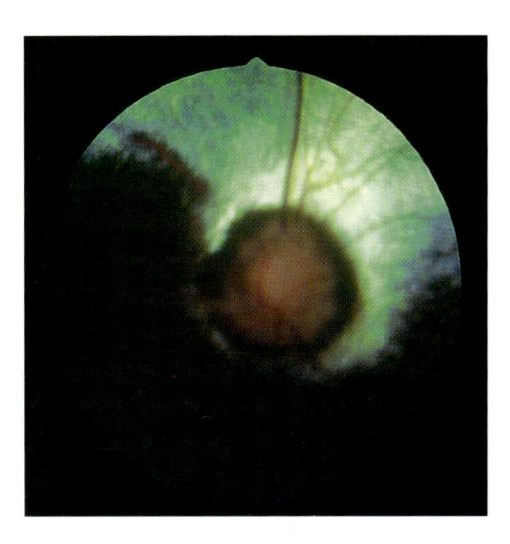

Fig. 10.28 Advanced optic disc cupping and vascular attenuation in chronic glaucoma associated with ocular melanosis in a Cairn Terrier.

of affected dogs. The aetiology of the condition remains unknown. Melanin accumulation in sclera and peripheral cornea can be remarkable and diagnosis is usually based on the pathognomonic clinical presentation (Figs 10.27 and 10.28).

TREATMENT

Treatment of glaucoma in the dog is one of the most difficult challenges encountered in veterinary ophthalmology and acute elevations in intraocular pressure are always an emergency requiring immediate intervention. Unlike in man, where primary open-angle glaucoma is the most common form of glaucoma seen, glaucoma in dogs is usually associated with angle closure and medical therapy alone is rarely successful in these cases. Even with the event of new agents for topical treatment such as prostaglandin analogues (latanoprost) and topical carbonic anhydrase inhibitors (dorzolamide and brinzolamide), surgical intervention in the form of laser transscleral cyclophotocoagulation (Cook *et al.*, 1997) and drainage implant procedures (Cook, 1997) should be considered. The introduction of cytostatic agents (Glover *et al.*, 1995; Tinsley *et al.*, 1995) gives further hope for better long-term success for the maintenance of safe intraocular pressure levels.

It has also become well recognised that damage to the retinal cells, and especially the optic nerve head, does not stop with the reduction in intraocular pressure but that the release of excitotoxic substances such as glutamate from dying retinal cells will continue to lead to axon destruction even after normal pressure levels are established (Brooks *et al.*, 1997). For this reason it is evident that lowering and maintaining intraocular pressure to a safe and acceptable level is not the only aspect of treatment for this condition, but that optic nerve neuroprotection may also be of importance (Brooks *et al.*, 1999).

See also Appendix IV for a table of drugs to be used for the symptomatic treatment of glaucoma.

REFERENCES

Bedford PG (1973) A practical method of gonioscopy and goniophotography in the dog and cat. *Journal of Small Animal Practice* **14**: 601–606.

Bedford PG (1977) Gonioscopy in the dog. *Journal of Small Animal Practice* **18**: 615–629.

Brooks DE, Garcia GA, Dreyer EB, Zurakowski D, Franco-Bourland RE (1997) Vitreous body glutamate concentration in dogs with glaucoma. *American Journal of Veterinary Research* **58**: 864–867.

Brooks DE, Komaromy AM, Kallberg ME (1999) Comparative optic nerve physiology: implications for glaucoma, neuroprotection, and neuroregeneration. *Veterinary Ophthalmology* **2**: 13–25.

Cook CS (1997) Surgery for glaucoma. *Veterinary Clinics of North America Small Animal Practice* **27**: 1109–1129.

Cook C, Davidson M, Brinkmann M, Priehs D, Abrams K, Nasisse M (1997) Diode laser transscleral cyclophotocoagulation for the treatment of glaucoma in dogs: results of six and twelve month follow-up. *Veterinary and Comparative Ophthalmology* **7**: 148–154.

Deehr AJ, Dubielzig RR (1998) A histopathological study of iridociliary cysts and glaucoma in Golden Retrievers. *Veterinary Ophthalmology* **1**: 153–158.

Gelatt KN, MacKay EO (1998) Distribution of intraocular pressure in dogs. *Veterinary Ophthalmology* **1**: 109–114.

Glover TL, Nasisse MP, Davidson MG (1995) Effects of topically applied mitomycin-C on intraocular pressure, facility of outflow, and fibrosis after glaucoma filtration surgery in clinically normal dogs [published erratum appears in *Am J Vet Res* 1995 **56**(11): 1533]. *American Journal of Veterinary Research* **56**: 936–940.

Gum GG, Gelatt KN, Knepper PA (1993) Histochemical localization of glycosaminoglycans in the aqueous outflow pathways in normal Beagles and Beagles with inherited glaucoma. *Progress in Veterinary and Comparative Ophthalmology* **3**: 52–57.

Lazarus JA, Pickett JP, Champagne ES (1998) Primary lens luxation in the Chinese Shar Pei: clinical and hereditary characteristics. *Veterinary Ophthalmology* **1**: 101–107.

REFERENCES

Peiffer RL Jr, Gelatt KN (1980) Aqueous humor outflow in Beagles with inherited glaucoma: gross and light microscopic observations of the iridocorneal angle. *American Journal of Veterinary Research* **41**: 861–867.

Peiffer RL Jr, Wilcock BP, Yin H (1990) The pathogenesis and significance of preiridal fibrovascular membrane in domestic animals. *Veterinary Pathology* **27**: 41–45.

Petersen-Jones SM (1991) Abnormal ocular pigment deposition associated with glaucoma in the Cairn Terrier. *Journal of Small Animal Practice* **32**: 19–22.

Read RA, Wood JLN, Lakhani KH (1998) Pectinate ligament dysplasia (PLD) and glaucoma in flat coated retrievers. I. Objectives, technique and results of a PLD survey. *Veterinary Ophthalmology* **1**: 85–90.

Smith RIE, Peiffer RL, Wilcock BP (1993) Some aspects of the pathology of canine glaucoma. *Progress in Veterinary and Comparative Ophthalmology* **3**: 16–28.

Tinsley DM, Niyo Y, Tinsley LM, Betts DM (1995) In vivo clinical trial of perioperative mitomycin-C in combination with a drainage device implantation in normal canine globes. *Veterinary and Comparative Ophthalmology* **5**: 231–241.

Wood JLN, Lakhani KH, Read RA (1998) Pectinate ligament dysplasia and glaucoma in flat coated retrievers. II. Assessment of prevalence and heritability. *Veterinary Ophthalmology* **1**: 91–99.

11 LENS

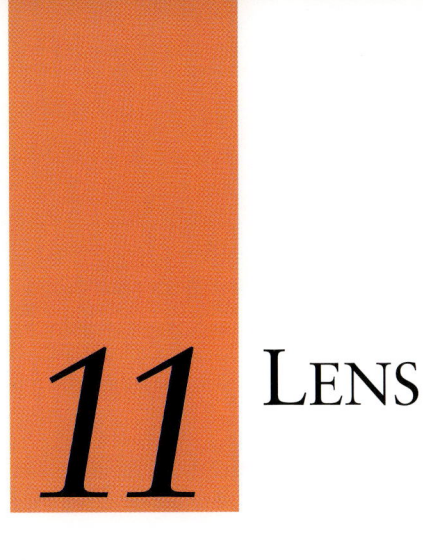

INTRODUCTION

The crystalline lens is a biconvex, transparent, avascular, refractive structure consisting of a nucleus (embryonic, fetal and adult), cortex and capsule suspended by many and dense zonular ligaments, attached to the capsule and connecting the ciliary body with the lens equator. With mydriasis and magnification these zonular fibres are visible in life. In the dog both lens surfaces have a similar curvature; the lens size varies from 9 to 11.5 mm in diameter, 7 mm thick from anterior to posterior surfaces and the volume is 0.5 ml. Anteriorly the iris rests on, and is supported by, the anterior lens surface, and posteriorly the lens is set into the fossa patellaris, a depression in the anterior vitreous. There is firm attachment between posterior capsule and vitreous, an important factor in lens luxation, particularly anterior luxation.

The lens is composed mainly of hexagonal fibres which increase in number with age as the lens nucleus increases in size and density. The primary lens fibres differentiate from the posterior epithelial cells and the secondary lens fibres by division from the anterior epithelial cells, the former during lens development and the latter during the life of the animal. The secondary fibres stretch from the anterior to the posterior cortex. The suture lines are sheets of amorphous material to which the ends of the fibres are attached. The anterior sutures are in the form of a 'Y-shaped' pattern and the posterior ones in the posterior cortex as an inverted 'Y'. These suture lines are an important site for the formation of some cataracts; they can be detected with careful examination in the live animal and are more apparent in some than others. It is important to note that the confluence of the suture lines is not where the hyaloid artery, or remnant, attaches to the posterior capsule, but to one side.

The elastic lens capsule varies considerably in thickness, the posterior capsule being thinner than the anterior and thinnest at the posterior pole. Beneath the anterior capsule is a single layer of epithelial cells, thickest at the equator and absent from beneath the posterior capsule except during early development.

The adult lens has no blood supply and nutrition is mainly via the aqueous which bathes the anterior face of the lens, less via the vitreous. Accommodation is the change in the refractive power (approximately 40 dioptres in the dog) to focus light onto the retina; it is poorly developed in the dog and reduces with age as the lens hardens; change in the lens shape is due to contraction of the ciliary body muscles and is also dependent upon the elasticity of the capsule.

The lens is derived from surface ectoderm which, with the optic vesicle, forms the lens placode, occurring early in embryogenesis. Invagination of the lens placode forms a hollow lens vesicle which is initially filled with primary lens fibres, the future embryonic lens nucleus in which sutures are absent. The secondary fibres differentiate from epithelial cells at the lens equator after birth, a process which continues throughout life. During development the hyaloid artery and the tunica vasculosa lentis supply the lens. It is remnants of both these vascular structures which may persist into adult life.

Nuclear sclerosis of the lens occurs in all dogs from the age of about 7 years, increasing in density with age. It is a normal ageing change and not a cataract – it is not an opacity. Sclerosis appears clinically as a bluish-white opalescence with the edge of the nucleus more apparent. It is due to lens fibre formation occurring throughout life causing compression of the older fibres in the nucleus (Figs 11.1 and 11.2).

Disorders of the lens can be classified into congenital anomalies, cataract and luxation.

CONGENITAL ANOMALIES

Aphakia (complete absence of the lens) is very rare but has been recorded in the dog associated with microphthalmos. Microphakia (small lens) is also rare but has been reported in cases of multiocular defects (MOD) and persistent hyperplastic primary vitreous (PHPV). Spherophakia (spherically-shaped lens) has been reported with abnormality of the

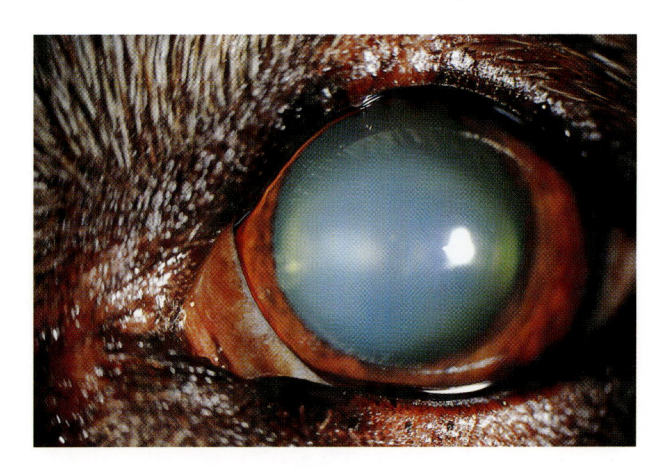

Fig. 11.1 Senile nuclear sclerosis.

LENS

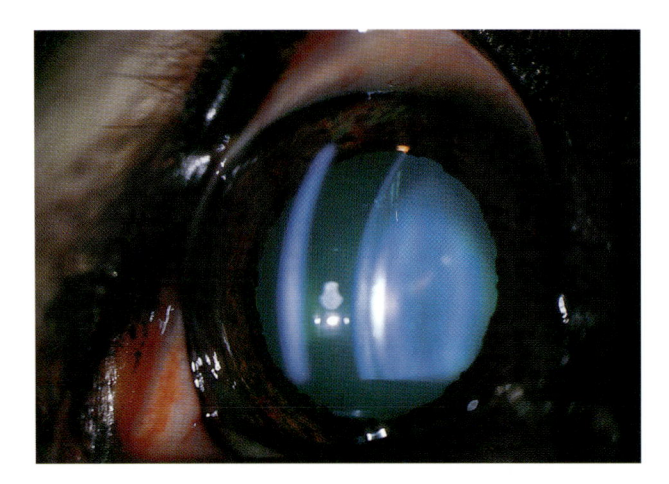

Fig. 11.2 Senile nuclear sclerosis (slit-lamp photograph).

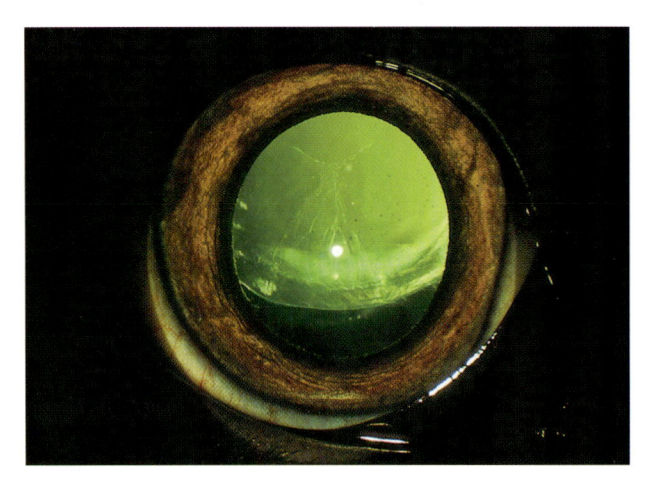

Fig. 11.3 Typical lens coloboma with partial cataract in a German Shepherd Dog.

ciliary processes. Lens colobomas appear as a notch or flattening of the lens equator and may be in the typical (ventral) or atypical position; they may also be associated with coloboma of the uvea and with partial cataract (Fig. 11.3).

Lenticonus (see Figs 11.26 and 11.27) and the more severe lentiglobus (deformities of the lens surface with resultant protrusion) may occur as a sporadic condition or together with hereditary microphthalmos and cataract in the Miniature Schnauzer and hereditary PHPV in the Dobermann.

Abnormalities, in particular persistence of the embryonic vascular supply of the lens, may involve the lens, e.g. persistent pupillary membranes and persistent hyaloid artery (see Chapters 12 and 13).

CATARACT

Cataract is simply defined as an opacity of the lens (capsule, cortex, nucleus) – the definition of 'opacity' is more difficult. Cataract is a common eye condition in the dog – many cataracts are inherited in this species (primary cataract), unlike the cat but similar to the human; several are associated with another eye condition (secondary cataracts); some are associated with systemic disease; some still have an unknown aetiology.

Cataract may be classified in many ways including the following:

- *Aetiology* – congenital (developmental); hereditary; secondary to another eye disease; metabolic; traumatic; toxic; dietary.
- *Age of onset* – juvenile (often incorrectly implies primary hereditary types); senile.
- *Location within the lens* – capsular; subcapsular; cortical; perinuclear; nuclear; equatorial; polar (axial); suture-line. May be further subdivided into anterior and posterior, e.g. cortical, polar.
- *Appearance* – wedge-shaped; vacuolar; spoke; stellate; punctate; purverulent (steelwool-like appearance, particularly of the nucleus) (Fig. 11.4).
- *Stage of progression or development* – incipient (early with no effect on vision); immature (tapetal reflex still visible); mature or complete (whole lens involved with no tapetal reflex visible); hypermature (resorption of lens material through capsule leading to decrease in size of lens with a flatter anterior surface, therefore an increase in anterior chamber depth, wrinkled capsule, often with metallic-like particles, areas of clearing with visible tapetal reflex in parts and a return of some, often useful, vision (Figs 11.5–11.7). During cataract development the immature and mature stages may imbibe fluid leading to a larger lens with clearer clefts particularly along the suture lines – known as intumescence. Resorption usually occurs in younger dogs. A Morgagnian cataract is a type of hypermature cataract in which the dense remains of the nucleus sink to a ventral position in a fluid cortex within the capsule. The leakage of lens material often leads to a usually mild uveitis with resultant darkened iris and possibly uveal cysts around the pupillary border and even posterior synechiae.

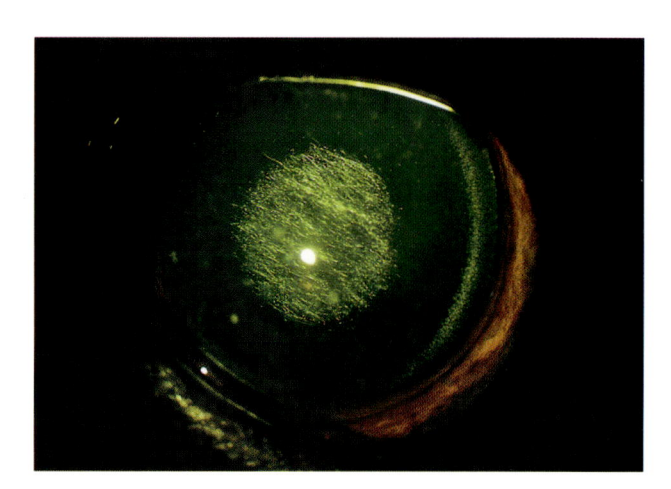

Fig. 11.4 Purverulent cataract.

CATARACT

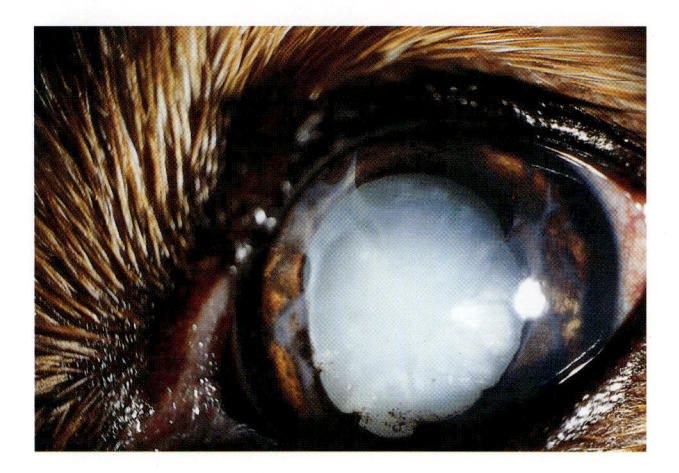

Fig. 11.5 Hypermature cataract. Note escape of lens material and posterior synechiae around 6 o'clock.

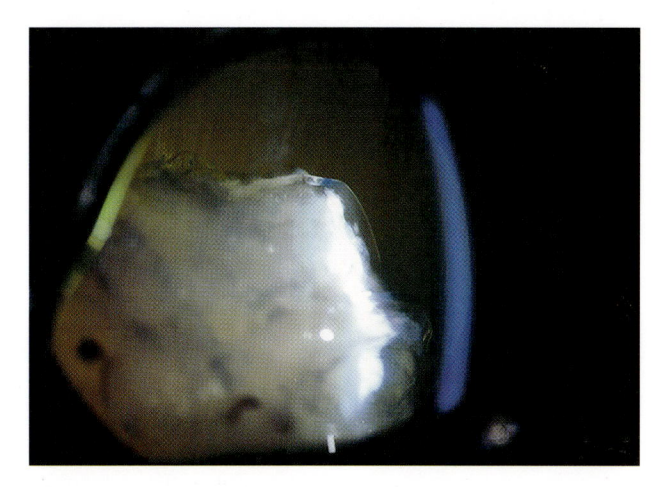

Fig. 11.6 Hypermature cataract with lens resorption. Note shrunken lens with wrinkled capsule.

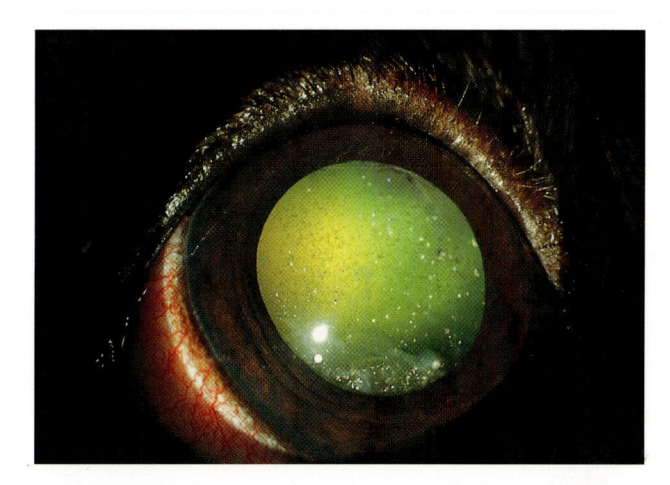

Fig. 11.7 Hypermature cataract and marked lens resorption. Note metallic particles of lens material, tapetal reflex and dull, dark thickened iris (post uveitis).

Cataracts may be partial or complete; bilateral or unilateral; symmetrical between the two eyes or not; progressive (often appears as vacuoles in the cortex) or stationary or temporary or undergoing resorption.

The diagnosis of cataract should not present any problem with the use of a pen torch, ophthalmoscopy and slit-lamp biomicroscopy (see Chapter 1). The differential diagnosis of cataract from other causes of leucoria (white pupil) includes corneal opacities, opacities in the anterior chamber such as hypopyon, and certain retinal detachments where the retina occupies a position just behind the lens, for example in cases of total retinal dysplasia. The most important differential diagnosis is between cataract and senile nuclear sclerosis and misdiagnosis is common in such cases. Although with direct illumination the lens may appear grey, or even opaque, in senile sclerosis, using distant direct ophthalmoscopy should easily distinguish it from true cataract.

Cataract may be classified by the cause into three main groups: primary hereditary; secondary; and other causes.

PRIMARY HEREDITARY CATARACTS

Primary hereditary cataracts are a large group in the dog, with a variable age of onset from puppies to young adults, the majority are not congenital and although most can be diagnosed in young adults there is sometimes a later manifestation. These cataracts differ considerably between the breeds but have a characteristic appearance for each breed together with age of onset and progression; they are usually, but not invariably, bilateral and symmetrical. The American College of Veterinary Ophthalmologists lists 97 breeds, some of which do not occur in the United Kingdom, in which inheritance is suspected, i.e. there is a breed predisposition. However, only 15 additional breeds are named as having proven hereditary cataract with a known mode of inheritance, the majority being autosomal recessive. Currently the British Veterinary Association/Kennel Club/International Sheepdog Society (BVA/KC/ISDS) Hereditary Eye Disease Scheme lists 17 breeds in its Schedule I of inherited ocular diseases, and a further 14 in Schedule III (conditions under investigation). A few breeds in both British schedules are not included in the American lists and there are further breeds in Europe with presumed or proven inherited cataract. This type of cataract, i.e. primary hereditary, can therefore affect an extremely large number of breeds and the appearance is often breed specific. The following are some examples.

Golden Retriever

The common form of hereditary cataract in the Golden Retriever (Curtis and Barnett, 1989) (Figs 11.8–11.10) is an opacity in the posterior cortical or subcapsular region at the posterior pole, not associated with the hyaloid artery or its remnant, that is ventro-medial to the confluence of the suture lines at the pole. The cataracts vary in appearance taking the form of an inverted 'Y' or triangle sometimes with extensions along the suture lines, or roughly circular, or irregular. They

LENS

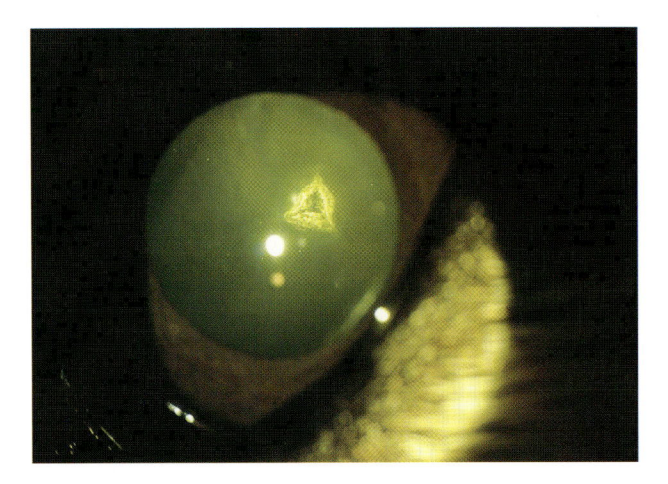

Fig. 11.8 Posterior polar cataract in a Golden Retriever.

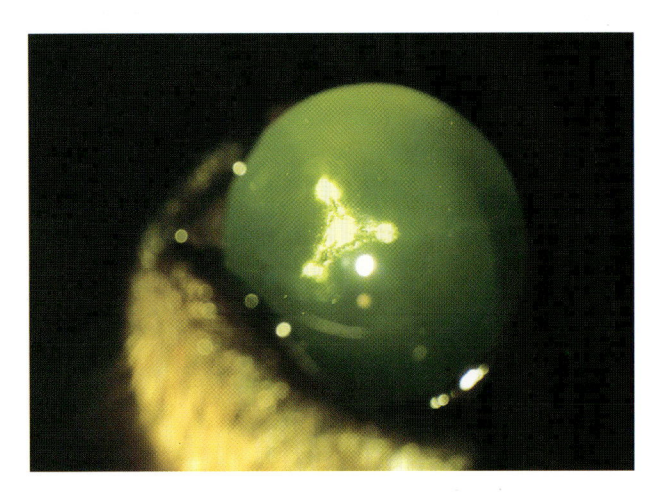

Fig. 11.9 Posterior polar cataract in a Golden Retriever.

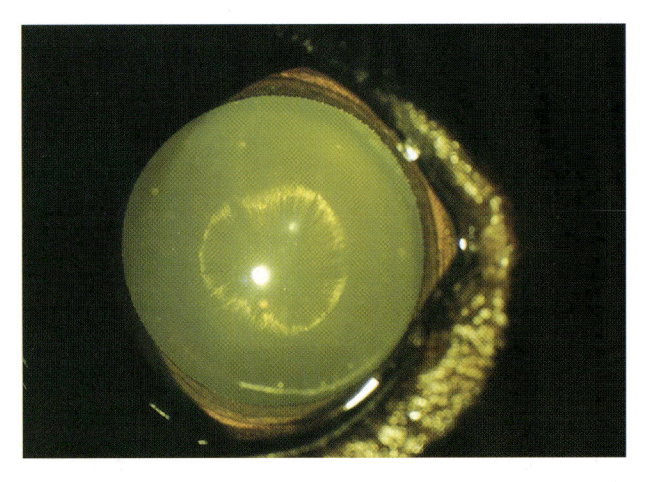

Fig. 11.10 Posterior polar cataract in a Golden Retriever.

are usually, but not invariably, bilateral and similar, although the opacity may occur in one eye before the other. Commonly they are small with no effect on vision and may remain stationary or be very slowly progressive for months to years, the dog retaining good vision all its life. These cataracts may be diagnosed as early as 6 months of age, are usually apparent between 1 and 2 years of age, but occasionally do not appear until the dog is several years of age, for example 8 or more. There does not seem to be any relationship between the early and late cases, sometimes the cataract in the parent generation appearing some years after its diagnosis in the offspring. It is this late manifestation in some cases that has led to a belief that this cataract is due to a recessive gene.

Another form of cataract in the Golden Retriever, but related to the posterior polar opacity, is a cortical cataract progressing to total cataract with complete loss of vision. This form is much less common than the posterior polar; it occurs in young adult dogs usually between 1 and 3 years of age; it is often accompanied by evidence of uveitis and sometimes lens resorption.

Primary hereditary cataract in the Golden Retriever is considered to be due to an autosomal dominant gene. Evidence is based on the reduction in incidence when not breeding from affected dogs, and the eradication from certain strains of Golden Retrievers which were affected with posterior polar as well as total cataract but have now remained clear for several generations. Further evidence is the occurrence of these forms of cataract in first-cross Golden Retrievers with breeds in which this form of cataract does not occur, e.g. the Border Collie and the Flat-coated Retriever, as well as the Labrador Retriever in which these forms of cataract do occur (see below).

A quite different form of cataract has also been reported in this breed. It appears as a bilateral perinuclear opacity, or halo, in young adult dogs, often under 12 months of age. It is unrelated to the posterior polar cortical and total forms of cataract described above and, although there is no proof of inheritance, its occurrence in the Golden Retriever does exhibit a strong breed predisposition and therefore possible hereditary factor.

Labrador Retriever

Posterior polar subcapsular, cortical and total forms of cataract in the Labrador (Curtis and Barnett, 1989) (Figs 11.11–11.14) seem to be identical to those described above in the Golden Retriever. The appearance, age of onset, stationary or progressive nature and inheritance are all similar in the two breeds. Several cases of posterior polar cataract have been observed in Labrador/Golden Retriever first crosses, but as the condition occurs in both breeds this information is of little value in proving the mode of inheritance.

Chesapeake Bay Retriever

Very similar forms of cataract have also been described in the Chesapeake Bay Retriever and again an autosomal dominant inheritance has been proposed but not proven.

Large Munsterlander

Similar forms of cataract also occur in the Large Munsterlander, but few descriptions have appeared. This

CATARACT

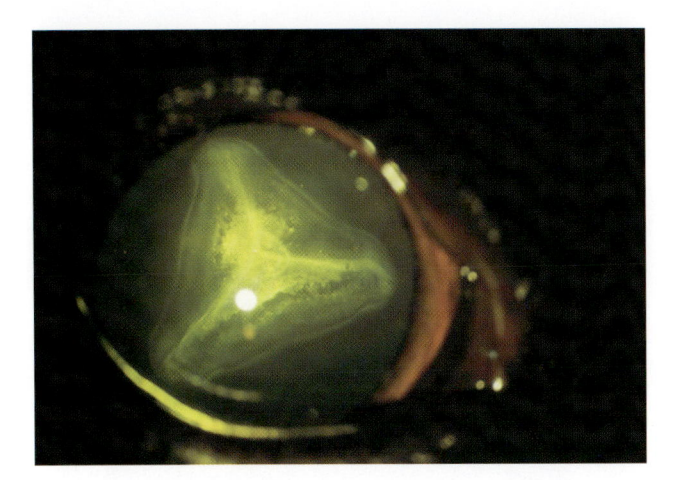

Fig. 11.11 Posterior polar cataract with suture line extensions in a Labrador Retriever.

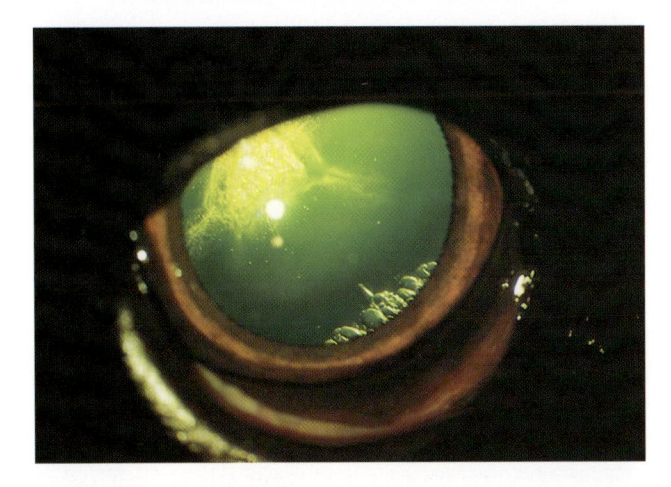

Fig. 11.12 Posterior polar and peripheral cortical cataract in a 1-year-old Labrador Retriever.

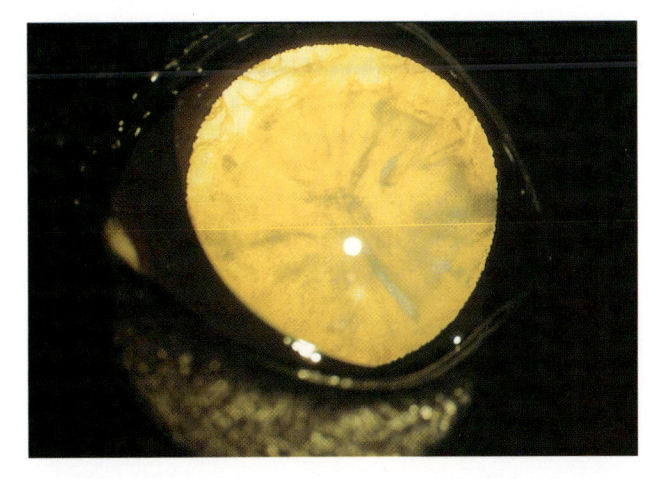

Fig. 11.13 Immature total cataract in a Labrador Retriever.

breed is included in Schedule I in the BVA/KC/ISDS eye scheme but is not included in the American lists.

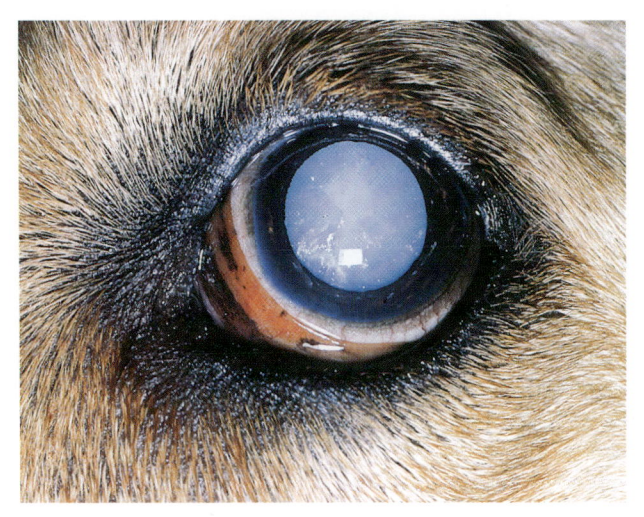

Fig. 11.14 Total mature cataract in a Labrador Retriever.

Irish Red and White Setter

The Irish Red and White Setter is another breed in Schedule I of the BVA/KC/ISDS scheme but not included in the American lists. Hereditary cataract in this breed commonly takes the form of a posterior polar subcapsular opacity, similar to the Golden and Labrador Retrievers, with occasional cases of progression. Inheritance is not known.

Boston Terrier

The Boston Terrier exhibits two distinct forms of hereditary cataract (Barnett, 1978; Curtis, 1984) (Figs 11.15–11.17) occurring at different ages; they are different in their appearance and progression.

The first form is apparent as early as 8 weeks of age but is not congenital. Both eyes are always affected equally and progress symmetrically. The first signs may affect the suture lines and the nucleus becomes opaque although the lens periphery initially remains clear. By 6 months most of the lens is involved with some areas showing greater density than others. Defective vision and obvious cataract occur usually

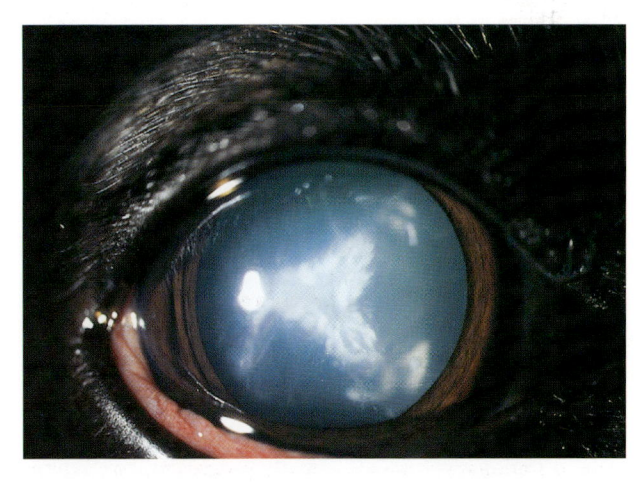

Fig. 11.15 Immature cataract in a Boston Terrier.

LENS

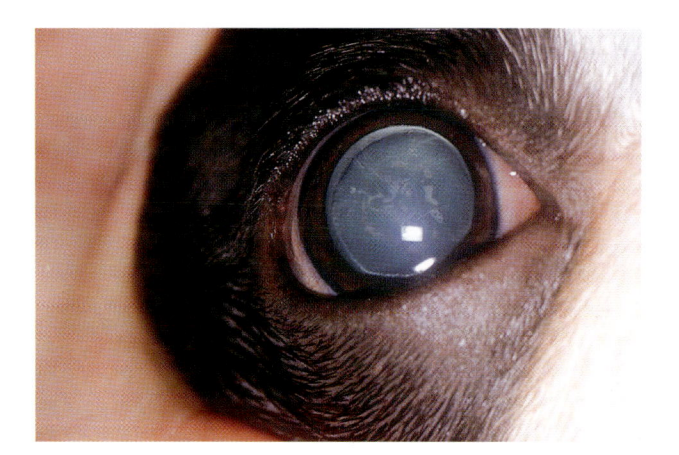

Fig. 11.16 Immature cataract in a Boston terrier.

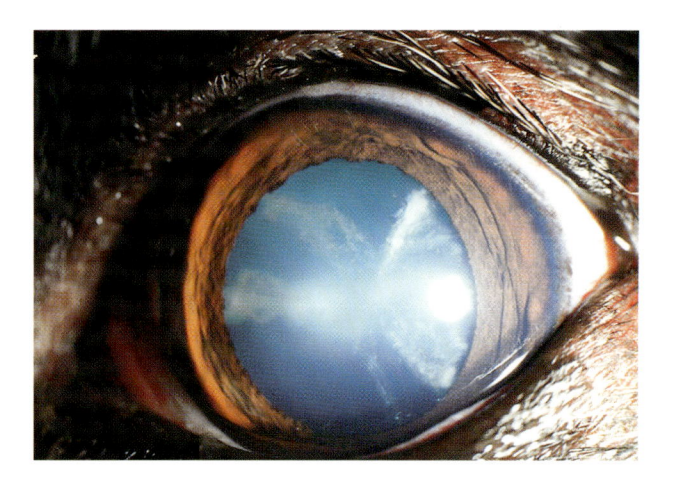

Fig. 11.17 Late-onset cataract in a Boston Terrier. Note different appearance to cataract in Figs 11.15 and 11.16.

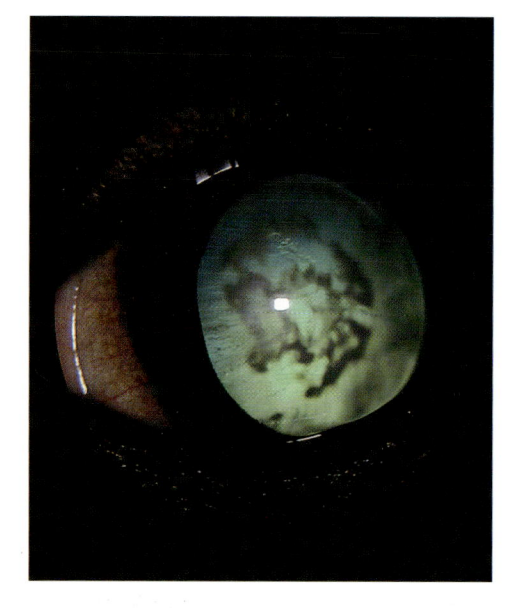

Fig. 11.18 Immature cataract in a Staffordshire Bull Terrier. Note similarity to the Boston Terriers in Figs 11.15 and 11.16.

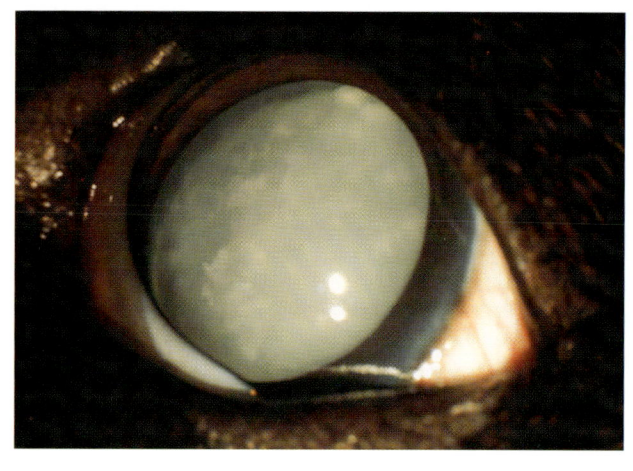

Fig. 11.19 Mature cataract in a Staffordshire Bull Terrier.

from 9 to 15 months of age with further progression and maturity of the cataract between 2 and 4 years of age. The inheritance of this form of cataract is due to a simple autosomal recessive gene proved by a test mating programme carried out in the 1970s. The incidence in the United Kingdom in this, numerically small, breed was high in the 1970s following the importation from Canada of an affected and popular stud dog. However, by breeding away from known affected lines the incidence was considerably reduced although odd cases still appear, possibly associated with other imported lines.

The other form of primary hereditary cataract in this breed is late-onset, occurring from 3 to 10 years of age mainly involving the equator and anterior cortex as radial wedges or spokes. The two eyes are usually affected but not symmetrically, and progression is slow or very slow and vision rarely affected. The mode of inheritance is unknown.

Staffordshire Bull Terrier

Cataract in the Staffordshire Bull Terrier (Barnett, 1978) (Figs 11.18 and 11.19) is very similar in appearance, bilateral nature and progression to the first form described above in the Boston Terrier. Again the cataract is not congenital but is always present under 1 year of age and affected dogs exhibit defective vision by 3 years of age. It is thought that inheritance is via a simple autosomal recessive gene and it is likely that the incidence will increase in the near future because of the involvement of a popular show strain.

American Cocker Spaniel

A variable form of hereditary cataract has been known in the American Cocker Spaniel for several years (Yakely *et al.*, 1971; Yakely, 1978) (Figs 11.20–11.22), the first reports appearing in 1971. In this breed the cataract does not show a characteristic form as it does in most other breeds. The cataract is usually bilateral although the appearance of the two eyes may differ considerably. Anterior and posterior

CATARACT

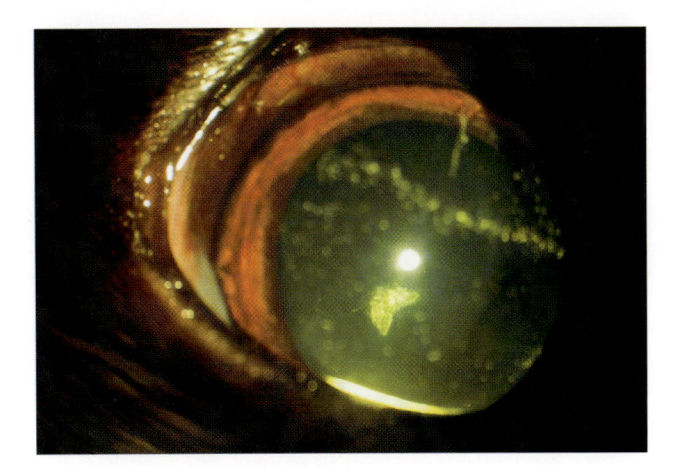

Fig. 11.20 Posterior polar and several small focal cataracts in a 17-month-old American Cocker Spaniel.

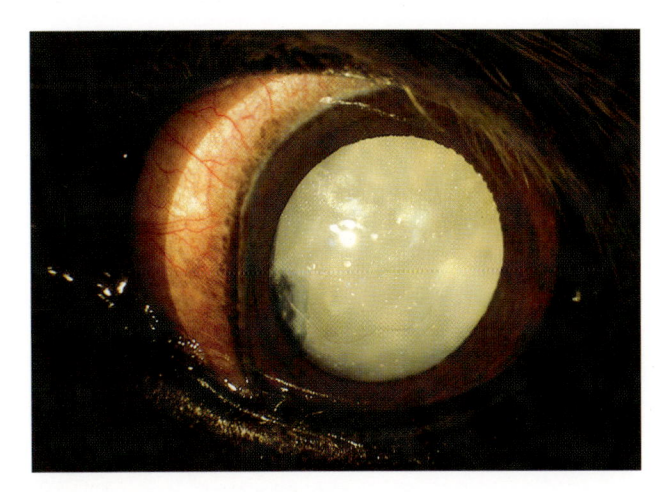

Fig. 11.21 Hypermature cataract in a 4-year-old American Cocker Spaniel. Note the dark iris and small uveal cysts on pupil border.

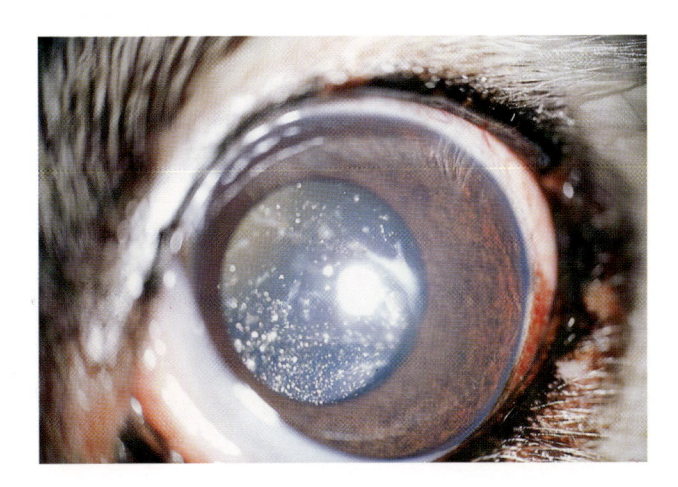

Fig. 11.22 Hypermature cataract with resorption in an American Cocker Spaniel. Note deep anterior chamber, flat anterior face of lens and shadow of pupil on lens and dark iris.

cortices are involved, with one or more foci of cataract; progression is very variable; the cataracts may remain stationary for several months or become total and dense with rapid progression, particularly in young dogs. In such cases a lens-induced uveitis is common, followed later by lens resorption and in some cases return of vision. The age incidence varies from 6 months to a few years and inheritance is again via a simple autosomal recessive gene.

Welsh Springer Spaniel

Cataract is bilateral and symmetrical in the Welsh Springer Spaniel (Barnett, 1980) (Fig. 11.23) and first appears at about 8 weeks of age as radiating lines of cortical vacuoles. Progression in both is rapid so that by 5 months of age the cataract is extensive and by 18 months of age is total and dense with complete loss of vision, although some resorption may occur. Inheritance is due to a simple autosomal recessive gene proved by test mating, including the back-cross.

German Shepherd Dog

Cataract is reported only in Europe in the German Shepherd Dog (Hippel, 1930; Barnett, 1986) and is of two forms. The first was reported in 1930 in Germany and was congenital and inherited as a dominant character. The second form is not congenital but is apparent by slit-lamp biomicroscopy as early as 8 weeks of age although not in all cases. Progression occurs mainly affecting the nucleus but with a clear subcapsular equatorial zone. The cataract is bilateral with minor differences between the two eyes. Progression to total cataract does not seem to occur and although vision is defective, complete blindness is not the rule. Test matings proved an autosomal recessive gene responsible.

The German Shepherd Dog is a popular breed but hereditary cataract has remained of low incidence in this breed in the United Kingdom. However, cases of a purverulent, bilateral cataract is not uncommon in ageing German Shepherd Dogs but with little or no apparent effect on vision.

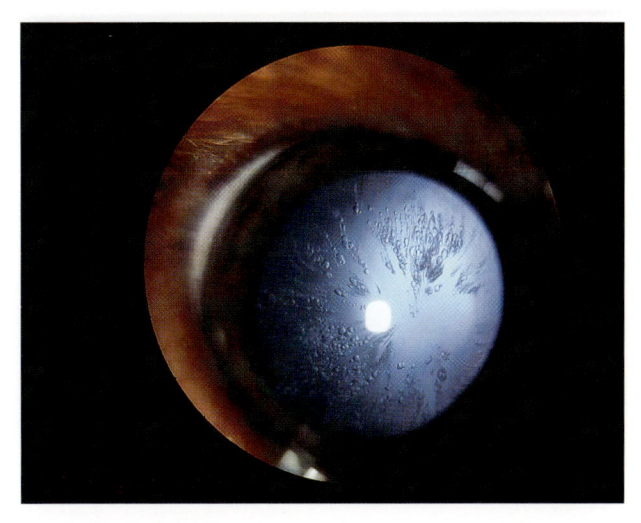

Fig. 11.23 Incipient cataract (cortical vacuole) in an 8-week-old Welsh Springer Spaniel.

LENS

Miniature Schnauzer

Cataract in the Miniature Schnauzer (Rubin *et al.*, 1969; Barnett, 1985b) (Fig. 11.24) is both congenital and hereditary and is associated with mild microphthalmos. When cataract was first recorded in this breed in the USA the cataract was considered primary and described as bilateral, symmetrical and progressive and there was no mention of microphthalmos. More recent reports of the Miniature Schnauzer in both the United States and the UK describe a congenital bilateral cataract, usually similar but not necessarily exactly symmetrical, and essentially nuclear in position, but occasionally with small extensions into the cortex which may slowly progress. A clear peripheral part and the absence of any anterior capsular involvement are typical of cataract in this breed and therefore unlike the congenital cataract with microphthalmos seen in a number of other breeds (see Chapter 4). As new and clear lens material is laid down with growth the opaque nucleus becomes smaller in relation to the size of the lens and fair vision can be retained. Affected eyes are microphthalmic but not markedly so. This fact may not be noticed particularly in young puppies unless compared with normal littermates. Other accompanying ocular signs include lenticonus and microphakia together with an intermittent, mainly rotary, ocular nystagmus. The anterior segment and fundus have proved to be normal, again unlike the microphthalmos and cataract described in other breeds (Chapter 4).

Test mating, including the back-cross, has proved a simple autosomal recessive mode of inheritance in the UK, the same as that described in the USA.

Cavalier King Charles Spaniel

The Cavalier King Charles Spaniel is another breed with two distinctly different types of cataract (Barnett, 1985a) (Figs 11.25–11.29); one congenital, the other not present at birth and progressing to total cataract.

The congenital form is similar to that described above in the Miniature Schnauzer and is also associated with

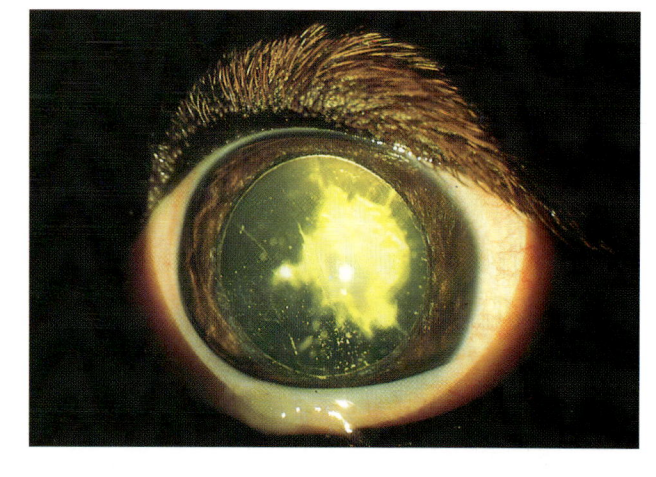

Fig. 11.25 Nuclear cataract with extensions but clear cortex in a Cavalier King Charles Spaniel. Note microphthalmos and similarity to Fig. 11.24.

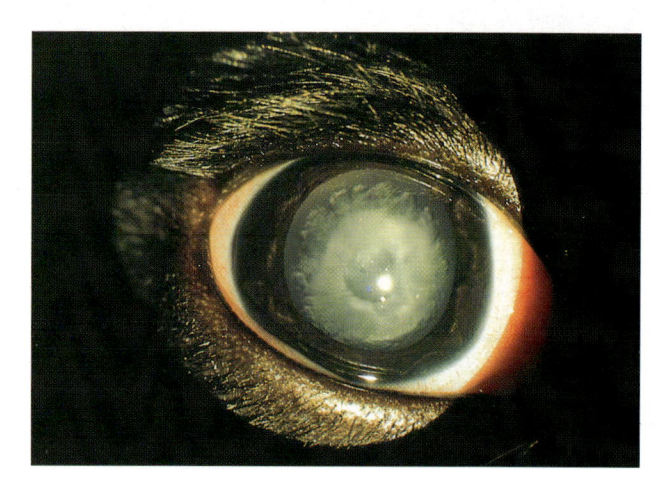

Fig. 11.26 Nuclear cataract and microphthalmos with lenticonus (central clearer area within the cataract and protruding into the vitreous) in a 7-week-old Cavalier King Charles Spaniel.

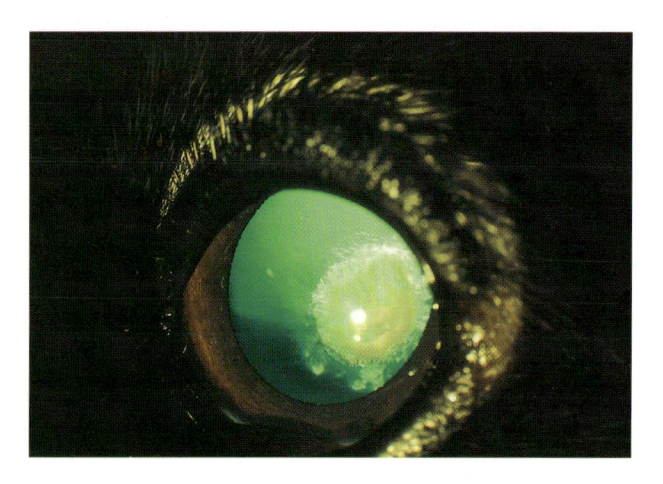

Fig. 11.24 Microphthalmos and nuclear cataract in a Miniature Schnauzer. Note clear lens cortex.

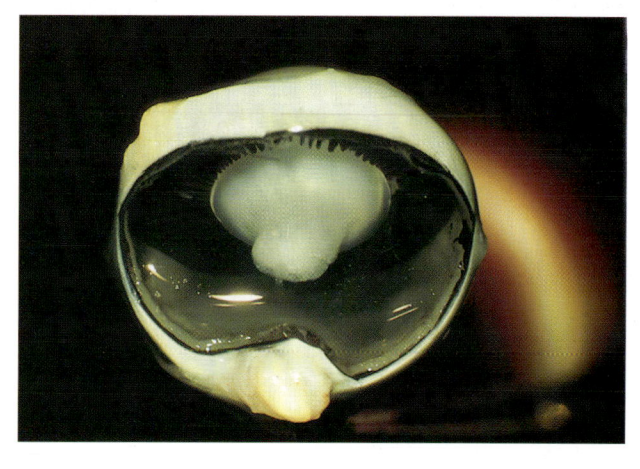

Fig. 11.27 Posterior lenticonus in a 7-week-old Cavalier King Charles Spaniel.

CATARACT

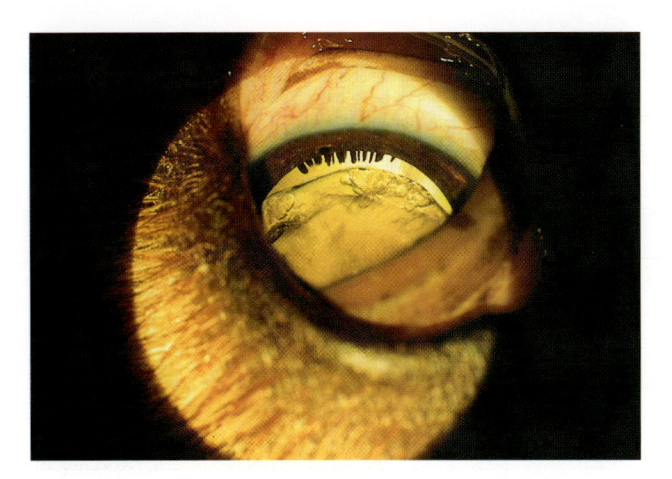

Fig. 11.28 Cataract, microphthalmos and zonular abnormality (multiocular defects) in a Cavalier King Charles Spaniel.

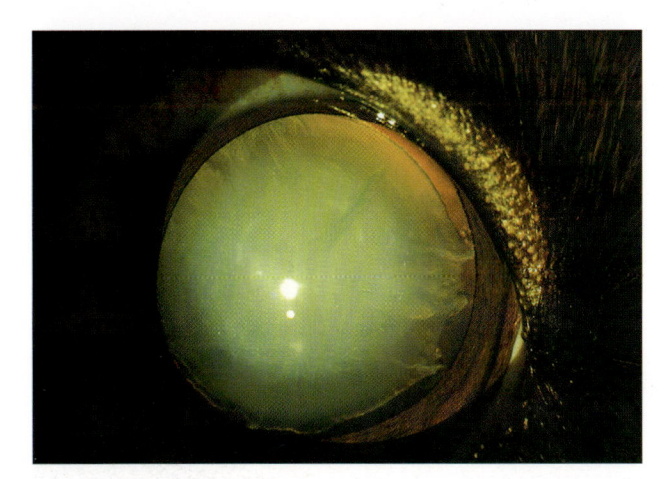

Fig. 11.29 Mature non-congenital cataract in a 4-year-old Cavalier King Charles Spaniel.

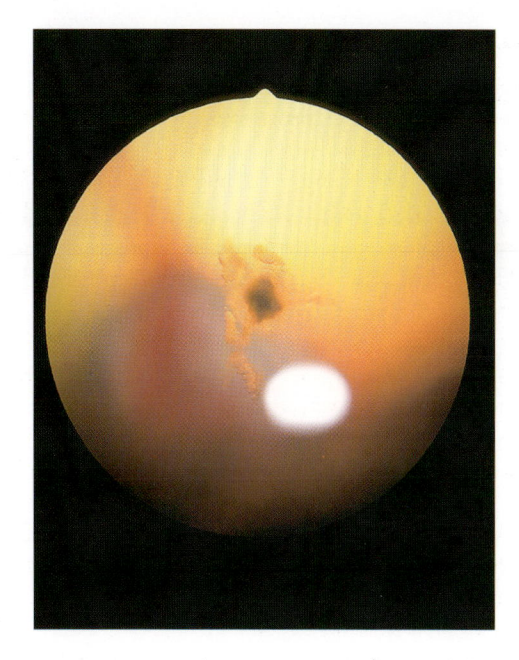

Fig. 11.30 Posterior polar cataract in a $5\frac{1}{2}$-year-old Leonberger.

microphthalmos; it is bilateral but rarely symmetrical, mainly nuclear with both capsular and cortical opacities, the latter may progress but the former do not. Additional anomalies include abnormalities of the ciliary body, iris hypoplasia and both lenticonus and lentiglobus.

The non-congenital cataract is not associated with microphthalmos or any other ocular anomaly; it is bilateral, symmetrical and progressive to become total in young adult dogs. It may be classed as a true primary cataract.

An initial study indicates that both forms of cataract in this breed are due to autosomal recessive genes.

Leonberger

Forms of hereditary cataract have recently been studied in the Leonberger (Heinrich, 1999) (Fig. 11.30). Posterior polar subcapsular cataract is the most common, but is often not as symmetrical as in the gundog breeds and is sometimes progressive with a variable age of onset. Pedigree analysis is suggestive of dominant inheritance. Nuclear cataract also occurs in this breed varying from mild to extensive with an effect on vision. Again there is variable age of onset and progression. A posterior nuclear type has also been described.

Other breeds

Primary hereditary cataract is classed as a Schedule I condition in the BVA/KC/ISDS eye scheme in the following breeds additional to those described above: Belgian Shepherd Dog, Norwegian Buhund (Fig. 11.31), Old English Sheepdog, Siberian Husky and Standard Poodle (Rubin and Flowers, 1972; Barnett and Startup, 1985). A further 14 breeds appear in Schedule III (conditions under investigation) as being suspected of inheritance.

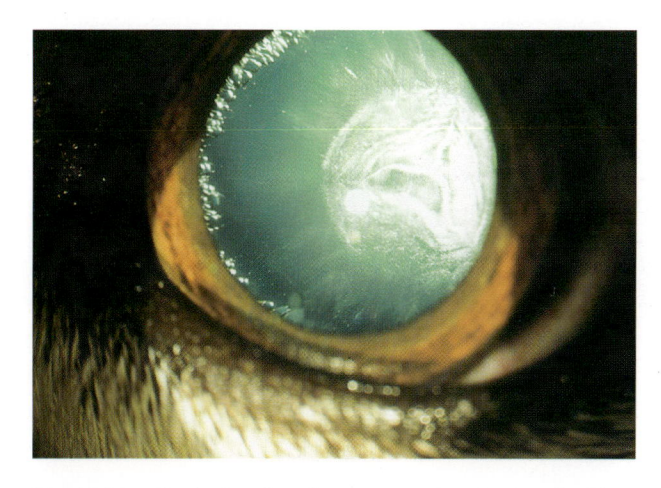

Fig. 11.31 Cortical and nuclear cataract in a 21-month-old Norwegian Buhund.

LENS

SECONDARY CATARACT

Secondary cataracts are cataracts secondary to another eye disease which may often prove to be hereditary.

Generalised progressive retinal atrophy

Secondary cataract (Figs 11.32 and 11.33) is a frequent, possibly invariable, sequel to generalised progressive retinal atrophy in most, if not all, breeds affected with this hereditary retinopathy, whether it be a rod or cone dysplasia or degeneration (see Chapter 14). The cataract commences as a usually posterior cortical type with wedges of vacuoles radiating towards the centre from the lens periphery and progressing to total cataract. It is not infrequently the presenting sign in affected breeds in which affected individuals may retain a surprisingly good pupillary light reflex in spite of their retinal degeneration. In these breeds an assessment of retinal activity by electroretinography should always be contemplated prior to surgery on the lens.

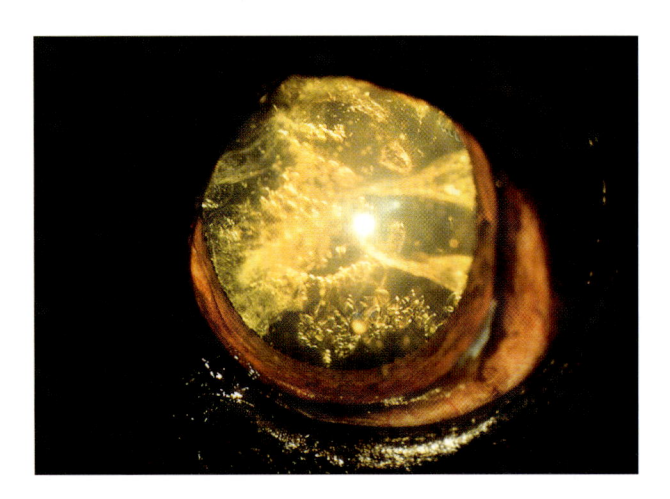

Fig. 11.32 Anterior and posterior cortical secondary cataract (generalised progressive retinal atrophy) in a 6-year-old Tibetan Terrier.

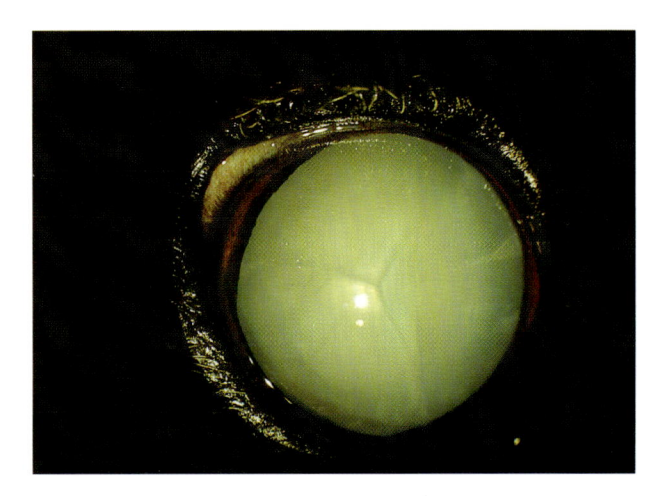

Fig. 11.33 Mature secondary cataract (generalised progressive retinal atrophy) in a Miniature Poodle.

Central progressive retinal atrophy (pigment epithelial dystrophy)

Secondary cataract, both cortical and large areas involving the posterior pole, occurs in conjunction with this form of retinal degeneration and secondary cataract can be seen with other forms of extensive, post-inflammatory, retinal degeneration in older dogs.

Retinal dysplasia

The total form of retinal dysplasia with infundibular retinal detachment may be accompanied by quite extensive forms of cortical cataract in breeds such as the Labrador Retriever, Sealyham Terrier and English Springer Spaniel. Cataract has not so far been described in cases of multifocal retinal dysplasia. Cataract may also occur with other forms of retinal detachment.

Glaucoma

Both primary and secondary glaucoma (see Chapter 10) in their advanced stages may be accompanied by cataract.

Lens luxation

The luxated lens when allowed to remain in the eye often becomes cataractous, particularly affecting the posterior part of the lens, no doubt because of its abnormal position and probably also because of the secondary glaucoma that will be present. It should be noted that mature cataractous lenses, due to degeneration of the zonule, may also luxate.

Uveitis

Anterior uveitis (iritis), whatever the aetiology, may cause cataract, usually anterior subcapsular and with or without posterior synechiae formation. This is an important cause of cataract, and possibly the commonest cause of secondary cataract, which may vary considerably in extent. Iris changes are invariably present, the commonest being darkening of the iris (see Chapter 12). Phakolytic uveitis due to a hypermature cataract is another example of the association between lens and iris – the accurate diagnosis of the primary condition is of particular importance in ophthalmology, a further case in this group of secondary cataracts being lens luxation and cataract; it is important to decide which came first prior to commencing treatment.

Persistent pupillary membranes

Persistent pupillary membranes may be attached to the posterior cornea or to the anterior lens capsule and be the cause of focal stationary opacities in either position, the latter being classed as a cataract. The extent of the opacity depends upon the severity of the persistent pupillary membrane but these opacities are not progressive and rarely interfere with vision. Isolated cases of this congenital anomaly may occur in any breed and are usually uniocular. However, they are inherited in the Basenji as a bilateral condition (see also Chapter 12).

CATARACT

Persistent hyaloid artery

Persistence of the hyaloid artery is often associated with a usually small capsular opacity, referred to as Mittendorf's dot, on the posterior capsule of the lens. The hyaloid remnant can be seen protruding into the vitreous and this condition should not be confused with a posterior polar cataract; the hyaloid artery meets the lens in a position ventromedial to the confluence of the suture lines, the site of posterior polar subcapsular cataracts inherited in several breeds (see above).

Persistent hyperplastic primary vitreous

Secondary cataract, together with occasional posterior lentiglobus and sometimes intralenticular haemorrhage, plaque and persistent hyaloid artery occur as odd uniocular cases as well as bilateral cases, inherited in the Dobermann and Staffordshire Bull Terrier (see also Chapter 13).

Multiocular defects

Congenital anomalies can affect all parts of the eye and are often present together (Figs 11.34 and 11.35). The primary lesion is probably microphthalmos (see Chapter 4) and in these cases the commonest defect is cataract.

OTHER CAUSES OF CATARACT

Trauma (Figs 11.36–11.38)

Cataract may result from either a blunt, i.e. non-penetrative, injury to the eye causing contusion, which is usually anterior subcapsular in position, or from a penetrating injury to cornea or sclera causing perforation of the anterior capsule with resultant focal to diffuse cataract, which may remain focal or progress. In such cases the escape of lens material may be apparent and there may also be an associated anterior uveitis. Often other signs of ocular injury are present, e.g. haemorrhage, or there may be no obvious signs; traumatic cataracts are usually uniocular; common causes of penetrating injury are cat claws, bites and gunshot wounds.

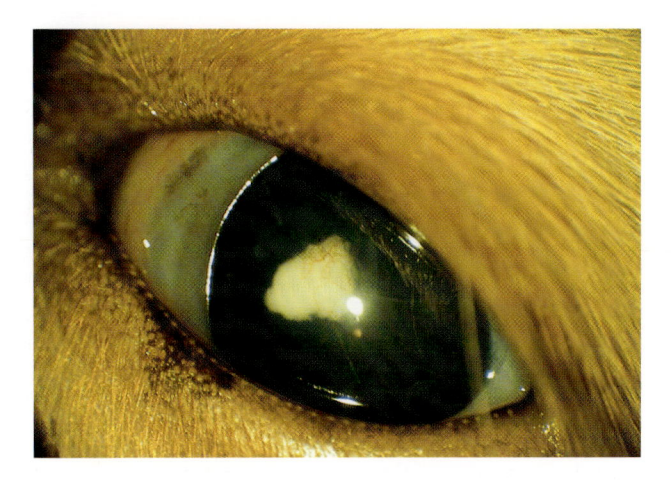

Fig. 11.35 Cataract with multiocular defects. Note dense paramydial cataract with small blood vessels from pupillary membranes and microphthalmos.

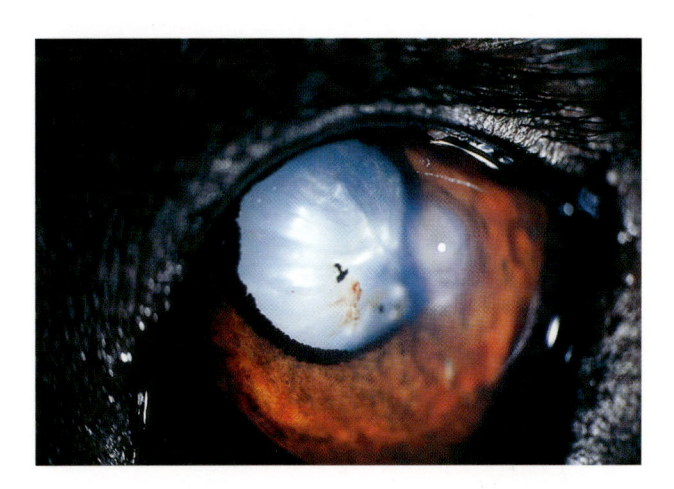

Fig. 11.36 Traumatic cataract due to penetrating corneal injury in a German Shepherd Dog. Note herniation of uveal tissue around pupil plus small posterior synechiae and haemorrhage on anterior capsule.

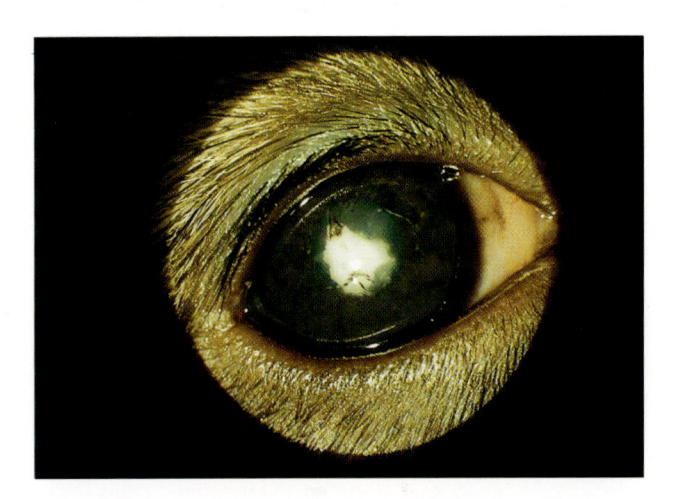

Fig. 11.34 Cataract with multiocular defects in a German Shepherd Dog puppy. Note microphthalmos with prominence of third eyelid, iris hypoplasia and pupillary membranes.

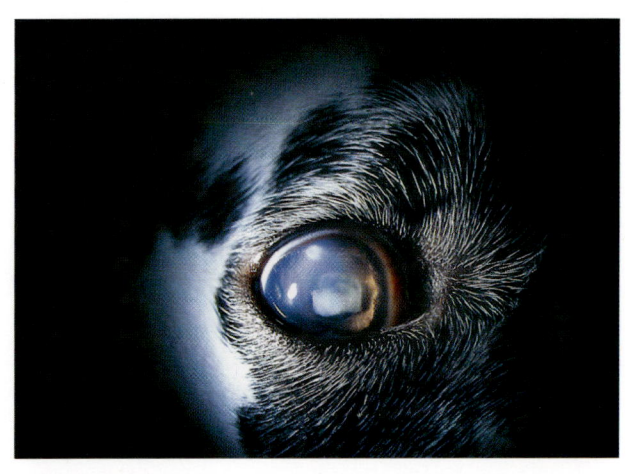

Fig. 11.37 Traumatic cataract due to cat claw injury in a Dalmatian.

LENS

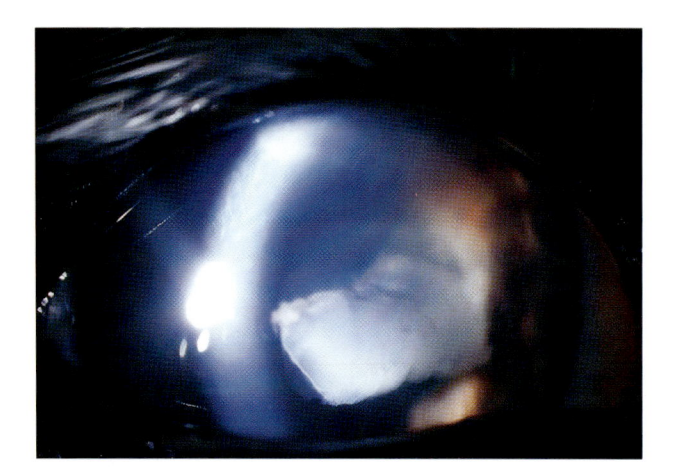

Fig. 11.38 Slit-lamp photograph of the same case as Fig. 11.37.

Diabetes mellitus

Diabetic cataract (Fig. 11.39) is always bilateral, symmetrical, total and irreversible. It may be extremely rapid in onset; it is not uncommon and it may be the first presenting sign of this systemic disease. It occurs particularly in cases which have not been adequately stabilised and in dogs in which the diabetes is controlled the lens may remain clear for several years. Two types of diabetic cataract occur; the first is acute with sudden onset, rapid progression and total; the second, described as pre-senile, is slower in onset and more dense in the nuclear portion. Both types typically show clear water clefts on their anterior face.

Hypercalcaemia

Multifocal punctate opacities in the cortex occur symmetrically in both eyes. It is rare.

Toxic

Many substances are known to be cataractogenic and cataract is a very important sign in ophthalmic toxicology (Fig. 11.40). Any part of the lens may be involved, often equatorial, cortical or suture line. The cataract is bilateral but not always symmetrical, as might be expected. An unusual lens change due to dimethylsulfoxide toxicity has been described.

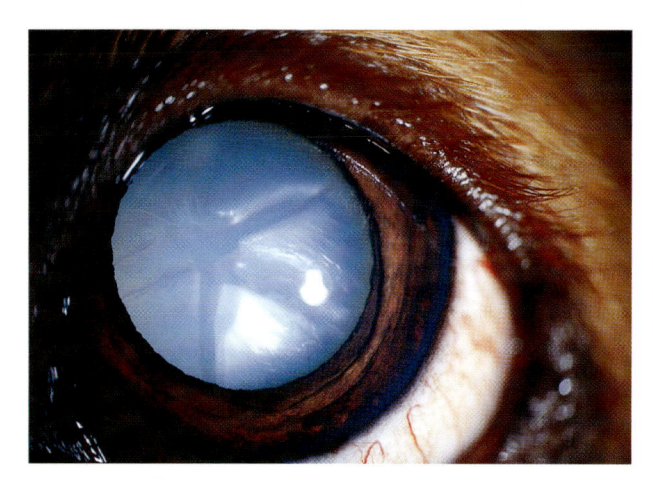

Fig. 11.39 Mature diabetic cataract. Note water clefts on anterior lens face.

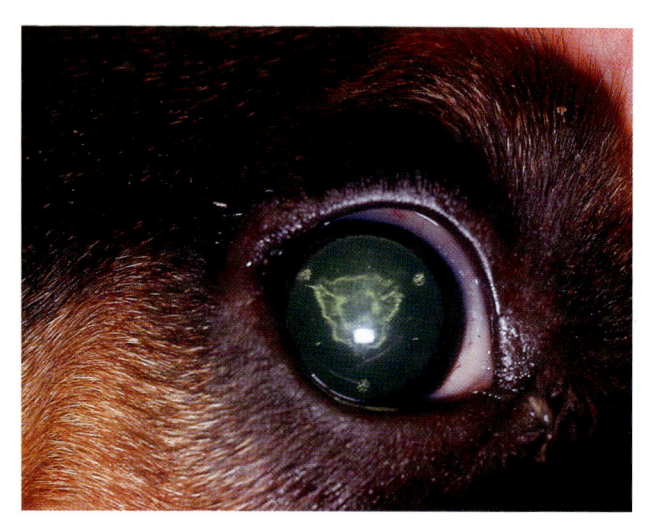

Fig. 11.40 Toxic cataract in young adult Beagle. Posterior polar and suture line opacities.

Deficiencies

Bilateral cataract in puppies fed an oral milk replacement diet and also a diet deficient in vitamin B complex in Foxhound puppies have been recorded, but deficiency cataracts in this species, except under exceptional circumstances, must be rare.

Radiation

Radiation therapy for neoplasia of the head region can cause cataract.

Senile or age-related cataract

The actual cause is unknown; the cataract has a slow and variable progression and involves the nucleus and cortex with multifocal opacities. These are true cataracts and occur together with nuclear sclerosis, which is a normal age change due to compression and an increase in density of the older fibres in the nuclear region, producing a well demarcated, less translucent and more opalescent central zone which gives the lens an opaque appearance in direct illumination but no true opacity in reflected light.

TREATMENT

In spite of several attempts at the medical treatment of cataract, surgery currently is the only successful method; the advent of phacoemulsification has significantly improved the prognosis.

LENS LUXATION

Lens luxation, or dislocation, is an important condition in the dog, particularly primary, or inherited, lens luxation

LENS LUXATION

which often requires immediate surgical treatment because of the often severe secondary glaucoma which frequently follows. Subluxation of the lens refers to partial dislocation from its patella fossa. Primary lens luxation is essentially a bilateral condition although rarely do both lenses luxate simultaneously; the dog usually presents with one obviously dislocated lens, the other eye showing earlier signs of luxation or at the time being normal, but if the condition is primary the second eye will always become involved, possibly in days or several months later. Primary lens luxation carries a strong breed incidence, basically the terrier breeds; although sporadic cases may occur in any breed they can almost invariably be classed as lens luxation secondary to some other eye disease, often following glaucoma or cataract, or are caused by trauma. Congenital lens luxation does occur in the dog but is rare and is associated with other lens or ocular congenital anomalies.

Clinical signs

The clinical signs of primary lens luxation can be conveniently divided into two groups, the first associated with the position of the lens, the second relating to the secondary glaucoma which follows the lens luxation (Curtis and Barnett, 1980; Curtis *et al.*, 1983).

With breakdown of the suspensory ligament of the lens, the zonule, which occurs first at the dorsolateral quadrant, vitreous and sometimes zonular fragments appear at the pupillary margin over the anterior lens capsule (Figs 11.41–11.43); this may occur prior to any actual movement of the lens. With early luxation or partial luxation of the lens the pathognomonic sign of iridodonesis, trembling of the iris on eye movement, occurs possibly accompanied by irregularity of the pupil and local bulging of the iris due to a shift in the position of the underlying lens. Changes in the depth of the anterior chamber, both decrease and increase, the latter with posterior luxation, may occur. Lens displacement is usually ventral leading to the appearance of an aphakic crescent and visible lens margin

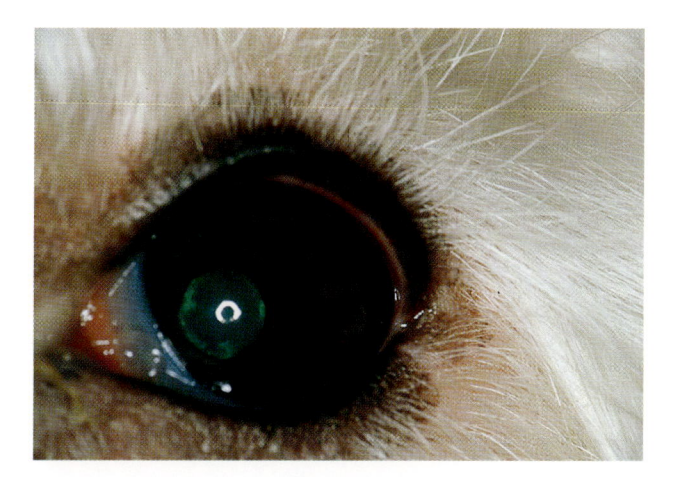

Fig. 11.41 Early lens luxation in a Sealyham Terrier. Vitreous around pupil in otherwise quiet eye.

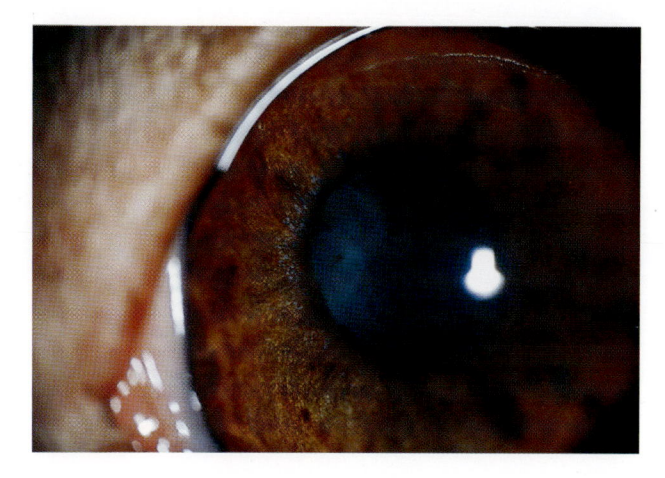

Fig. 11.42 Early lens luxation in a Jack Russell Terrier. Vitreous cloud at medial border of pupil.

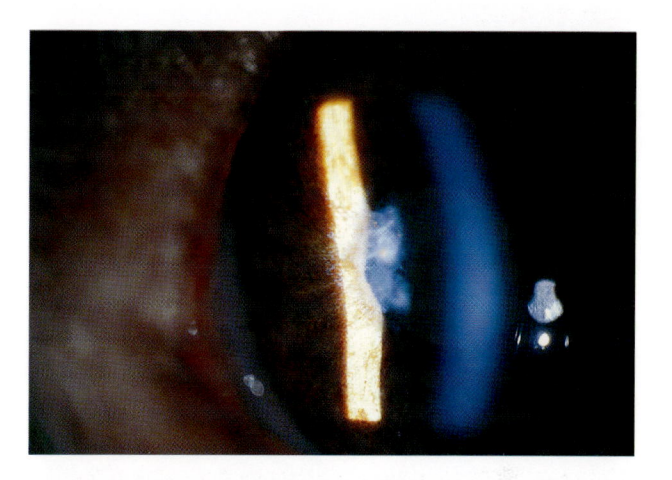

Fig. 11.43 Early lens luxation in the same dog as in Fig. 11.42. Vitreous in pupil (slit-lamp photograph).

in the pupil, particularly when dilated (Figs 11.44–11.48). Dislocation of the lens may be anterior (Fig. 11.49) or posterior, the former being more common. In anterior luxation the large lens comes to lie in front of the iris, pressing against the posterior cornea and producing a permanent subcentral oval corneal opacity (Fig. 11.50). In posterior luxation the lens moves backwards and, because of gravity, lies in the ventral part of the posterior segment of the eye in a more fluid and degenerate vitreous. The whole pupil is now aphakic and the anterior chamber is deeper than normal (Fig. 11.51). The lens can easily move between the anterior and posterior parts of the eye through the pupil, and back again, and the use of miotics to constrict the pupil, and trap the lens in the posterior segment, is never permanently successful. With posterior luxation the oval subcentral corneal opacity previously described is often present indicating previous anterior luxation. Occasionally the lens may become stuck in the pupil, so producing pupil block and severe secondary glaucoma due to narrowing of the angle of filtration with bulging forwards of the iris root and subsequent anterior ring synechiae. Occasionally signs of secondary uveitis may be present with lens luxation.

LENS

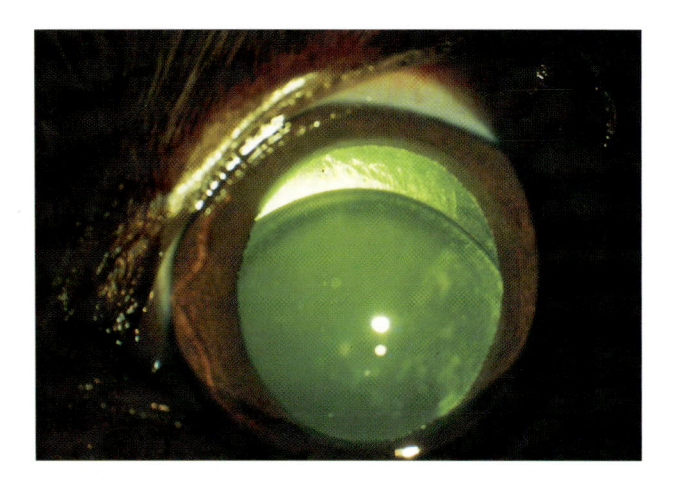

Fig. 11.44 Lens luxation with aphakic crescent superiorly (pupil dilated) in a Tibetan Terrier. Note vitreous swirling above and in front of lens.

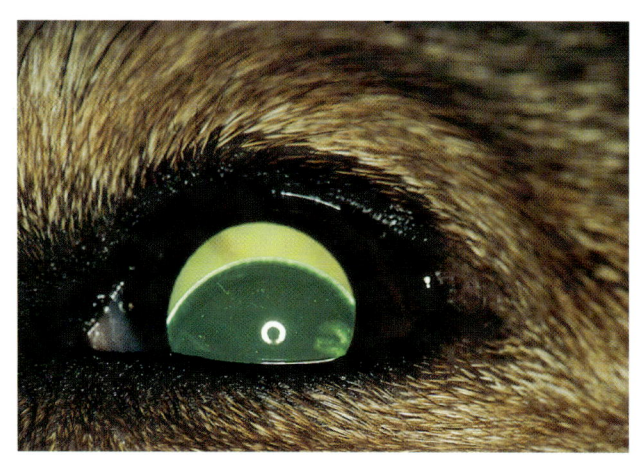

Fig. 11.47 Aphakic crescent.

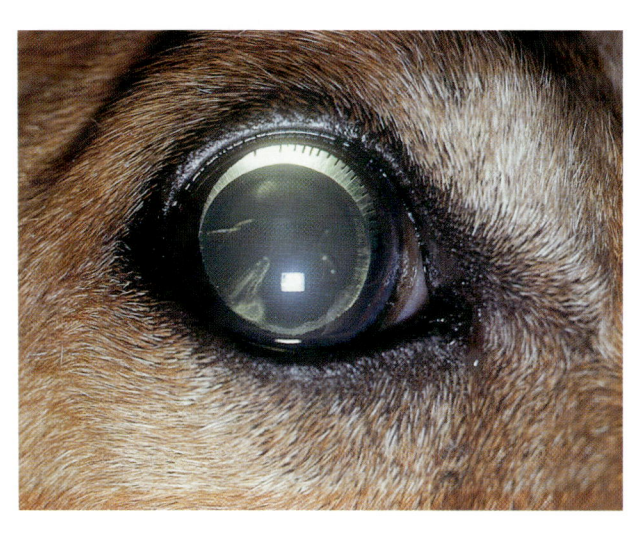

Fig. 11.45 Lens luxation in a Jack Russell Terrier. Note breakdown of zonule with vitreous in lower part of pupil.

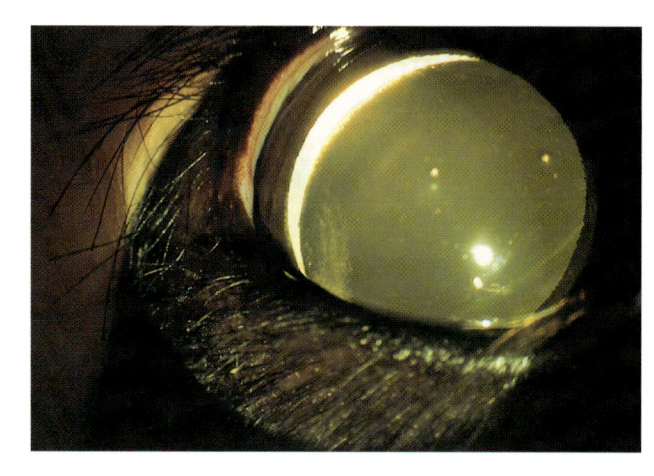

Fig. 11.48 Aphakic crescent in a Tibetan Terrier.

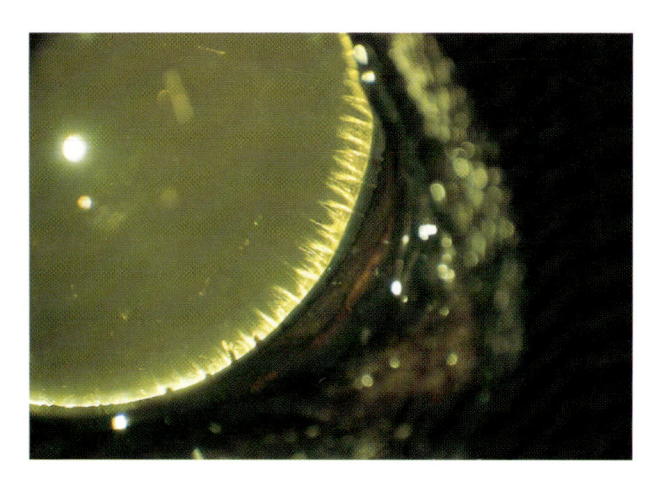

Fig. 11.46 Early breakdown of zonule (pupil dilated) in a Tibetan Terrier.

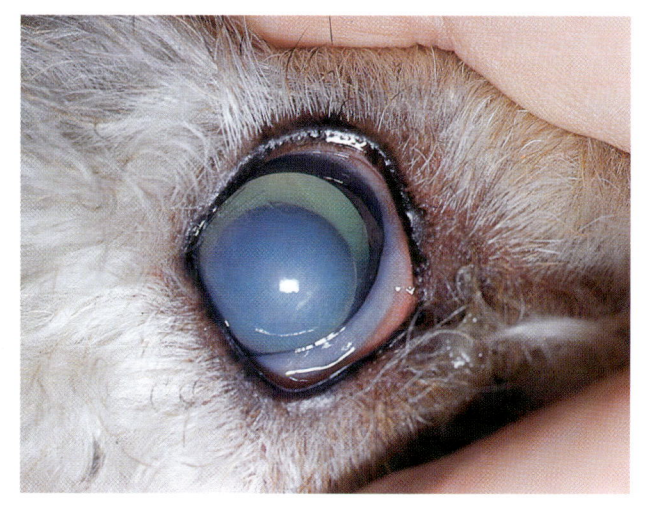

Fig. 11.49 Anterior luxation with early corneal oedema in a Sealyham Terrier.

LENS LUXATION

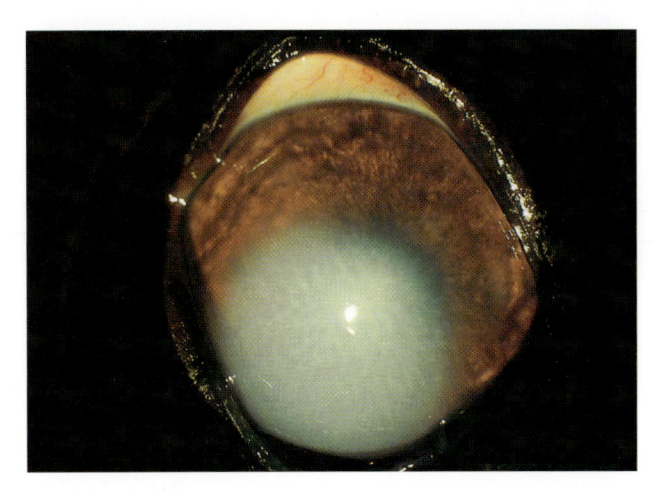

Fig. 11.50 Posterior luxation with typical corneal opacity due to previous anterior luxation in a Tibetan Terrier.

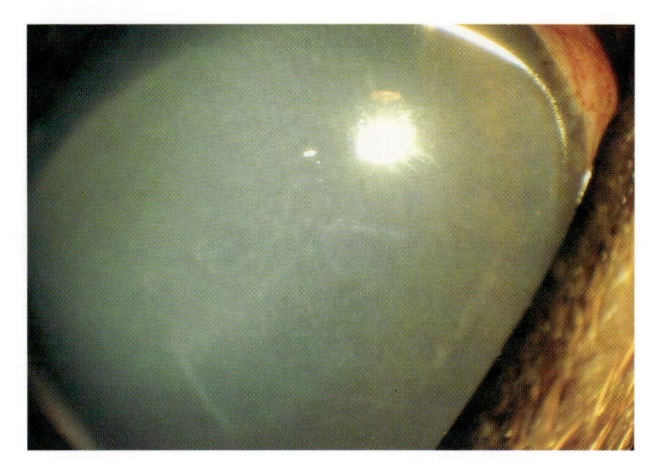

Fig. 11.52 Steamy cornea (corneal oedema) due to severe secondary glaucoma in a Jack Russell Terrier.

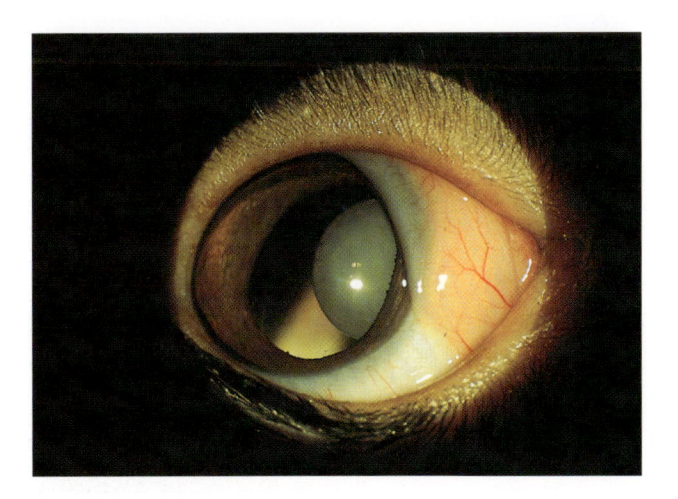

Fig. 11.51 Posterior lens luxation of long-standing in a Lancashire Heeler. Note lens now cataractous.

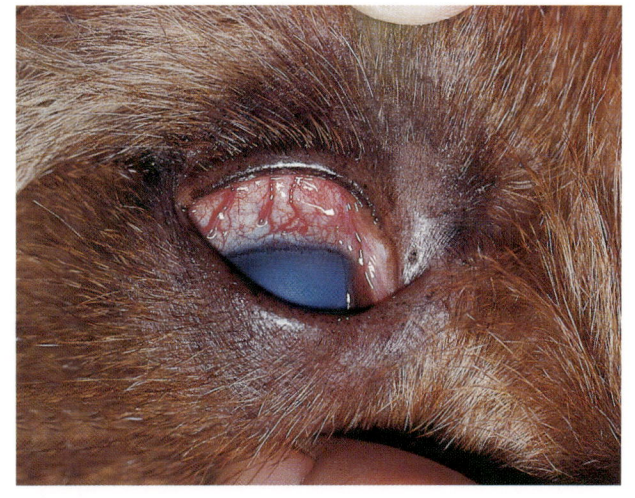

Fig. 11.53 Severe conjunctival congestion and corneal oedema (secondary glaucoma).

The use of a short-acting mydriatic may assist diagnosis, particularly in early cases to reveal vitreal tags, the edge of the lens and early and narrow aphakic crescents.

The glaucoma associated with lens luxation is undoubtedly secondary (Figs 11.52 and 11.53) although the opposite, i.e. primary glaucoma as a cause of the lens luxation, has been suggested (also see later). Evidence for the former includes a normal intraocular pressure in early cases and in eyes prior to lens luxation, gonioscopy revealing an open angle initially, and the breed and the age incidence (see later). The ocular signs of glaucoma are episcleral congestion, pupil dilation, corneal oedema of the whole cornea, lacrimation, blepharospasm and pain, often severe. When luxation of the lens occurs there is always a vitreal attachment to the posterior capsule. If the lens passes anteriorly and through the pupil this vitreal attachment is forced into the angle of filtration, so blocking it, by the normal flow of aqueous. This fact can be confirmed at surgery to remove the dislocated lens because, when first entering the eye on the corneal side of the limbus, a blob of vitreous often presents prior to the escape of aqueous.

INCIDENCE AND INHERITANCE

It is usually the terrier breeds that suffer from lens luxation, both in the UK and also in other countries. Historically, Fox Terriers and Sealyham Terriers were the breeds mainly cited (Formston, 1945), but these breeds are no longer as popular as they were and it is now the Jack Russell Terrier in which most cases occur. Breeds involved are as follows: Jack Russell Terrier, Sealyham Terrier, Wire-haired Fox Terrier, Smooth-haired Fox Terrier, Tibetan Terrier, Lakeland Terrier, Welsh Terrier, Norwich Terrier, Norfolk Terrier, Miniature Bull Terrier and most recently the Lancashire Heeler. Primary lens luxation has also been reported in the Border Collie (Foster et al., 1986).

The incidence in the Miniature Bull Terrier is of considerable concern, certainly in both the UK and Australia, in that several cases are known in this, numerically small, breed. The condition has never been recorded in the standard Bull Terrier and the occurrence of this hereditary eye condition in the Miniature Bull Terrier is probably another example of an inherited condition being introduced into a breed by crossing that breed with another; in this case during the miniaturisation of the Bull Terrier with smooth-coated Jack Russell and Fox Terriers.

Hereditary lens luxation is not a congenital condition but occurs typically in middle age, usually between 3 and 8 years with a mean at 4–5 years. Both the breed and age incidence are different from secondary lens luxation.

Lens luxation is an autosomal condition. Both sex-linked and sex-limited theories may be discounted. However, a preponderance of females to males has been recorded by a number of authors.

Recessive inheritance has been shown in the Tibetan Terrier (Willis et al., 1979) and the mating of two affected individuals was consistent with this opinion. Recessive inheritance has also been shown to be most likely in the few cases recorded in the Border Collie and autosomal recessive inheritance is also indicated in the Miniature Bull Terrier. However, dominant inheritance has been suggested by some authors and the number of cases currently occurring in what are obviously cross-bred terriers is difficult to explain by recessive inheritance.

Secondary lens luxation

Secondary lens luxation may follow glaucoma, cataract (Fig. 11.54) or trauma. Primary glaucoma with pressure on the zonule or tearing of the zonule in early hydrophthalmos can lead to partial or total dislocation of the lens (Fig. 11.55). The lens is usually displaced medially and behind the iris (lateral aphakic crescent) and the condition may remain unilateral.

Secondary luxation of a cataractous lens, probably caused by degeneration in the zonule associated with cataract formation, occurs with various types of cataract. Trauma producing lens luxation is comparatively rare.

Lens luxation (bilateral) has also been reported in the Ehlers–Danlos syndrome (Barnett and Cottrell, 1987), an hereditary connective tissue disease with skin fragility, joint laxity and hyperextensibility.

The breed incidence of secondary lens luxation is much broader and quite different from that seen with primary luxation (see above). The age incidence is also different, secondary luxation occurring in older dogs, usually over the age of 8 years.

Treatment

Surgical extraction of the dislocated lens is the treatment of choice particularly in early cases; the earlier the case the better the prognosis, subluxation with no increase in intraocular pressure being the ideal. Later cases with an obvious secondary glaucoma and possibly peripheral ring synechiae may also require treatment for the glaucoma. The removal of

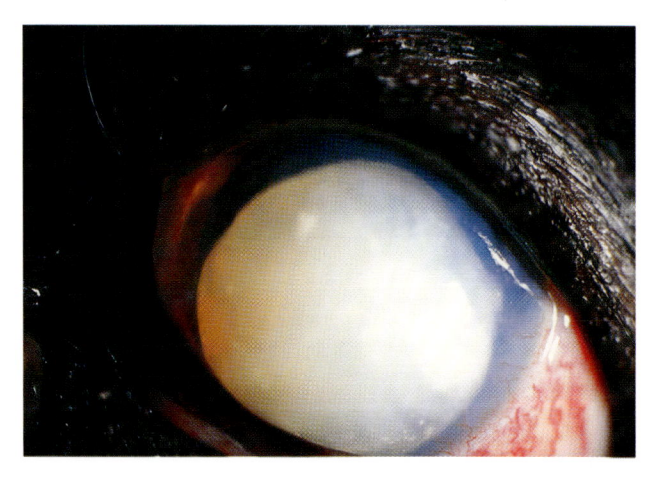

Fig. 11.54 Secondary luxation of a mature cataract with subsequent glaucoma in a Cavalier King Charles Spaniel.

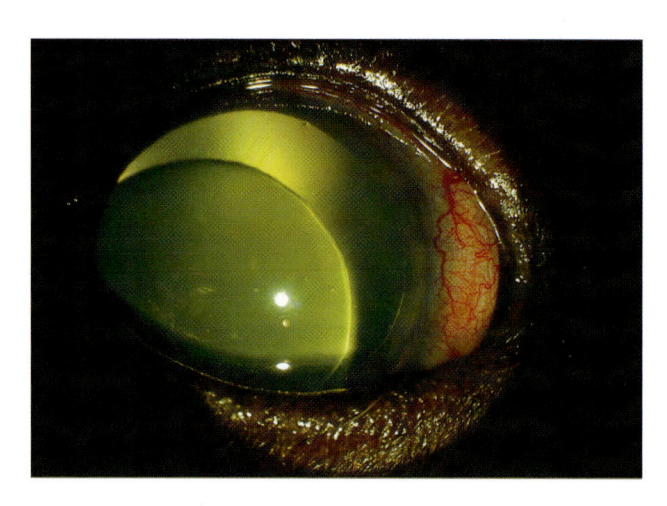

Fig. 11.55 Primary glaucoma with secondary lens luxation in a Dachshund.

a posteriorly dislocated lens with some liquefaction of the vitreous may easily have complications, but to keep the posteriorly dislocated lens in the posterior segment and prevent it coming through the pupil, even with miotics, for any practical period of time is not possible. Therefore, removal of the lens is the better option.

References

Barnett KC (1978) Hereditary cataract in the dog. *Journal of Small Animal Practice* **19**: 109–120.

Barnett KC (1980) Hereditary cataract in the Welsh Springer Spaniel. *Journal of Small Animal Practice* **21**: 621–625.

Barnett KC (1985a) The diagnosis and differential diagnosis of cataract in the dog. *Journal of Small Animal Practice* **26**: 305–316.

Barnett KC (1985b) Hereditary cataract in the Miniature Schnauzer. *Journal of Small Animal Practice* **26**: 635–644.

Barnett KC (1986) Hereditary cataract in the German Shepherd Dog. *Journal of Small Animal Practice* **27**: 387–395.

REFERENCES

Barnett KC, Cottrell BD (1987) Ehlers–Danlos syndrome in a dog: ocular, cutaneous and articular abnormalities. *Journal of Small Animal Practice* **28**: 941–946.

Barnett KC, Startup FG (1985) Hereditary cataract in the standard poodle. *Veterinary Record* **117**: 15–16.

Curtis R (1984) Late-onset cataract in the Boston terrier. *Veterinary Record* **115**: 577–578.

Curtis R, Barnett KC (1980) Primary lens luxation in the dog. *Journal of Small Animal Practice* **21**: 657–668.

Curtis R, Barnett KC (1989) A survey of cataracts in golden and labrador retrievers. *Journal of Small Animal Practice* **30**: 277–286.

Curtis R, Barnett KC, Lewis SJ (1983) Clinical and pathological observations concerning the aetiology of primary lens luxation in the dog. *Veterinary Record* **112**: 238–246.

Formston C (1945) Observations on subluxation and luxation of the crystalline lens in the dog. *Journal of Comparative Pathology* **55**: 168.

Foster SJ, Curtis R, Barnett KC (1986) Primary lens luxation in the Border Collie. *Journal of Small Animal Practice* **27**: 1–6.

Heinrich C (1999) A survey of cataract in the Leonberger. Dissertation RCVS DVOphthal.

Hippel EV (1930) Embryologische Untersuchungen uber Vererbung angeborener Katarakt, uber Schichtstar des Hundes sowie uber eine besondere Form von Kapselkatarakt. *v. Graefes Archive fur Ophthalmologic* **124**: 300.

Rubin L, Flowers R (1972) Inherited cataract in a family of Standard Poodles. *Journal of the American Veterinary Medical Association* **161**: 207–208.

Rubin LF, Koch SA, Huber RJ (1969) Hereditary cataracts in Miniature Schnauzers. *Journal of the American Veterinary Medical Association* **154**: 1456–1458.

Willis MB, Curtis R, Barnett KC, Tempest WM (1979) Genetic aspects of lens luxation in the Tibetan terrier. *Veterinary Record* **104**: 409–412.

Yakely WL (1978) A study of the heritability of cataracts in the American Cocker Spaniel. *Journal of the American Veterinary Medical Association* **172**: 814–817.

Yakely WL, Hegreberg GA, Padgett GA (1971) Familial cataracts in the American Cocker Spaniel. *Journal of the American Animal Hospital Association* **7**: 127–135.

12 UVEAL TRACT

INTRODUCTION

The uveal tract is divided into three geographically separate parts, namely the iris, the ciliary body and the choroid (Fig. 12.1). Both iris and ciliary body are referred to as the anterior uvea whereas the choroid represents the posterior uvea. The uvea is the most vascular tunic of the eye and is responsible for the vast majority of the ocular metabolism with the ciliary body as the site of aqueous humour formation and the choroid in its essential role for retinal nutrition. The anterior uvea is the site of the blood–aqueous barrier and breakdown of this barrier during uveal inflammation is responsible for many of the clinical signs of anterior uveitis.

Embryologically, the uveal tract has both neuroectodermal and mesenchymal origins and, in addition, the vascular endothelium of the uveal vessels is derived from mesodermal cells. The bilayered epithelia of posterior iris and ciliary body originate from the anterior aspect of the neuroectodermal optic cup and the iris sphincter and dilator muscle are the only mammalian muscles of neuroectodermal origin. The stroma of iris, ciliary body and choroid is derived from migrated neural crest cells, as are the ciliary muscles and the endothelium of the trabecular meshwork.

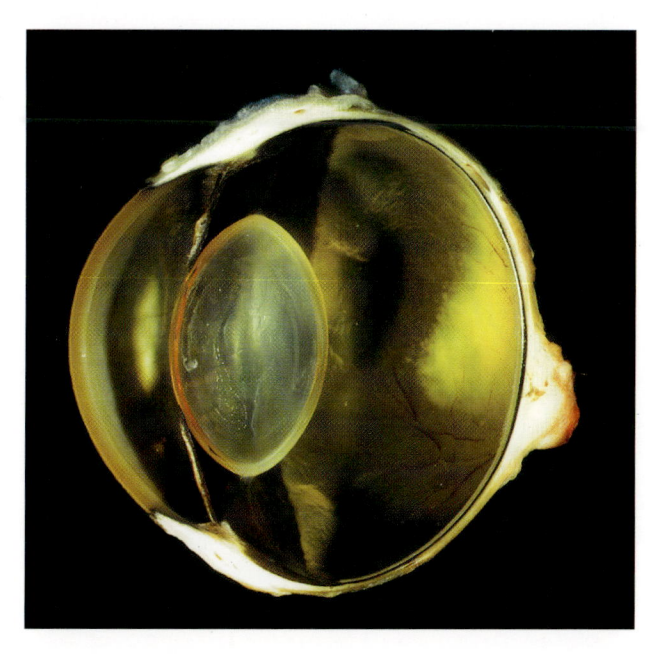

Fig. 12.1 Post-mortem view of iris, ciliary body and choroid. (Courtesy of J Mould.)

The iris is the anteriormost part of the uveal tract. It forms an incomplete contractile diaphragm, which divides the anterior ocular compartment, or anterior segment, into an anterior and a posterior chamber that communicate via the pupil. The iris is supported by the lens and any change in lens position will lead to anterior or posterior displacement of the iris plane. Lacking iris support, seen as iridodonesis (iris-wobble), is pathognomonic for lens instability. The round canine pupil is the central iris opening and pupil size is determined by the balance between iris dilator and iris sphincter muscles. The iris surface can be divided into a central pupillary zone and a peripheral, ciliary zone. The border between the two zones is named the iris collarette. The major vascular supply to the iris is via the long posterior ciliary arteries that form the major iridal circle. This structure is visible towards the iris base and is not entirely complete in the dog. Small radial arteries leave the arterial circle towards the pupil, supplying small vessels in the iris stroma. The anterior iris surface does not consist of a continuous epithelial layer but the fibroblasts and the melanocytes of the anterior iris stroma are arranged in the fashion of a pseudoepithelium, the 'anterior border layer'. The iris sphincter muscle, a thin band of circular, non-striated muscles, is situated in the pupillary portion of the iris stroma. The principle of dual innervation applies to both dilator and sphincter muscle, which are innervated sympathetically and parasympathetically (Yoshitomi and Ito, 1986). However, parasympathetic innervation dominates in the sphincter muscle whereas sympathetic innervation predominates in the dilator muscle. A bilayered pigmented epithelium forms the posterior aspect of the iris. The anterior epithelial layer gives rise to the iris dilator muscle. This muscle, which consists of a well-developed single layer of unstriated muscles, can be considered as a myoepithelium. The densely pigmented posterior iris epithelium is directly continuous with the non-pigmented outer epithelium of the ciliary body, whereas the anterior epithelial layer is continuous with the pigmented inner layer of the ciliary body epithelium.

The function of the iris is to control the amount of incoming light by adjusting the pupil size. Pupillary constriction is mediated by parasympathetic fibres in the oculomotor nerve whereas pupillary dilation is controlled by postganglionic sympathetic nerve fibres. Injury to the sympathetic fibres leads to miosis as seen in Horner's syndrome (Chapter 15).

The ciliary body is located between iris and choroid and consists of a highly vascular stroma, poorly developed ciliary muscles for limited accommodation and a bilayered posterior epithelium. It provides nourishment for avascular ocular structures by production of the aqueous humour and gives anchorage to the lens zonules via the ciliary body processes. The ciliary body can be divided into an anterior pars plicata with around 74 blade-like ciliary body processes and a posterior pars plana. The anteriormost aspect of the ciliary body forms an essential part of the iridocorneal angle (see Chapter 10). The posterior, unpigmented epithelium of the ciliary body is continuous with the neurosensory retina whereas the inner, pigmented epithelium is continuous with the retinal pigment epithelium. The area of transition between pars plana of the ciliary body and the neuroretina is termed ora ciliaris retinae and is an important landmark for surgical access into the posterior segment.

The ciliary body processes are the main sites of aqueous humour formation. Aqueous humour is a clear fluid with a refractive index of 1.335. It is formed by a combination of ultrafiltration, diffusion and active secretion. The latter is the most important mechanism and accounts for the majority of aqueous humour production. Active secretion takes place in the posterior, non-pigmented ciliary epithelium. Both Na/K-ATPase and carbonic anhydrase are enzymes highly involved in the production of aqueous humour. Medical intervention to reduce the rate of aqueous humour formation is directed at modifying carbonic anhydrase function. The rate of aqueous humour formation equals the rate of outflow under physiologically normal circumstances and the intraocular pressure is maintained at a constant level. The aqueous humour resembles an ultrafiltrate of plasma with markedly lower protein levels (0.38 mg/100 ml in the aqueous humour compared with 6.5 mg/100 ml in plasma). During breakdown of the blood–aqueous barrier, protein levels in the aqueous humour are dramatically increased, which can be clinically appreciated as aqueous flare (see below).

The tight junctions of the non-pigmented ciliary body epithelium form the blood–aqueous barrier, prohibiting free diffusion of protein and low molecular weight (above 40 Å) solutes into the aqueous humour. No barrier exists between blood and vitreous body and large fenestrations in the ciliary body vasculature allow leakage of most plasma components up to a size of 250 Å into the stroma. This gives the ciliary body tissue fluid a plasmoid appearance. This anterior part of the blood–ocular barrier is not as efficient as the blood–retinal barrier and some protein does pass into the aqueous humour (see above). Furthermore, tight junctions of the endothelium of the iris vessels prohibit free diffusion of solutes larger than 40 Å, as the large intracellular spaces of the anterior iris stroma are in free contact with the aqueous humour in the anterior chamber.

The highly vascularised and heavily pigmented choroid is situated between retina and sclera. Histologically, the choroid can be divided into five layers including Bruch's membrane, the choriocapillaris, the cellular tapetum (which can be absent occasionally), the stroma and the suprachoroid. The arterial blood supply for the choroid comes from the long and short posterior ciliary arteries and from the anterior ciliary arteries. Venous drainage of the choroid occurs via the vortex veins. The choroid is essential for the function of the posterior retinal layers and choroidal blood flow is extremely rapid. Unlike retinal vessels, choroidal vessels lack all autoregulation in the dog and are therefore extremely prone to systemic blood pressure alterations. The choroidal capillaries are highly permeable and allow nutrients to diffuse readily into the retinal pigment epithelium, whose tight junctions act as the blood–retinal barrier. The plasmoid character of the choroidal tissue fluid with its high osmotic pressure assists in keeping the retina dehydrated and aligned to the outer ocular tunics.

Congenital and developmental anomalies

Colour variations

Iris colour is due to the amount of melanocytes in the iris stroma and the thickness of the anterior border layer. It can vary considerably between individuals (Figs 12.2–12.4 and 12.8) and even between the two eyes of an individual (Fig. 12.5). Animals with colour dilution often have blue irides (Fig. 12.4) as a result of lack of pigment in the iris stroma. True ocular albinism with lack of all pigment has not been reported in the dog. The difference in iris colour in the same eye or between the two eyes of an individual is termed heterochromia iridis (Figs 12.5 and 12.6). Iris colour is inherited and related to coat colour and fundus colour (see Chapter 14).

Aniridia, iris hypoplasia and iris coloboma

Aniridia, the total absence of the iris, is extremely rare in the dog, whereas iris hypoplasia has been reported alone or in conjunction with other defects associated with merle ocular dysgenesis (Gelatt and McGill, 1973; Cook et al., 1991). Iris hypoplasia may affect part or the whole iris and can be partial (Fig. 12.7) or complete (Fig. 12.8). A coloboma is the focal total absence of iris tissue and only rarely found in the dog (Figs 12.8 and 12.9). Typical colobomata are situated in the

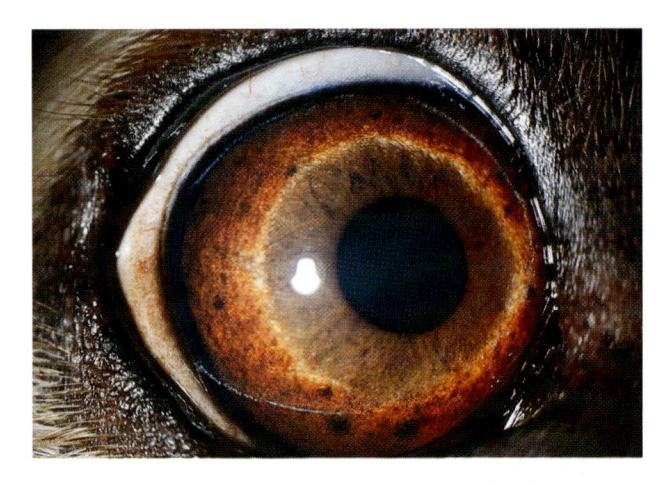

Fig. 12.2 Brown pigmented iris in a 5-year-old Labrador Retriever (yellow coat colour).

CONGENITAL AND DEVELOPMENTAL ANOMALIES

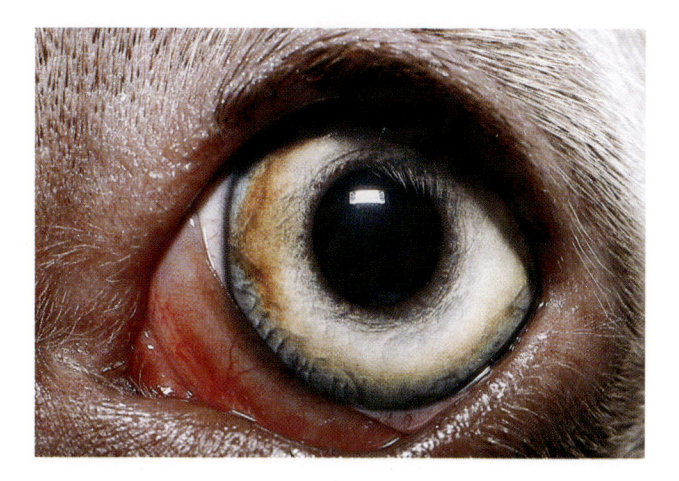

Fig. 12.3 Yellow iris in a silver-grey Weimaraner.

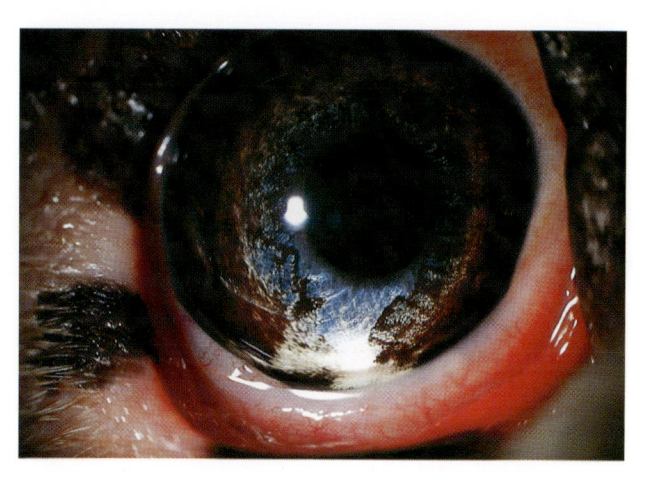

Fig. 12.6 Heterochromia iridis in a 3-year-old English Bulldog ('parti-coloured' iris).

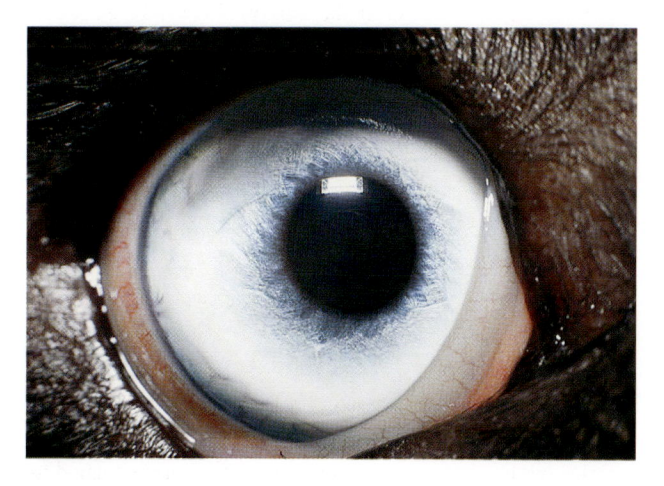

Fig. 12.4 Blue iris ('wall eye' or 'China eye') in a Bernese Mountain Dog. (Courtesy of PW Renwick.)

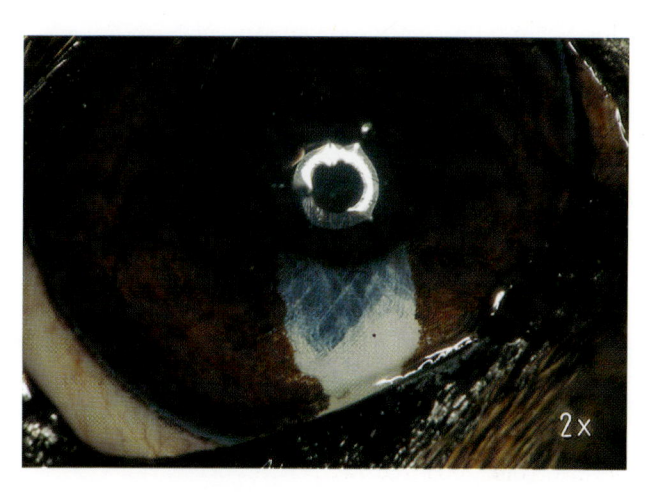

Fig. 12.7 Partial iris hypoplasia in a 1-year-old Tibetan Spaniel resulting in heterochromia iridis. Both eyes were identical, a condition recognised in this breed.

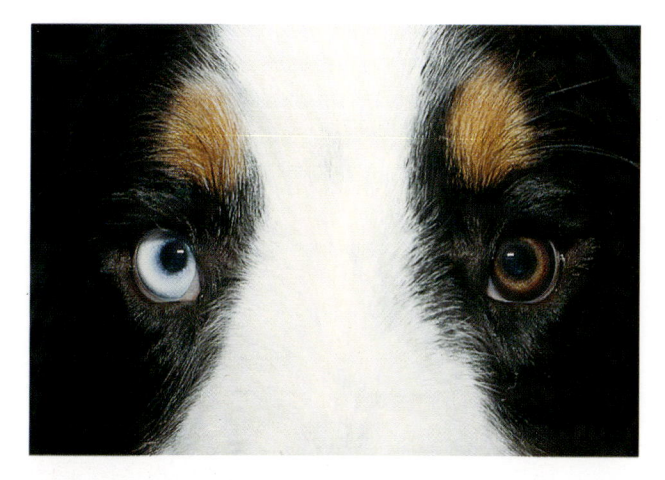

Fig. 12.5 Heterochromia iridis in a Bernese Mountain Dog (same dog as in Fig. 12.4). (Courtesy of PW Renwick.)

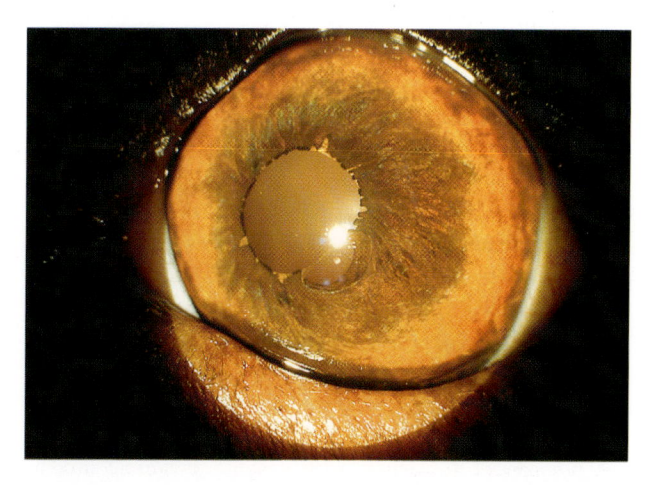

Fig. 12.8 Mild iris hypoplasia and small iris coloboma from 4–6 o'clock in an English Springer Spaniel. Note bright brown iris colour associated with liver coat colour.

129

UVEAL TRACT

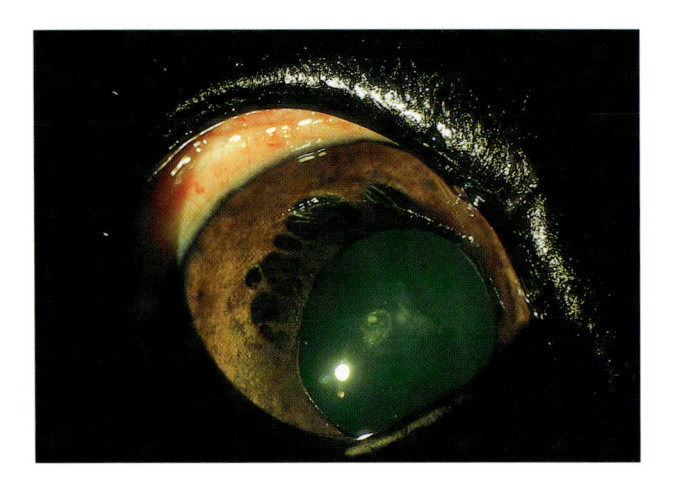

Fig. 12.9 Multiple small iris colobomata.

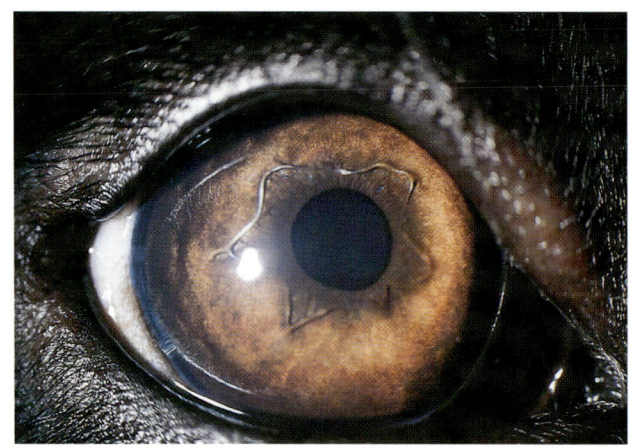

Fig. 12.10 Persistent pupillary membranes in a young Leonberger – typical star-shaped appearance.

6 o'clock position and are thought to be the result of an incomplete fusion of the optic fissure. Atypical coloboma can affect any part of the iris. Iris coloboma can be associated with other ocular colobomata such as lens coloboma and zonular defects.

CHOROIDAL HYPOPLASIA

Choroidal hypoplasia is seen as the mildest form of collie eye anomaly and presents as a hypopigmented patch lateral to the optic disc. This condition is discussed in more detail in Chapter 14 (see Figs 14.19 and 14.22).

PERSISTENT PUPILLARY MEMBRANES

Persistent pupillary membranes (PPMs) are remnants of the anterior pupillary membrane (see Chapter 11), which should have receded by approximately 8 weeks of age. However, fine remnants may take up to 6 months to regress fully and a diagnosis of PPM should not be made before this age. PPMs are common in the dog but fortunately of little clinical significance in the majority of affected individuals. Clinically, PPMs present as tissue strands originating from the iris collarette (Fig. 12.10). This detail is important in distinguishing between anterior and posterior synechiae, with the latter usually involving the pupillary margin. The majority of PPMs are avascular and the tissue strands can be seen extending blind into the anterior chamber or spanning from one point on the iris surface (Fig. 12.10), sometimes across the pupil (Fig. 12.11), to another point on the iris surface. Occasionally, PPMs can attach to the corneal endothelium (Figs 12.12 and 12.13) or the anterior lens surface (Fig. 12.14), causing focal opacities at their points of insertion. These opacities histologically resemble areas of dysplasia of lens epithelium or corneal endothelium and Descemet's membrane. Clinically, anterior capsular and subcapsular cataract formation or corneal oedema are seen on slit-lamp biomicroscopy. Extensive PPM formation with ensuing blindness due to corneal opacification has been described in the Basenji (Roberts and Bistner, 1968; Barnett and Knight, 1969), a breed in which this condition is believed to be inherited. PPMs

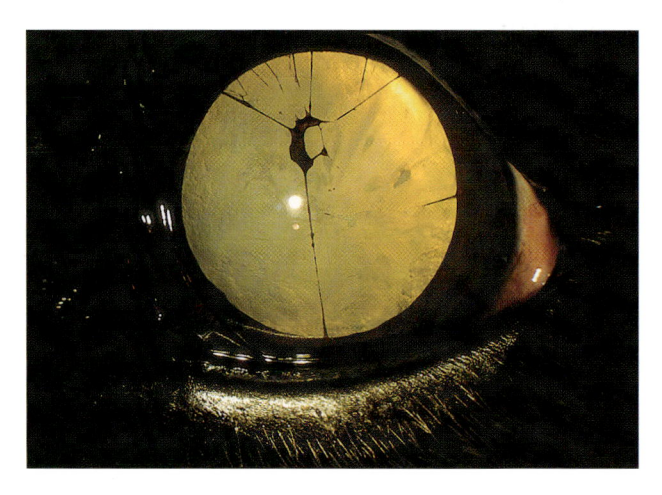

Fig. 12.11 Fine persistent pupillary membranes highlighted against the tapetal reflex spanning across the pupil. Note extensive cataract formation.

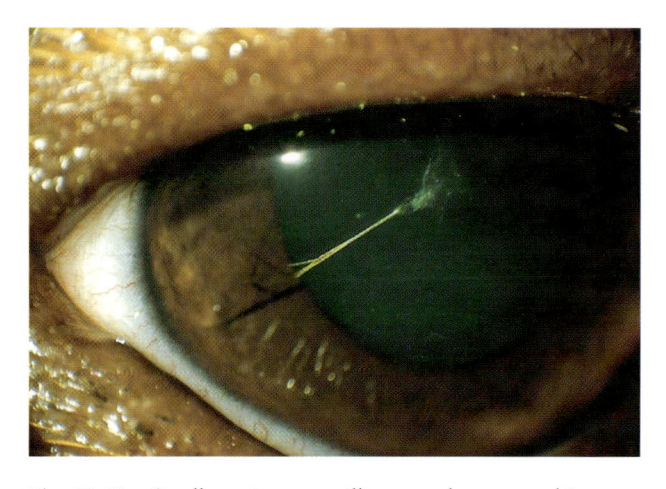

Fig. 12.12 Small persistent pupillary membrane attaching to the corneal endothelium causing a focal corneal opacity in a Basenji puppy.

ACQUIRED CONDITIONS OF THE IRIS

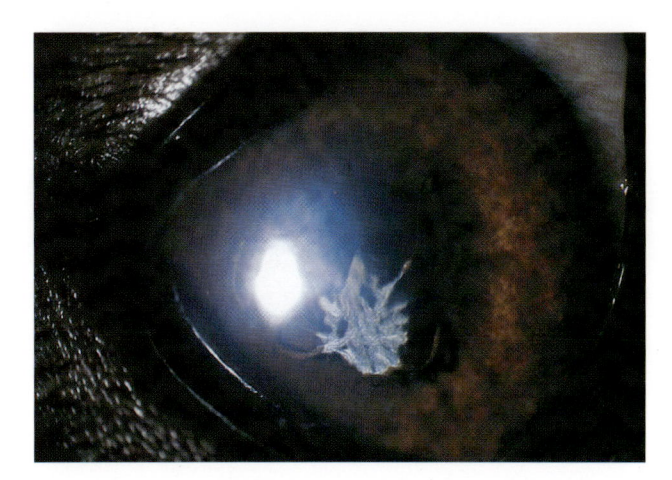

Fig. 12.13 More extensive corneal opacity with persistent pupillary membrane adhesion to the corneal endothelium.

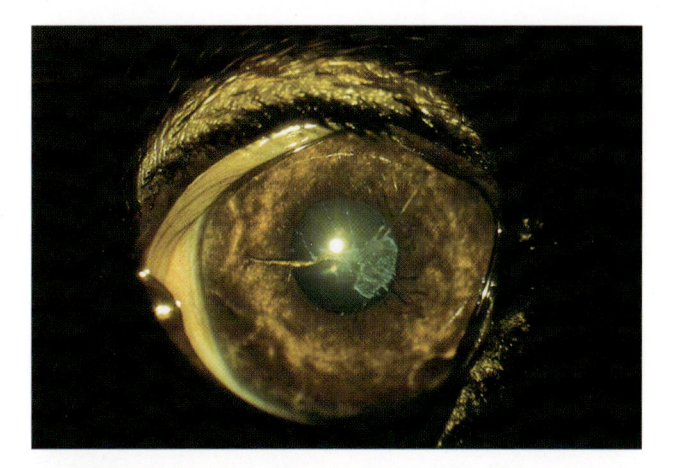

Fig. 12.14 Multiple persistent pupillary membranes adherent to anterior lens surface in association with multiple ocular defects including microphthalmia and cataract in an English Bullmastiff.

have also been described in the Cocker Spaniel (Strande *et al.*, 1988) and are a common finding in eyes with multiocular defects (Fig. 12.14) (Collins *et al.*, 1992).

ANTERIOR SEGMENT DYSGENESIS

Failure of the normal formation of the anterior chamber with the regression of the mesenchymal tissue may lead to several abnormalities such as goniodysgenesis (see Chapter 10) or anterior segment dysgenesis syndrome. The latter has been described in the Doberman Pinscher (Peiffer and Fischer, 1983) and affected puppies suffer from severe and multiple ocular anomalies, including malformation of cornea, lens and anterior uvea. Affected puppies are blind from birth.

ACQUIRED CONDITIONS OF THE IRIS

BENIGN IRIS PIGMENTATION

Discrete foci of hyperpigmentation (freckles) are commonly seen in the canine iris and must be distinguished clinically from melanocytic neoplasms. Iris freckles are well-circumscribed clusters of hyperpigmented melanocytes that do not protrude above the iris surface as seen on slit-lamp examination (Fig. 12.15). Once pigmented areas protrude above the iris surface or lead to a distortion of the normal iris architecture, an increase in cellularity of the pigmented cells must be assumed and the presence of a neoplastic process such as a benign iris melanoma must be considered (see below).

Diffuse iris melanosis is also occasionally seen and can be the earliest indicator of a chronic low-grade uveitis (Figs 12.47 and 11.7). Diffuse iris thickening and darkening is a key feature of the ocular melanosis syndrome described for the Cairn Terrier and occasionally seen in other breeds (Fig. 12.16). Affected dogs show infiltration of the uveal tract, sclera, and drainage angle with hyperpigmented melanocytes, and the condition does eventually lead to loss of sight due to glaucoma.

IRIS ATROPHY

Both senile and secondary iris atrophy have been reported in the dog (Belkin, 1975).

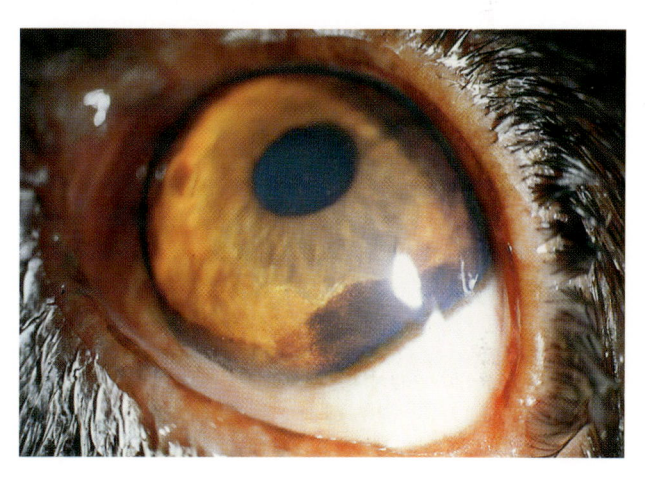

Fig. 12.15 Focal iris hyperpigmentation in an English Springer Spaniel.

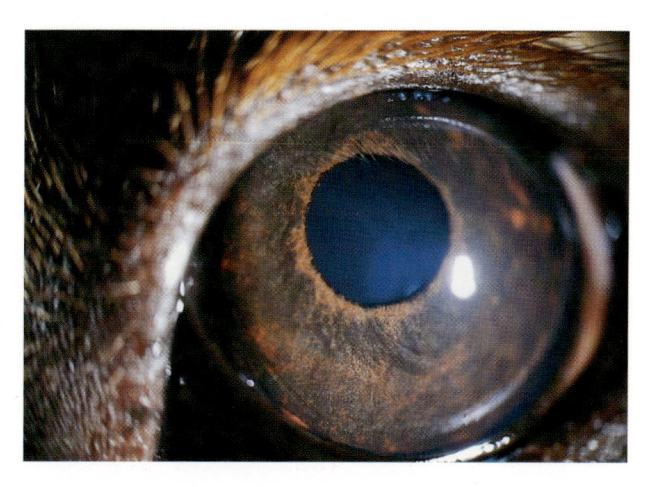

Fig. 12.16 Diffuse iris hyperpigmentation in a Golden Retriever. Both eyes were affected in this case with the changes more advanced in the left eye.

131

UVEAL TRACT

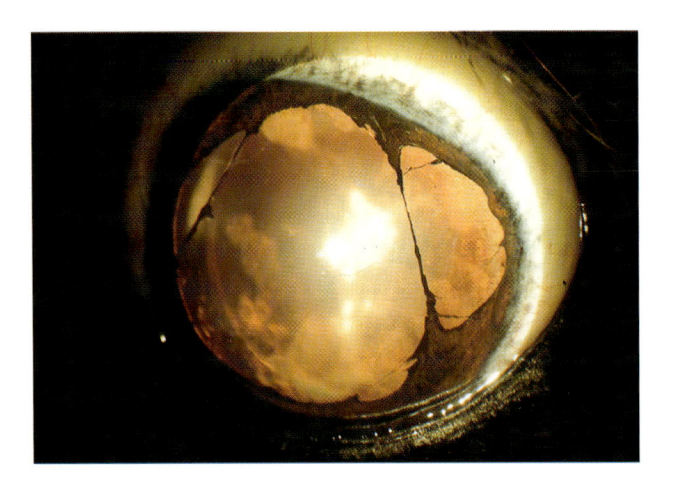

Fig. 12.17 Advanced iris atrophy in a 9-year-old Shih Tzu and concurrent incipient cataract.

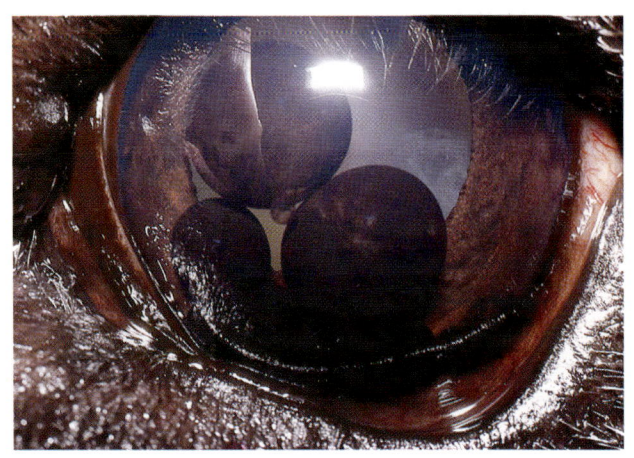

Fig. 12.19 Multiple free-floating iris cysts in a 9-year-old Labrador Retriever. (Courtesy of PW Renwick.)

Senile iris atrophy is a condition commonly seen in older dogs and the resultant loss of sphincter muscle function can result in a dilated pupil with a poor pupillary light response. The poodle breeds appear especially predisposed to this condition, which can be so extensive that full-thickness defects similar to iris coloboma can occur (Fig. 12.17). Essentially of no clinical importance, senile iris atrophy can complicate the assessment of vision with the help of pupillary light responses.

In contrast to senile iris atrophy, secondary iris atrophy due to iritis or glaucoma can be associated with visual deficits.

IRIS CYSTS

Iris cysts are pigmented spheres that can be found free-floating in the anterior chamber or attached to the pupillary margin (Corcoran and Koch, 1993). Single (Fig. 12.18) or multiple (Fig. 12.19) cysts are found and frequently both eyes of the same individual are affected. Large cysts can become stuck between iris and cornea (Fig. 12.18) or rupture (Fig. 12.20), sometimes leaving pigmented remnants on the

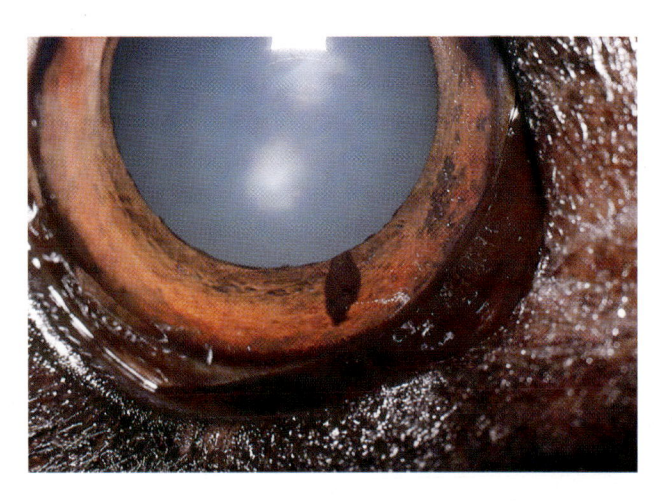

Fig. 12.20 Ruptured iris cyst still adhering to the posterior iris epithelium at the pupillary margins.

corneal endothelium. Size, position and the fact that they can be transilluminated (Fig. 12.21) allow differentiation of cysts from melanocytic iris neoplasms. Occasionally, cysts can contain blood (Figs 12.22 and 12.23). The aetiology of iris cyst formation is unclear and although some may be congenital, underlying inflammatory disease must be considered (Fig. 12.24). Surgical intervention is not required in the majority of cases although obstruction of the visual axis may justify removal in some dogs (guide dogs). A more severe condition with glaucoma as a result of the formation of ciliary body cysts has been described in the Golden Retriever (Deehr and Dubielzig, 1998) and the Great Dane (Spiess et al., 1998) (see Chapter 10). However, in neither breed has the presence of ciliary body cysts been associated with glaucoma in the United Kingdom.

SYNECHIAE

Adhesions between iris and corneal endothelium (anterior synechiae) or iris and lens (posterior synechiae) are usually the result of anterior uveal inflammation or trauma (Figs 12.25

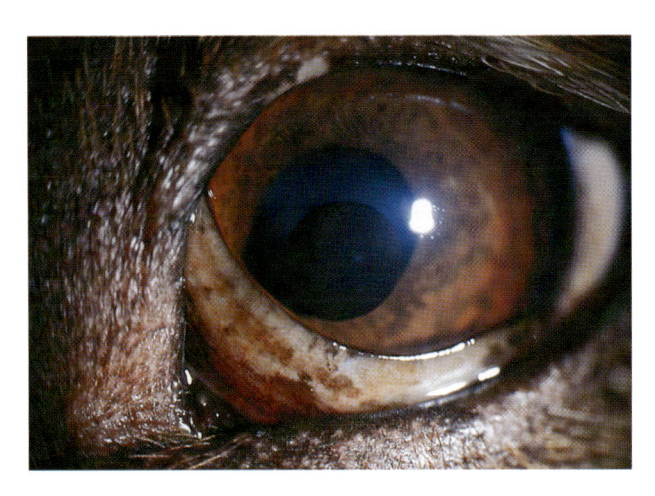

Fig. 12.18 Iris cyst wedged between iris and corneal endothelium in the pupillary aperture in an adult Labrador Retriever.

ACQUIRED CONDITIONS OF THE IRIS

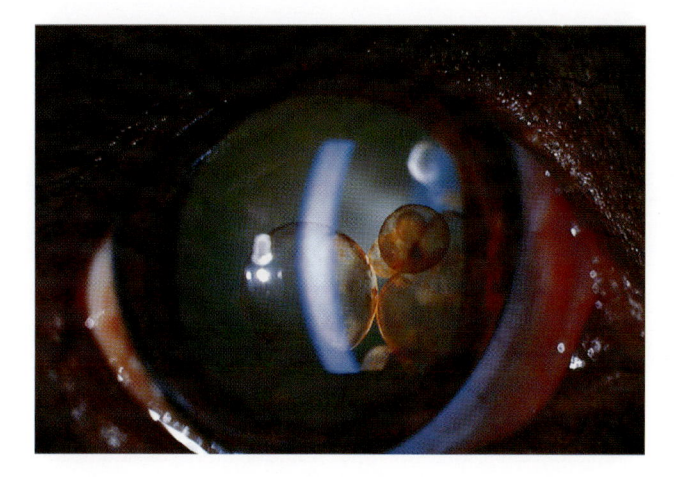

Fig. 12.21 Transillumination of iris cysts with the help of a slit beam. Transillumination is helpful to distinguish iris cysts from pigmented uveal neoplasms.

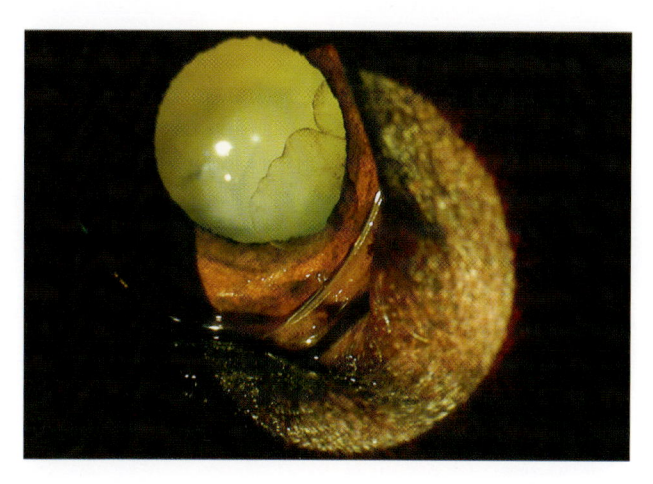

Fig. 12.24 Iris cyst formation associated with cataract formation. Note the cysts originate in the posterior chamber where they are still attached to the pigmented iris epithelium.

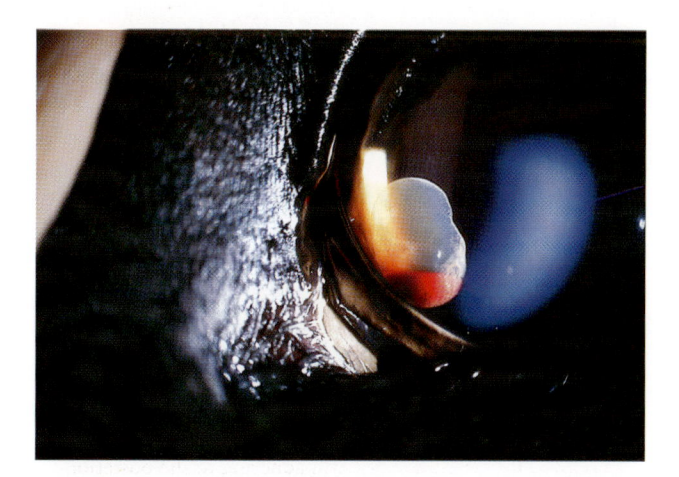

Fig. 12.22 Blood-filled iris cyst in an adult female Standard Poodle.

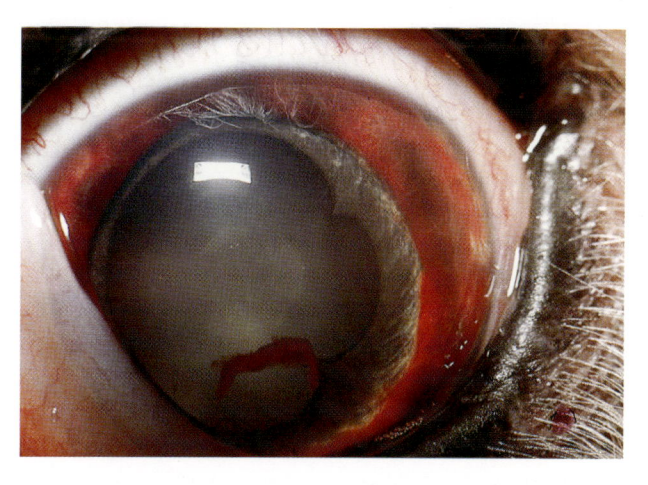

Fig. 12.25 Posterior synechiae and haemorrhage on the anterior lens capsule as the result of a chronic anterior uveitis in a 10-year-old Old English Sheepdog. Note the iris swelling and colour change (originally blue iris) described as rubeosis iridis.

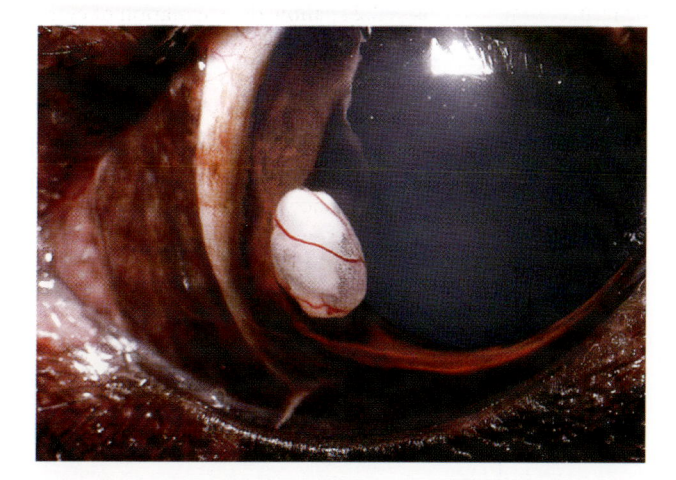

Fig. 12.23 Unusual, vascularised and possibly calcified iris cyst. Note the ectropion uveae to both sides of the cyst indicating a chronic inflammatory process in the anterior chamber.

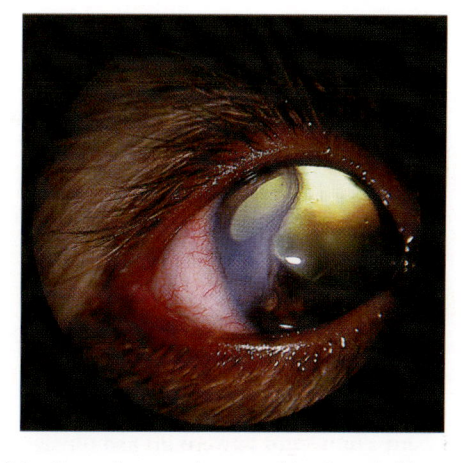

Fig. 12.26 Extensive anterior synechiae in a Golden Retriever puppy following cat scratch injury with iris prolapse.

UVEAL TRACT

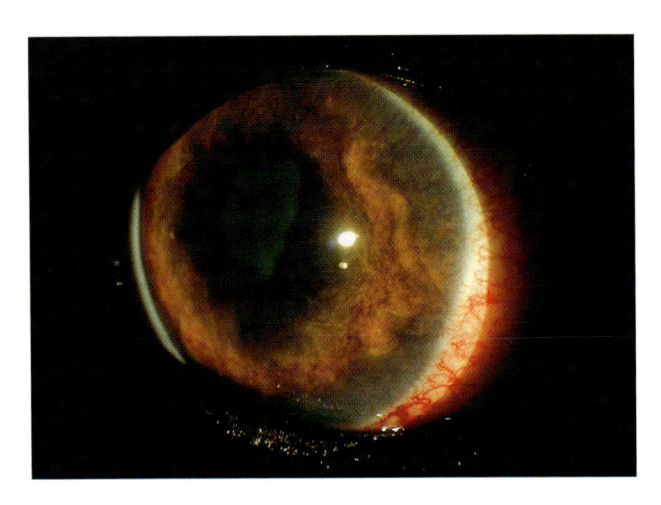

Fig. 12.27 Iris bombé formation and glaucoma as the result of total posterior synechiae in a chronic uveitis of unknown aetiology.

and 12.26). Extensive synechia formation does not only interfere with a clear visual axis but can impair aqueous humour circulation and cause glaucoma. Iris bombé formation is the result of a total posterior synechia, and the increased aqueous humour pressure in the posterior chamber leads to a forward billowing of the iris tissue with resultant peripheral anterior synechia formation and obstruction of the iridocorneal angle (Fig. 12.27).

UVEITIS

Inflammation of the uveal tract can be divided into anterior uveitis (iritis and iridocyclitis), intermediate uveitis (pars planitis) and posterior uveitis (choroiditis). Retinal involvement is common in choroiditis due to the close proximity between retina and choroid, and the term chorioretinitis is preferred. In panuveitis, the entire uveal tract is involved in the inflammatory process. The ocular irritative response involves the breakdown of the blood–ocular barrier (Bellhorn, 1991). This breakdown usually takes place at the level of the iris vascular endothelium, which contracts in response to chemical mediators and creates gaps in the vascular wall through which both proteins and cells can leak into the aqueous humour. The tight junctions of the non-pigmented ciliary epithelium tend to break down later as the result of ciliary body swelling and it may be months before these anterior components of the blood–ocular barrier can be restored. The disruption of the blood–eye barrier allows exposure of ocular antigens to the systemic immune system, which leads to an overwhelming of the usually existing low-dose tolerance mechanisms against these antigens.

A wide variety of both exogenous and endogenous aetiologies exist including traumatic, infectious, neoplastic, metabolic, parasitic and toxic causes. Systemic aetiologies must be considered, especially in bilateral cases of uveal inflammation, and every effort must be made to identify and treat the underlying cause. In addition to the routine ophthalmic examination, further diagnostic aids including haematology and biochemistry profiles, clotting assays, ocular ultrasonography and intraocular pressure assessment should be employed. Serological tests are available for a number of conditions that are known causes of uveitis including antibody titre assays for *Toxoplasma*, *Leishmania*, *Borrelia* and *Ehrlichia*. However, even with extensive investigations, the aetiology of the uveal inflammation remains unidentified in a large proportion of cases. Although these cases are often grouped together as idiopathic, immune-mediated disease must be suspected.

Clinical signs of uveitis vary according to severity, type and duration of the inflammation. A strict classification according to the type of cellular infiltrate in neutrophilic, lymphocytic–plasmacytic and granulomatous is, clinically, usually not possible as, especially with time, combinations of the different types of inflammation are common. Unlike in the cat, low-grade chronic lymphocytic–plasmacytic uveitis with only mild clinical symptoms is less common and it is often the dramatic and sudden onset clinical signs of an acute uveitis that raises the owner's concern. Blepharospasm and epiphora, conjunctival hyperaemia, episcleral congestion and corneal oedema are common presenting signs (Fig. 12.28). Depending on the degree of severity, sudden loss of vision occurs. The hyperaemia of the deep perilimbal anterior ciliary vessels, also termed 'ciliary flush', can be readily distinguished from simple conjunctival hyperaemia with the application of a drop of 10% phenylephrine. This drug will blanch the conjunctival vessels but will not affect the deeper vessels. The iris can change colour and become lighter (Fig. 12.29) or darker (Figs 12.25 and 12.47) and iris thickness can increase both focally or diffusely (Fig. 12.29).

Miosis is commonly seen in uveitis and is the result of a prostaglandin-mediated spasm in iris sphincter and ciliary body musculature (Fig. 12.30). Miosis is a common feature in reflex uveitis, where corneal erosion leads to iris contraction via axon reflex. Relief of the ocular pain caused by this muscle spasm with the help of cycloplegic drugs is one of the

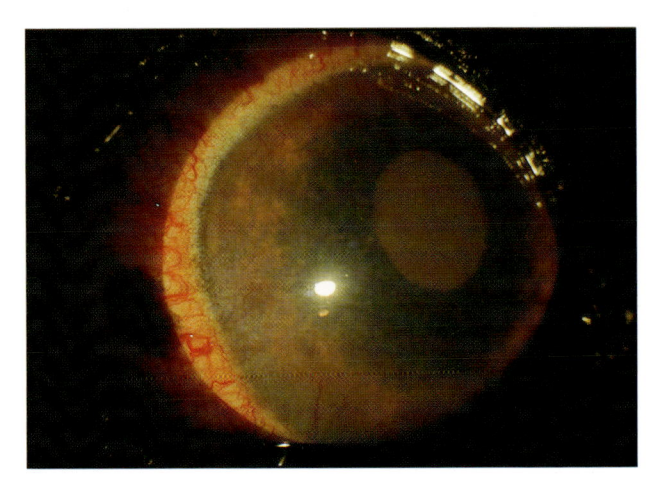

Fig. 12.28 Anterior uveitis of unknown aetiology with ciliary flush, miosis, corneal oedema and corneal vascularisation in an adult Collie cross.

ACQUIRED CONDITIONS OF THE IRIS

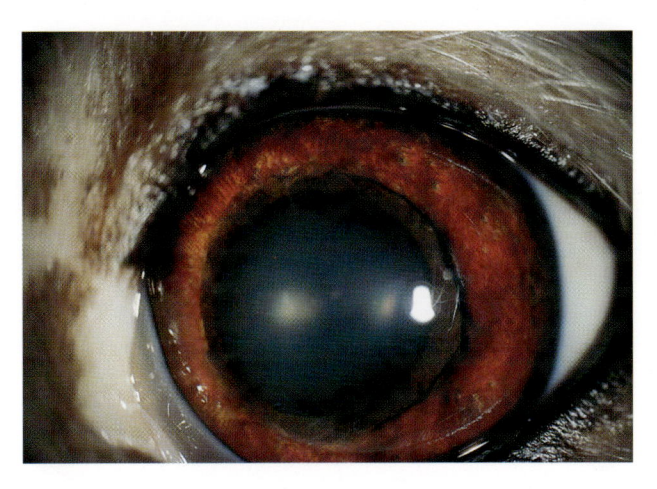

Fig. 12.29 Dramatic swelling and rubeosis iridis in a 10-year-old English Springer Spaniel.

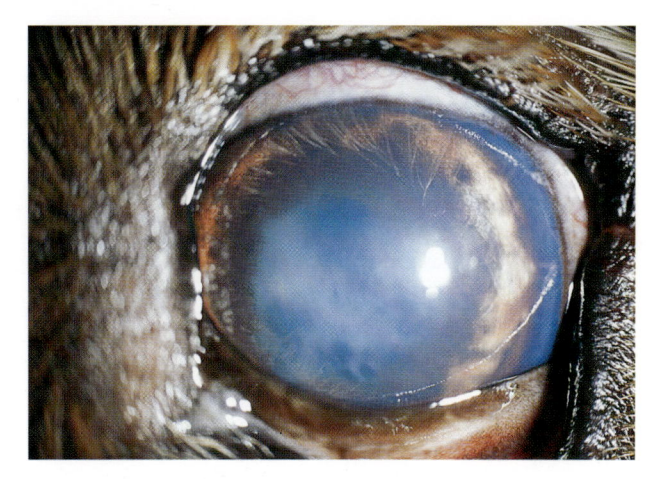

Fig. 12.31 Chronic uveitis with extensive posterior synechiae and incipient cataract formation in a 5-year-old Golden Retriever.

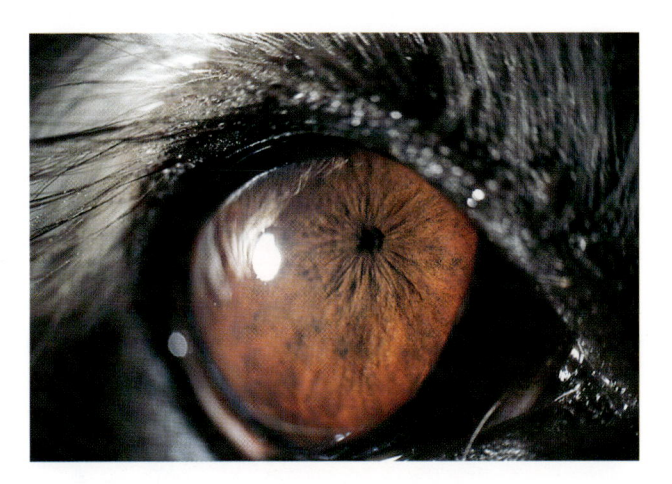

Fig. 12.30 Extreme miosis mediated by prostaglandin 2 alpha.

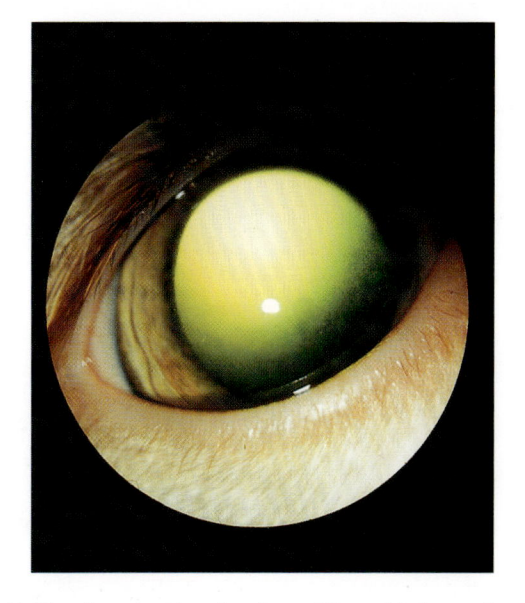

Fig. 12.32 Anterior chamber flare. (Note: this is a cat's eye.)

mainstays of uveitis therapy. However, pupillary constriction is not found in all cases of uveitis as iris mobility can be impaired by the formation of posterior synechiae (Fig. 12.31). Furthermore, inflammation-related increases in intraocular pressure can result in paralysis of the iris sphincter muscle and mydriasis ensues.

In general, uveitis is associated with ocular hypotension due to a reduction in aqueous humour formation. For this reason, tonometry can be a helpful diagnostic tool in cases of mild or subclinical uveitis where a reduction in intraocular pressure may be the only symptom found. The pupillary border of the iris can be seen to fold forward to adhere to the anterior iris surface (ectropion uveae) (see Fig. 12.23) or backwards to adhere to the posterior iris epithelium (entropion uveae). Increased amounts of cells and protein in the aqueous humour are visible on slit-lamp examination of the anterior chamber as aqueous flare (see Chapter 10) (Fig. 12.32). In severe cases, fibrin clots can form in the anterior chamber (Fig. 12.33). Quantification of the degree of aqueous flare in anterior chamber laser flaremetry and fluorophotometry is a helpful diagnostic aid to quantify the

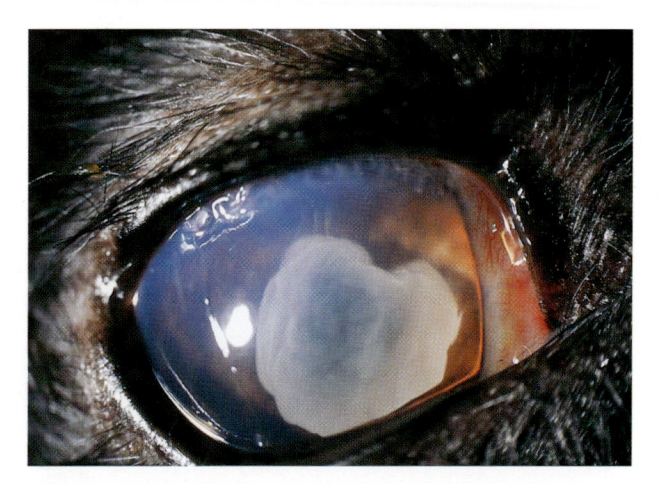

Fig. 12.33 Fibrin clot in the anterior chamber of a Tibetan Terrier following intracapsular lendectomy for primary lens luxation and extensive corneal vascularisation.

UVEAL TRACT

severity of the ocular irritative response (Krohne et al., 1995) under experimental circumstances. Cells and debris (including protein and pigment) that become adherent to the corneal endothelium are described as keratic precipitates. The colour of keratic precipitates is variable depending on the main constituent of the deposit. Waxy-yellow deposits have been described as 'mutton-fat' precipitates (Fig. 12.34) and are believed to consist of macrophages and plasma cells, whereas lymphocytic–plasmacytic deposits appear fine and granular (Fig. 12.35). The majority of keratic precipitates are located at the inferior endothelium due to thermal convection currents. As this area of cornea is often obscured by the third eyelid, keratic precipitates are readily overlooked. The presence of keratic precipitates in an otherwise quiet eye is suggestive of a previous episode of uveitis, as are posterior synechiae or remaining patches of pigment on the anterior lens capsule. Cataract formation is a common sequel of uveitis as the changes in aqueous humour composition may have adverse effects on the metabolism of the avascular lens.

The accumulation of white blood cells in the ventral part of the anterior chamber is termed hypopyon. Hypopyon can be the result of a sterile reflex uveitis in response to corneal ulceration (Fig. 12.36) or due to an infectious endophthalmitis (Fig. 12.37). Large accumulations of neoplastic white blood cells are seen in ocular lymphosarcoma (Fig. 12.38). Occasionally, uveitis results in anterior chamber haemorrhage, described as hyphaema (Fig. 12.39).

Inflammation of the posterior uveal tract can be seen alone or in association with anterior uveal inflammation. Subretinal effusions associated with choroiditis appear as hyporeflective, grey and dull patches in the tapetal fundus and as areas of lighter pigmentation in the non-tapetal fundus. Extensive subretinal effusions can lead to serous retinal detachment with resultant loss of vision (Fig. 12.40). Mild to severe infiltration of the vitreous with inflammatory cells and plasma components becomes clinically manifest as vitritis (see Fig. 13.13). Ocular ultrasonography is an essen-

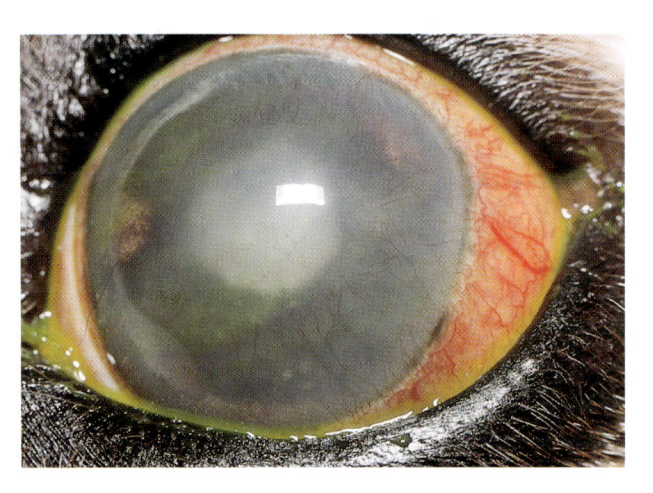

Fig. 12.34 'Mutton-fat' keratic precipitates in a chronic untreated lens-induced uveitis in a diabetic Boxer cross. Note also corneal oedema.

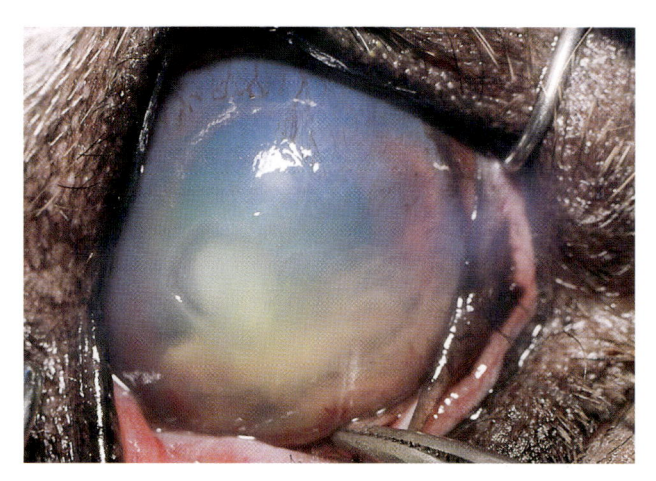

Fig. 12.36 Sterile hypopyon secondary to deep corneal ulceration in a 9-year-old Shih Tzu.

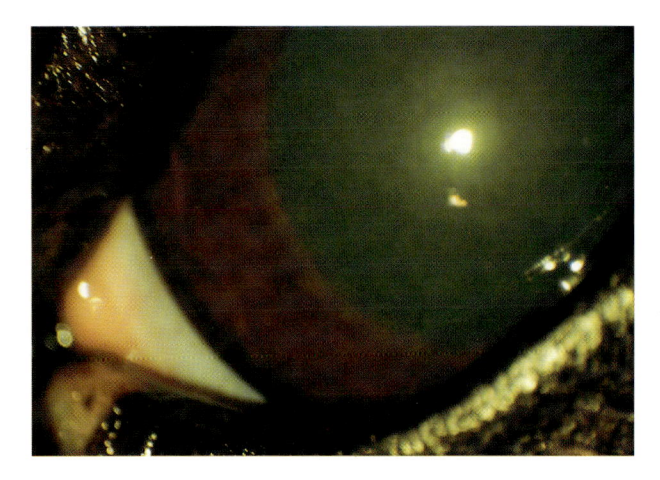

Fig. 12.35 Fine granular keratic precipitates in chronic, uncontrolled lens-induced uveitis.

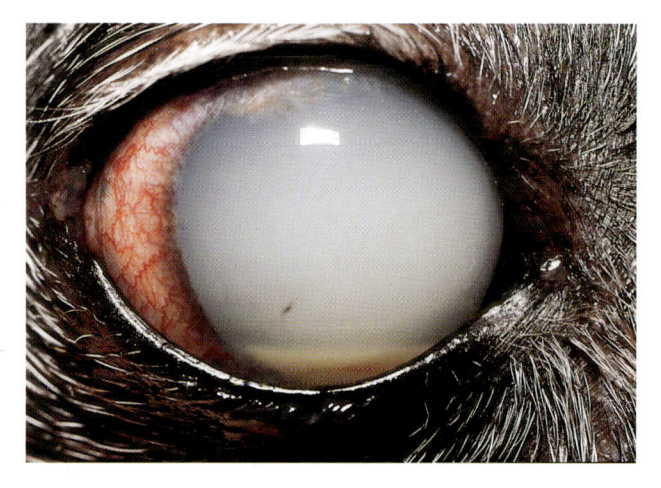

Fig. 12.37 Possibly infectious endophthalmitis with hypopyon 12 months following phacoemulsification in a 12-year-old Jack Russell Terrier.

ACQUIRED CONDITIONS OF THE IRIS

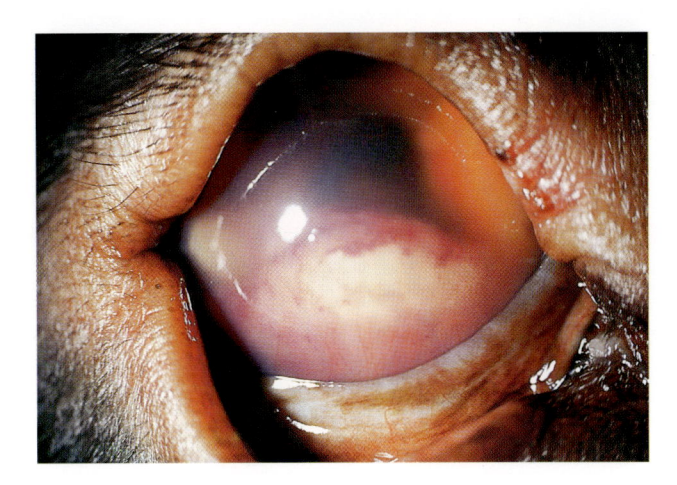

Fig. 12.38 Uveitis and hypopyon in multicentric lymphoma in a young adult Labrador Retriever.

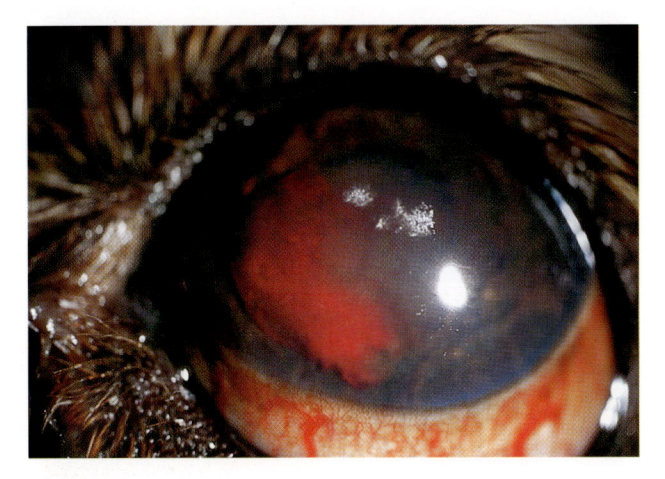

Fig. 12.39 Mild anterior uveitis and intraocular haemorrhage in a Cavalier King Charles Spaniel with pyometra. The ocular lesions were the presenting complaint.

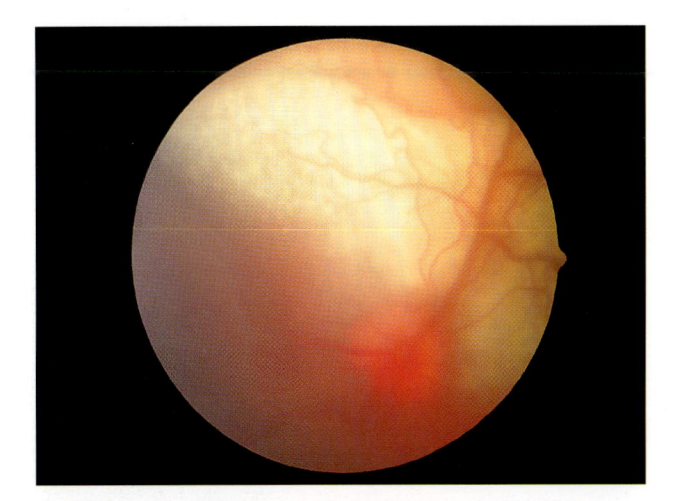

Fig. 12.40 Posterior uveitis with subretinal effusion and partial retinal detachment of unknown aetiology in a 9-year-old Pointer cross Spaniel. The dog also had anterior uveitis at the time of presentation.

tial diagnostic procedure in cases of posterior segment inflammation and can demonstrate choroidal thickening.

Complications of uncontrolled uveal inflammation are serious and can result in permanent loss of vision through corneal oedema, cataract formation, glaucoma, retinal detachment and phthisis bulbi (Fig. 12.41 and see Fig. 4.21).

Traumatic uveitis (see also Chapter 3) can be the result of direct involvement of the uveal tract or secondary to injury to other ocular structures. Traumatic uveitis is usually limited to one eye and the severity of the inflammation is related to the type of injury. Generally, sharp trauma is better tolerated than blunt trauma and whereas uveal involvement is readily assessed in perforations of the anterior segment (Fig. 12.42), it is difficult to assess uveal trauma in scleral ruptures. Reflex uveitis is commonly seen following corneal abrasions (cat scratch!) and does usually readily respond to medical treatment. More severe signs of anterior uveitis are associated with perforating ocular injuries and retained intraocular foreign bodies. Infection and disruption of the

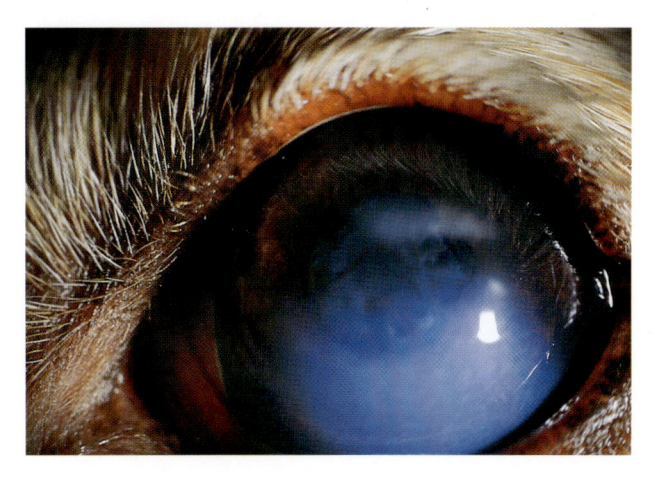

Fig. 12.41 Permanent corneal oedema, posterior synechiae and cataract formation as the result of chronic uveitis in an 8-year-old Labrador Retriever.

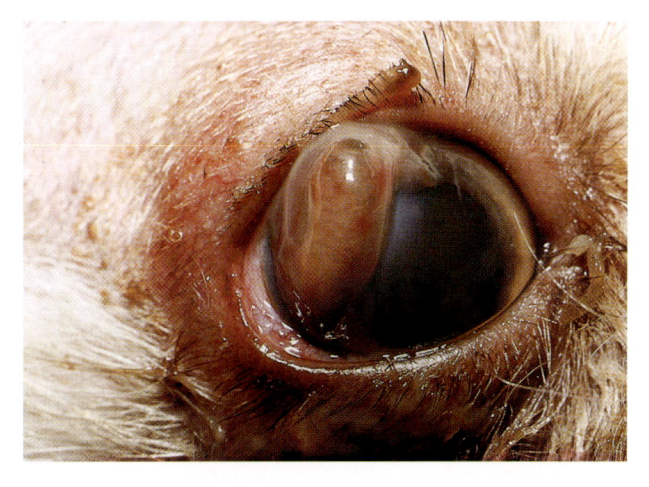

Fig. 12.42 Extensive prolapse of uveal tissue following large limbal perforation in a young Jack Russell Terrier.

anterior lens capsule can lead to treatment-resistant deleterious inflammation (see below)(Fig. 12.43). Blunt trauma to the eye causes a shock wave, which can result in extensive intraocular haemorrhage as it reverberates through iris and ciliary body. A guarded prognosis must be given especially for ocular shotgun injuries where both perforation and severe intraocular haemorrhage are combined (see Fig. 3.23).

Infectious uveitis is rare in the UK but commonly seen in the more southern European countries and the US. However, with the changes in quarantine regulations and with the introduction of pet travel schemes, veterinary surgeons must be aware of the increasingly frequent presentation of such 'exotic' conditions.

Infectious uveitis can be the result of damage caused directly by the pathogen, by immune-mediated responses or by circulating endotoxins.

Corneal oedema as the result of uveitis due to infection with canine adenovirus (CAV)1 and as a response to the CAV1 vaccine (see Fig. 9.42) is only occasionally seen following the introduction of a CAV2 vaccine (Curtis and Barnett, 1983). Whereas the acute clinical phase is characterised by a subclinical lymphocytic–plasmacytic anterior uveitis, it is the delayed type hypersensitivity reaction against intraocular antigen that damages the corneal endothelium (Aguirre *et al.*, 1975) 2–3 weeks following initial viraemia, leading to the characteristic corneal oedema. Total recovery and corneal clearing occurs in the majority of animals within 2–3 weeks and only 3% of affected individuals retain permanent corneal damage. Sight-hounds, especially Afghans are reported to carry an increased risk for complications of CAV1 uveitis including permanent corneal oedema and glaucoma (Curtis and Barnett, 1981). Diagnosis is based on history (young dog with recent illness or vaccination) and paired serum titres for CAV1 and CAV2. Canine distemper is a less common cause of posterior uveitis, and choroidal inflammation is usually secondary to virus-related retinal inflammation (see Chapter 14).

The tick-borne rickettsia *Ehrlichia canis* has been reported as a cause of uveitis in the dog in the UK (Gould *et al.*, 2000). Dogs that fail to eliminate the organism after the acute phase may become subclinically infected and it may be several years before chronic disease develops. Chronic ehrlichiosis is characterised by bleeding tendencies as a result of thrombocytopenia, platelet function deficits and serum hyperviscosity. Uveitis associated with vasculitis and haemorrhage is the most common ophthalmological sign and is seen with chronic forms of the disease (Fig. 12.44). Diagnosis is based on serology or PCR techniques and treatment with systemic tetracyclines is indicated in addition to routine anti-inflammatory medication (see Appendix IV).

Disseminated bacterial disease including tuberculosis (Zeiss *et al.*, 1994), brucellosis (Gwin *et al.*, 1980) and borreliosis (Munger, 1990) has been associated with uveitis in the dog. Both septicaemia and toxaemia are causes of uveitis (see Fig. 12.39) and intact bitches especially should be investigated for pyometra (Schwink and Barstad, 1986). Mycotic agents and algae as the cause of uveitis in the dog are rare in the UK but common in the US, especially infection with blastomycosis, histoplasmosis and coccidiodomycosis. However, aspergillosis, cryptococcosis and protothecosis are occasionally seen in European countries as causes of severe uveitis in the dog (Fig. 12.45). All the above listed mycotic infections can affect the eye following ingestion or inhalation of the organism. Although ocular symptoms may be the only signs found in some dogs, disseminated disease is common. Vitreal paracentesis is required to allow positive diagnosis by cytological examination and a poor prognosis must be given.

Cryptococcosis, caused by *Cryptococcus neoformans*, can involve any part of the body but a predilection for the brain and the meninges exists. Ocular cryptococcosis is seen as the result of extension from the central nervous system along the meningeal sheath of the optic nerve or following

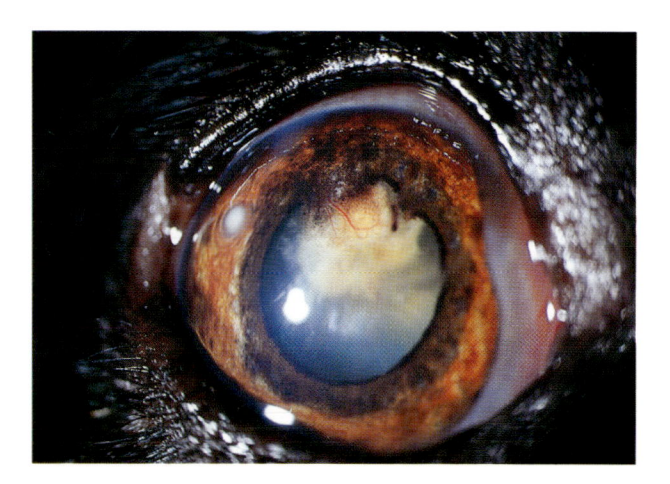

Fig. 12.43 Endophthalmitis in an adult Border Collie following a perforating cat scratch injury. Surgical treatment involving synechiolysis and phacoemulsification together with aggressive antibacterial and anti-inflammatory treatment was successful in preserving eye and vision.

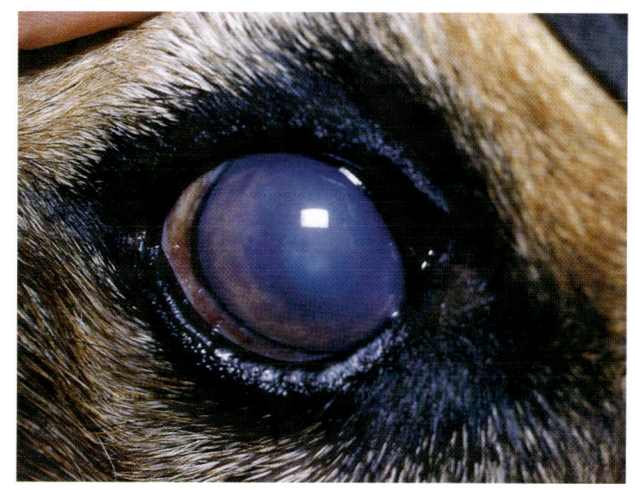

Fig. 12.44 Uveitis and corneal oedema associated with chronic ehrlichiosis in a 3-year-old German Shepherd Dog.

ACQUIRED CONDITIONS OF THE IRIS

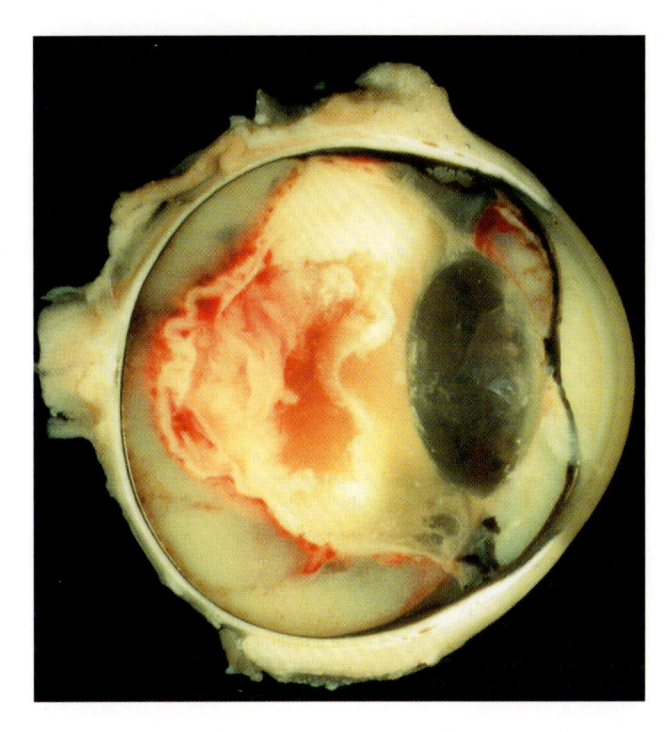

Fig. 12.45 Granulomatous panuveitis in disseminated aspergillosis in a 5-year-old German Shephered Dog. (Courtesy of JRB Mould.)

haematogenous spread. Ocular signs of cryptococcosis are retinitis with choroidal involvement and anterior uveitis. Despite adequate treatment with itraconazole, a poor long-term prognosis must be given (Jergens *et al.*, 1986).

Blastomycosis is caused by *Blastomyces dermatitidis* and is a very common problem in endemic areas in the US (Buyukmihci, 1982). The fungal organism causes systemic disease after inhalation and spread from the lungs in immune-compromised individuals. Ocular involvement is common and may be the only presenting sign. Pyogranulomatous lesions in the choroid are usually the first changes and progression to clinically visible subretinal granulomas with resultant detachment follows. The anterior segment is involved later in the disease process and anterior uveitis is only rarely believed to be caused by direct presence of the organism but rather through inflammatory mediators from the posterior segment. Dogs with posterior segment disease alone carry a better prognosis for response to treatment with systemic antifungals such as itraconazole than dogs with concurrent anterior segment inflammation (Brooks *et al.*, 1991). This may reflect the natural progression of the disease process with regards to time or the fact that the aggressive host immune response to the posterior segment disease may be adverse instead of protective. Blind eyes should be enucleated as they may present a reservoir for the organism.

Histoplasma capsulatum is the cause for histoplasmosis, a fungal uveitis endemic to the river valleys of the Ohio, Missouri and Mississippi. The life cycle of this parasite is similar to *Blastomyces dermatitidis* and young dogs of large hunting breeds are predisposed. The choroid appears to be the ocular target organ and a pyogranulomatous chorioretinitis is the classic lesion. Anterior uveitis is seen but is usually non-granulomatous. Diagnosis via vitreal aspirate is difficult as the organism is sparse in numbers, but serology is available. The prognosis for dogs with ocular lesions is poor even with adequate therapy.

Leishmania and *Toxoplasma* are protozoal organisms that are a known cause of uveitis in the dog (Ciaramella *et al.*, 1997). The dog is a reservoir for *Leishmania* sp. in endemic areas and the natural cycle of infection is a zoonosis with blood-sucking sandflies of the genus *Phlebotomus*. Clinical pathology in leishmaniasis is caused by the over-exuberant host immune response, which is non-protective and detrimental through the formation of large amounts of circulating immune complexes. Anterior uveitis and chorioretinitis with lymphocytic–histiocytic infiltrates are found in approximately 15% of affected dogs and can present together with keratitis and adnexal lesions (Fig. 12.46). Diagnosis is made by serology or by direct identification of the organism in lymph node aspirates. Uveitis resolution in response to antiprotozoal (N-methylyglucamine antimonate and allopurinol) and anti-inflammatory therapy (see below) is reported as good. However, in some cases, antimicrobial therapy seems to shift the immune-pathological status from anergic to allergic without achieving a definitive cure, resulting in a persistent granulomatous iridocyclitis.

Acute toxoplasmosis as a cause of uveitis in the dog is rare but should be considered differentially diagnostically as a cause for anterior and posterior segment inflammation especially in young or immune-suppressed patients. Serology with paired serum samples 2 weeks apart demonstrating a four-fold increase in *Toxoplasma* IgM antibodies is considered as diagnostic. Clindamycin is the antibiotic of choice but topical and systemic anti-inflammatory treatment must be given concurrently.

Migrating larvae, including *Toxocara canis*, *Dirofilaria immitis* and *Angiostrongylus vasorum*, are a known cause of uveitis. The uveitis associated with these organisms is postulated to be a combination of mechanical damage, toxic

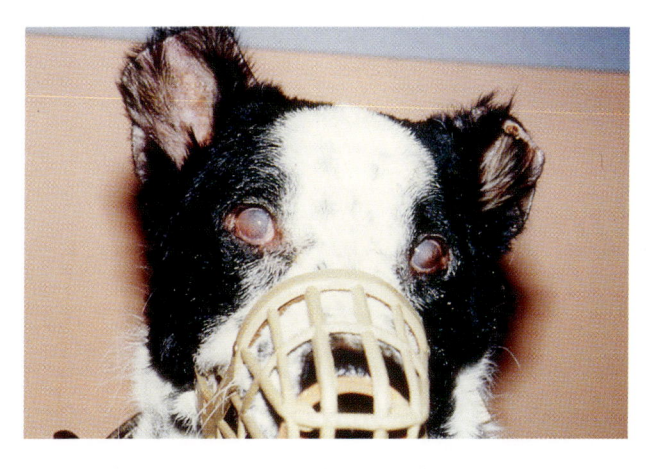

Fig. 12.46 Keratouveitis, blepharitis and ear-tip necrosis in a Greek Shepherd Dog that was imported to the UK.

139

UVEAL TRACT

metabolic by-products from the organism or immune mediated. Dirofilariasis is not endemic in the UK but may be seen in dogs imported from southern European countries. Larvae are most commonly seen in the anterior chamber, and surgical intervention is required (Carastro *et al.*, 1992). Aberrant migration of *Toxocara* larvae into the eye is usually seen as focal chorioretinal granuloma formation in young dogs (Johnson *et al.*, 1989). Routine hygienic measures, feeding of cooked meat and regular worming should limit this disease to a minimum. Angiostrongyliasis is endemic to areas in England and Wales and ingestion of infected snails leads to infection with colonisation of heart and pulmonary arteries. Aberrant migrating larvae can occasionally be seen as free nematodes in the anterior chamber or within the vitreous (King *et al.*, 1994). Mild to severe granulomatous uveitis can result and treatment with levamisole is indicated.

LENS-INDUCED UVEITIS

Lens-induced uveitis is a common finding in dogs (van der Woerdt *et al.*, 1992) and two distinct forms can be distinguished (Wilcock and Peiffer, 1987). Leakage of liquefied lens protein that associates rapidly maturing and hypermature cataracts leads to a generally mild, lymphocytic–plasmacytic anterior uveitis termed phacolytic uveitis. Clinical signs are iris darkening, conjunctival hyperaemia and poor response mydriatics (Fig. 12.47). More severe forms of phacolytic uveitis may accompany cataracts of extremely rapid onset, especially in young animals and in diabetic patients. In these cases, anterior chamber flare, loss of iris surface detail and more marked photophobia and ocular discomfort can be seen. With intumescence of a rapidly forming cataract, a shallow anterior chamber is seen, whereas the hypermaturing cataracts leads to a decrease in lens volume, seen as a flattened anterior lens surface and deepened anterior chamber. It is not clear whether this type of ocular inflammation is due to a breakdown of the normal low dose tolerance to lens

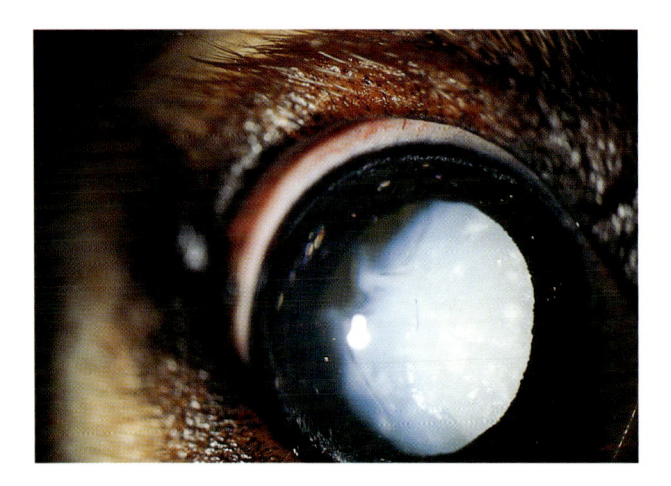

Fig. 12.47 Mild lens-induced uveitis accompanying the hypermature diabetes induced cataract in a 6-year-old diabetic Labrador Retriever. Note wrinkling of the anterior lens capsule and peripheral total lens clearance.

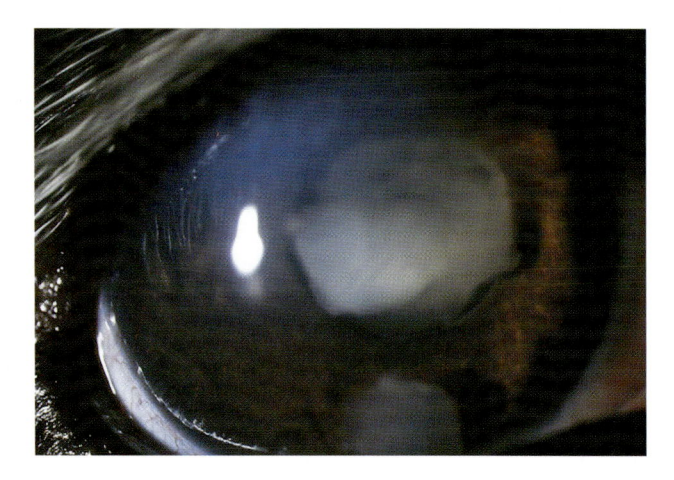

Fig. 12.48 Phacoclastic uveitis following perforating corneal injury and anterior lens capsule rupture in a Dalmation puppy 1 week after the injury. Surgical intervention in the form of phacoemulsification was not successful and glaucoma necessitated enucleation.

proteins, which are potentially very antigenic, or whether non-immunological, direct chemotactic properties of the denatured lens protein are involved. Lens-induced uveitis has been associated with a high incidence of pre- and postoperative complications of phacoemulsification such as glaucoma and retinal detachment, and control of the inflammation must be attempted prior to surgery (Paulsen *et al.*, 1986).

The second form of lens-induced uveitis is a severe intraocular inflammation following the rupture of the capsular bag with resultant exposure of large amounts of lens proteins (Fig. 12.48). This inflammation, termed phacoclastic uveitis, is histologically characterised by intralenticular neutrophils and perilenticular fibroplasia of the lens capsule. The clinical signs of this detrimental inflammation are usually delayed by up to 2 weeks after the initial injury, which very commonly involves penetrating trauma to the anterior ocular segment. Only early surgical intervention to remove the exposed lens material with the help of phacoemulsification carries a favourable prognosis (Davidson *et al.*, 1991).

A severe form of pigmentary uveitis of unknown aetiology has been reported in the Golden Retriever (see Fig. 12.31). Initially usually unilateral, both eyes are affected in the majority of dogs and extensive posterior synechia formation commonly results in glaucoma. A relationship between this condition and glaucoma as the result of iridociliary cyst formation has been suggested (Deehr and Dubielzig, 1998).

IMMUNE-MEDIATED UVEITIS (UVEODERMATOLOGIC SYNDROME)

Uveodermatologic syndrome (UDS) is an immune-mediated disease that closely resembles the human Vogt–Koyanaga–Harada syndrome and is often referred to as VKH-like syndrome in the dog. It predominantly affects young adult Japanese Akitas, Siberian Huskies and Samoyeds but has also been reported in a number of other breeds (Kern *et al.*,

ACQUIRED CONDITIONS OF THE IRIS

1985; Herrera and Duchene, 1998). Bilateral varying degrees of anterior and posterior uveitis (Figs 12.49–12.51) together with skin lesions are the presenting signs. Symmetrical facial leucoderma can be associated with erythema, crusting alopecia and leukotrichia (Fig. 12.52). Neurological disease is absent unlike in man where dysacousis and tinnitus are the signs of a concurrent meningitis. Laboratory parameters are normal. The aetiology of the condition is not entirely understood but it is assumed that UDS represents an autoimmune disease where humoral and cellular components are directed against melanocytes (Morgan, 1989) and neuronal antigens (Murphy et al., 1991). Modification of the normal immune response following integration of viral nucleic acid into the host genome has been discussed as a possible mechanism for the autoimmune disease, but no proof for this suggestion has been found in either dog or man to date. The ocular changes are usually first apparent and can vary from a mild anterior or posterior uveitis to a severe panuveitis with sequelae such as corneal oedema, synechia, cataract and glaucoma form-

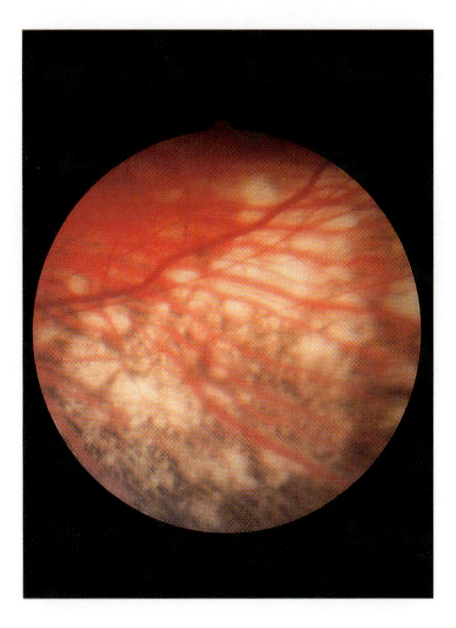

Fig. 12.51 Patchy choroidal depigmentation in chronic uveodermatological syndrome in a 4-year-old German Shepherd Dog.

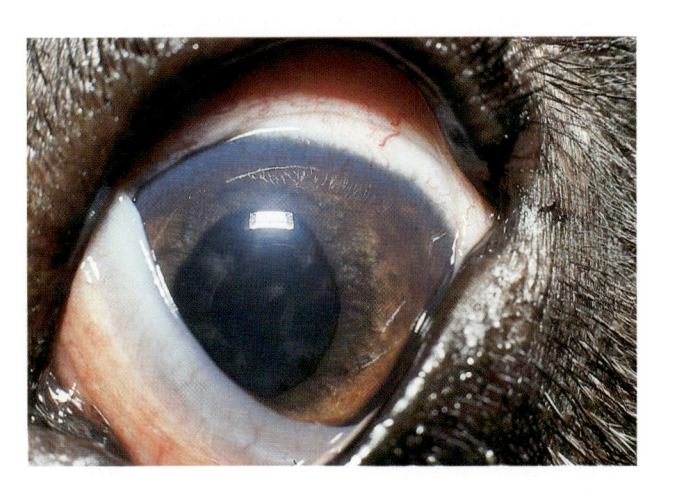

Fig. 12.49 Acute anterior uveitis in a Japanese Akita with uveodermatological syndrome. (Courtesy of PW Renwick.)

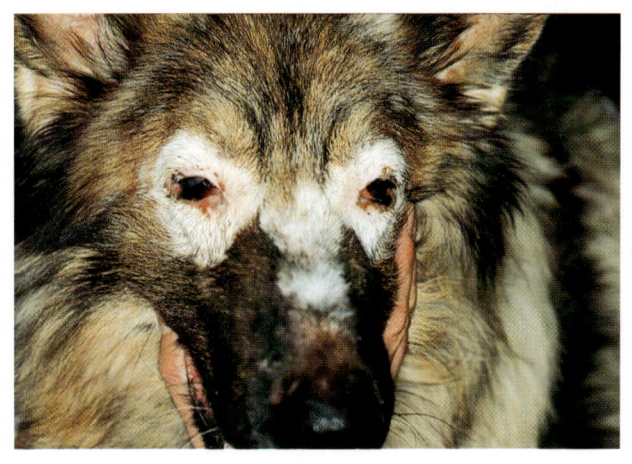

Fig. 12.52 Skin lesions in UDS with symmetrical facial leukotrichosis and crusting dermatitis in a 4-year-old German Shepherd Dog.

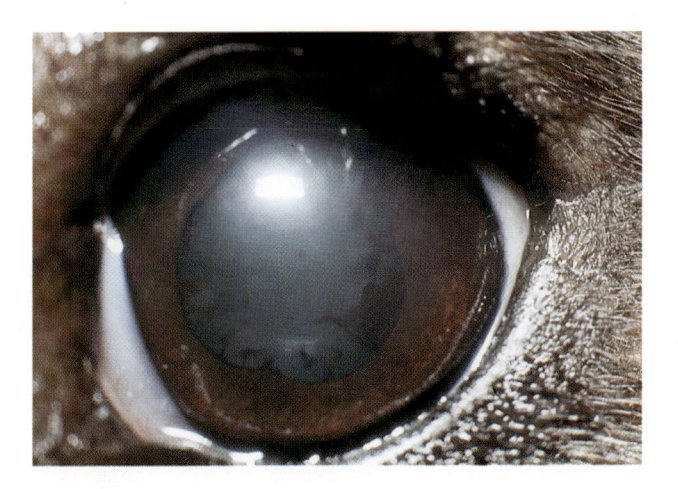

Fig. 12.50 Chronic anterior uveitis in a Japanese Akita with uveodermatological syndrome. (Courtesy of PW Renwick.)

ation. Retinal detachment is common and ocular ultrasonography must be carried out if the degree of anterior uveitis does not allow visual inspection of the fundus. Skin lesions are occasionally not present until convalescence. The diagnosis of UDS is based on signalment, clinical presentation and skin biopsies, which show an interface dermatitis with a lichenoid pattern. Histological examination of affected globes shows a uveitis of the granulomatous type and destruction of the retinal pigment epithelium, together with the presence of pigment-laden macrophages. The prognosis for salvage of vision in UDS is guarded even with adequate immunosuppressive therapy with high dose steroids and azathioprin. The condition is characterised by relapses and remittances and life-long therapy is usually required.

UVEAL TRACT

UVEITIS ASSOCIATED WITH NEOPLASIA

All primary and secondary intraocular tumours can release neoplastic cells into the eye, causing a more or less severe inflammatory response. Uveitis can also be the result of a tumour-related phenomenon such as hyperviscosity in multiple myeloma, which has been associated with retinal haemorrhages and anterior uveitis (Hendrix *et al.*, 1998). Uveitis is the most common presentation of ocular lymphoma and also a common finding in multicentric lymphoma (see Fig. 12.38) (Krohne *et al.* 1994).

UVEITIS ASSOCIATED WITH LIPID-LADEN AQUEOUS

Canine lipoproteins range from 50–350 Å in diameter and are thereby excluded from the aqueous humour by the blood–aqueous barrier. However, breakdown of this barrier in anterior uveitis can lead to a lipid-laden aqueous humour in animals with transient chylomicronaemia (see Fig. 3.42) (Olin *et al.*, 1976).

HYPHAEMA

Hyphaema is the accumulation of blood in the anterior chamber. The intraocular blood may indicate bleeding from iris, ciliary body or retinal vessels and a vast number of aetiologies must be considered (Komaromy *et al.*, 1999, 2000). Traumatic hyphaema is common in the dog (see Figs 3.23 and 3.25), rarely bilateral and usually associated with periorbital trauma and conjunctival haemorrhages. Systemic disease must be considered if evidence of haemorrhage is found in both eyes and a careful general examination to detect haemorrhages in other sites (oral and genital mucosa, skin) must be carried out (Figs 12.53 and 12.54). Congenital dysplastic lesions such as persistent hyaloid arteries or abnormal retinal vessels in association with chorioretinal dysplasia must be considered and the fellow eye should be carefully examined for any evidence of similar lesions. Systemic hypertension is not a common disease in the dog but can lead to haemorrhages from damaged choroidal and retinal vessels. Clotting disorders, both endogenous and exogenous, are not uncommonly seen in the dog and clotting assays, including platelet number and function, should be assessed if bilateral hyphaema is found (Figs 12.53–12.56). Large intraocular haemorrhages can be associated with intraocular neoplasms and ocular ultrasonography is required if examination of intraocular detail is obscured by the presence of blood. Haemorrhage from pre-iridal fibrovascular membranes has been reported in association with chronic retinal detachments, uveitis and glaucoma (Fig. 12.57) (Peiffer *et al.*, 1990). Plain haemorrhage in the anterior chamber does not always clot and often clears uneventfully in relatively short time (Figs 12.55 and 12.56). Apart from aetiological therapy, symptomatic treatment with topical and systemic anti-inflammatories is indicated. The use of cycloplegic drugs such as atropine is not without risk as, whilst reducing the chance of central posterior synechiae formation, pupillary

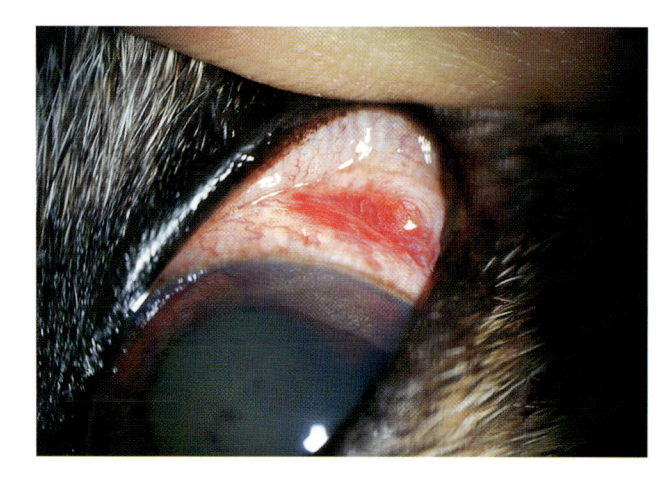

Fig. 12.54 Same eye as in Fig. 12.53. The presence of a subconjunctival haemorrhage together with bilateral intraocular haemorrhage should raise suspicion of a generalised clotting defect.

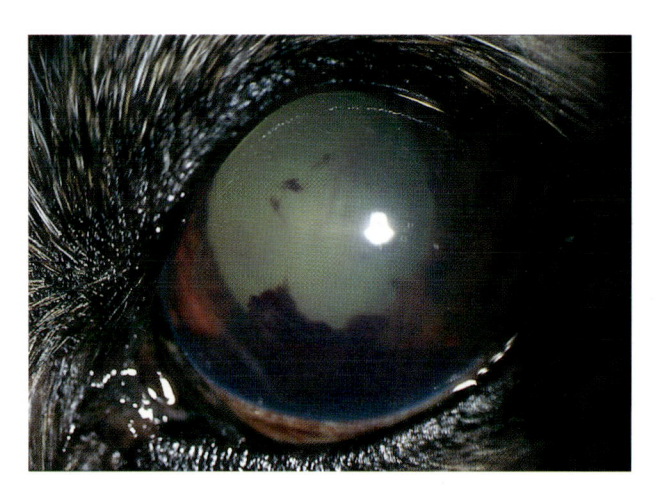

Fig. 12.53 Hyphaema due to immune-mediated thrombocytopaenia in a female crossbred. Note the intraocular haemorrhage is only partially clotted.

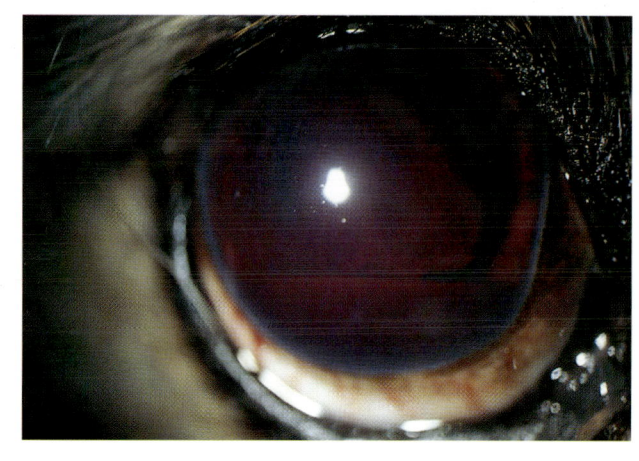

Fig. 12.55 The other eye of same dog as in Fig. 12.53 on initial presentation.

ACQUIRED CONDITIONS OF THE IRIS

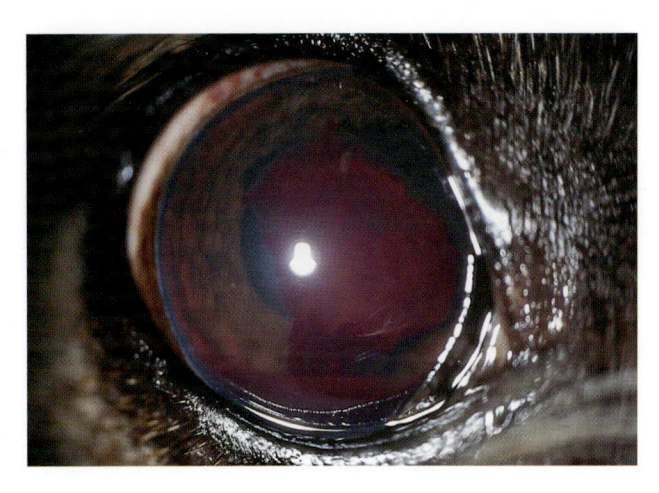

Fig. 12.56 The same eye as in Fig. 12.53 after 2 days on treatment for immune-mediated thrombocytopaenia. Uncomplicated hyphaema usually clears within several days.

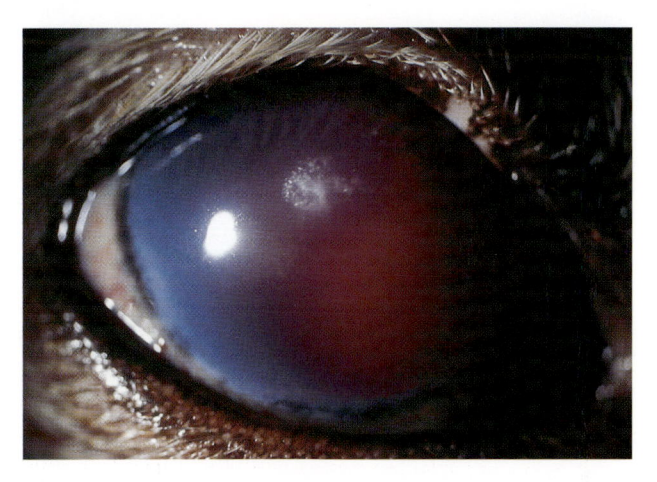

Fig. 12.57 'Eight-ball' formation of clotted intraocular blood leading to an increase in intraocular pressure in an 8-year-old Labrador Retriever. The cause for the haemorrhage was chronic primary glaucoma.

dilation may further impair the iridocorneal angle, which is already compromised by the presence of red blood cells, free haemoglobin, inflammatory cells and debris. Careful monitoring of the intraocular pressure is required during hyphaema treatment and concern is especially raised if the blood in the anterior chamber clots, leading to the so-called 'eight ball' formation (Fig. 12.57). Surgical intervention in the form of a tissue plasminogen activator injection into the anterior chamber (Martin *et al.*, 1993) to dissolve the fibrin clot may be required in order to prevent ocular hypertension.

UVEAL NEOPLASIA

Uveal melanoma

Uveal melanomas are the most common canine intraocular tumour and the majority of canine uveal melanomas arise in the anterior uvea (Wilcock and Peiffer, 1986). Unlike in people, choroidal melanomas are rare. Clinically, it may be difficult to distinguish between iris (Figs 12.58 and 12.59) or ciliary body melanoma (Figs 12.60 and 12.61) and ciliary body melanomas can extend into the choroid (Fig. 12.62). Darkly pigmented breeds such as the German Shepherd Dog (Giuliano *et al.* 1999) and the Boxer have been reported to have a higher incidence of uveal melanomas than other breeds, and inherited iris melanoma has been proposed in a family of Labrador Retrievers (Attali-Soussay *et al.*, 2001). Clinically, focal or diffuse growth can be seen and although diffuse spread is sometimes obvious (Fig. 12.63), it cannot always be excluded clinically. Large masses can displace the pupil resulting in dyscoria (Fig. 12.64) and contact with the corneal endothelium can present as focal corneal oedema (see Fig. 9.12). Free pigment is frequently found in the anterior chamber and haemorrhage and inflammation are usually late-stage sequelae of uveal melanomas. Most melanomas are heavily pigmented but amelanotic melanomas can occur (Fig. 12.65). Whereas growth of most iris melanomas is slow, more rapid growth

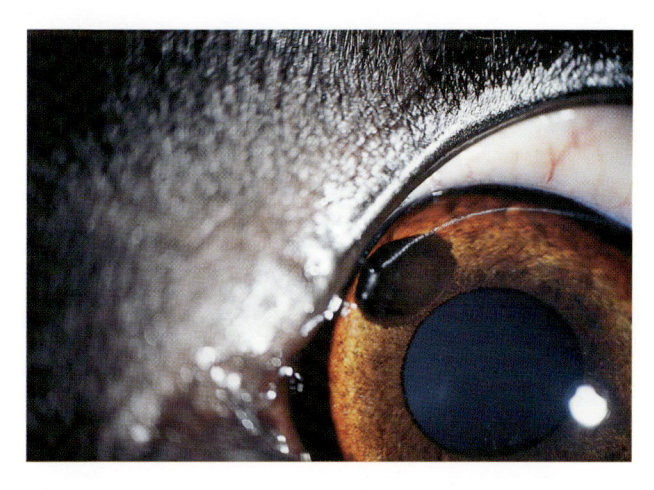

Fig. 12.58 Iris melanoma in a Labrador Retriever. The tumour had been monitored for over 12 months and was extremely slow growing.

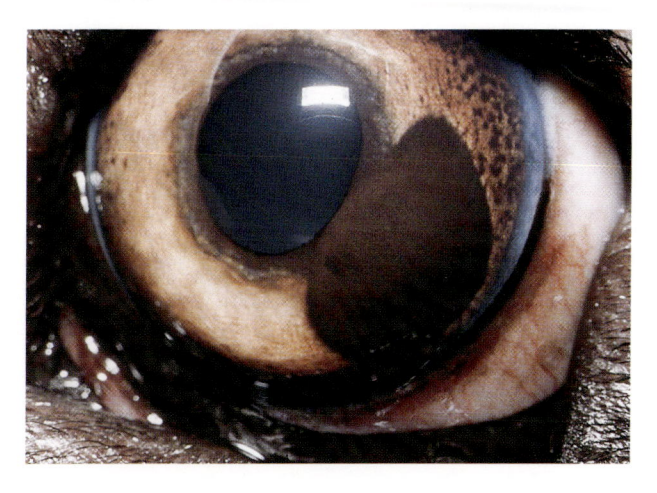

Fig. 12.59 Iris melanoma in a 6-month-old Neapolitan Mastiff. Note the diffuse spread of pigmented cells on the iris surface. (Courtesy of PW Renwick.)

UVEAL TRACT

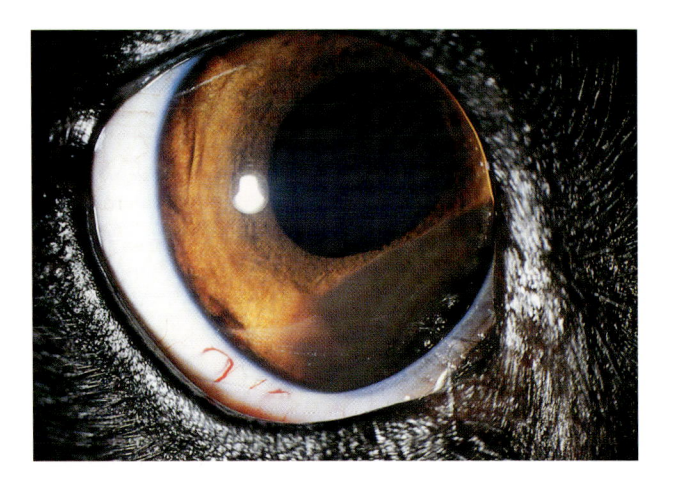

Fig. 12.60 Ciliary body melanoma in a 3-year-old Labrador Retriever cross.

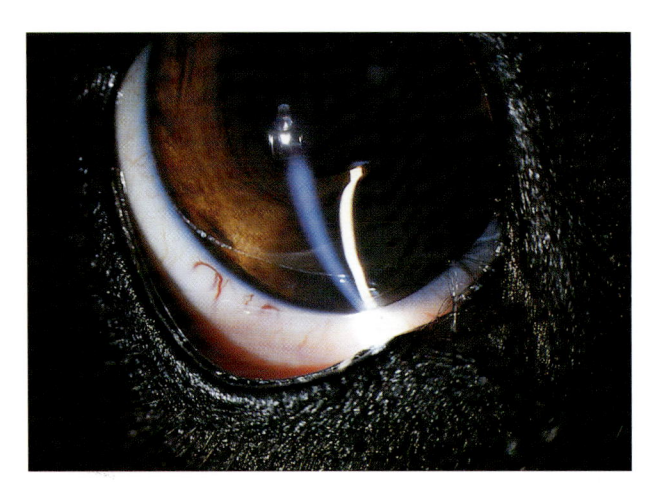

Fig. 12.61 Slit beam depicting three-dimensional extension of the mass in Fig. 12.60.

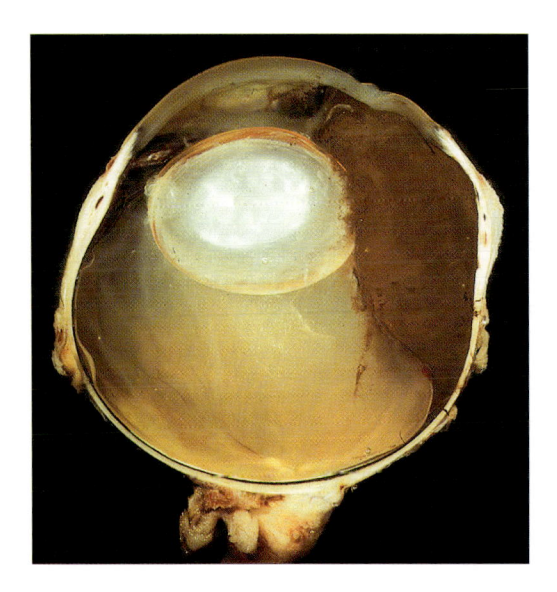

Fig. 12.62 Anterior uveal melanoma extending into the choroid. Post-enucleation specimen in a 12-year-old English Springer Spaniel. (Courtesy of JRB Mould.)

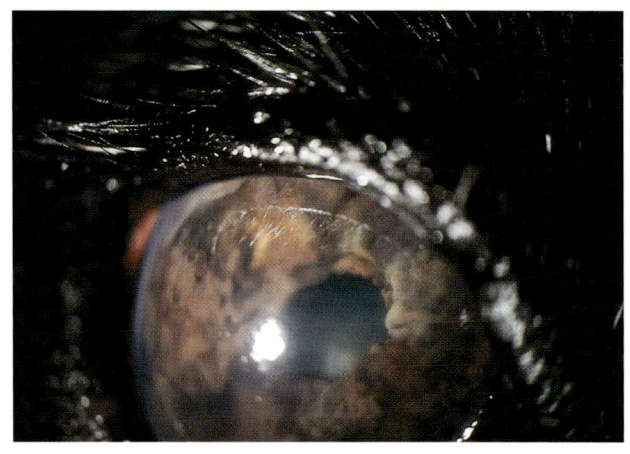

Fig. 12.63 Diffuse iris melanoma in a 10-year-old Boxer.

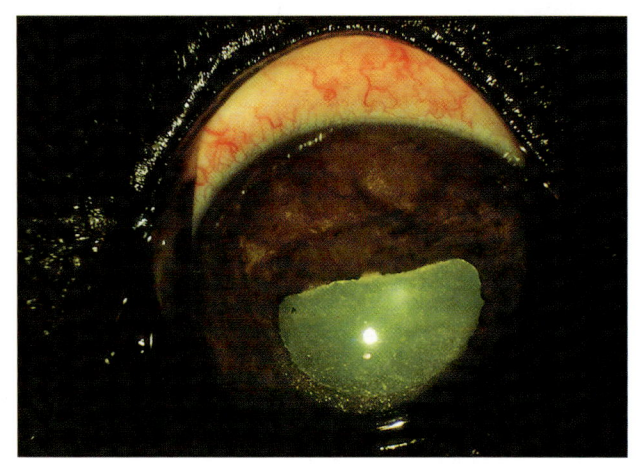

Fig. 12.64 Large anterior uveal melanoma in a Labrador Retriever resulting in dyscoria.

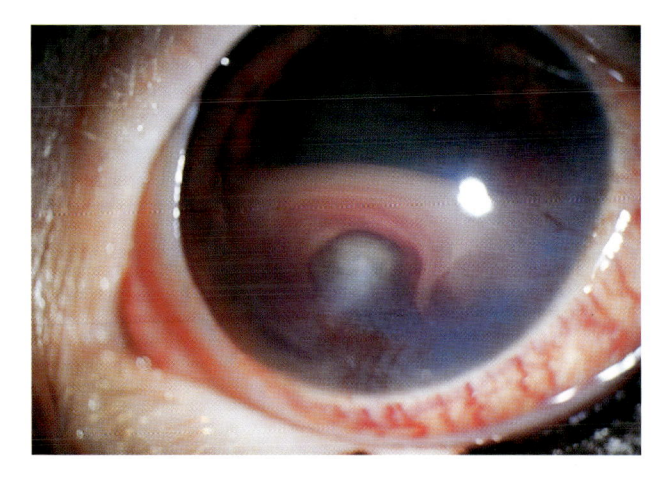

Fig. 12.65 Amelanotic melanoma in a 9-year-old white Boxer.

with scleral invasion and globe perforation (Fig. 12.66) can be seen in anterior uveal melanomas. Even benign melanomas can be destructive to the eye by displacement of other ocular structures and interference with aqueous humour drainage pathways.

ACQUIRED CONDITIONS OF THE IRIS

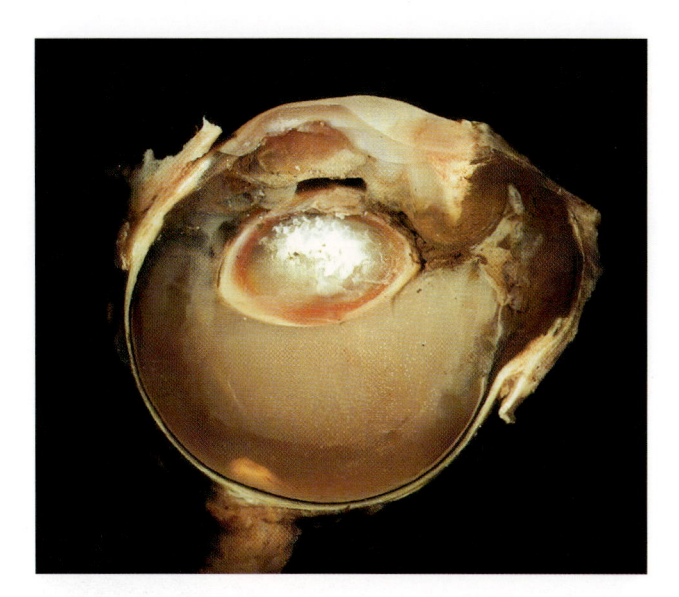

Fig. 12.66 Anterior uveal melanoma with aggressive scleral invasion resulting in globe perforation in an Airedale Terrier. (Courtesy of JRB Mould.)

Uveal melanomas must be distinguished from limbal melanomas as the treatment of the two tumour types differs considerably (see Chapter 8). Morphologically, anterior uveal melanomas range from well-differentiated spindle cell tumours to more anaplastic spindle cell or epithelioid cell tumours, whereas choroidal melanomas usually consist of benign appearing, plump polyhedral cells (Dubielzig et al., 1985). Diagnosis of a uveal melanoma can be aided by ocular ultrasonography and, if required, surgical biopsy. Care must be taken with the interpretation of needle aspirates as these may not be representative for the entire tumour cell population. Enucleation remains the treatment of choice for the majority of choroidal and ciliary body melanomas whereas laser ablation of focal iris melanomas appears to be a successful alternative (Cook and Wilkie, 1999). Enucleation should be followed by histopathology to allow confirmation of the clinical diagnosis and grading for prognostic purposes. Histopathological grading is based on cell types found and histological indices, including nuclear to cytoplasmic ratio, mitotic index and nuclear pleomorphism. The majority of canine anterior uveal melanomas are believed to be benign and metastasis is reported to occur in less than 5% of confirmed cases.

Epithelial ciliary body neoplasms

Ciliary body neoplasms are the second most common primary intraocular neoplasm in the dog. According to their different embryological origin, ciliary body adenomas/adenocarcinomas and medulloepitheliomas must be distinguished.

Ciliary body adenomas originate from the posterior unpigmented epithelium and occasionally from the inner pigmented epithelium of the ciliary body and can be differentiated into adenomas and adenocarcinomas histologically (Dubielzig et al., 1998). Both tumours may be seen as usually unpigmented masses protruding into the pupil (Figs 12.67 and 12.68). A high incidence of secondary glaucoma formation has been associated with this tumour and it has been suggested that even small adenomas can cause extensive pre-iridal fibrovascular membrane formation with impairment of the iridocorneal angle (Peiffer et al., 1990). Surgical resection of ciliary body adenomas has been performed successfully (Clerc, 1996) and both adenomas and adenocarcinomas have been reported to have a low metastatic potential.

Medulloepitheliomas of the ciliary body are neuroepithelial tumours that are occasionally found in young dogs.

Secondary uveal neoplasia

Extraocular neoplasms have been reported to metastasise to the eye both via haematogenous spread and via direct invasion from structures adjacent to the eye. In contrast to

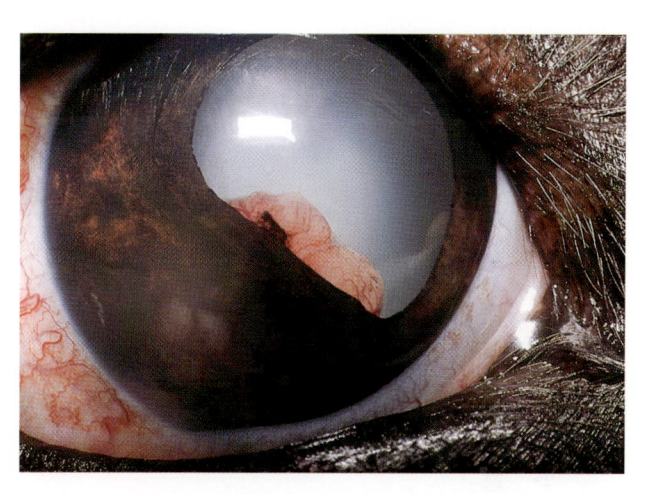

Fig. 12.67 Large unpigmented ciliary body adenoma protruding behind the pupil in an 11-year-old Border Collie. Note the associated thinning of the ciliary body at 7 o'clock. (Courtesy of PW Renwick.)

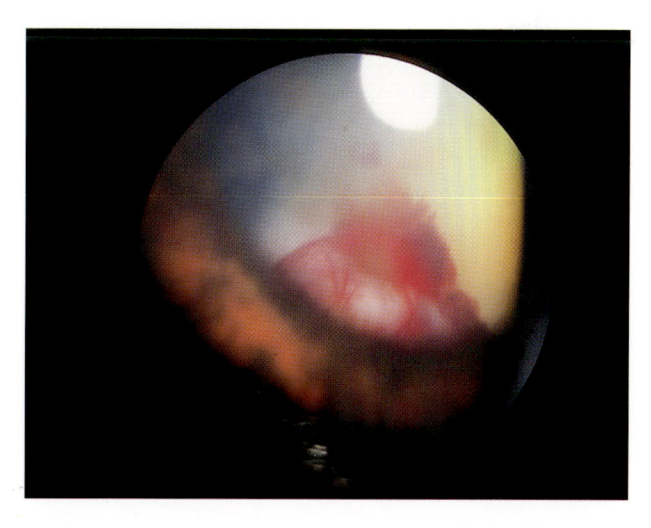

Fig. 12.68 Tip of a ciliary body adenoma with associated vitreal haemorrhage seen through pupillary opening in a 7-year-old female Greyhound.

UVEAL TRACT

primary ocular neoplasia, haematogenous spread of neoplasia to the eye is often bilateral. Ocular metastasis can present as a focal mass (Fig. 12.69) or disseminated spread resulting in diffuse uveitis (Figs 12.70 and 12.71). Careful search of the primary tumour is required and especially mammary adenocarcinoma must be considered in the bitch (Fig. 12.72).

The most common secondary uveal neoplasm is intraocular lymphosarcoma (Dubielzig, 1990). Primary ocular lymphosarcoma is thought to be extremely rare. Severe anterior uveitis and hypopyon, caused by the accumulation of neoplastic leukocytes, is also seen (Figs 12.70 and 12.71). Uveal inflammation in multicentric lymphoma is not always due to direct involvement of the eye in the neoplastic process by infiltration with neoplastic cells but can be the result of tumour-related phenomena such as hyperviscosity (see Fig. 13.12) and bleeding tendencies. Distinct masses are rarely observed in ocular lymphosarcoma and diffuse uveal infiltration with neoplastic lymphocytes is more commonly found on histology. Although clinical disease in the form of generalised lymphadenopathy is apparent on general examination of most cases of multicentric lymphosarcoma, ocular lesions may occasionally be the only presenting sign. Dogs diagnosed with multicentric lymphoma that have concurrent uveitis and retinal haemorrhages usually suffer from bone marrow involvement and should be graded clinically as advanced stages (stage 5) (Krohne et al., 1994).

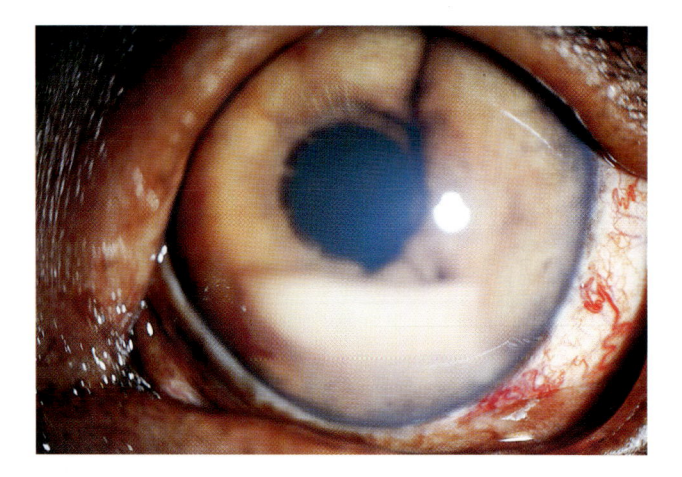

Fig. 12.71 Uveitis associated with lymphosarcoma in a 4-year-old Labrador Retriever. Notice the large accumulation of suspected neoplastic leukocytes in the anterior chamber.

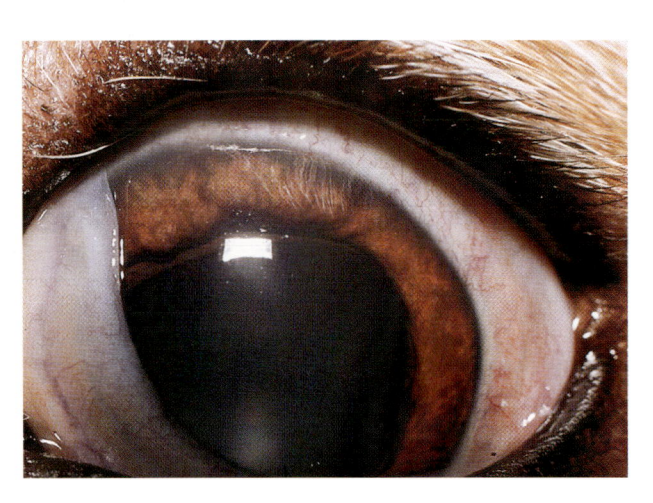

Fig. 12.69 Iris swelling in a 10-year-old Beagle with suspected multicentric neoplasia.

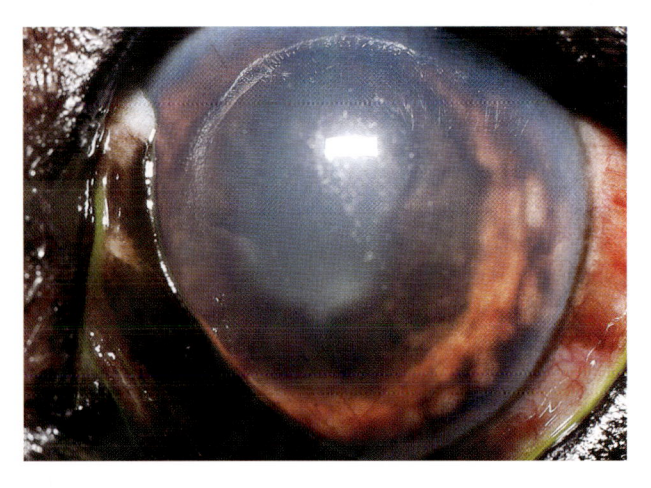

Fig. 12.70 Uveitis in an 8-year-old Flat-coated Retriever with multicentric lymphoma. Marked generalised lymphadenopathy was present.

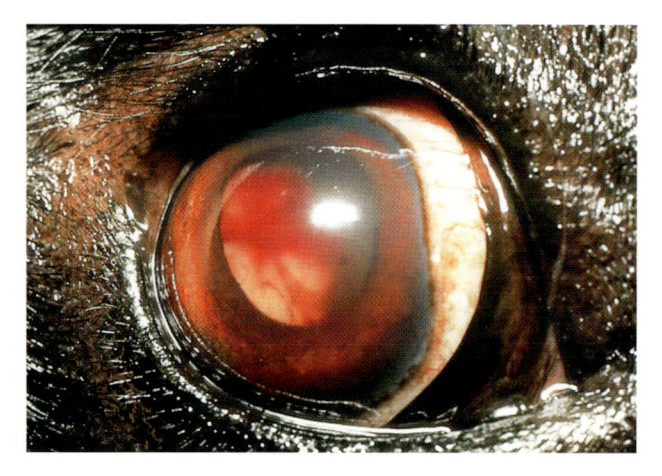

Fig. 12.72 Intraocular metastasis of a mammary adenocarcinoma in a Rottweiler. (Courtesy of PW Renwick.)

References

Aguirre G, Carmichael L, Bistner S (1975) Corneal endothelium in viral induced anterior uveitis. Ultrastructural changes following canine adenovirus type 1 infection. *Archives of Ophthalmology* 93: 219–224.

Attali-Soussay K, Jegou JP, Clerc B (2001) Retrobulbar tumours in dogs and cats: 25 cases. *Veterinary Ophthalmology* 4:1:19–28.

Barnett KC, Knight GC (1969) Persistent pupillary membrane and associated defects in the Basenji. *Vaterinary Record* 85: 242–248.

REFERENCES

Belkin PV (1975) Iris atrophy in a dog. *Modern Veterinary Practice* 56: 259.

Bellhorn RW (1991) An overview of the blood–ocular barriers. *Progress in Veterinary and Comparative Ophthalmology* 1: 205–211; 214–217.

Brooks DE, Legendre AM, Gum GG, Laratta LJ, Abrams KL, Morgan RV (1991) The treatment of canine ocular blastomycosis with systemically administered itraconazole. *Progress in Veterinary and Comparative Ophthalmology* 1: 263–268.

Buyukmihci N (1982) Ocular lesions of blastomycosis in the dog. *Journal of the American Veterinary Medical Association* 180: 426–431.

Carastro SM, Dugan SJ, Paul AJ (1992) Intraocular dirofilariasis in dogs. *Compendium on Continuing Education for the Practicing Veterinarian* 14: 209–217.

Ciaramella P, Oliva G, Luna RD et al. (1997) A retrospective clinical study of canine leishmaniasis in 150 dogs naturally infected by *Leishmania infantum*. *Veterinary Record* 141: 539–543.

Clerc B (1996) Surgery and chemotherapy for the treatment of adenocarcinoma of the iris and ciliary body in five dogs. *Veterinary and Comparative Ophthalmology* 6: 265–270.

Collins BK, Collier LL, Johnson GS, Shibuya H, Moore CP, da Silva Curiel JM (1992) Familial cataracts and concurrent ocular anomalies in Chow Chows. *Journal of the American Veterinary Medical Association* 200: 1485–1491.

Cook CS, Wilkie DA (1999) Treatment of presumed iris melanoma in dogs by diode laser photocoagulation: 23 cases. *Veterinary Ophthalmology* 2: 217–225.

Cook CS, Burling K, Nelson EJ (1991) Embryogenesis of posterior segment colobomas in the Australian Shepherd dog. *Progress in Veterinary and Comparative Ophthalmology* 1: 163–170.

Corcoran KA, Koch SA (1993) Uveal cysts in dogs: 28 cases (1989–1991). *Journal of the American Veterinary Medical Association* 203: 545–546.

Curtis R, Barnett KC (1981) Canine adenovirus-induced ocular lesions in the Afghan hound. *Cornell Veterinarian* 71: 85–95.

Curtis R, Barnett KC (1983) The 'blue eye' phenomenon. *Veterinary Record* 112: 347–353.

Davidson MG, Nasisse MP, Jamieson VE, English RV, Olivero DK (1991) Traumatic anterior lens capsule disruption. *Journal of the American Animal Hospital Association* 27: 410–414.

Deehr AJ, Dubielzig RR (1998) A histopathological study of iridociliary cysts and glaucoma in Golden Retrievers. *Veterinary Ophthalmology* 1: 153–158.

Dubielzig RR (1990) Ocular neoplasia in small animals. *Veterinary Clinics of North America: Small Animal Practice* 20: 837–848.

Dubielzig RR, Aguirre GD, Gross SL, Diters RW (1985) Choroidal melanomas in dogs. *Veterinary Pathology* 22: 582–585.

Dubielzig RR, Steinberg H, Garvin H, Deehr AJ, Fischer B (1998) Iridociliary epithelial tumors in 100 dogs and 17 cats: a morphological study. *Veterinary Ophthalmology* 1: 223–231.

Gelatt KN, McGill LD (1973) Clinical characteristics of microphthalmia with colobomas of the Australian Shepherd Dog. *Journal of the American Veterinary Medical Association* 162: 393–396.

Giuliano EA, Chappell R, Fischer B, Dubielzig RR (1999) A matched observational study of canine survival with primary intraocular melanocytic neoplasia. *Veterinary Ophthalmology* 2: 185–190.

Gould DJ, Murphy K, Rudorf H, Crispin SM (2000) Canine monocytic ehrlichiosis presenting as acute blindness 36 months after importation into the UK [In Process Citation]. *Journal of Small Animal Practice* 41: 263–265.

Gwin RM, Kolwalski JJ, Wyman M, Winston S (1980) Ocular lesions associated with *Brucella canis* infection in a dog. *Journal of the American Animal Hospital Association* 16: 607–610.

Hendrix DVH, Gelatt KN, Smith PJ, Brooks DE, Whittaker CJG, Chmielewski NT (1998) Ophthalmic disease as the presenting complaint in five dogs with multiple myeloma. *Journal of the American Animal Hospital Association* 34: 121–128.

Herrera HD, Duchene AG (1998) Uveodermatological syndrome (Vogt-Koyanagi-Harada-like syndrome) with generalized depigmentation in a Dachshund. *Veterinary Ophthalmology* 1: 47–51.

Jergens AE, Wheeler CA, Collier LL (1986) Cryptococcosis involving the eye and central nervous system of a dog. *Journal of the American Veterinary Medical Association* 189: 302–304.

Johnson BW, Kirkpatrick CE, Whiteley HE, Morton D, Helper LC (1989) Retinitis and intraocular larval migration in a group of Border Collies. *Journal of the American Animal Hospital Association* 25: 623–629.

Kern TJ, Walton DK, Riis RC, Manning TO, Laratta LJ, Dziezyc J (1985) Uveitis associated with poliosis and vitiligo in six dogs. *Journal of the American Veterinary Medical Association* 187: 408–414.

King MCA, Grose RMR, Startup G (1994) *Angiostrongylus vasorum* in the anterior chamber of a dog's eye. *Journal of Small Animal Practice* 35: 326–328.

Komaromy AM, Ramsey DT, Brooks DE, Ramsey CC, Kallberg ME, Andrew SE (1999) Hyphema. Part I. Pathophysiologic considerations. *Compendium on Continuing Education for the Practicing Veterinarian* 21: 1064–1069; 1091.

Komaromy AM, Brooks DE, Kallberg ME, Andrew SE, Ramsey DT, Ramsey CC (2000) Hyphema. Part II. Diagnosis and treatment. *Compendium on Continuing Education for the Practicing Veterinarian* 22: 74–79.

Krohne SG, Henderson NM, Richardson RC, Vestre WA (1994) Prevalence of ocular involvement in dogs with multicentric lymphoma: prospective evaluation of 94 cases. *Veterinary and Comparative Ophthalmology* 4: 127–135.

Krohne SG, Krohne DT, Lindley DM, Will MT (1995) Use of laser flaremetry to measure aqueous humor protein concentration in dogs. *Journal of the American Veterinary Medical Association* 206: 1167–1172.

Martin C, Kaswan R, Gratzek A, Champagne E, Salisbury MA, Ward D (1993) Ocular use of tissue plasminogen activator in companion animals. *Progress in Veterinary and Comparative Ophthalmology* 3: 29–36.

Morgan RV (1989) Vogt–Koyanagi–Harada syndrome in humans and dogs. *Compendium on Continuing Education for the Practicing Veterinarian* 11: 1211–1214; 1216; 1218.

Munger RJ (1990) Uveitis as a manifestation of *Borrelia burgdorferi* infection in dogs [letter; comment]. *Journal of the American Veterinary Medical Association* 197: 811.

Murphy CJ, Bellhorn RW, Thirkill C (1991) Anti-retinal antibodies associated with Vogt–Koyanagi–Harada-like syndrome in a dog. *Journal of the American Animal Hospital Association* 27: 399–402.

Olin DD, Rogers WA, MacMillan AD (1976) Lipid-laden aqueous humor associated with anterior uveitis and concurrent hyperlipemia in two dogs. *Journal of the American Veterinary Medical Association* 168: 861–864.

Paulsen ME, Lavach JD, Severin GA, Eichenbaum JD (1986) The effect of lens-induced uveitis on the success of extracapsular cataract extraction: a retrospective study of 65 lens removals in the dog. *Journal of the American Animal Hospital Association* **22**: 49–56.

Peiffer RL Jr, Fischer CA (1983) Microphthalmia, retinal dysplasia, and anterior segment dysgenesis in a litter of Doberman Pinschers. *Journal of the American Veterinary Medical Association* **183**: 875–878.

Peiffer RL Jr, Wilcock BP, Yin H (1990) The pathogenesis and significance of pre-iridal fibrovascular membrane in domestic animals. *Veterinary Pathology* **27**: 41–45.

Roberts SR, Bistner SI (1968) Persistent pupillary membrane in Basenji dogs. *Journal of the American Veterinary Medical Association* **153**: 533–542.

Schwink K, Barstad R (1986) Uveitis as the presenting clinical sign in a bitch with pyometra. *Compendium on Continuing Education for the Practicing Veterinarian* **8**: 9–11.

Spiess BM, Bolliger JO, Guscetti F, Haessig M, Lackner PA, Ruehli MB (1998) Multiple ciliary body cysts and secondary glaucoma in the Great Dane: a report of nine cases. *Veterinary Ophthalmology* **1**: 41–45.

Strande A, Nicolaissen B, Bjerkas I (1988) Persistent pupillary membrane and congenital cataract in a litter of English cocker spaniels. *Journal of Small Animal Practice* **29**: 257–260.

van der Woerdt A, Nasisse MP, Davidson MG (1992) Lens-induced uveitis in dogs: 151 cases (1985–1990). *Journal of the American Veterinary Medical Association* **201**: 921–926.

Wilcock BP, Peiffer RL Jr (1986) Morphology and behavior of primary ocular melanomas in 91 dogs. *Veterinary Pathology* **23**: 418–424.

Wilcock BP, Peiffer RL Jr (1987) The pathology of lens-induced uveitis in dogs. *Veterinary Pathology* **24**: 549–553.

Yoshitomi T, Ito Y (1986) Double reciprocal innervations in dog iris sphincter and dilator muscles. *Investigative Ophthalmology and Visual Science* **27**: 83–91.

Zeiss CJ, Jardine J, Hychzermeyer H (1994) A case of disseminated tuberculosis in a dog caused by *Mycobacterium avium-intracellulare*. *Journal of the American Animal Hospital Association* **30**: 419–424.

13 Vitreous

Introduction

The vitreous is a transparent hydrogel that occupies the posterior segment of the globe. It consists of approximately 99% of water and only 1% of its volume is made up of collagen fibrils, vitreal cells (hyalocytes) and proteoglycans. While acting as a clear medium for the transmittance of light between lens and retina, the vitreous also provides mechanical support for the eye during movement. As a nutrient reservoir the vitreous is involved in the metabolism of the retina and adjacent tissues.

The vitreous is bound anteriorly by the lens, its zonules and the ciliary body and posteriorly by the retinal cup. Filling most of the posterior cavity of the globe, the vitreous shape closely resembles a sphere. A depression within the anterior vitreous, the fossa hyaloidea, supports the lens. The vitreous can be divided into a cortical zone, which is characterised by a more dense arrangement of collagen fibrils and a central zone with a more liquid character.

Collagen fibrils form a skeleton for the vitreal gel by entrapping large coiled hyaluronic acid molecules. Depending on the concentration of sodium hyaluronate, the vitreous gel is approximately 2–4 times as viscous as water. The cortical vitreous is attached by the condensation of the fine collagen fibrils to the peripheral retina and the pars plana (vitreous base), the posterior lens capsule (hyaloidocapsular ligament), the margins of the optic disc (at the base of the hyaloid canal) and the internal limiting membrane. A small number of macrophage-derived cells named hyalocytes are found in the vitreous, the highest number being in the cortical zone. The exact function of these cells is not fully understood but they are believed to have phagocytic functions and take part in vitreal hyaluronic acid production (Forrester *et al.*, 1996).

The development of the vitreous has traditionally been divided into three stages (Boeve *et al.*, 1988). In the first stage, the relatively small retrolental space is filled by the primary vitreous, consisting of the hyaloid artery and its branches. Atrophy of the tunica vasculosa lentis occurs from around day 45 of gestation and is usually completed 2–4 weeks post partum.

In the second phase, secondary or adult vitreous fills the increasing space of the posterior optic cavity. The atrophying primary vitreous becomes condensed in the centre of the posterior segment and forms Cloquet's Canal. The area of previous hyaloid artery attachment on the posterior lens capsule remains visible in the adult dog as Mittendorf's dot ventromedial to the confluence of the posterior suture lines. A fine remnant of the atrophied vessel is usually visible on slit-lamp examination within the anterior vitreous. In the third stage of vitreal development the collagen condensations of the vitreal base and the zonular fibres are formed.

Incomplete regression of the structures of the primary vitreous gives rise to several congenital vitreal abnormalities (Cook, 1995).

Congenital anomalies

Failure of the normal regression of the hyaloid vascular system is a relatively rare and usually sporadic congenital ocular anomaly in the dog. The most common clinical presentation is as a small vascular remnant, protruding from the surface of the posterior lens capsule into the anterior vitreous (Fig. 13.1) (Leon, 1988). Occasionally a patent vessel is present and haemorrhage into the lens accompanied by cataract formation can occur.

Persistence of the posterior part of the hyaloid vasculature can be associated with vitreal haemorrhage.

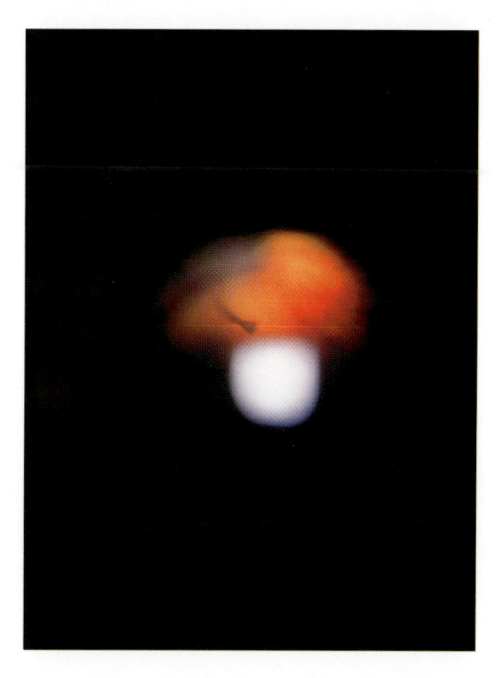

Fig. 13.1 Persistent hyaloid artery, anterior remnant visible attached to posterior lens capsule.

VITREOUS

Persistent hyperplastic primary vitreous (PHPV)/persistent hyperplastic tunica vasculosa lentis (PHTVL)

In PHPV/PHTVL, the hyaloid system and the tunica vasculosa lentis become hyperplastic during early embryological development and continue to proliferate after birth. Clinically visible lesions vary in severity from fine pigment spots to a marked fibrovascular plaque on the posterior lens capsule (Figs 13.2–13.4). Persistent capsulopupillary vessels, presenting as pigmented strands or indeed patent vessels, are described in the Staffordshire Bull Terrier (Leon *et al.*, 1986) (Figs 13.5 and 13.6), and can be found coursing from the anterior iris over the lens equator and back to the anterior lens and iris surface. Lens coloboma and elongated ciliary processes are occasionally seen (Fig. 13.7) Persistent hyaloid artery and extensive cataract formation with intralenticular haemorrhage and pigment deposition occur in severely affected dogs (Fig. 13.8).

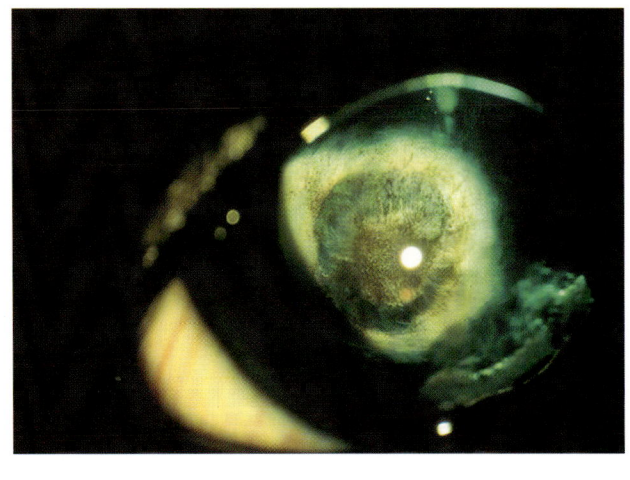

Fig. 13.4 PHPV/PHTVL. Typical retrolental fibrovascular plaque with posterior lenticonus in a Staffordshire Bull Terrier.

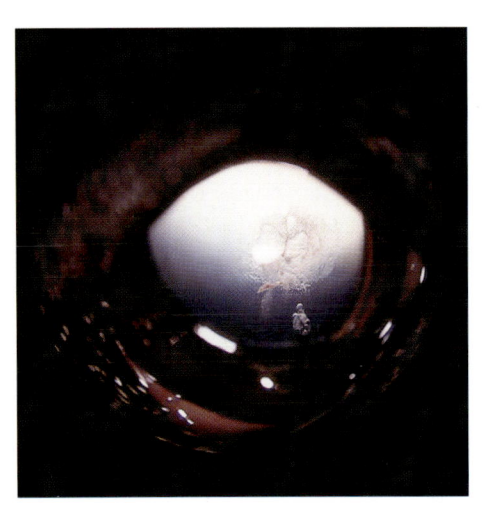

Fig. 13.2 PHPV/PHTVL. Unilateral retrolental fibrovascular plaque in a 4-month-old Dobermann. (Courtesy of PW Renwick.)

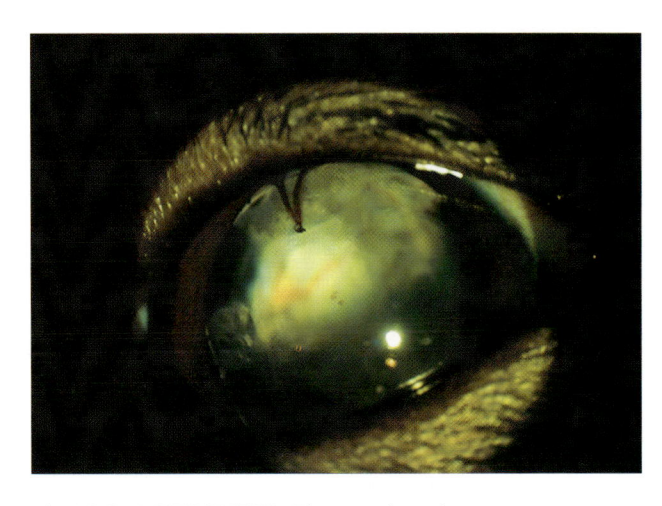

Fig. 13.5 PHPV/PHTVL. Pigmented persistent capsulopupillary loop in a Staffordshire Bull Terrier.

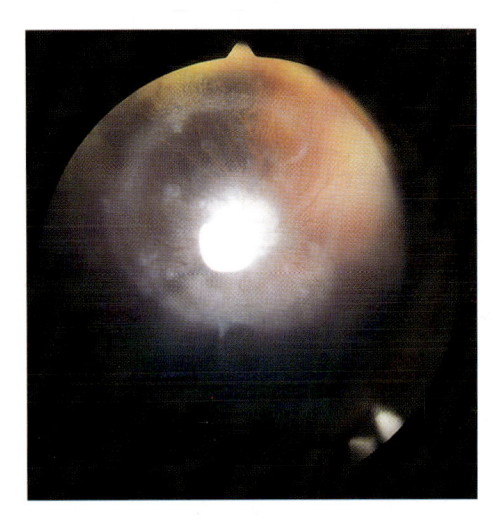

Fig. 13.3 PHPV/PHTVL. Unilateral retrolental fibrovascular plaque in a 6-month-old Cocker Spaniel.

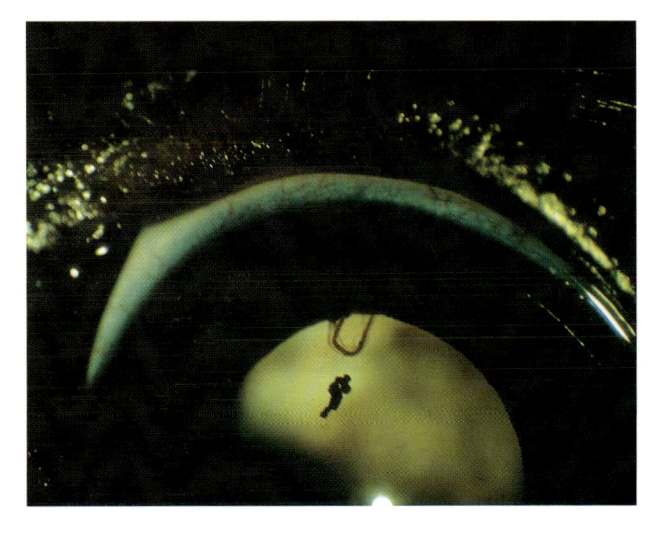

Fig. 13.6 PHPV/PHTVL. Persistent capsulopupillary vessel plus pigment on anterior lens capsule in a Staffordshire Bull Terrier.

VITREAL HAEMORRHAGE

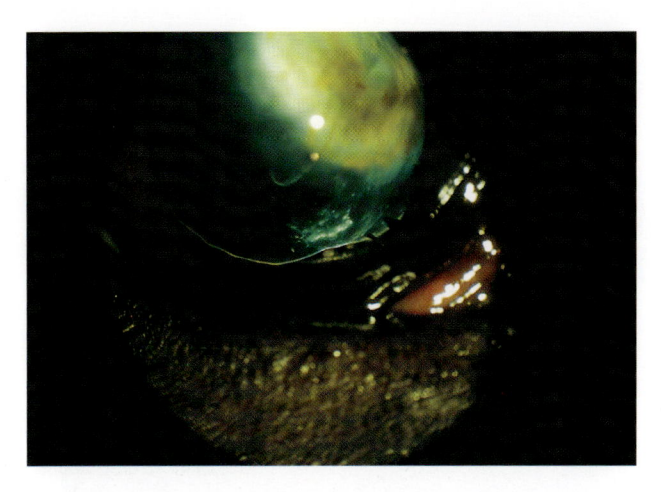

Fig. 13.7 PHPV/PHTVL. Lens coloboma and elongated ciliary processes in a Staffordshire Bull Terrier.

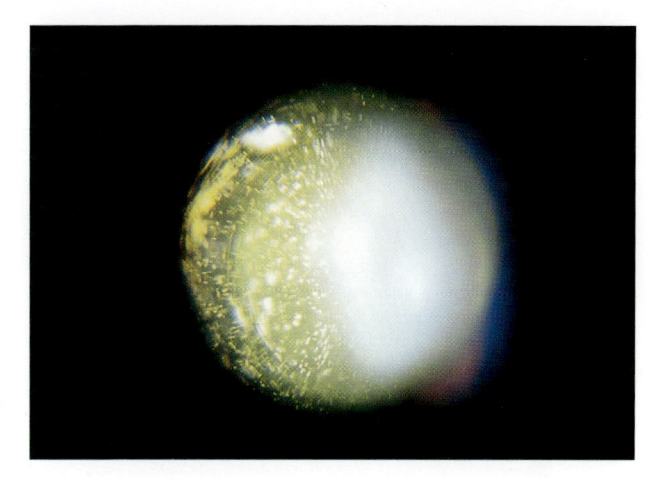

Fig. 13.9 Asteroid hyalosis.

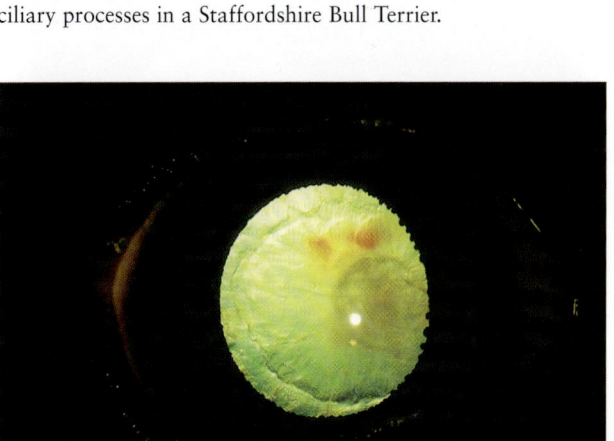

Fig. 13.8 PHPV/PHTVL. Progressive cataract secondary to intralenticular haemorrhage in a Staffordshire Bull Terrier. Note the fine cysts lining the pupillary aperture indicating uveitis.

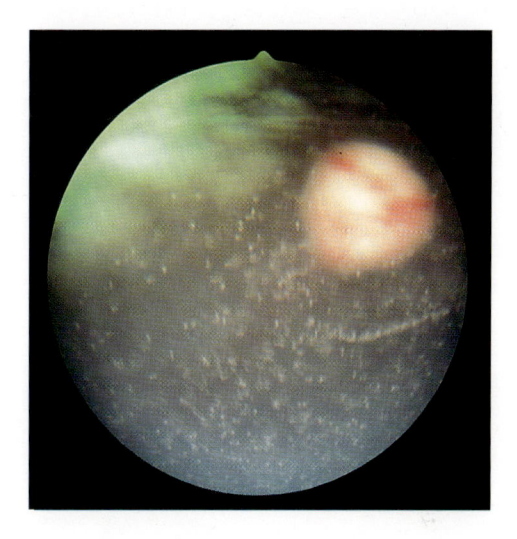

Fig. 13.10 Asteroid hyalosis in a Miniature Longhaired Dachshund. (Courtesy of PW Renwick.)

This condition has been reported as a bilateral and inherited trait in the Staffordshire Bull Terrier (Leon et al., 1986) and the Doberman Pinscher (Stades, 1980; Boeve et al., 1992), and has been studied extensively in the latter breed where the responsible gene is thought to be incomplete dominant (Stades, 1983). Unlike the Dobermann, where dogs with anomalies from grade 2 to 6 will develop progressive cataract and blindness, extensive cataracts are rare in association with the typical fibrovascular plaque on the posterior lens capsule seen in the Staffordshire Bull Terrier.

VITREAL DEGENERATIONS

Degenerative vitreal conditions are common in the dog and are seen not only in association with concurrent ocular disease but also as an age-related phenomenon. The most commonly seen vitreal degenerations are syneresis, asteroid hyalosis and synchysis scintillans. Syneresis is the liquefaction of the vitreal gel and occurs as a result of a breakdown of the collagen framework. The liquefied vitreous can be seen swirling during ocular movement and clumps of collagen present as distinct vitreal floaters. In synchysis scintillans, a large number of fine scintillating particles containing cholesterol are found in the liquefied vitreous. The particles settle out ventrally while the eye is at rest but become dispersed throughout the vitreous following rapid ocular movement.

Asteroid hyalosis is a form of endogenous vitreal degeneration in which, in contrast to synchysis scintillans, the vitreous does not become liquefied. Clinically, a myriad of fine refractive particles can be seen dispersed within the vitreous (Figs 13.9 and 13.10) and the opacities remain in position during ocular movement.

VITREAL HAEMORRHAGE

As the vitreous is primarily avascular, vitreal haemorrhage is always the result of a pathological process from neighbouring ocular tissue. It is commonly seen in clotting disorders,

VITREOUS

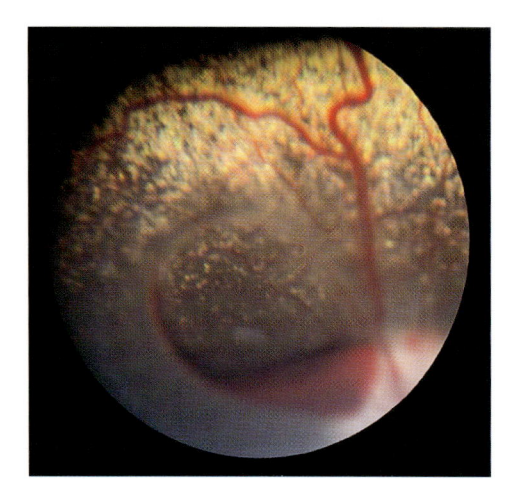

Fig. 13.11 Keel-boat shaped preretinal haemorrhage in a 4-year-old Cavalier King Charles Spaniel.

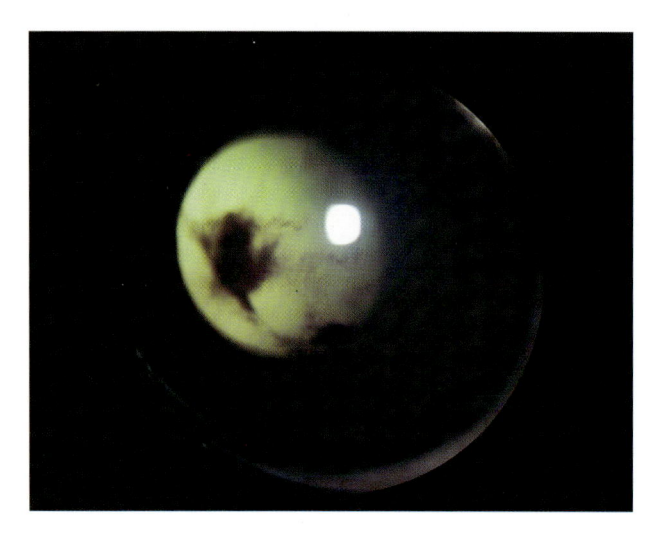

Fig. 13.12 Intravitreal haemorrhage in a 4-year-old Chihuahua with hyperviscosity secondary to polycythaemia.

into the vitreous and destroy the gel structure. Hyalitis presents clinically as generalised 'blurring' of fundus detail on ophthalmoscopy (Fig. 13.13) and severe hyalitis may render fundus examination impossible. Occasionally, more localised infiltrates or vitreal membranes can be seen (Fig 13.14). The most severe form of hyalitis is seen in infectious endophthalmitis following surgery, penetrating injuries or spread from systemic disease; both bacterial and fungal aetiologies must be considered. Rare in the UK, endophthalmitis due to ocular mycoses such as blastomycosis, cryptococcosis and histoplasmosis is seen in other geographic areas.

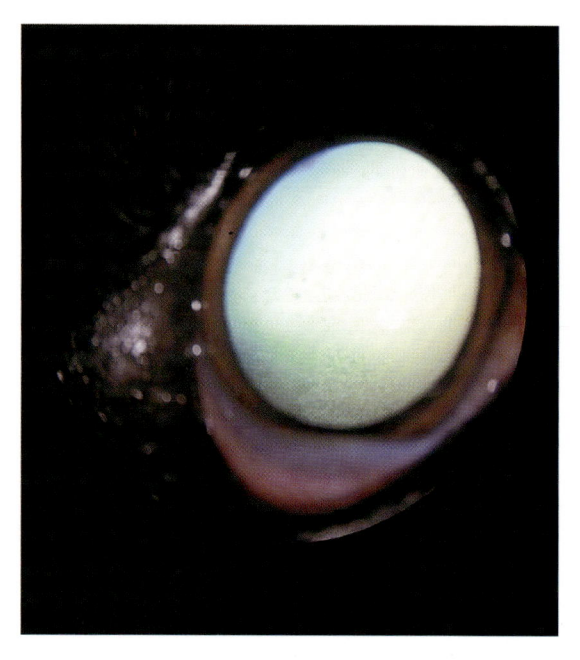

Fig. 13.13 Hyalitis with diffuse vitreal flare and anterior vitreal deposits in a 3-year-old crossbred dog. (Courtesy of P.W. Renwick.)

intraocular neoplasia, uveitis, collie eye anomaly and glaucoma (Smith *et al.*, 1993). The location of a vitreal haemorrhage can be classified into pre-retinal (between posterior vitreal face and internal limiting membrane) and intravitreal. Whereas preretinal haemorrhages are usually keel-boat shaped (Fig. 13.11) and resorb rapidly, haemorrhage into the vitreal body is generally diffuse (Fig. 13.12) and will clear only very slowly over weeks and months. Proliferative vitreoretinopathy and vitreoretinal traction band formation can ensue.

HYALITIS

Primary vitreal inflammation is rare because of the lack of vascular supply and the low number of resident cells. However, the vitreous can become involved in inflammation of the neighbouring tissue and, with the breakdown of the intraocular barriers, inflammatory cells and proteins leak

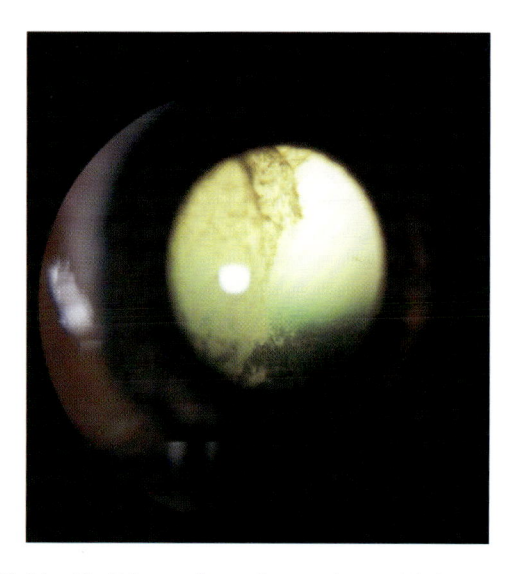

Fig. 13.14 Cyclitic membrane in anterior uveitis in a Labrador Retriever.

VITREAL PROLAPSE AND HERNIATION

FOREIGN BODIES

Vitreal foreign bodies are generally associated with severe ocular trauma. Possibly the most commonly seen intraocular foreign bodies both in dog and cat are airgun pellet or lead shot, the next most common being intraocular plant material. Ocular ultrasound examination of the posterior segment is advised and removal of the foreign body if possible. Ocular foreign bodies can result in intractable endophthalmitis and enucleation may be necessary.

CYSTS

Uveal cysts can sometimes be found on examination of the vitreous and present as more or less pigmented, semitransparent spherical structures floating in the vitreous body. They can vary in size and usually have no effect on vision (Figs 13.15 and 13.16).

NEOPLASIA

Primary vitreal neoplasia has not been reported, but the involvement of the vitreous is seen in neoplasia of the adjacent tissues, by infiltration with neoplastic cells, tumour-related haemorrhage and displacement of the vitreous by solid tumours (Fig. 13.17). Metastatic spread of a distant tumour must also be considered. Clinically, hyalitis, intravitreal haemorrhage, retinal detachment or masses within the vitreal cavity may be observed; further diagnostic aids such as ocular ultrasonography and vitreocentesis should be considered. Treatment will depend on the type of tumour present but most eyes with solid intraocular neoplasms will require enucleation. Cytology of a vitreal aspirate may aid in diagnosis of systemic metastasis, especially if the primary tumour site has not been identified.

VITREAL PROLAPSE AND HERNIATION

Extraocular prolapse of vitreous can be seen in traumatic ocular injuries with scleral or corneal lacerations or during intraocular surgery, i.e. when the posterior lens capsule is perforated in cataract surgery. Herniation of degenerate vitreous through the pupil into the anterior chamber (Fig. 13.18 and see Figs 11.41–11.43) is often the first sign of lens instability. As a result of zonular breakdown, the anchoring collagen fibril arrangements at the hyaloidocapsular ligament weaken and the anterior vitreous undergoes syneresis. In severe cases, the herniated vitreous can obstruct the iridocorneal angle leading to intraocular pressure increase (secondary glaucoma). Herniated vitreous is often present on first incision into the anterior chamber in a case of lens luxation, and closure of the anterior chamber should not be carried out until all vitreous has been removed from the anterior segment.

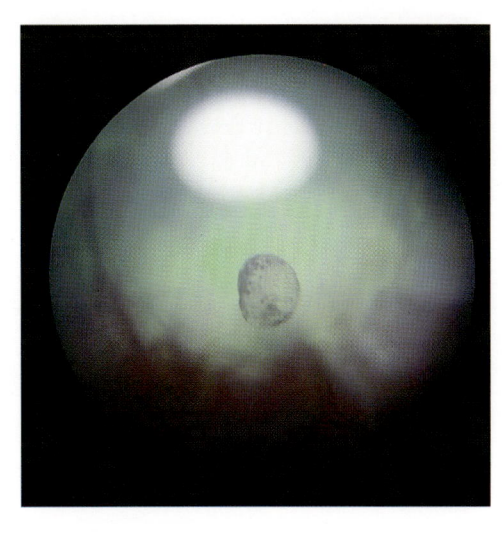

Fig. 13.15 Small vitreal cyst in a crossbred dog.

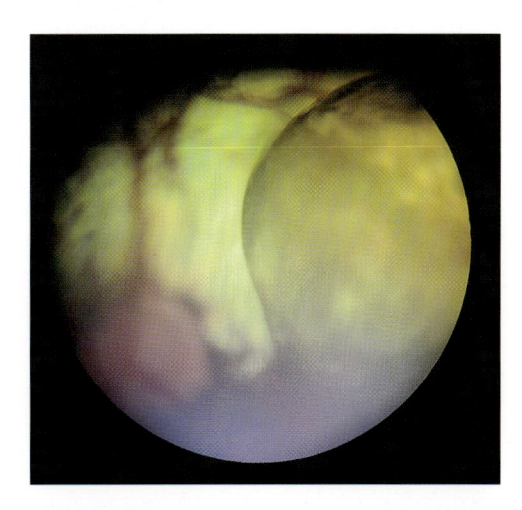

Fig. 13.16 Large vitreal cyst in a 13-year-old Jack Russell Terrier.

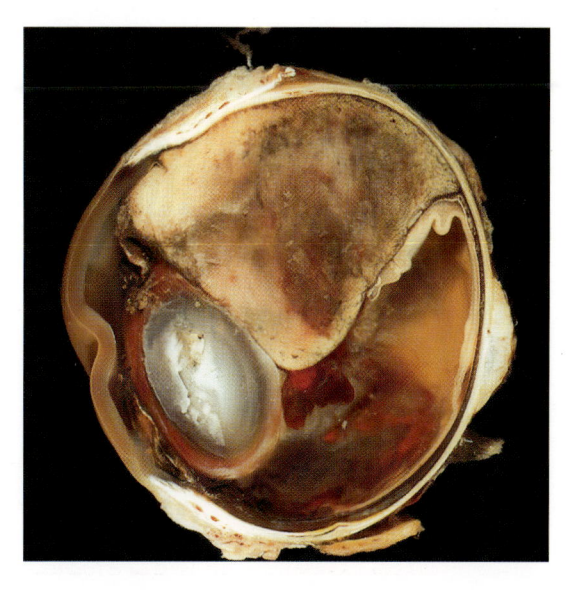

Fig. 13.17 Post-mortem photograph of vitreal haemorrhage and vitreal displacement by uveal melanoma in a Collie cross.

VITREOUS

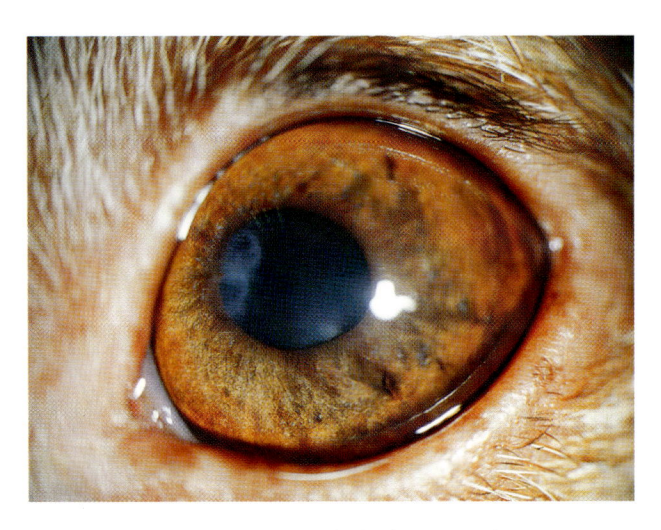

Fig. 13.18 Vitrael tags in pupil, the first sign of a primary lens luxation, in a 3-year-old Jack Russell Terrier.

REFERENCES

Boevé MH, van der Linde-Sipman JS *et al.* (1988) Early morphogenesis of the canine lens, hyaloid system, and vitreous body. *Anatomical Record* **220**: 435–441.

Boevé MH, S.F.C. *et al.* (1992) Persistent hyperplastic tunica vasculosa lentis and primary vitreous in the dog: A comparative review. *Veterinary and Comparative Ophthalmology* **2**(4): 163–172.

Cook CS (1995) Embryogenesis of congenital eye malformations. *Veterinary and Comparative Ophthalmology* **5**(2): 109–122.

Forrester JV, Dick AD, *et al.* (1996) *The Eye – Basic Sciences in Practice*. WB Saunders, Edinburgh.

Leon A (1988) Disease of the vitreous in the dog and the cat. *Journal of Small Animal Practice* **29**: 448.

Leon A, Curtis R, *et al.* (1986) Hereditary persistent hyperplastic primary vitreous in the Staffordshire Bull Terrier. *Journal of the American Animal Hospital Association* **22**: 765–774.

Smith RIE, Peiffer RL *et al.* (1993) Some aspects of the pathology of canine glaucoma. *Progress in Veterinary and Comparative Ophthalmology* **3**(1): 16–28.

Stades FC (1980) Persistent hyperplastic tunica vasculosa lentis and persistent hyperplastic primary vitreous (PHTVL/PHPV) in 90 closely related Doberman Pinschers. Clinical aspects. *Journal of the American Animal Hospital Association* **16**: 739–751.

Stades FC (1983) Persistent hyperplastic tunica vasculosa lentis and persistent hyperplastic primary vitreous in Doberman Pinschers: Genetic aspects. *Journal of the American Animal Hospital Association* **19**: 957–964.

14 FUNDUS

Introducton

The ocular fundus is the inner aspect of the posterior segment of the eye viewed ophthalmoscopically; it comprises the optic disc, the retina and retinal vasculature together with the tapetum, choroid and sclera where visible.

The retina and optic nerve develop from neural ectoderm, the outermost layer (retinal pigment epithelium) from the outer layer of the two-layered optic cup, following invagination of the optic vesicle, and the inner nine layers of the sensory retina from the inner layer of the optic cup. The retina extends from the edge of the optic disc to the ora ciliaris retinae.

The classification of canine retinal disease is complex and may be approached in different ways. Hereditary retinal diseases, both congenital and the abiotrophies, are of great importance in this species and have received the greatest interest and study but are by no means the only canine retinopathies. Post-inflammatory retinopathies undoubtedly occur but are infrequently presented to the veterinary surgeon and little is known of their aetiology, particularly in the United Kingdom. Retinal disease associated with systemic disease is also unusual although hypertensive retinopathy is becoming more understood and diabetic retinopathy has been described. For the correct diagnosis of any retinal disease a thorough knowledge of the wide variations of the normal canine fundus must be recognised and understood.

The normal fundus

There is a huge variation in the ophthalmoscopic appearance of the canine fundus and much more so than in any other of the domestic species. This fact is hardly surprising when one considers the marked differences in the appearance of the breeds from the Chihuahua and Papillon to the Great Dane and Irish Wolfhound. Differences in size, shape, weight and coat colour type and length are all considerable. There are certain connections between coat and eye (iris) colour, and even coat length, and fundus appearance. There are also some breeds that show distinct similarities and even some strains or families within a breed with colours or patterns that are inherited in that particular line.

Each part of the fundus will be described separately and it should be recalled that the puppy fundus is not fully developed until around 3 months (see Chapter 2). The two eyes of a dog are often mirror images of each other, except in cases of subalbinism.

The tapetum, tapetum lucidum or tapetal fundus is a semicircular to triangular reflective and brightly coloured structure in the dorsal half of the fundus (Fig. 14.1) and is surrounded by the dark and dull non-reflective non-tapetal fundus. The size of the tapetum varies from breed to breed and is best developed in the gaze hounds, i.e. those dogs that hunt by sight such as the Greyhound. It is poorest developed in the toy breeds; in fact only half the normal tapetum may be present, in which case it is always the lateral (temporal) part which is present. In a show-winning strain of Labrador Retriever, as well as in other breeds (Fig. 14.2), the tapetal region is often represented by a pale fawn non-reflective background, through which the choroidal vessels are not visible and in which some individuals have a sparse scattering of reflective tapetal spots over the area (Figs 14.3 and 14.4). In certain dogs the tapetum is absent (Fig. 14.5), mainly in dogs with a merle coat colour but also a few others. The bright colours of the tapetum are orange, yellow, green and blue and usually more than one colour is present in an eye. The commonest colour combination is a mainly yellow tapetum with a green border becoming blue at its junction with the non-tapetal fundus (Fig. 14.6). However, mainly yellow (Fig. 14.7), green, blue (Fig. 14.8) or orange tapetal fundi do occur and there is no strict relationship between the colour of the tapetum and the coat colour or breed. The tapetum may appear granular with tiny blocks of individual colours or less granular with the colours merging

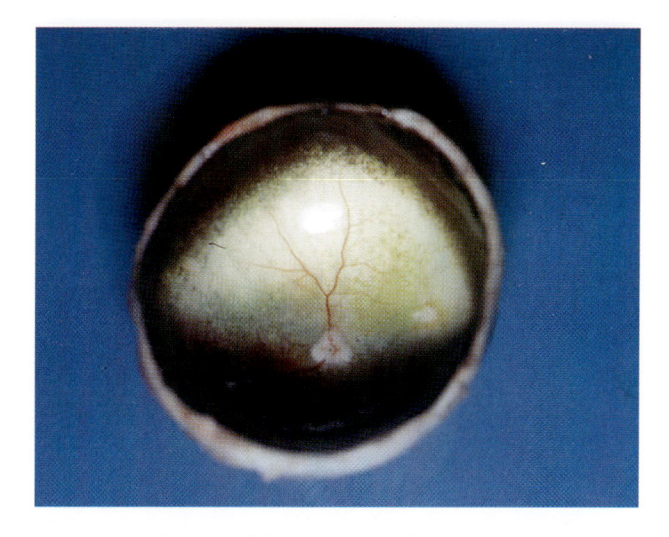

Fig. 14.1 The tapetal fundus surrounded by non-tapetal fundus in an adult Greyhound.

FUNDUS

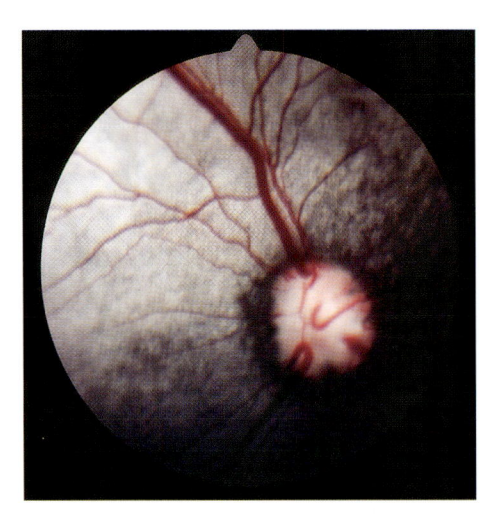

Fig. 14.2 Pale tapetal region in a young adult Miniature Longhaired Dachshund. Compare with Fig. 14.5.

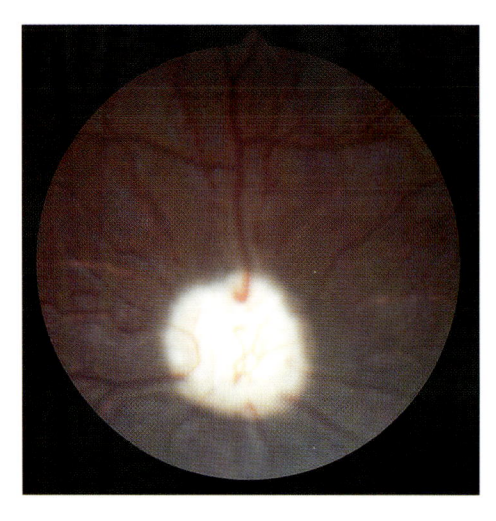

Fig. 14.5 Total absence of any tapetal area in a brindle Boston Terrier.

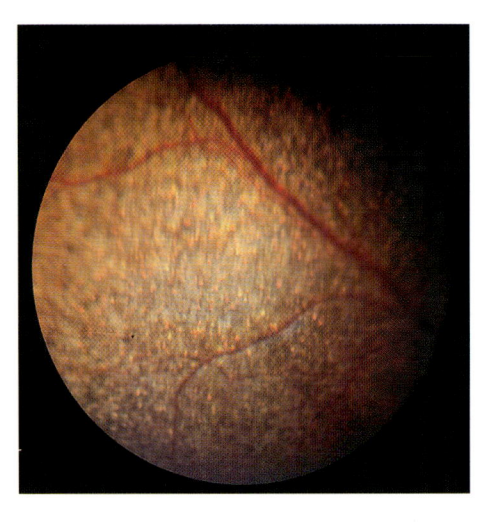

Fig. 14.3 Pale fawn tapetum with sparse scattering of tapetal colours in a yellow Labrador.

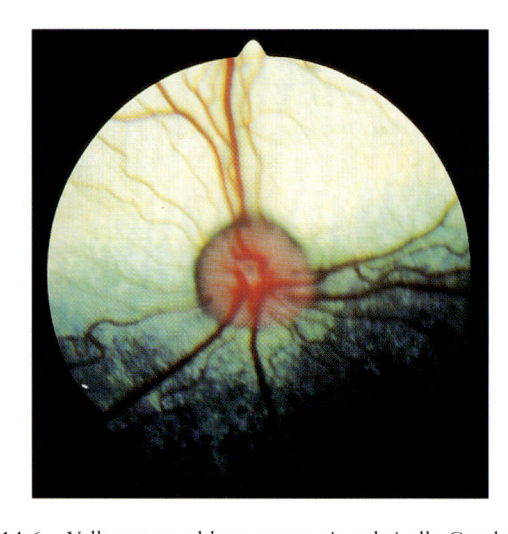

Fig. 14.6 Yellow-green-blue tapetum in a brindle Greyhound.

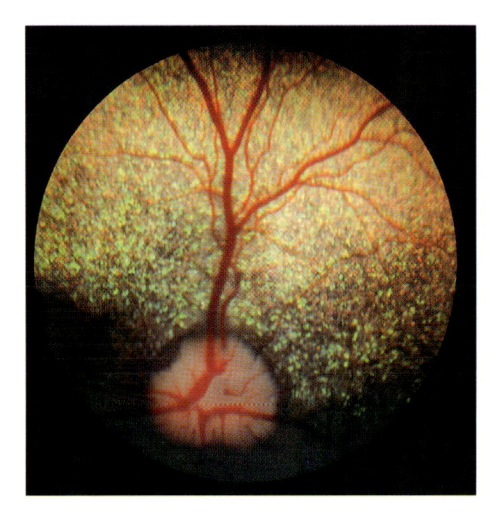

Fig. 14.4 Scattering of tapetal colours more pronounced than in Fig. 14.3 in the same strain of Labrador as in Fig. 14.3.

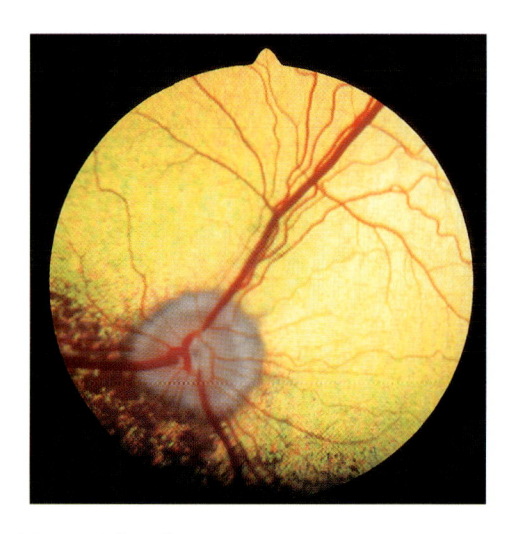

Fig. 14.7 Mainly yellow tapetum.

THE NORMAL FUNDUS

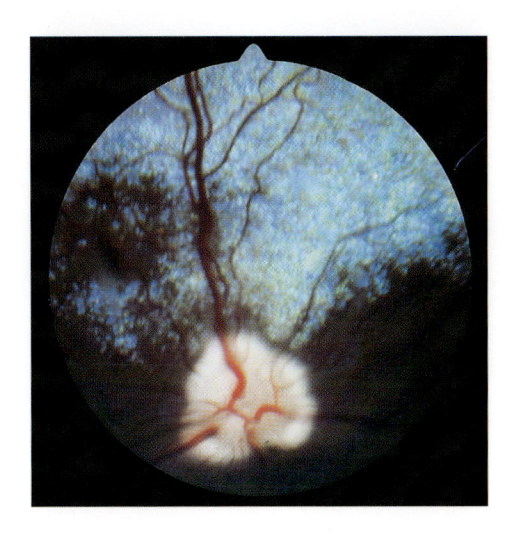

Fig. 14.8 Mainly blue tapetum.

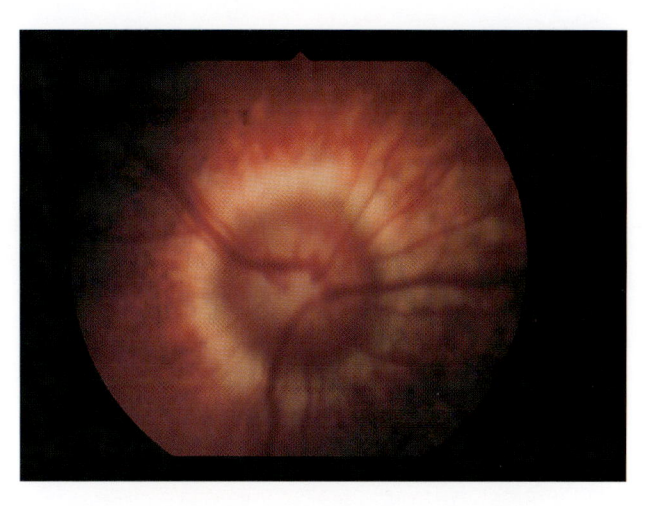

Fig. 14.10 Subalbinotic fundus in a blue merle dog. Note the unusual halo around the optic disc.

more diffusely from one to the other. In the dog with a merle coat colour and heterochromic or parti-coloured iris, randomly situated, variously sized segments of subalbinism appear in both tapetal and non-tapetal areas. In these subalbinotic areas the tapetum is absent and the choroidal vessels are visible against a white background of sclera (Fig. 14.9). These segments may be quite extensive, occupying the greater part of the fundus, and any tapetal structure is invariably absent (Fig. 14.10).

The tapetum nigrum or non-tapetal fundus is more extensive than the tapetal fundus and surrounds it on all sides. It is dark grey to brown in colour and non-reflective although the area below the base of the tapetal fundus is often paler brown in colour. In dogs with a brown, chocolate or liver coat colour, coupled with a more golden brown iris, the non-tapetal fundus is less heavily pigmented, and often the underlying choroidal circulation is visible as radiating orange-red branching vessels in a regular pattern and sometimes referred to as tigroid (Figs 14.11 and 14.12). The

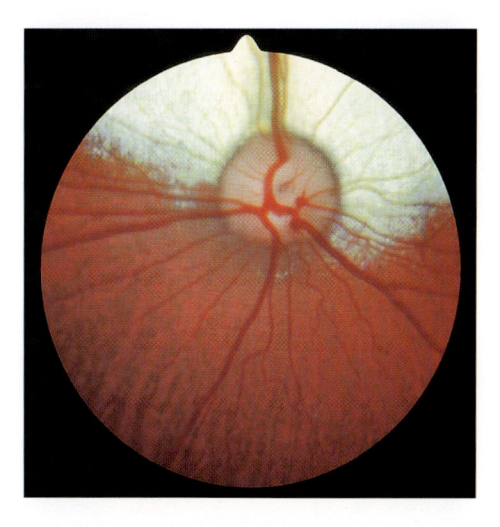

Fig. 14.11 Tigroid non-tapetal fundus in a liver/white Pointer. Note the sudden change from tapetal to non-tapetal fundus.

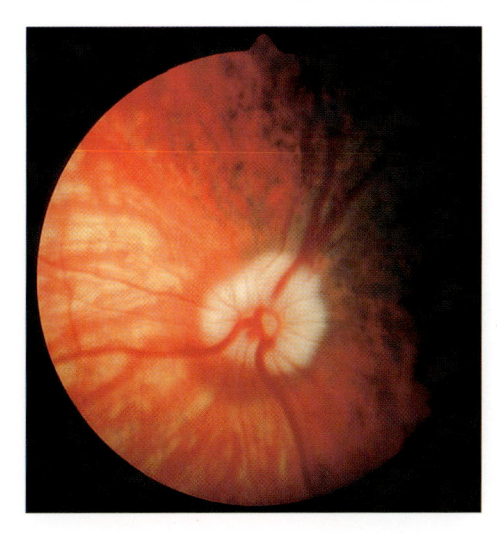

Fig. 14.9 Subalbinotic fundus in a blue merle dog.

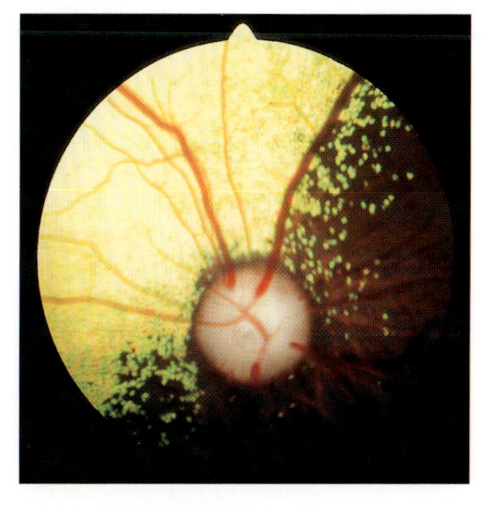

Fig. 14.12 Less pronounced tigroid non-tapetal fundus in a brown Miniature Poodle. Note the gradual transition from tapetum to non-tapetum.

157

FUNDUS

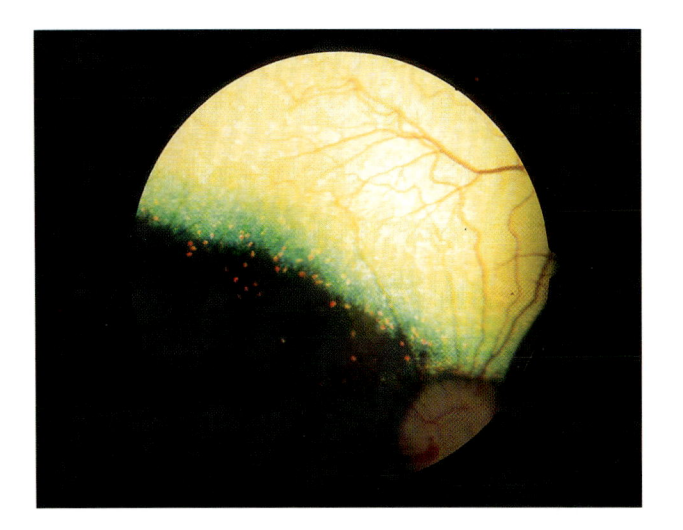

Fig. 14.13 Islets of tapetum inside non-tapetum.

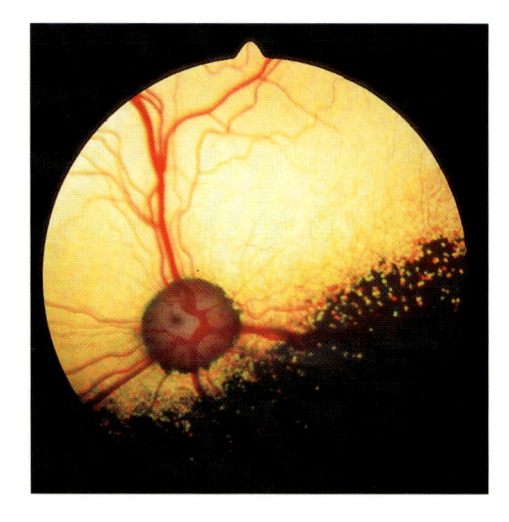

Fig. 14.14 Micropapilla in an Irish Setter.

junction between tapetal and non-tapetal fundus appears as a distinct line of demarcation in short-coated dogs (Fig. 14.11), e.g. Labrador Retriever, but as a gradual transition with scattered foci of tapetal colours in long-coated dogs (Fig. 14.12), e.g. Golden Retriever. This remarkable difference occurs even in varieties of the same breed, e.g. Smooth-haired and Rough-haired or Longhaired Dachshunds. In some dogs, islets of tapetum occur in the non-tapetal fundus (Fig. 14.13) and, similarly, patches of non-tapetal fundus are occasionally present in the tapetal region.

The optic disc, papilla or nerve head also varies considerably in its ophthalmoscopic appearance. The disc is usually located about the junction between tapetal and non-tapetal regions but it may appear completely within the tapetum lucidum or completely within the tapetum nigrum, a fact which depends upon the size of the tapetum and not the position of the optic nerve. However, the appearance of the disc does differ somewhat according to its background. The size of the disc is again very variable and not dependent on the size of the dog or on the degree of myelination. A small but functional disc can be referred to as micropapilla (Fig. 14.14) and can be difficult to distinguish, in appearance but not function, from the pathological condition of optic nerve hypoplasia (see later). The shape of the disc may be circular, triangular or oval and may be indented on one or more edges. The colour of the disc varies from white to deep pink according to degrees of myelination (Fig. 14.15) and blood in the venous circulation. Myelination of the optic disc is common in the dog and may expand the size of the disc into the surrounding fundus quite considerably (Fig. 14.16). Due to myelination the edge of the disc may be raised, the size increased and the outline made less distinct; the term 'pseudopapilloedema' (Fig. 14.17) has been applied to this condition, which is a normal variant and does not change with time. This appearance of the disc is common in the German Shepherd Dog and Golden Retriever and often the Boxer. In the centre of some discs a small grey pit may be

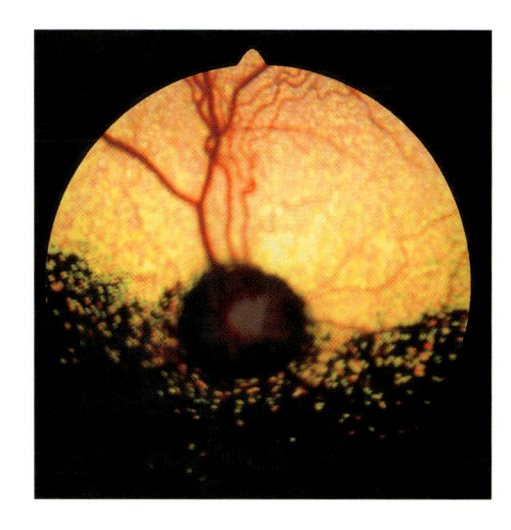

Fig. 14.15 Poor myelination in a Golden Retriever.

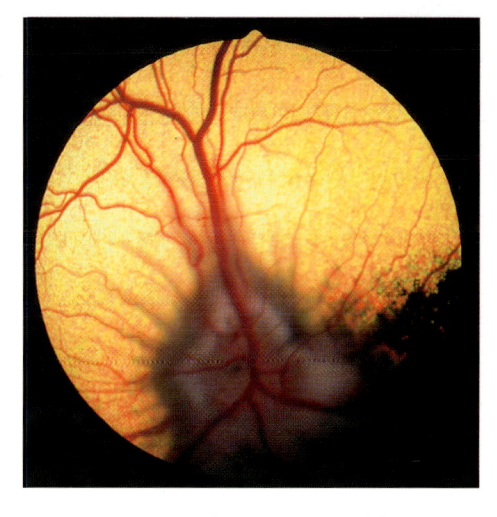

Fig. 14.16 Excessive myelination in a Golden Retriever.

COLLIE EYE ANOMALY

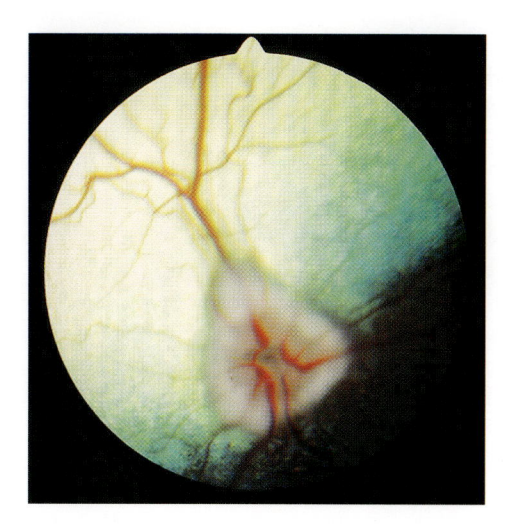

Fig. 14.17 Pseudopapilloedema in a Golden Retriever.

visible; this is the physiological cup and the origin of the hyaloid vasculature. The disc may be surrounded by a pigmented ring where the tapetum is absent or a hyper-reflective ring, known as conus, where the retina has not reached.

Retinal blood vessels or vasculature is described as holangiotic (direct visible blood supply) and consists of 15–20 retinal arterioles, which leave the disc just inside its edge to cross the fundus, and usually three or four larger, darker, less tortuous veins (Fig. 14.18) that empty into a venous circle on the disc which may be partially embedded within disc tissue and may exhibit pulsations at certain times. In the dog it may be difficult to distinguish artery from vein over the fundus away from the disc. There is no central retinal artery or vein in the dog. The area centralis, of greatest cone density, is an area devoid of retinal vessels but encircled by fine branches, lateral (temporal) and slightly dorsal to the optic disc.

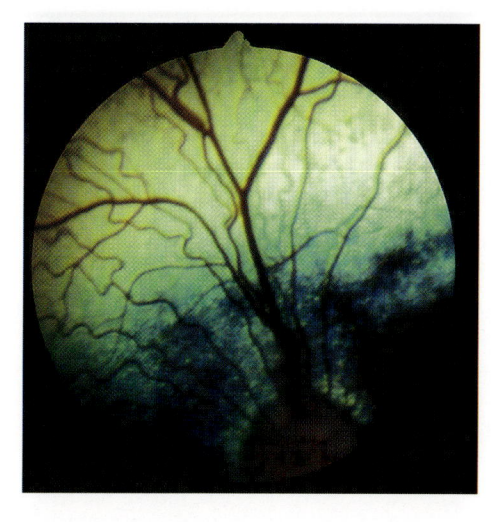

Fig. 14.18 Retinal blood vessels – larger straighter veins and smaller more tortuous arterioles (exaggerated case).

COLLIE EYE ANOMALY

Collie eye anomaly (CEA) is a congenital and hereditary syndrome caused by abnormal mesodermal differentiation resulting in defects of the sclera, choroid, retina, optic disc and retinal blood vessels. The condition is essentially bilateral but rarely symmetrical, often the two eyes showing considerable differences in severity. Like many congenital conditions the degree of abnormality varies considerably from mild to severe, and similarly the effect on vision varies from no apparent defect to total blindness in one or both eyes. This condition is not progressive but the ophthalmoscopic appearance of the commonest clinical sign (chorioretinal dysplasia, CRD) does change with age in mild cases, leading to some confusion in diagnosis (see later).

Collie eye anomaly was first described as congenital anomaly of the optic nerve by Magrane in America in 1953 and since that time several names have been attached to this condition, the latest being congenital posterior segment anomaly (PGC Bedford, personal communication). CEA occurs in the collie breeds (Rough, Smooth and Shetland Sheepdog). At one time 'sheltie eye anomaly' was used for the latter breed but it is now accepted that it is the same condition. CEA, in all its forms, also occurs in the Border Collie in the UK but at a lower, although increasing, frequency. The latter fact is probably due to the advent of the Border Collie as a show dog. Single cases of an ophthalmoscopically identical anomaly have been recorded in several other breeds but with no breed predisposition until Bedford (1998) described an identical condition in the Lancashire Heeler. The Lancashire Heeler, although it may look like a terrier, is actually a herding dog. CEA occurs in all coat colours, although initially it was thought to be related to the merling gene, and there is no difference in the frequency or severity between the different coat colours. CEA is autosomal, there being no difference between the sexes.

CEA is an inherited condition with a very high incidence – over 90% affected recorded in collies in certain parts of the USA. This remarkable frequency perhaps indicates, albeit unwittingly, some selection for CEA along with another breed point, for example eye size or skull shape (Barnett and Stades, 1979). In 1968 (Yakely et al., 1968) established CEA as an autosomal recessive condition although dominant inheritance was suggested by some to account for the colobomas. However, recessive inheritance of a pleomorphic condition has been accepted by many until a recent paper (Wallin-Håkanson et al., 2000), based on the ophthalmoscopic examination of over 8000 Rough Collies in Sweden between 1989 and 1997, questioned the hypothesis of simple (monogenic) autosomal recessive inheritance and suggested that CRD and coloboma were inherited as separate traits or by polygenic transmission. It is worth pointing out that Yakely's original report (1968) on the genetic transmission of an ocular fundus anomaly in collies was based on crossing affected collie bitches with a male Doberman Pinscher, a breed in which the condition has never been described. They studied F1 (18 puppies in three litters), F2 and back-cross generations and a further report (Yakely, 1972) described a decreased prevalence from 97 to 59%, through selective breeding, in a three-year period. However, the criteria for 'affected' were not as well-defined or rigorous as with the Wallin-Håkanson report, particularly with regard to the age at examination and the specific lesion of the collie eye anomaly that categorised the animal as affected or not; it was not a simple comparison between CRD and coloboma.

Chorioretinal dysplasia, or choroidal hypoplasia (CH), is the essential lesion of collie eye anomaly and may be described as pathognomonic (Figs 14.19 and 14.20). The lesion is always bilateral but often asymmetrical. It is always lateral (temporal) to the optic disc, varying from immediately adjacent to the disc to 2–3 disc diameters away. It is this position of CRD that is a most important sign for ophthalmoscopic diagnosis of CEA. In the affected area the choroidal vessels are abnormal in form and distribution, being fewer and broader. Furthermore, these vessels can be viewed ophthalmoscopically due to the absence of pigment in the overlying retinal pigment epithelium, together with a focal absence of the tapetum. Because of this and the visible white sclera beneath, the lesion was once called a 'pale area'. The severity of CRD varies from mild, in which a small area is affected on the temporal side of the disc, to severe, in which the affected area extends to both sides of the disc but is always more extensive on the temporal side. Because of the absence of the tapetum and the presence of areas of sub-albinism in the fundus, and consequent visibility of the choroidal vasculature, in dogs with a merle coat colour, the diagnosis of CRD in these animals is more difficult and may be assisted by comparing choroidal circulation on both sides of the disc. CRD, or CH, exhibit the unfortunately termed 'go normal' phenomenon in which mildly affected areas are no longer visible ophthalmoscopically due to fundus, including tapetal, development during the first few weeks of life (Figs 14.21–14.23). For this reason it is advised that for any control scheme to eradicate or reduce the incidence of CEA, puppies should be examined ideally at 5–7 weeks before this situation develops (see also Chapter 2). It is now thought that the 'go normal' situation is more frequent than was first realised, further adding to the problem of control.

Colobomas are the other main lesion in CEA (Figs 14.24–14.30). They are fairly common, posterior polar in position, appearing ophthalmoscopically to involve the optic disc or the peripapillary region, sometimes bilateral but mostly unilateral. According to their position they may be described as typical or atypical (on the medial or lateral border of the disc) or may involve the whole disc. They vary in extent, both size and depth, the larger ones distorting the area of the disc, and in colour from pink to grey to black depending upon depth. Recognition is aided by the disappearance of retinal blood vessels over the edge of the coloboma.

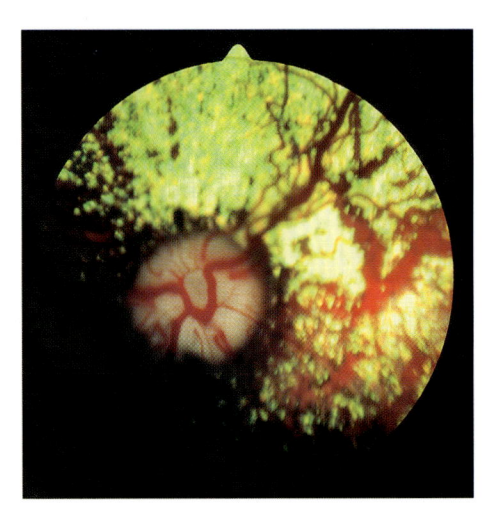

Fig. 14.19 Mild chorioretinal dysplasia lateral to disc in a Border Collie.

Retinal detachment is usually unilateral (Fig. 14.31), occasionally bilateral and may be partial, often over an area of CRD, or total sometimes with disinsertion (Figs 14.32 and 14.33), the retrolental folds being visible ophthalmoscopically. Retinal detachment usually occurs in young puppies but can develop later in life.

Intraocular haemorrhage is an occasional finding associated with CEA, and CEA should always be suspected in a young collie presenting with hyphaema (Fig. 14.34). Haemorrhage also occurs in the posterior segment in a few cases and may be related to retinal detachments and preretinal vascular loops, which can occasionally be seen ophthalmoscopically.

Other ocular signs: excessive tortuosity of the retinal blood vessels was originally thought to be part of CEA but is now no longer considered pathognomonic; vermiform streaks,

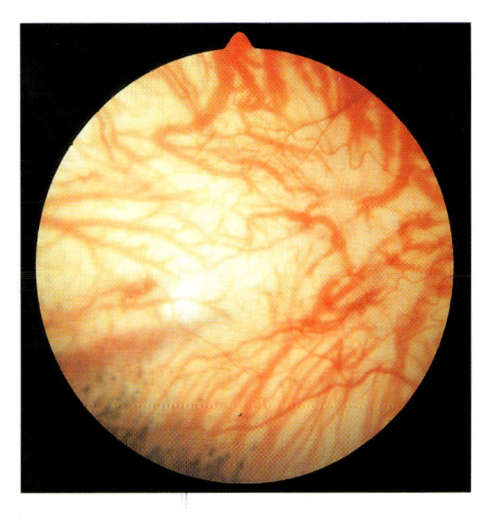

Fig. 14.20 Severe chorioretinal dysplasia in a blue merle Rough Collie.

COLLIE EYE ANOMALY

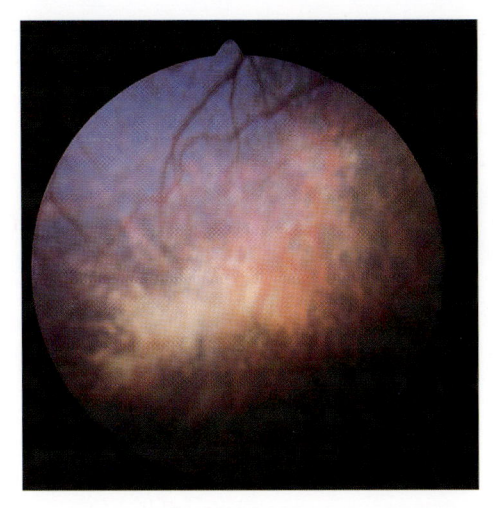

Fig. 14.21 The 'go-normal' phenomenon. Chorioretinal dysplasia lateral to optic disc in a 5-week-old Border Collie.

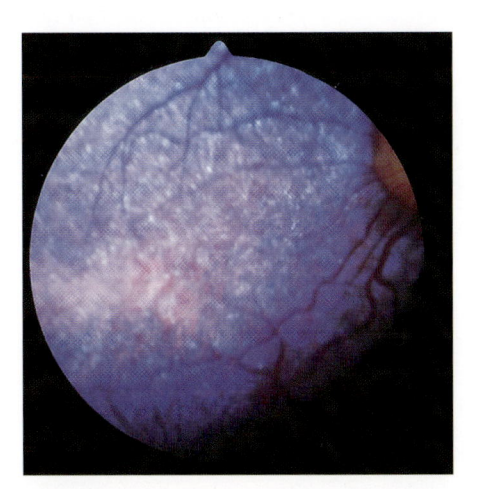

Fig. 14.22 The 'go-normal' phenomenon. Chorioretinal dysplasia lateral to optic disc in the same puppy as in Fig. 14.21 at 6 weeks old.

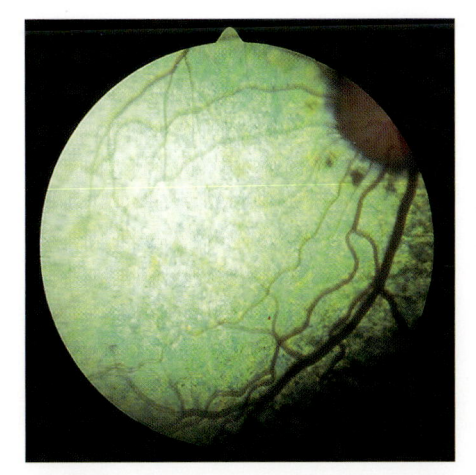

Fig. 14.23 The 'go-normal' phenomenon. Disappearance of chorioretinal dysplasia due to tapetal development in the same puppy as in Fig. 14.21 at 14 weeks. Note the identical retinal blood vessels in Figs 14.21–14.23.

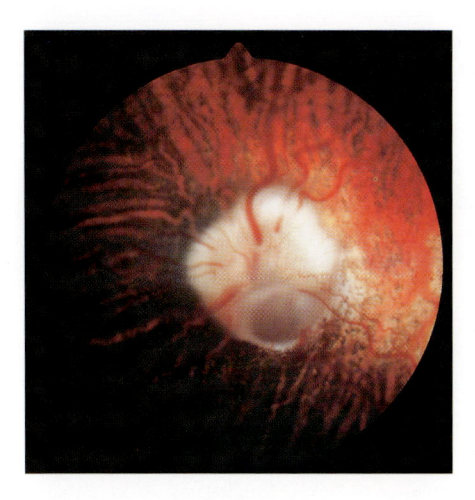

Fig. 14.24 Chorioretinal dysplasia adjacent to the disc and small typical coloboma in the ventral part of the disc.

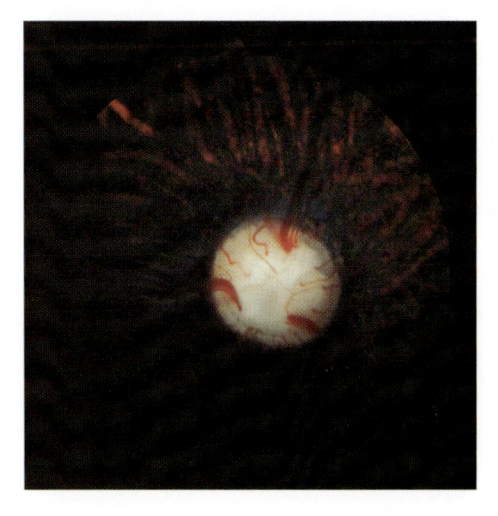

Fig. 14.25 Coloboma in centre part of disc. Note the main retinal veins disappearing over the edge of the coloboma.

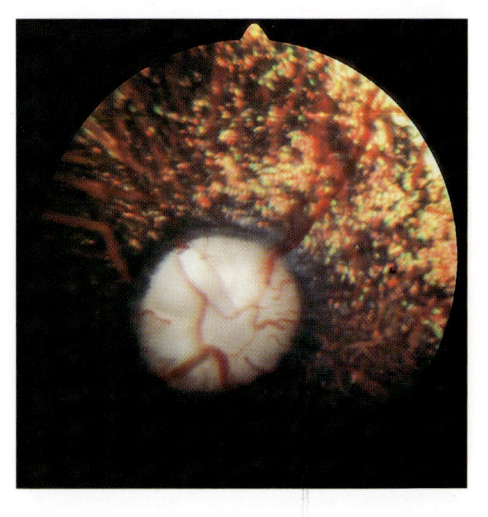

Fig. 14.26 Shallow coloboma in medial part of disc.

FUNDUS

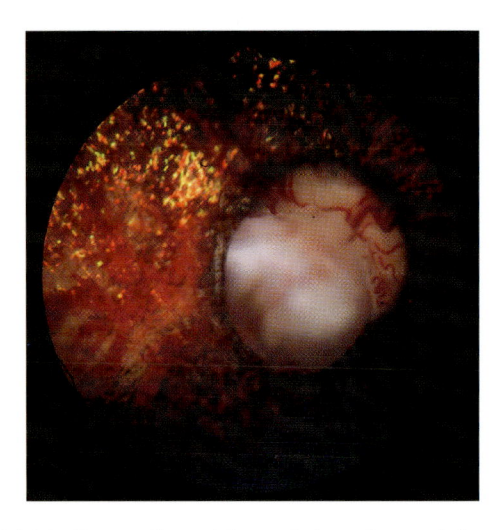

Fig. 14.27 Larger disc coloboma in lateral part of disc, together with mild chorioretinal dysplasia.

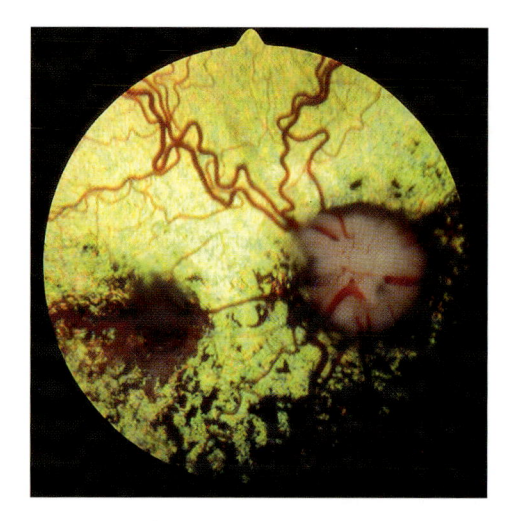

Fig. 14.30 Atypical coloboma away from the optic disc. Note the excessive tortuosity of retinal blood vessels.

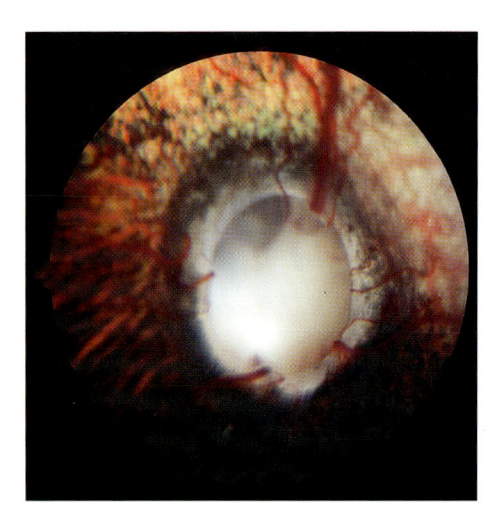

Fig. 14.28 Large disc coloboma affecting the whole disc. Note the disappearance of retinal blood vessels over the edge of the coloboma.

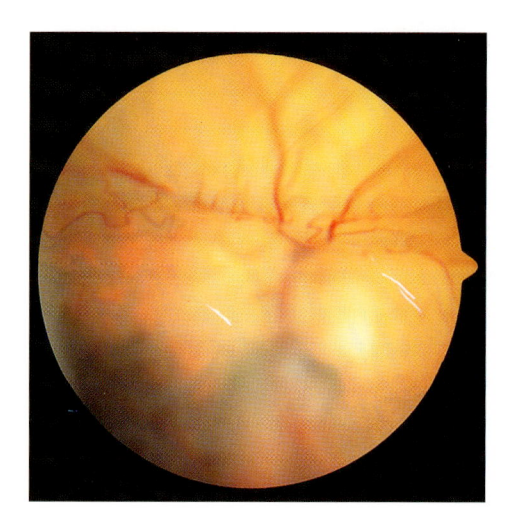

Fig. 14.31 Total retinal detachment.

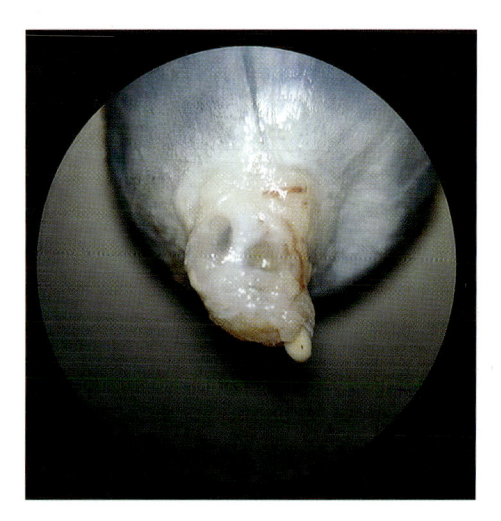

Fig. 14.29 External appearance of posterior segment coloboma. Note the optic nerve pushed to one side.

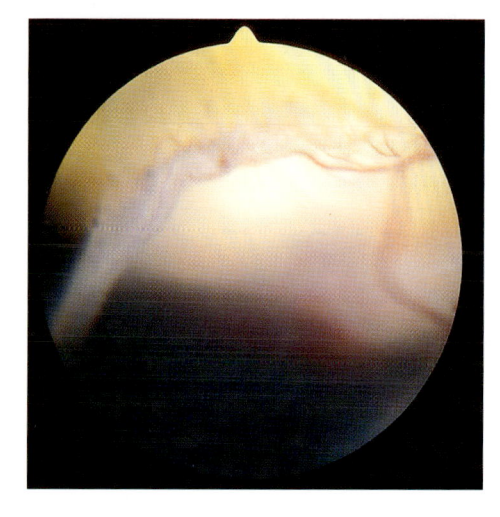

Fig. 14.32 Retinal detachment and disinsertion.

RETINAL DYSPLASIA

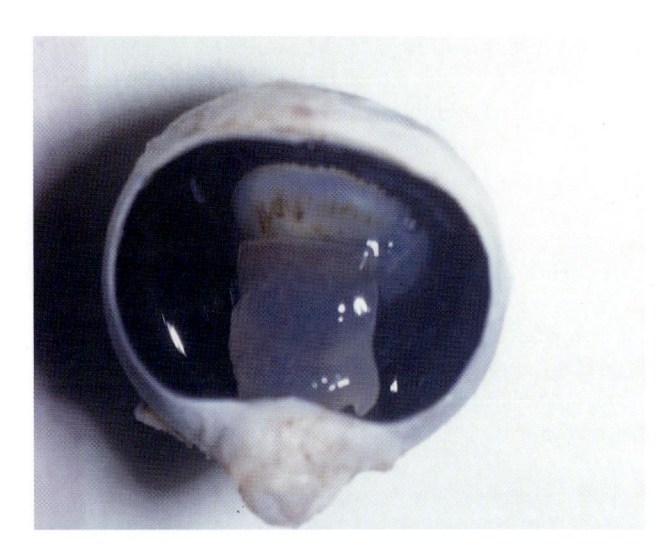

Fig. 14.33 External appearance of total detachment and disinsertion.

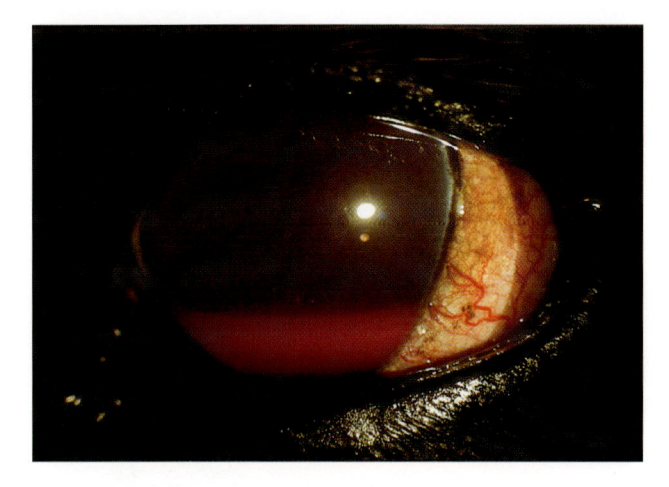

Fig. 14.34 Hyphaema in collie eye anomaly.

short, sometimes branching, retinal folds, appearing pale grey in the non-tapetal fundus and darker in the tapetal fundus, are only temporary and disappear during the first few months of life (see also retinal dysplasia); small corneal opacities were originally, but are no longer, considered as part of CEA; microphthalmos is common in the collie breeds but also is no longer considered as part of CEA.

The effect on vision of CEA varies from minor (CRD), usually not apparent to an owner, to more severe (larger colobomas and partial detachments) to total blindness (intraocular haemorrhage and total detachments).

Retinal dysplasia

Retinal dysplasia may be defined as abnormal retinal differentiation resulting in the formation of rosettes and multifocal disorganisation. Retinal folds, without rosette formation, can result from unequal growth of the inner and outer layers of the optic cup and may not be permanent. Retinal folds do not represent abnormal differentiation and are not, therefore, true retinal dysplasia. However, this difference cannot be distinguished ophthalmoscopically, and hence retinal folds are frequently diagnosed clinically as retinal dysplasia. Retinal dysplasia has a variable aetiology and a variable pathogenesis. It may appear in conjunction with other ocular, and sometimes systemic, abnormalities. The clinical (ophthalmoscopic) appearance is similar whatever the cause – in other words hereditary retinal dysplasia cannot be distinguished from that due to other (non-hereditary) causes although histopathologically there may be differences.

The first report in the dog of bilateral retinal dysplasia and total retinal detachment was in the Sealyham Terrier, with an autosomal recessive mode of inheritance and no apparent associated abnormalities (Ashton et al., 1968) (Figs 14.35–14.37). However, there had been a previous report of hereditary retinal detachment in the Bedlington Terrier (Rubin, 1963) that described a clinically similar condition, later to be called retinal dysplasia (Rubin, 1968). This was also proved, by test mating and cross breeding with mongrel dogs, to be due to a simple recessive factor. A similar form of hereditary retinal dysplasia in the Labrador Retriever in England and Sweden was next recorded (Barnett et al., 1970). In this breed, puppies were first presented with reduced vision at 6–8 weeks of age, sometimes later. Both eyes were always affected, some puppies showed a degree of microphthalmos and in the majority there was an accompanying, rapid, intermittent nystagmus. Pupils were dilated and there were no pupillary light reflexes. Several affected animals showed cortical cataract at an early age and this was progressive. Retrolental retinal folds of extensive detachment were visible by ophthalmoscopy and even naked-eye examination, presenting as a leukocoria. Macroscopic examination of enucleated globes showed total retinal detachment of a cystic retina, infundibular in type and sometimes with disinsertion. Histopathological examination revealed retinal folds and rosette formation. Analysis of the frequency

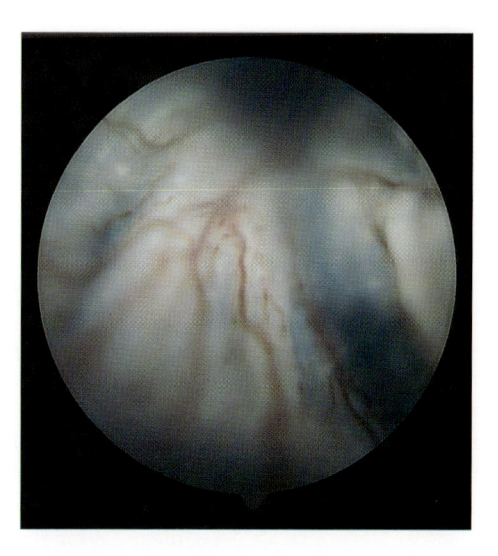

Fig. 14.35 Total retinal dysplasia – retinal detachment viewed ophthalmoscopically in a Labrador Retriever.

FUNDUS

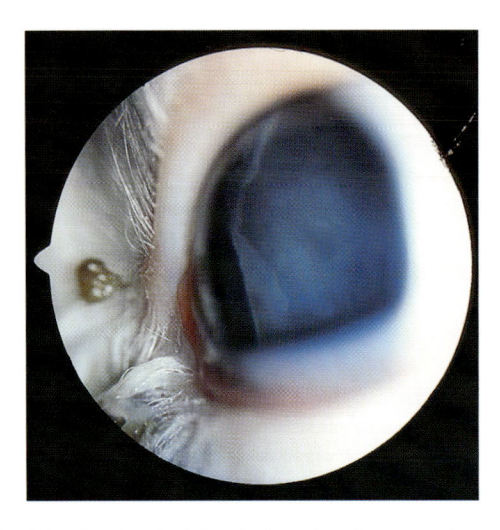

Fig. 14.36 Total retinal dysplasia – detachment and disinsertion in a Sealyham Terrier.

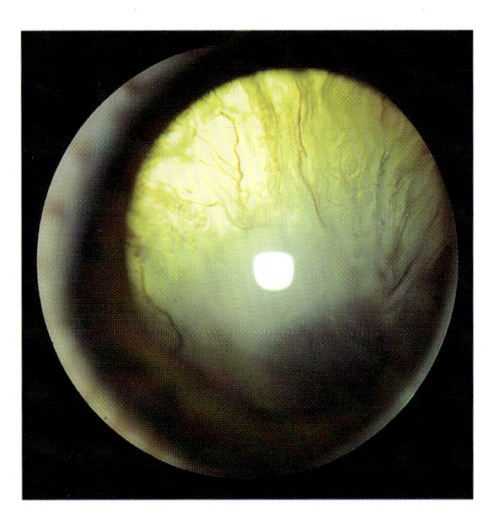

Fig. 14.37 Total retinal dysplasia – retinal folds viewed against tapetal reflex in an English Springer Spaniel.

in 15 litters in Sweden, all born from clinically normal parents, showed the defect was due to a single autosomal recessive gene; pedigree analysis revealed that all cases, in both England and Sweden, could be traced on both sire and dam side of the pedigree to one dog born in 1934. Retinal dysplasia with detachment has also been recorded in the Yorkshire Terrier (Stades, 1978).

Retinal dysplasia associated with skeletal abnormalities (shortening of limb bones and abnormal joint development) has also been described in Labrador Retrievers, in the United States but not elsewhere (Carrig et al., 1977). Puppies were affected by 8 weeks of age with marked skeletal maldevelopment and severely defective vision, dilated pupils and lens opacity. Other ocular findings included central corneal opacity, persistent hyaloid, central retinal degeneration and funnel-shaped total retinal detachment, similar to the Labrador puppies in England and Sweden described above. Carrig et al. (1988) studied 124 affected puppies and deduced that the ocular and skeletal lesions were inherited together and were the results of a single gene with recessive effects on the skeleton but incomplete dominant effects on the eye. However, a similar condition (short-limbed dwarfism and retinal detachment) in the Samoyed was thought, from family studies and limited breeding experiments, to follow an autosomal recessive mode of inheritance (Meyers et al., 1983).

All the above reports of retinal dysplasia were of a total form with detachment, bilateral and the cause of complete blindness in puppies. The first report of a focal/multifocal retinal dysplasia (nine cases) was in the English Springer Spaniel in America (Lavach et al., 1978) and there is no doubt that this condition occurs in this breed in the UK, mainly in working strains, as a bilateral, but not necessarily symmetrical, congenital and hereditary condition. Differing degrees of severity occur varying from a few retinal folds, mainly in the tapetal fundus, to many retinal folds and focal areas of tapetal hyper-reflectivity in the adult usually just superior to the optic disc, to total retinal detachment similar to that reported above in the Sealyham and Bedlington Terriers and Labrador. Other ocular anomalies include corneal dystrophy and cortical cataract. Most important is the variation in vision from apparently normal (few retinal folds) to total blindness (retinal detachment). Schmidt et al. (1979) described the condition as a genetically determined defect due to an autosomal recessive trait. Light microscopy of the postnatal lesions was described by O'Toole et al. (1983). A multifocal retinal dysplasia was also described in field trial strains in the Labrador in America (Nelson and MacMillan, 1983). Both unilateral and bilateral cases occurred, the dysplastic foci were usually in the central tapetal fundus superior to the optic disc and dogs were not blind. These authors suggested that this multifocal retinal dysplasia was a lesser manifestation than the total retinal dysplasia with skeletal abnormalities, and reported the results of two test litters suggesting dominant inheritance with incomplete penetrance.

Hereditary focal/multifocal retinal dysplasia (Figs 14.38–14.51) has also been recorded in the American Cocker Spaniel (MacMillan and Lipton, 1978) and more recently in the UK in the Golden Retriever (Crispin et al., 1999; Long and Crispin, 1999). It also occurs in the UK in the Cavalier King Charles Spaniel and, in all these breeds, simple autosomal recessive inheritance is suggested and evidence presented. This is the same as in the English Springer Spaniel and similar to the total forms of retinal dysplasia in the Bedlington and Sealyham Terriers and Labrador Retriever, except in association with skeletal abnormalities where inheritance may be more complex. The retinal folds or rosettes may be single or multiple, linear or oval to round, sometimes 'V' or 'Y' shaped streaks, grey in colour and hyporeflective. They are more common in the tapetal fundus, particularly in the central area, and appear below the retinal blood vessels when viewed ophthalmoscopically. In the non-tapetal fundus they are pale grey in colour against the darker background and are sometimes

RETINAL DYSPLASIA

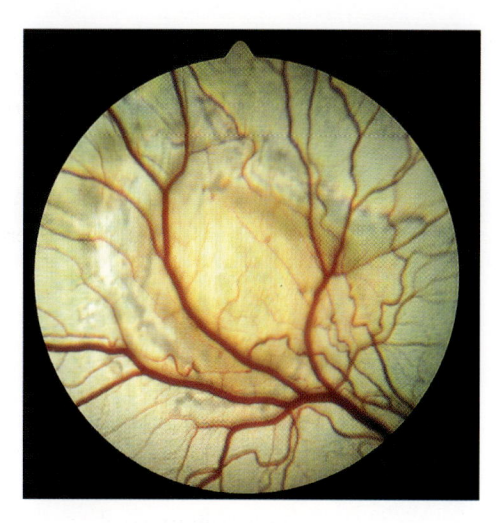

Fig. 14.38 Multifocal retinal dysplasia – geographic form in a 13-month-old Labrador Retriever.

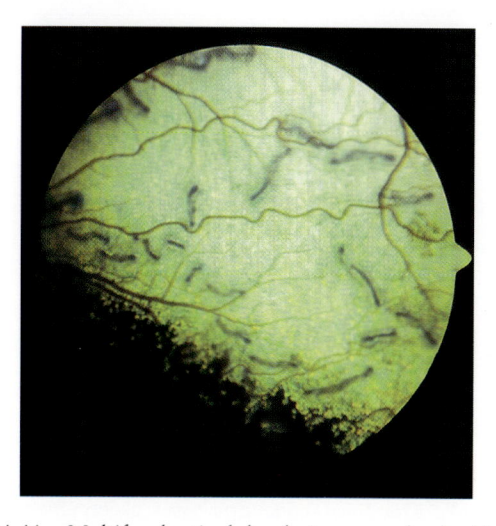

Fig. 14.41 Multifocal retinal dysplasia – note the double nature of some of the folds in the peripheral tapetum in a 15-week-old Golden Retriever.

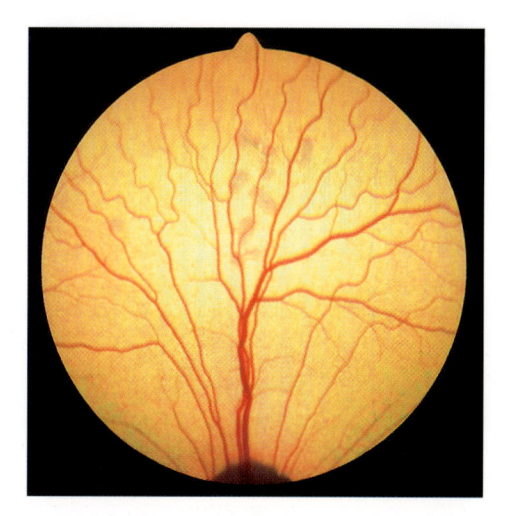

Fig. 14.39 Multifocal retinal dysplasia – few retinal folds in superior tapetal region in a 15-month-old Golden Retriever.

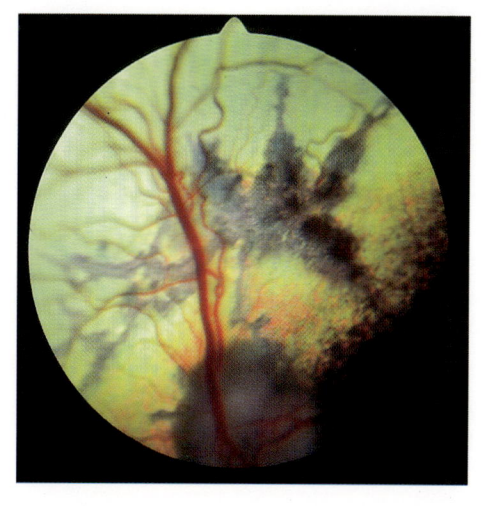

Fig. 14.42 Multifocal retinal dysplasia – more severe form than in Fig. 14.41 immediately above disc in a 6-month-old English Springer Spaniel.

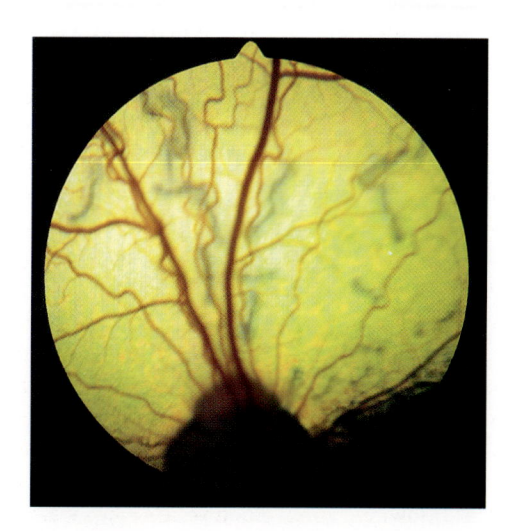

Fig. 14.40 Multifocal retinal dysplasia – more extensive folds than in Fig. 14.39, in a 12-month-old Golden Retriever.

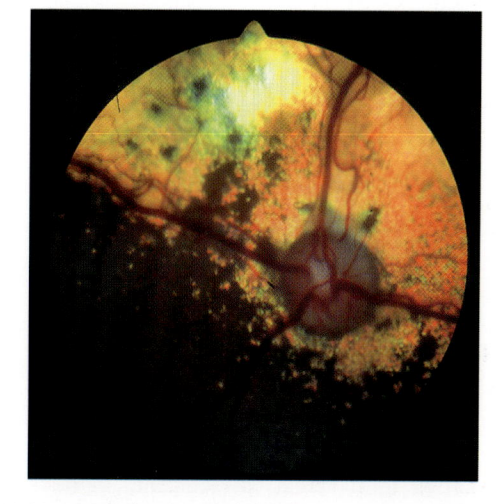

Fig. 14.43 Multifocal retinal dysplasia – severe changes superior to disc in a 2-year-old English Springer Spaniel.

FUNDUS

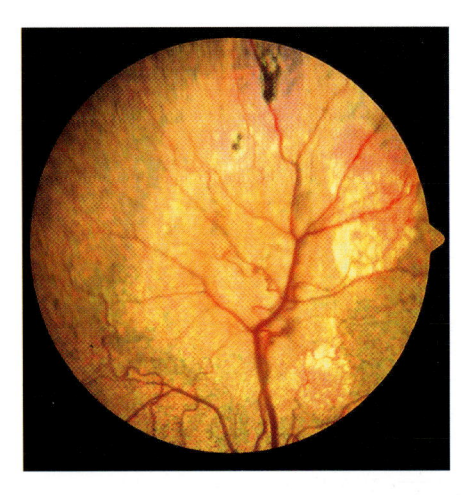

Fig. 14.44 Multifocal retinal dysplasia – geographic form in the superior central tapetal region surrounded by areas of hyper-reflectivity in an adult Cavalier King Charles Spaniel. Note excessive tortuosity of some of the fine arterioles.

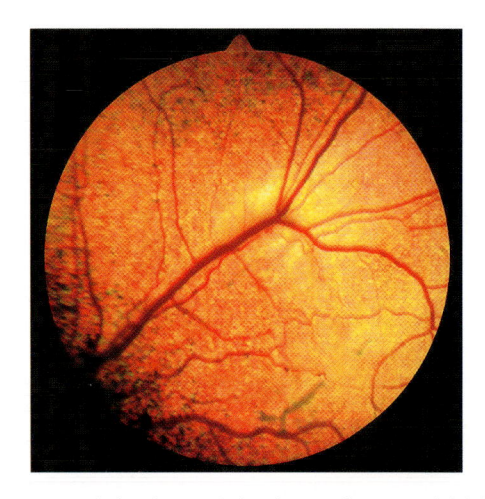

Fig. 14.47 Multifocal retinal dysplasia – few retinal folds in the superior tapetum in an 11-month-old Cavalier King Charles Spaniel.

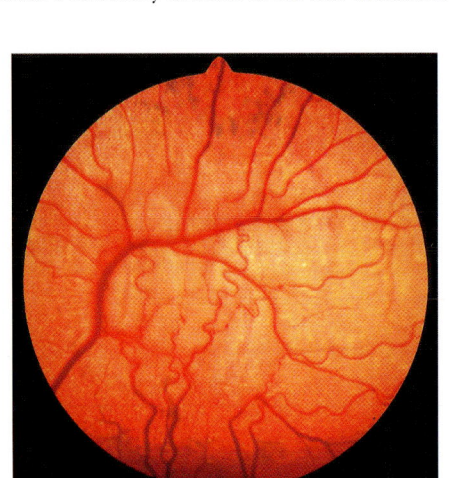

Fig. 14.45 Multifocal retinal dysplasia – folds and areas of detachment in a 2-year-old Cavalier King Charles Spaniel. Again note the excessive tortuosity of the retinal arterioles.

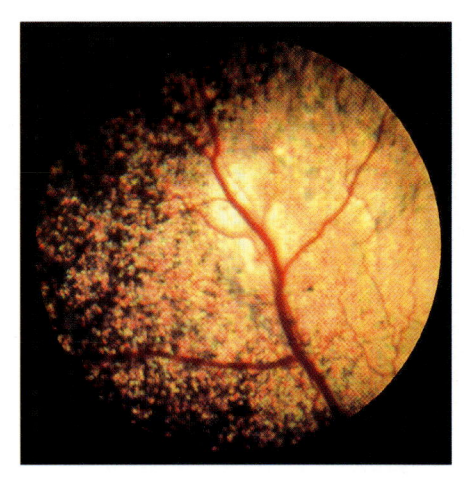

Fig. 14.48 Multifocal retinal dysplasia – area of increased reflectivity, few folds and small area of detachment in an 8-month-old Cavalier King Charles Spaniel.

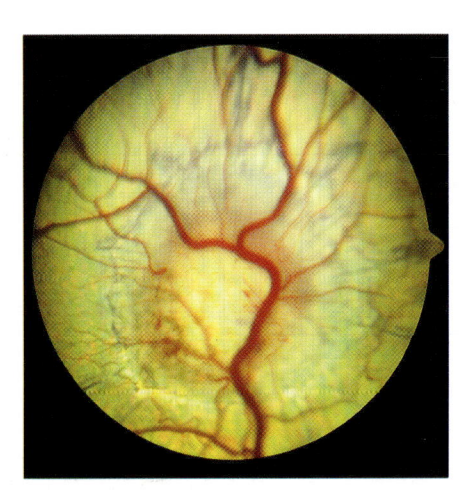

Fig. 14.46 Multifocal retinal dysplasia – geographic form, similar to Fig. 14.45 but in a 4-month-old Cavalier King Charles Spaniel.

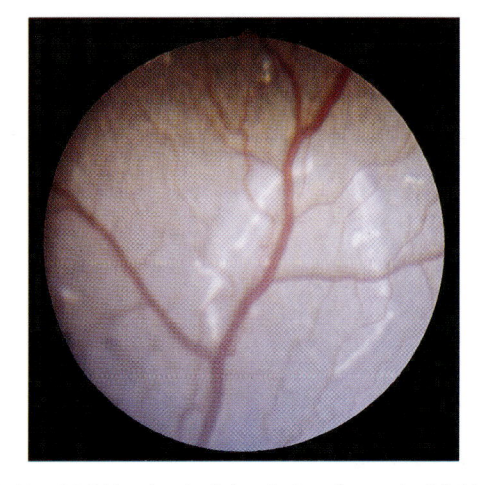

Fig. 14.49 Multifocal retinal dysplasia – few retinal folds appearing as pale areas in the superior developing tapetal region in a 7-week-old Cavalier King Charles Spaniel.

RETINAL DYSPLASIA

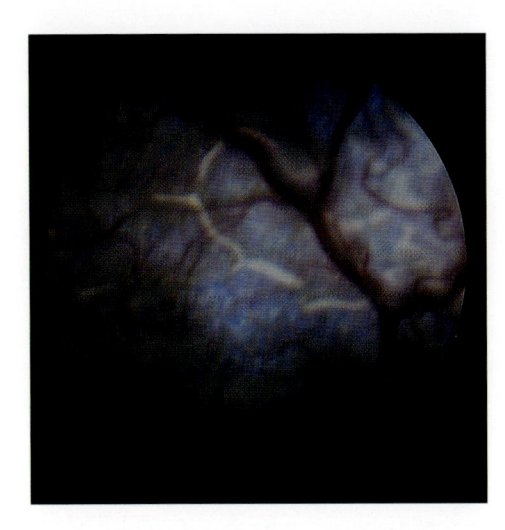

Fig. 14.50 Multifocal retinal dysplasia – pale branching folds in the tapetal region in a 6-week-old Cavalier King Charles Spaniel.

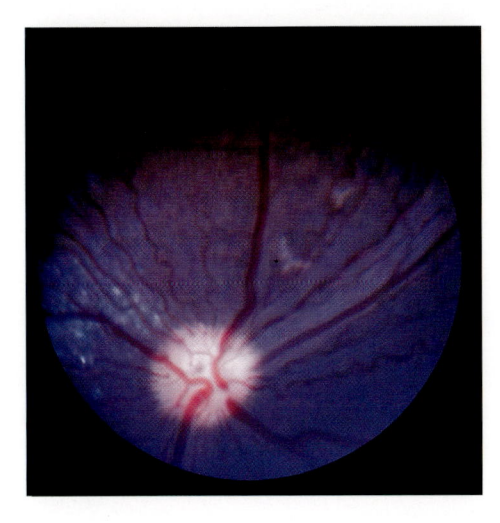

Fig. 14.51 Multifocal retinal dysplasia – few pale branching folds in the non-tapetal fundus in a 12-week-old Cavalier King Charles Spaniel.

more easily visible. In the Cavalier King Charles Spaniel, diagnosis by ophthalmoscopy can be made at a few weeks of age, although it may sometimes be easier following full tapetal development. The condition is pleomorphic and with variation in severity, i.e. the number of retinal folds, between individuals and between the two eyes of the same animal. Over one-third of cases examined, in a survey of over 1000 dogs of which over 8% were affected, have been unilateral and these were not necessarily minimally affected cases, although in this toy breed no dogs have been presented because of defective vision. Interestingly, there was a significantly higher incidence in solid-coloured (black/tan, ruby) Cavaliers than in particoloured (Blenheim, tri), demonstrating that certain strains in the same breed were more affected than others. The basic ophthalmoscopic lesion is the retinal fold, typically in the superior tapetal fundus several disc diameters above the optic disc, i.e. at the posterior pole of the eye, not immediately above the disc as frequently occurs in the English Springer Spaniel. These folds may be in the form of a roughly circular, plaque-like lesion with altered reflectivity and often a double border and folds around the margin. This third ophthalmoscopic appearance of retinal dysplasia, the other two forms being retinal folds (focal/multifocal) and total retinal detachment, has, unfortunately, been termed 'geographic'. These plaque-like lesions usually involve the major dorsal retinal blood vessels with detachment of the retina in the area involved; often minor blood vessels show increased tortuosity and sometimes small retinal haemorrhages are present. These lesions are usually unilateral and, in spite of the detachment, defective vision has not been a presenting sign; in fact cases are only diagnosed on routine ophthalmoscopic examination, usually in certification schemes for the control of hereditary eye abnormalities.

The focal/multifocal, including the so-called geographic forms, also occur in the Labrador Retriever in the UK, where it has also been reported in the Hungarian Puli, Rottweiler, Sussex Spaniel, Field Spaniel and Giant Schnauzer.

Retinal dysplasia as part of a congenital, and possibly inherited, multiple ocular defects syndrome has been recorded in the UK and elsewhere in the Akita, Old English Sheepdog and Dobermann (Lewis *et al.*, 1986). Retinal folds are often seen in microphthalmic eyes and temporary retinal folds, or vermiform streaks, have been recognised for many years in the collie breeds (Rough and Smooth Collie and Shetland Sheepdog) and were originally considered to be part of the collie eye anomaly. Temporary retinal folds, present in young puppies but disappearing ophthalmoscopically in the young adult around 12 months of age, have been seen in both the Labrador and Golden Retriever breeds, and this phenomenon was originally noted in the Beagle (Rubin, 1974). It is widely accepted that not all cases of retinal dysplasia (retinal folds) are hereditary in origin although certainly the majority, particularly in the breeds already implicated, are inherited. Other proven causes are canine adenovirus, canine herpes virus and irradiation.

Retinal dysplasia, particularly the milder focal/multifocal forms which rarely, if ever, are the cause of defective vision, presents difficulties in diagnosis in schemes for the control of hereditary eye abnormalities based only on ophthalmoscopic examination. These difficulties include the following (see Figs 14.52–14.54):

- Retinal dysplasia may be due to other non-hereditary causes indistinguishable ophthalmoscopically from inherited cases.
- Retinal folds disappear in puppies, even in breeds with proven hereditary multifocal retinal dysplasia.
- Minimal cases (single focal lesion unilaterally) occur in these same breeds.
- Retinal dysplasia is classed as a congenital condition but a recent report (Holle *et al.*, 1999) records the geographic form not visible ophthalmoscopically until 10 weeks of

FUNDUS

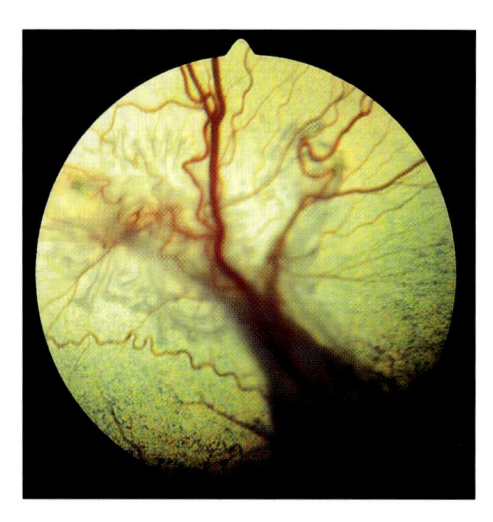

Fig. 14.52 Retinal dysplasia – folds, detachment and blood vessel anomalies above disc in a 5-year-old Golden Retriever. This dog was known to have had parvovirus infection.

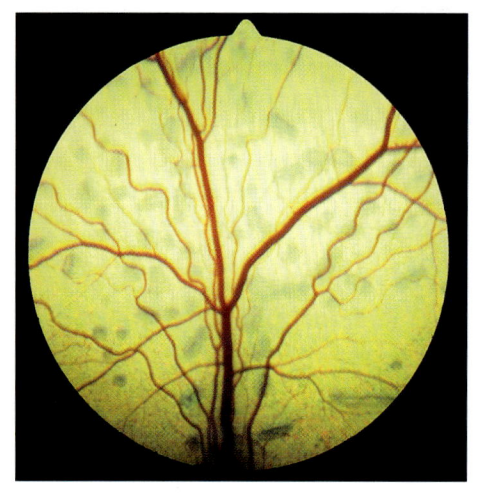

Fig. 14.53 Retinal dysplasia – folds and rosettes in the central tapetal region in a Labrador/Golden Retriever cross.

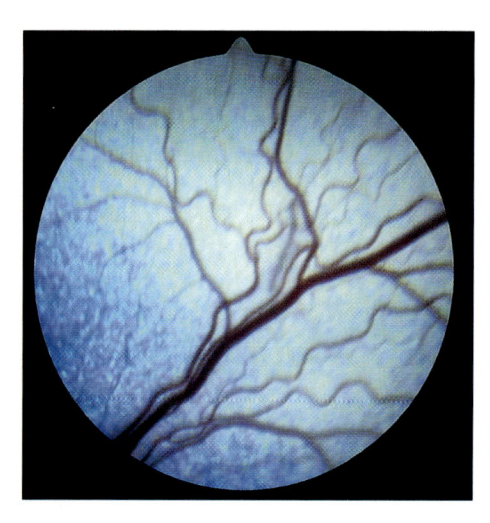

Fig. 14.54 Retinal dysplasia – retinal folds in a Golden Retriever/Border Collie cross.

age in most cases in implicated breeds and crossbreeds. However, this is not always the case (see Fig. 14.49).

CANINE RETINAL DYSTROPHIES

The first report of an inherited canine retinal degeneration leading to blindness came from Sweden in the Gordon Setter (Magnusson, 1911). The condition was called retinitis pigmentosa because of its similarity to an inherited retinal degeneration in man. It was later named progressive retinal atrophy, or simply referred to by the initials PRA, in both the canine and veterinary literature, and has since been recorded in several breeds in many parts of the world. This condition was later referred to as generalised progressive retinal atrophy (GPRA) to distinguish it from central progressive retinal atrophy (CPRA). GPRA has been further subdivided into a number of distinctly separate conditions, all primarily affecting the photoreceptors and classed as dysplasias or degenerations depending upon whether the rods and/or cones are affected prior to maturation (up to 6 weeks) or later in life. These separate conditions are inherited by different genes in some cases, e.g. rod–cone dysplasia in the Irish Setter, or by the same gene, e.g. rod–cone degeneration in the Miniature Poodle and Cocker Spaniel. However, and of particular importance to the veterinary clinician, all the GPRAs appear the same ophthalmoscopically and have the same effect on vision, ending ultimately in total blindness, but they occur at different ages which are breed-specific.

Generalised progressive retinal atrophy (Figs 14.55–14.61) is a bilaterally symmetrical and progressive inherited retinal degeneration (retinal dystrophy) occurring at a certain age in life, according to the breed. It is these points that are particularly helpful in distinguishing it from other retinal degenerations due to any other cause. Almost invariably the first clinical sign noted by an owner is impaired vision in dim light, or night blindness. This sign may be noticed following removal to a new home or in unfamiliar surroundings and occasionally some affected dogs prefer to be left in a lighted room. Night blindness proceeds to day blindness and ultimately total blindness, but the speed of progression over months or years, depending on the breed, does allow the dog to learn about its surroundings and some become remarkably adept at avoiding obstacles. Ophthalmoscopically the first sign is an increased reflectivity in the tapetal fundus due to degeneration, and therefore thinning, of the retina above the tapetum. Later in the course of the disease, depigmentation of the non-tapetal fundus occurs so that the area becomes paler grey in patches with darker areas between. Attenuation, or narrowing, of the retinal blood vessels is perhaps the most obvious ophthalmoscopic sign, but is secondary to those changes previously described. Pallor of the optic disc, due to vessel attenuation and later to optic nerve degeneration, becomes more evident in the later stages. Pupillary dilation and a sluggish pupillary light reflex occur, but the retention of some pupillary light reflex with GPRA is the rule and this fact can be

CANINE RETINAL DYSTROPHIES

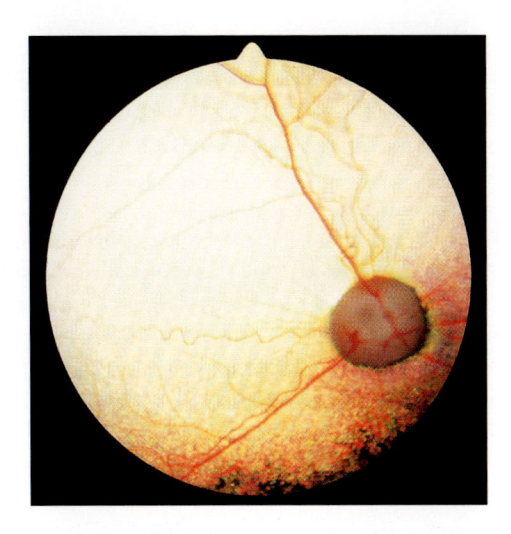

Fig. 14.55 Rod–cone dysplasia in a 3-month-old Irish Setter. Note the obvious narrowing of the blood vessels.

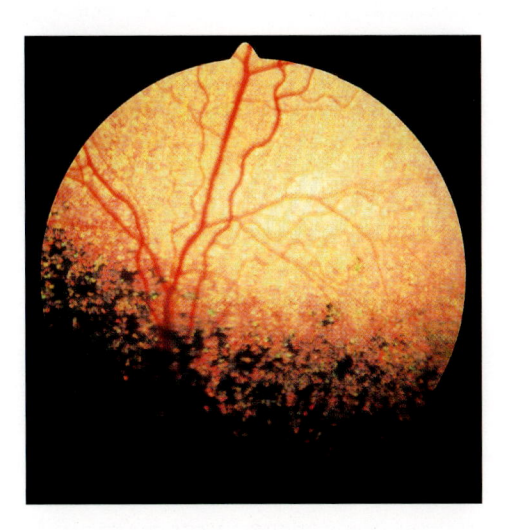

Fig. 14.56 Cone–rod degeneration in a 1-year-old Miniature Longhaired Dachshund showing early fundus changes.

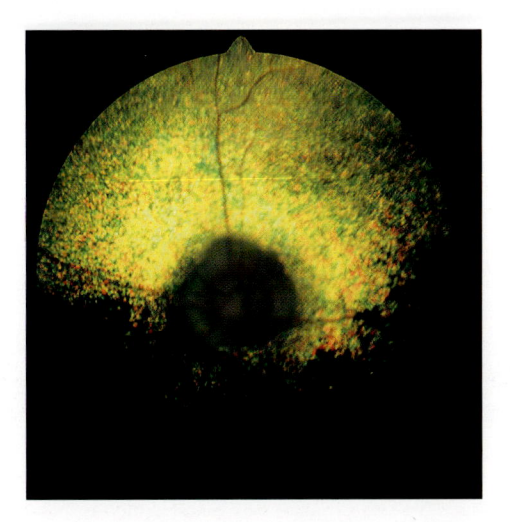

Fig. 14.57 Progressive retinal atrophy in an 18-month-old Tibetan Terrier. Note the typical tapetal hyper-reflectivity.

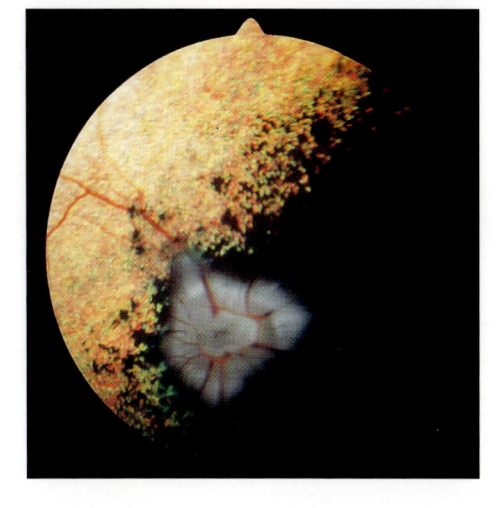

Fig. 14.58 Progressive rod–cone degeneration in a 5-year-old Miniature Poodle.

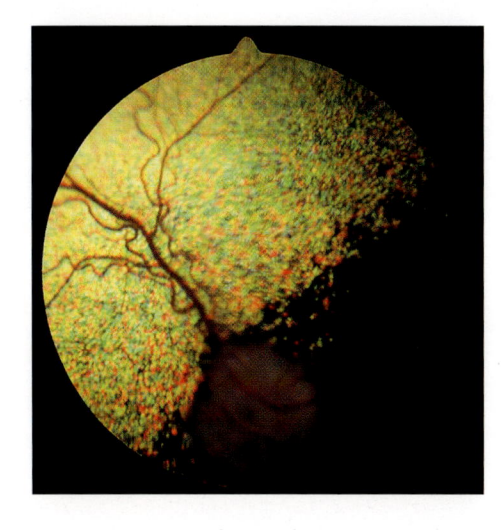

Fig. 14.59 Progressive rod–cone degeneration in a 3-year-old Golden Retriever.

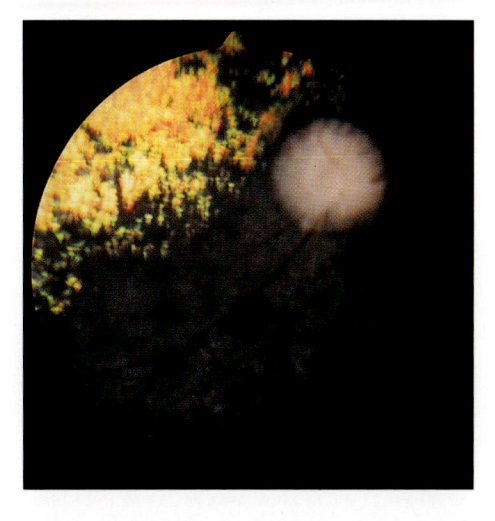

Fig. 14.60 Typical pigmentary changes in non-tapetal fundus in an 18-month-old Miniature Longhaired Dachshund.

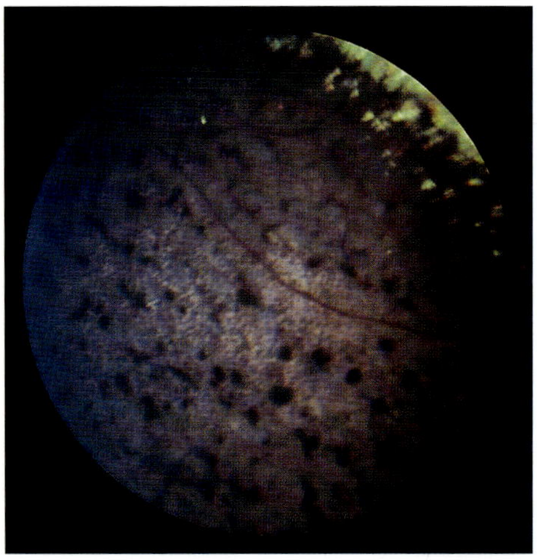

Fig. 14.61 Typical pigmentary changes in non-tapetal fundus in a 4-year-old Labrador Retriever.

Breeds affected with GPRA in the UK are listed in Table 14.1. However, several other breeds have been reported in other countries and there is no doubt that further breeds will be recorded in the future. All forms of GPRA, both the photoreceptor dysplasias and degenerations, are due to simple autosomal recessive inheritance with the single exception, to date, of the Siberian Husky which has been reported as X-linked in the USA (Acland *et al.*, 1994). Furthermore, by crossing affected dogs of different breeds it was originally thought that the same gene was involved in some of the breeds, for example the Miniature and Toy Poodle, the American Cocker Spaniel, the English Cocker Spaniel and the Labrador Retriever. However, with the recent progress in molecular genetics and the advent of DNA-based diagnostic tests for the presence of GPRA it may be shown that there are different gene defects in the same breed, i.e. two types of rod–cone degeneration in the same breed occurring at different ages. This has already been suspected in both the Labrador and Golden Retriever, and possibly others, by differences in age of onset and progression and by pedigree analysis.

Central progressive retinal atrophy (Figs 14.62–14.64), or retinal pigment epithelial dystrophy (RPED), was first described by Parry in 1954, the term being used to distinguish CPRA from GPRA as two distinctly different conditions, the former primarily affecting the retinal pigment epithelium and secondarily the photoreceptor layer. The condition was particularly prevalent in the UK but was also described in several other countries and from the first description (Parry, 1954a) showed a definite breed incidence.

useful in the differential diagnosis of other retinopathies. Secondary cataract to the retinal degeneration almost invariably occurs in the dog (but not in the cat). This is usually posterior cortical with vacuolation, but often becomes total quite rapidly so preventing ophthalmoscopic examination of the fundus and indicating the necessity for electroretinography before cataract surgery in any of the breeds affected with PRA. A number of these total cataracts may dislocate with time, no doubt due to the degeneration of the zonule, although secondary glaucoma in such cases is not as severe as with primary lens dislocation in the terrier breeds (see Chapter 11).

Table 14.1 Breeds affected with GPRA in the UK. All simple recessive inheritance.

Breed	Age*	Type of dystrophy
Irish Setter	6/8W–1Y	Rod–cone dysplasia type 1. Eradicated UK
Rough Collie	6/8W–1Y	Rod–cone dysplasia type 2. Not recorded UK
Miniature Longhaired Dachshund	6M–2Y	Cone–rod degeneration. UK
Cardigan Welsh Corgi	3M–1Y	Early onset progressive retinal atrophy. UK
Elkhound	6M–3/5Y	Rod dysplasia. UK. Also a separate early retinal degeneration in this breed but not UK
Miniature Schnauzer	2Y–5Y	Photoreceptor dysplasia. UK
Miniature or Toy Poodle	3Y–5/7Y	Progressive rod–cone degeneration. UK
English Cocker Spaniel	2Y–5Y	Progressive rod–cone degeneration. UK
American Cocker Spaniel	3/5Y–4/6Y	Progressive rod–cone degeneration. UK
Labrador Retriever	2/3Y–5/6Y	Progressive rod–cone degeneration. UK
Golden Retriever	2/3Y–5/6Y	Progressive rod–cone degeneration. UK
Tibetan Terrier	9M–2/3Y	Progressive retinal atrophy. UK
Tibetan Spaniel	2Y–5Y	Progressive retinal atrophy. UK
Papillon	4Y–8Y	Progressive retinal atrophy. UK

*Behavioural change (night blindness) to day or total blindness (approximate figures only, also variation between individuals). W, week; M, month; Y, year.

Note: Diagnosis by electroretinography is possible before fundus changes appear.

CANINE RETINAL DYSTROPHIES

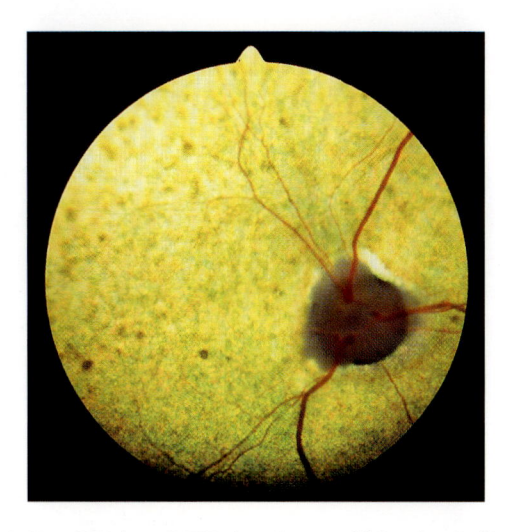

Fig. 14.62 CPRA or RPED in a 3-year-old Border Collie.

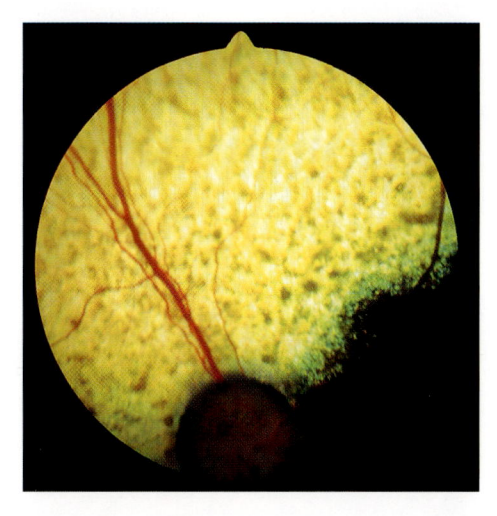

Fig. 14.63 CPRA or RPED in a 3-year-old Labrador Retriever.

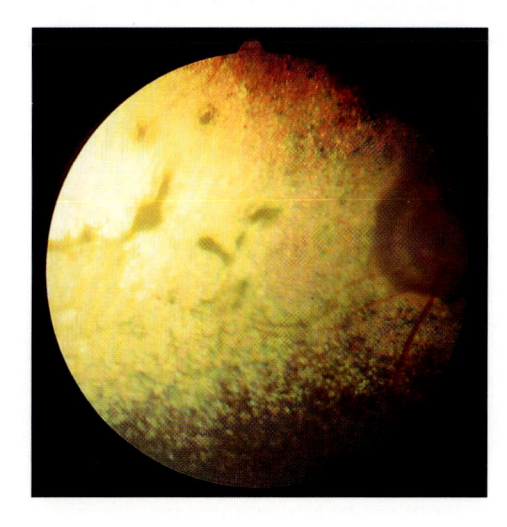

Fig. 14.64 CPRA or RPED in a 9-year-old Border Collie. Note the fewer and denser pigment spots with hyper-reflectivity in an advanced case.

The main breeds affected were the Labrador Retriever, Golden Retriever, Border Collie, Rough Collie, Shetland Sheepdog, English Springer Spaniel and English Cocker Spaniel. It was also particularly prevalent in the Briard (Bedford, 1984) and later in the Polish Lowland Sheepdog. A different form of a congenital and hereditary retinal dystrophy in the Briard has been described in Sweden (Narfström et al., 1989) but without any fundus changes ophthalmoscopically, at least in the early stages.

In recent years RPED seems to have disappeared from countries other than the UK and in the UK the incidence is considerably less, perhaps at least partially due to control schemes. CPRA, or RPED, was originally thought to be an inherited progressive retinal atrophy but always different from GPRA in its ophthalmoscopic appearance, effect on vision and breeds affected. The breed incidence and prevalence in certain strains within a breed led to investigation into the exact mode of inheritance, but this was never proved although both recessive and dominant modes were postulated. It is probable that this condition is not a simple inherited retinal degeneration, as is GPRA, but the undoubted breed incidence of naturally occurring cases strongly indicates some genetic predisposition in these breeds and strains. It is interesting that similar lesions have been produced experimentally in dogs where diets are deficient in vitamin E (Riis et al., 1981) and dogs affected with CPRA have been shown to have low plasma levels of vitamin E, so indicating some connection between RPED (CPRA) and vitamin E deficiency. A neurological syndrome with ataxia has been described in some cases of RPED, particularly in the Cocker Spaniel, but no such signs have occurred in other cases of CPRA in such working breeds as the Border Collie and Labrador Retriever, perhaps indicating various forms of this condition.

The ophthalmoscopic appearance of RPED is the presence of numerous light brown pigmented spots or foci scattered regularly in the tapetal region. These spots of lipopigment differ slightly between certain breeds in both colour and form and may appear as a reticulum or network with a hyper-reflective tapetum, indicating retinal thinning or degeneration, between them. The first signs of the disease occur in the area centralis region lateral to the optic disc but the condition is progressive and soon the whole tapetal area is affected, later spreading into the non-tapetal fundus. With progression the pigment spots coalesce becoming fewer in number and more dense in appearance on a highly reflective tapetal background. The pigment foci are due to cell nests of hypertrophied pigment-laden cells that have migrated from the pigment epithelium through the degenerate retina to the innermost layer. Secondary cataract to this retinal degeneration occurs in a number of cases but is not as regular in appearance or as frequent as with GPRA. Diagnosis by ophthalmoscopy is possible as early as 18 months in some cases but by no means in all. Defective vision may be noticed at 3–5 years but certain cases show no signs below 6–8 years.

FUNDUS

CPRA is also bilateral, symmetrical and progressive. Vision is affected but not as with GPRA. Night blindness is not an early sign. In fact poor vision is more noticeable in bright light than in dull light and total blindness does not occur in all cases in spite of the progression. The retention of peripheral vision allows the dog to pick up moving objects better than even quite large stationary objects.

OTHER RETINOPATHIES

Post-inflammatory retinopathies in the dog are not rare but, in comparison with the hereditary retinopathies, have received little attention or research and are seldom accurately diagnosed, particularly in the United Kingdom. In addition to the post-inflammatory retinopathies, and the retinal dystrophies previously described, there are a number of rare inherited lipid storage diseases presenting with blindness and neurological signs.

Post-inflammatory retinopathies are usually secondary to a choroiditis and should more accurately be described as chorioretinitis. They may be acute or active, or chronic and inactive. They may affect one or both eyes and, except in severe or advanced cases, are not bilaterally symmetrical. One or both eyes may show one or more lesions usually irregular in shape and well demarcated, particularly in the chronic cases. They may present with degrees of defective vision varying to complete blindness, but the ophthalmoscopic signs are not specific to any particular disease and further investigation as to aetiology is usually necessary for treatment of the particular systemic condition. The asymmetry, often sudden onset, together with the breed and age should distinguish these post-inflammatory retinopathies from the hereditary retinopathies.

For many years canine distemper has been a known cause of retinal degeneration (Parry 1954b). Other causes, most of which have not been reported in the UK, include rickettsial diseases (canine ehrlichiosis); mycotic diseases (blastomycosis, cryptococcosis and histoplasmosis); and protozoal diseases (toxoplasmosis).

Figs 14.65 to 14.70 illustrate cases of post-inflammatory retinopathies of unknown aetiology.

HYPERTENSIVE RETINOPATHY

It is only since about 1990 that hypertension has been diagnosed clinically in veterinary medicine, a fact mainly due to the unavailability of a satisfactory (non-invasive) and dependable method for the indirect measurement of blood pressure in the dog and, even more so, in the cat. However, sudden blindness with retinal haemorrhage and detachment was recognised in the dog many years ago (Keyes and Goldblatt, 1937) in experimentally induced hypertension models. Clinical cases of hypertension in the dog were originally considered to be mainly secondary to renal failure or hormonal imbalance. However, cases of essential, or primary, hypertension, presenting with ocular signs and with

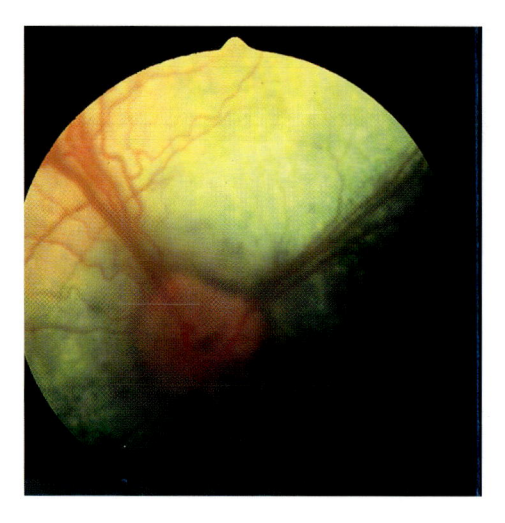

Fig. 14.65 Active chorioretinitis and optic neuritis in a 2-year-old crossbred. Note congestion of blood vessels, swelling of disc and hazy appearance of retina due to exudate, particularly in peripapillary region. Possible toxoplasmosis case. (Courtesy of SM Crispin.)

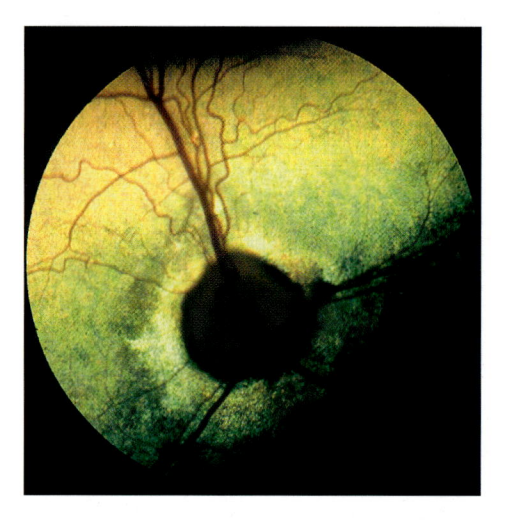

Fig. 14.66 Same dog as in Fig. 14.65 after treatment. Note less swollen disc, clearer appearance of fundus and hyper-reflective irregular peripapillary ring. (Courtesy of SM Crispin.)

sudden blindness have recently been documented (Bovee et al., 1989; Sansom and Bodey, 1997).

The ocular signs associated with hypertension in the dog are not pathognomonic in this species, as they are in man, but their presence when recognised ophthalmoscopically should lead to further investigation of some systemic condition. The basic fundus signs are haemorrhages and retinal detachment, both leading to sudden blindness. Increased or excessive tortuosity (Figs 14.71–14.73) of the retinal arterioles is often, possibly invariably, present but blood vessel tortuosity in the canine fundus is very variable, although it is interesting that a recent survey (A Bodey and KC Barnett – unpublished observations) of adult Deerhounds, a breed with a normal 'high' blood pressure, all exhibited marked

HYPERTENSIVE RETINOPATHY

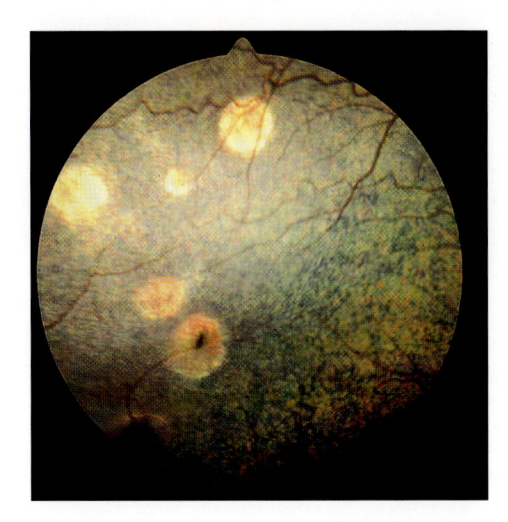

Fig. 14.67 Chorioretinitis – several small well-demarcated hyper-reflective areas, some with pigmented centres, together with more diffuse areas of hyper-reflectivity indicating retinal degeneration in a 5-year-old Golden Retriever. The dog had had a severe attack of gastroenteritis and pyrexia 2 years previously but no specific diagnosis was made.

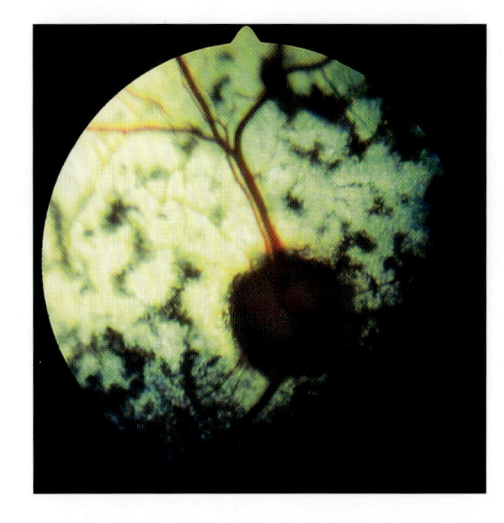

Fig. 14.69 Chorioretinitis and optic atrophy in a blind 5-year-old Border Collie. Note similarity of pigmentary changes to Fig. 14.68 and again at the junction of tapetal and non-tapetal fundus.

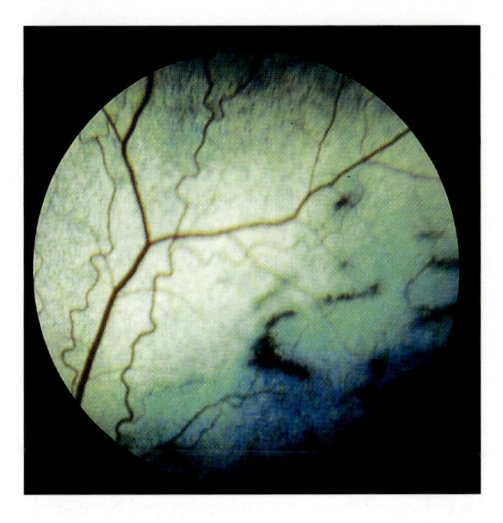

Fig. 14.68 Inactive pigmentary lesions of chorioretinitis at the junction of tapetal with non-tapetal fundus in a 3-year-old Lancashire Heeler. No history.

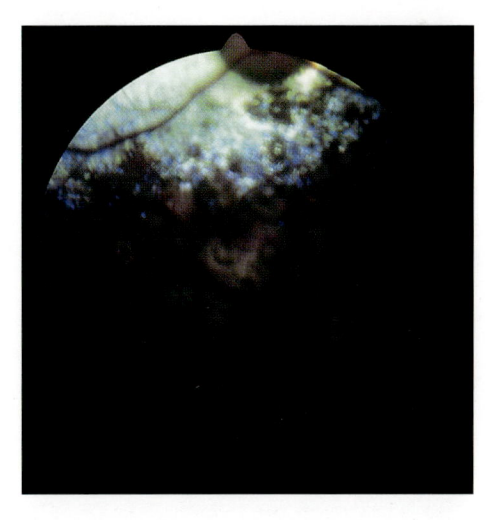

Fig. 14.70 Inactive chorioretinitis in the non-tapetal fundus in a young adult, unvaccinated Greyhound.

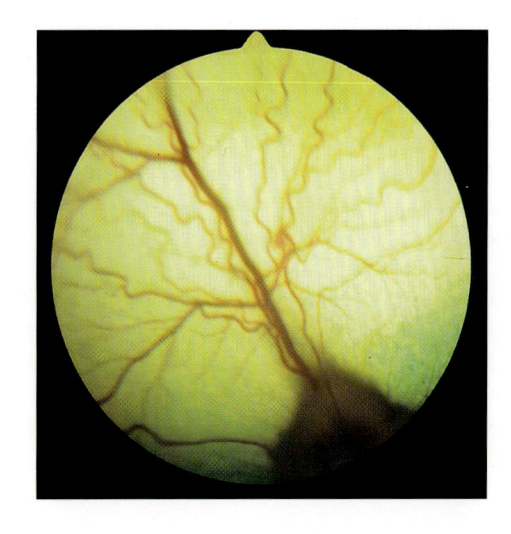

Fig. 14.71 Tortuosity of retinal arterioles plus one small haemorrhage in an 11-year-old Labrador cross Golden Retriever, spayed female. BP was 192/130 (systolic/diastolic mmHg); haematology and biochemistry were routine with nothing significant.

FUNDUS

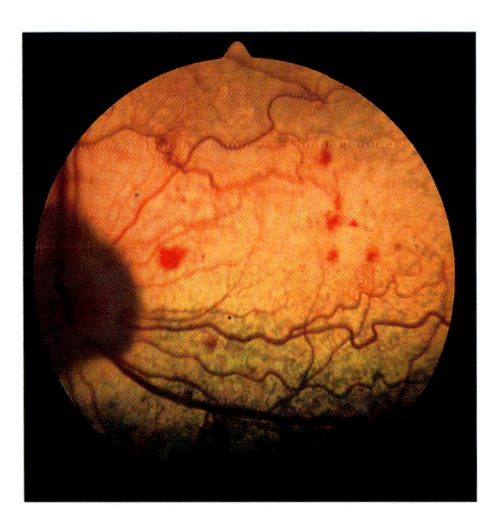

Fig. 14.72 Arteriolar tortuosity together with small dot/blot haemorrhages, particularly in area centralis, and an area of exudative retinal detachment in the upper part of the figure, in a 12-year-old Labrador cross Golden Retriever, female, right eye. BP was 165/103 (systolic/diastolic mmHg); haematology and biochemistry were routine with nothing significant.

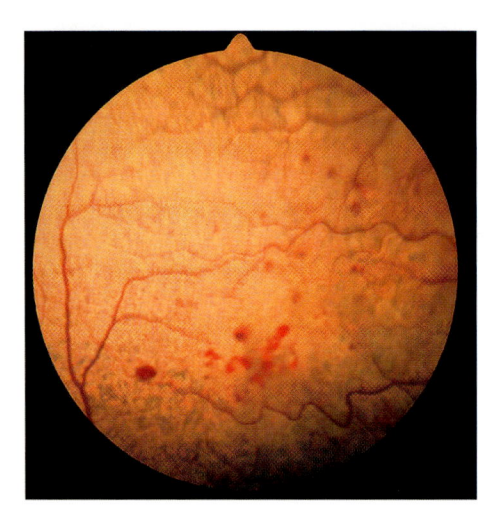

Fig. 14.73 Similar changes of tortuosity and small haemorrhages, particularly in area centralis, in the same dog as in Fig. 14.72, left eye.

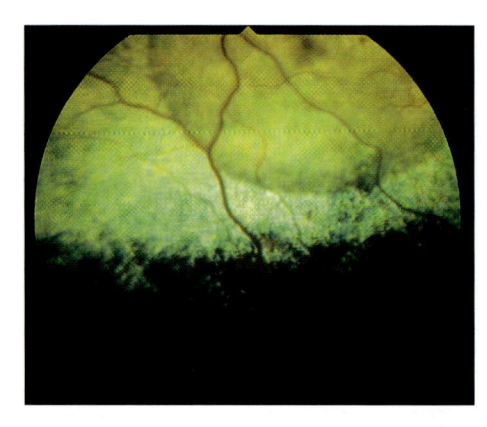

Fig. 14.74 Bullous retinal detachment in a 10-year-old Labrador, spayed female. BP was 182/93 (systolic/diastolic mmHg); haematology and biochemistry were routine with nothing significant.

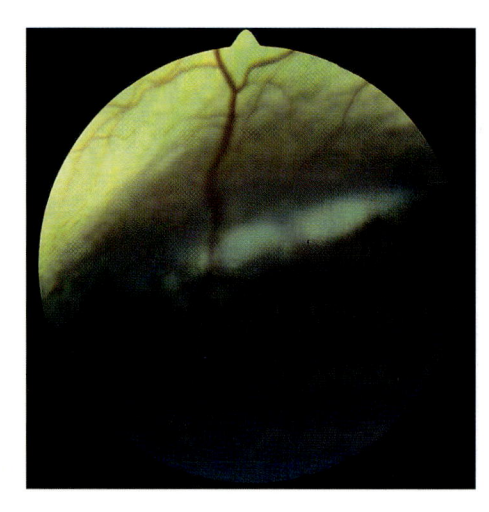

Fig. 14.75 Extensive retinal detachment in an 11-year-old Labrador cross Golden Retriever, spayed female. Note loss of tapetal reflex and altered course of blood vessel. BP was 210/130 (systolic/diastolic mmHg).

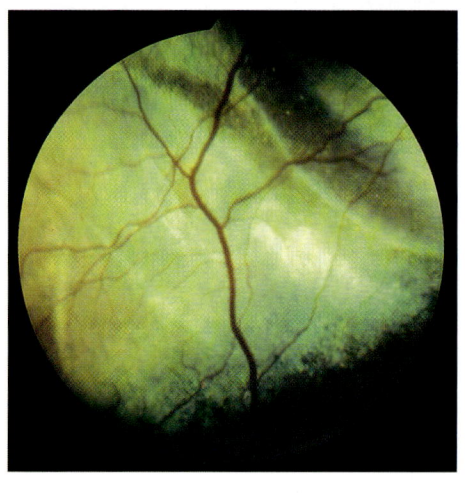

Fig. 14.76 Retina reattached with pigmentary change in tapetal area and patchy hyper-reflectivity in the same dog as in Fig. 14.75, 2 months later following treatment.

tortuosity. Small, round haemorrhages, often in groups, usually on the temporal side of the optic disc and interestingly in or near the area centralis, intraretinal and of the 'dot and blot' type (Figs 14.72 and 14.73), are a usual sign. Evidence of retinal degeneration may be seen in this area. Larger haemorrhages also occur. Small retinal bullae are occasionally seen which may coalesce to form larger bullae and finally total retinal detachment of the serous type (Fig. 14.74 and Figs 14.75–14.77). Similar fundus changes have been seen in cases of both Cushing's syndrome (Fig. 14.78) and diabetes mellitus (Fig. 14.79) of long standing. Both of these may be due to secondary hypertension, but in the latter case it was not possible to measure the blood pressure.

RETINAL HAEMORRHAGES

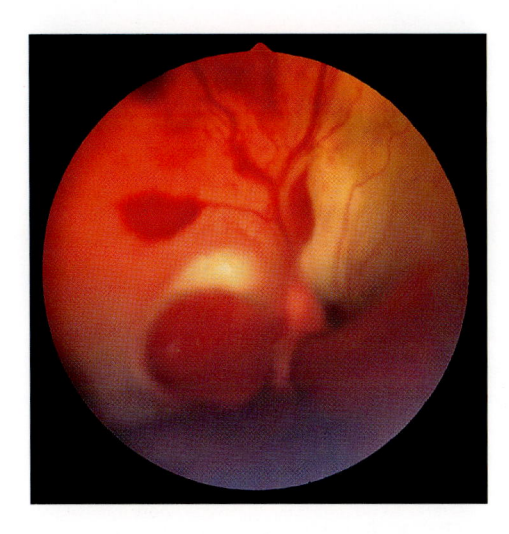

Fig. 14.77 Total retinal detachment partially obscuring optic disc together with retinal and vitreal haemorrhages in a 10-year-old obese Cocker Spaniel, male. No abnormalities were detected in the other eye. BP was 198/130 (systolic/diastolic mmHg); haematology and biochemistry were routine with nothing significant.

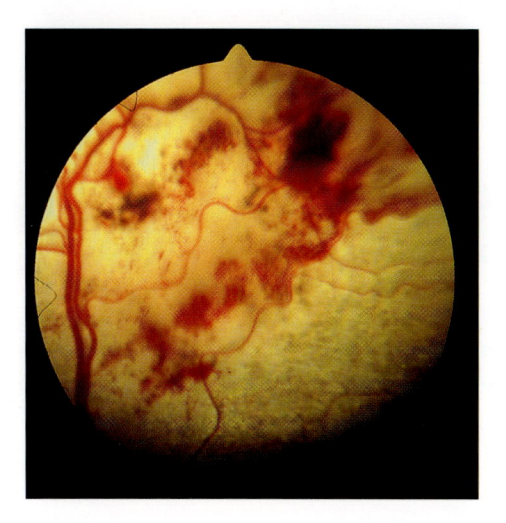

Fig. 14.79 Retinal haemorrhages and detachment in a 10-year-old Standard Poodle, male with diabetes mellitus of several years duration. Blood pressure not measured.

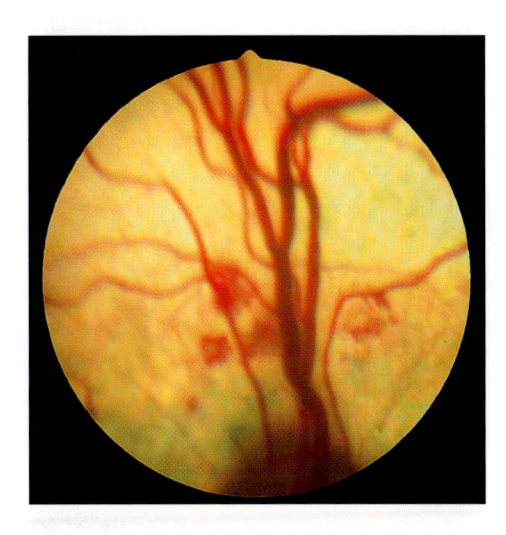

Fig. 14.78 Gross congestion of 12 o'clock vein and arteriole showing venous banking at first arteriovenous crossing plus haemorrhages and detachment; beading of arteriole on the right in a 9-year-old Beagle, male with Cushing's syndrome. Systolic BP was 170 mmHg.

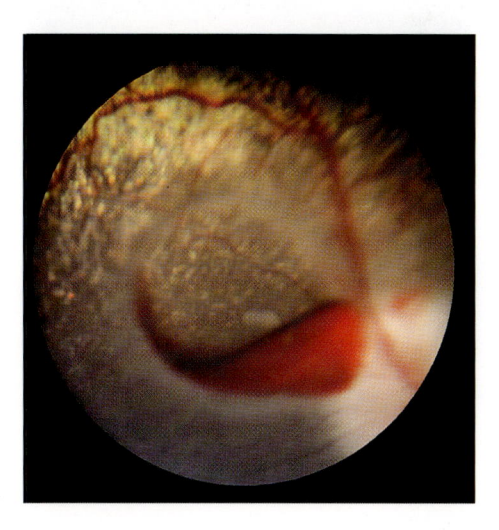

Fig. 14.80 Keel-boat shaped fundus with optic neuritis in a Cavalier King Charles Spaniel haemorrhage.

Retinal haemorrhages

Retinal haemorrhages are not rare in the dog and usually indicate some systemic disease requiring further investigation. A few small, round haemorrhages are quite often seen in the ageing dog with no history or evidence of disease including haematological and biochemical investigations and blood pressure measurement.

Haemorrhages may be described as flame-shaped, occurring in the nerve fibre layer and having a streaky appearance, dot and blot, small and round and in the deeper structures; or keel-boat shaped with a very typical appearance and situated between the outer retinal layer and vitreous (Fig. 14.80). For the exact location of haemorrhages fluoroscein angiography may be necessary.

Trauma is an obvious cause for some haemorrhages, which will resolve with time leaving no trace ophthalmoscopically, but whatever the cause, if not treated successfully, repeated haemorrhages may well occur. Figure 14.81 shows quite extensive haemorrhage beneath the superficial retinal blood vessels in a 43-day-old Border Collie puppy, presumably traumatic in origin, which completely resolved in a few weeks and did not recur.

Haemorrhages of the dot and blot type commonly occur in cases of hypertension (see Figs 14.71–14.73, 14.77 and 14.78) and diabetes (Fig. 14.79). Retinal haemorrhages may also occur with anaemia and in cases of haemostatic defects

FUNDUS

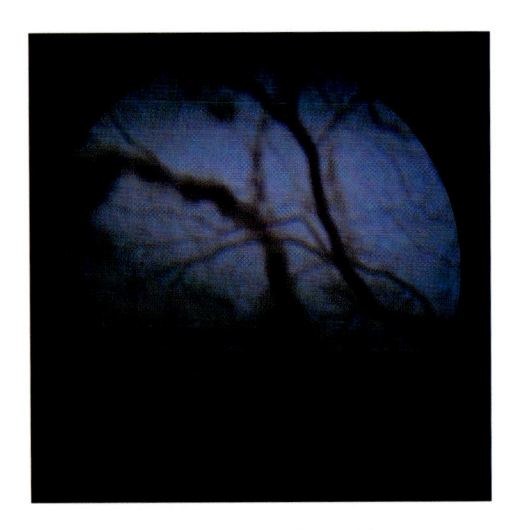

Fig. 14.81 Retinal haemorrhage of possible traumatic origin in a Border Collie puppy.

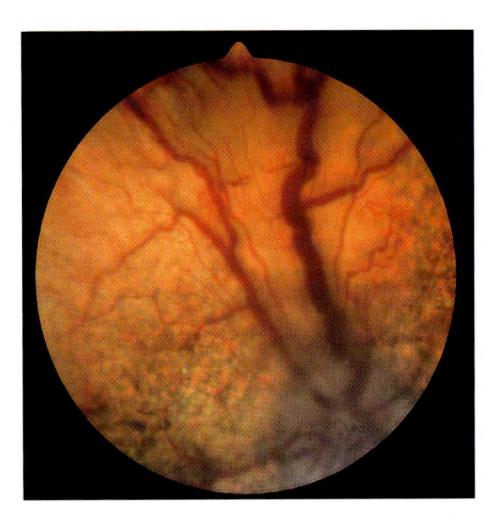

Fig. 14.82 Hyperviscosity syndrome in plasma cell myeloma in a 10-year-old Standard Poodle.

including inherited clotting factor defects, Warfarin poisoning, von Willebrand's disease and thrombocytopenias. In addition haemorrhages may be seen in the hyperviscosity syndrome together with grossly distended and tortuous blood vessels (Fig. 14.82).

Retinal detachments

Retinal detachment shows certain similarities to retinal haemorrhages and not infrequently accompanies retinal haemorrhages. Retinal detachment is more correctly a retinal separation, or retinoschisis, occurring between the retinal pigment epithelium (RPE) and the sensory or neuroretina (see development of the retina in the introductory paragraph). The loss of integrity between the RPE and the neuroretina leads to loss of function and secondary retinal degeneration and, obviously depending upon the size or extent of the detachment, to total or partial loss of vision.

Retinal detachment may be exudative, or serous, with fluid occupying the subretinal space. Removal of this fluid allows the retina to fall back into place with a return of vision if it occurs before secondary degeneration. Retinal detachment may also occur due to traction from forces in the vitreous, or may be associated with a tear, when it is known as a rhegmatogenous detachment. Total retinal detachment, with dialysis or disinsertion at the ora ciliaris retinae, allows the retina to hang down in folds obscuring the optic disc, it remaining attached around the optic nerve head.

Trauma, as with haemorrhage, is a cause of retinal detachment and hypertension is another important aetiology (see Figs 14.72, 14.74, 14.75 and 14.77–14.79). Idiopathic detachments also occur and retinal detachment following intraocular surgery is an unfortunate occasional sequel. Retinal detachment as part of the CEA may be congenital or occur later in life, in which case usually during the first few months (see Figs 14.31–14.33). Retinal detachment also occurs with hereditary retinal dysplasia of the total form in the Labrador, Sealyham and Bedlington Terrier and sometimes in the English Springer Spaniel (see Figs 14.35–14.37), as well as in the geographic form of multifocal retinal dysplasia in several breeds (see Figs 14.38, 14.45, 14.48 and 14.52). Another cause of retinal detachment is pressure on the globe, which may be a retrobulbar tumour (Fig. 14.83) or fluid due to abscess or infection (see Fig. 4.26), in either case usually accompanied by exophthalmos.

The optic disc

See also Chapter 15 Neuro-ophthalmology.

Optic nerve hypoplasia

Optic nerve hypoplasia (Fig. 14.84) is a congenital and hereditary condition in Miniature and Toy Poodles and isolated cases occur in many other breeds. It may be unilateral

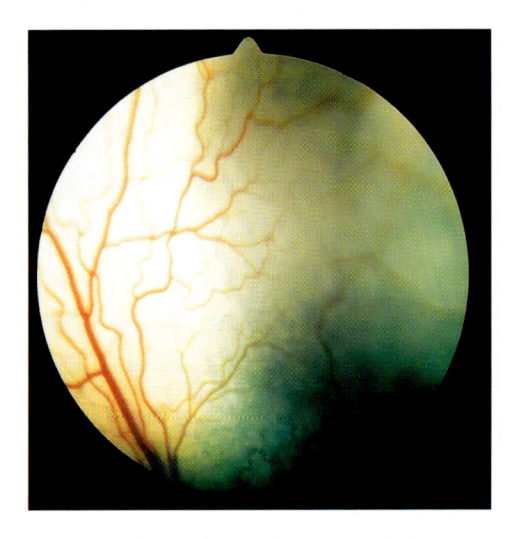

Fig. 14.83 Retinal detachment due to retrobulbar pressure caused by an optic nerve glioma in an 8-year-old Labrador.

THE OPTIC DISC

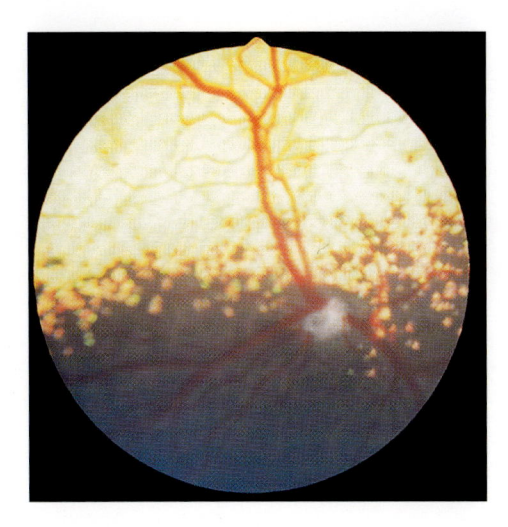

Fig. 14.84 Optic nerve hypoplasia in a 10-month-old Miniature Poodle.

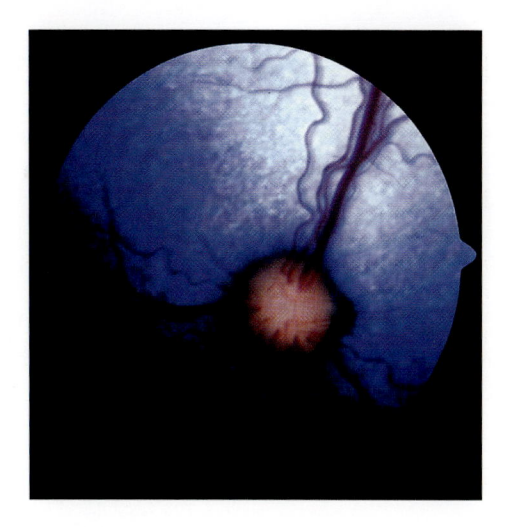

Fig. 14.86 Colobomatous cupping of the optic disc in a Basset Griffon Vendeen.

or bilateral and in the latter case the dog is blind. This hypoplasia is accompanied by a dilated pupil with no pupillary light reflex, the disc appearing very small, grey-white and with no myelinated fibres on the surrounding fundus; the retinal blood vessels appear particularly large in comparison with the disc but the rest of the fundus appears normal.

Micropapilla (see Fig. 14.14), a small but functional optic disc, also occurs in the dog and in some cases it may be difficult to distinguish between micropapilla and true optic nerve hypoplasia by ophthalmoscopy. However, the absence of vision and the pupillary light reflex, not always obvious in unilateral cases, should distinguish the two conditions.

Optic disc coloboma

Coloboma of the optic disc (Figs 14.85 and 14.86 and see Figs 14.25–14.29) is another congenital, and sometimes inherited, anomaly of the optic disc. Coloboma as part of CEA (see previous section) may or may not enlarge the size of the optic disc, varying in size and depth and in its effect on vision. It may be unilateral or bilateral and can occasionally appear in the collie breeds without ophthalmoscopic evidence of chorioretinal dysplasia.

Coloboma of the optic disc has also been described in the Basenji, together with colobomatous cupping of the optic disc, in association with persistent pupillary membranes, an inherited ocular abnormality in this breed. A similar situation has been seen in the Basset Griffon Vendeen.

Isolated cases of optic disc coloboma also occur, both typical and atypical in position.

Papilloedema

Papilloedema (Fig. 14.87) is swelling of the optic papilla without inflammation and associated with an increased intracranial pressure. Papilloedema is usually bilateral but rare unilateral cases do occur. Papilloedema is not a cause of blindness but, if the cause is not relieved, papilloedema will result in optic atrophy which is associated with blindness,

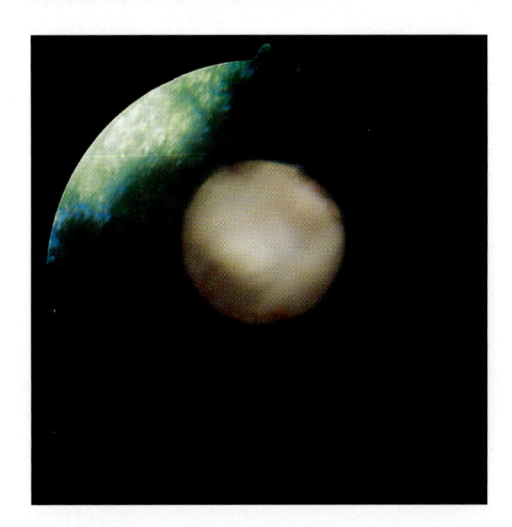

Fig. 14.85 Coloboma of the optic disc in a Basenji.

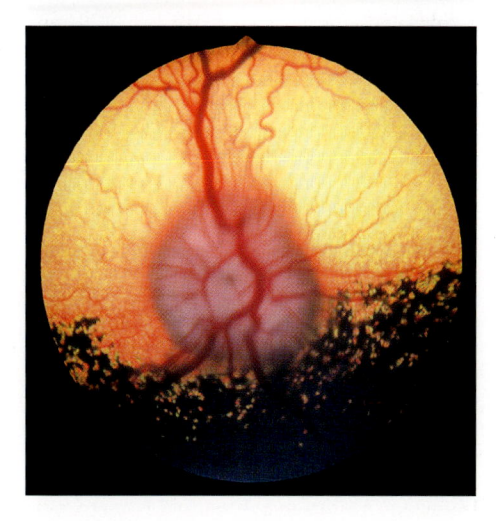

Fig. 14.87 Papilloedema in a 2½-year-old Golden Retriever. Frontal tumour was diagnosed by MRI.

FUNDUS

dilated pupils and absence of pupillary light reflex. In the dog, papilloedema is associated with brain tumours.

Diagnosis of papilloedema by ophthalmoscopy can be difficult, mainly due to the common medulation of optic nerve fibres present in the dog that give the disc a swollen appearance particularly in certain breeds (see Fig. 14.17). The disc with papilloedema is swollen and therefore enlarged in size, pinker in colour due to the venous congestion, the edge is indistinct and sometimes the smaller blood vessels can be seen dipping over the edge of the swollen disc onto the surrounding fundus. Small haemorrhages on or around the edge of the disc may be present.

OPTIC NEURITIS (PAPILLITIS)

Optic neuritis (Fig. 14.88) is inflammation of the optic nerve and may be retrobulbar, in which case ophthalmoscopic signs are not present. The condition is usually acute with sudden loss of vision (cf. papilloedema) and may be unilateral or bilateral. Most cases are idiopathic although there are some known causes in the dog. The pupils are fixed and dilated and the optic disc appears swollen, pink and with an indistinct edge. Frequently inflammatory exudate and oedema of the adjacent peripapillary retina and haemorrhages are present in this area. Blindness accompanies optic neuritis but the electroretinogram is not affected. Treatment with systemic corticosteroids can lead to the return of vision but recurrence is likely.

OPTIC ATROPHY

Atrophy of the optic nerve (optic disc) (Fig. 14.89) may follow trauma to the optic nerve, and in particular is apparent ophthalmoscopically several weeks or months following prolapse of the globe in spite of successful replacement and with no outward signs of other injury. Optic atrophy is the end stage of papilloedema and optic neuritis and also generalised progressive retinal atrophy, cases of chorioretinitis involving the disc (see Fig. 14.69) and both primary and secondary glaucoma.

Ophthalmoscopically the disc appears flat, grey and structureless, sometimes with an indented border. The pupil is dilated and there is loss of the pupillary light reflex. Optic atrophy may be unilateral or bilateral depending upon the primary cause.

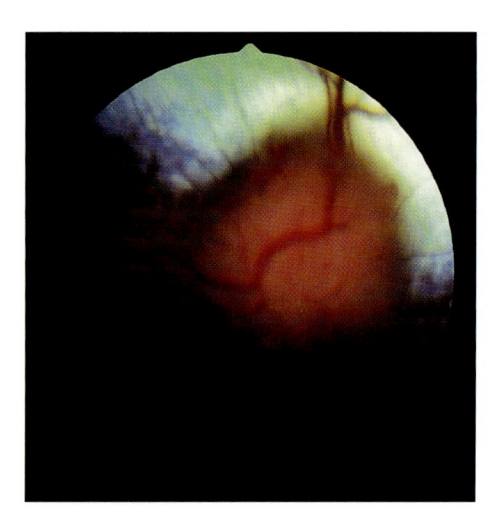

Fig. 14.88 Optic neuritis in a 4-year-old Border Collie with granulomatous meningoencephalitis. Note the small haemorrhages at 2 and 7 o'clock.

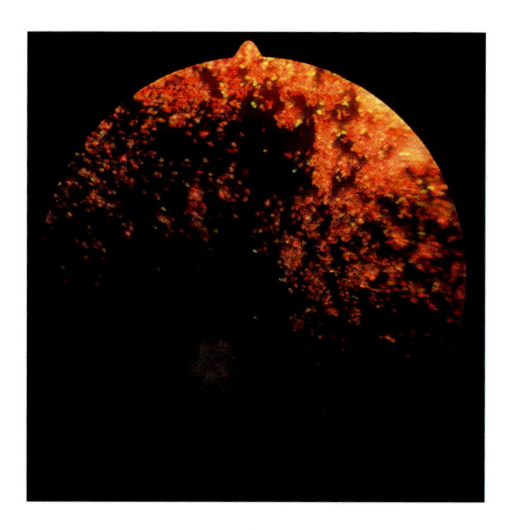

Fig. 14.89 Optic nerve atrophy several months after an apparently successful replacement of a prolapsed globe in an 18-month-old Lhasa Apso.

SUDDEN ACQUIRED RETINAL DEGENERATION

The cause of this unusual retinopathy is unknown and it is not rare in the United Kingdom. There is a sudden, possibly over a few days, loss of vision accompanied by dilated pupils and absent pupillary light reflexes. Ophthalmoscopic examination reveals no abnormality but the electroretinogram is flat. Weeks to months later ophthalmoscopic examination reveals typical signs of a bilaterally symmetrical retinal degeneration with hyper-reflectivity of the tapetal fundus and attenuation of the retinal blood vessels (Fig. 14.90). Adult dogs usually in middle-age are affected; there is no breed susceptibility and the condition occurs in crossbreds as well as pedigree dogs. The bilaterally symmetrical retinal degeneration is very similar ophthalmoscopically to generalised progressive retinal atrophy but the sudden onset, initially with no ophthalmoscopic changes, in adult dogs of any and mixed breeding should distinguish the two conditions.

NEOPLASIA OF THE FUNDUS

Primary tumours affecting all parts of the fundus are very rare in this species. Recorded are medulloepithelioma and choroidal melanoma. A retrobulbar meningioma of the optic nerve was suspected ophthalmoscopically and confirmed following enucleation. The most common secondary tumour is the malignant lymphoma.

REFERENCES

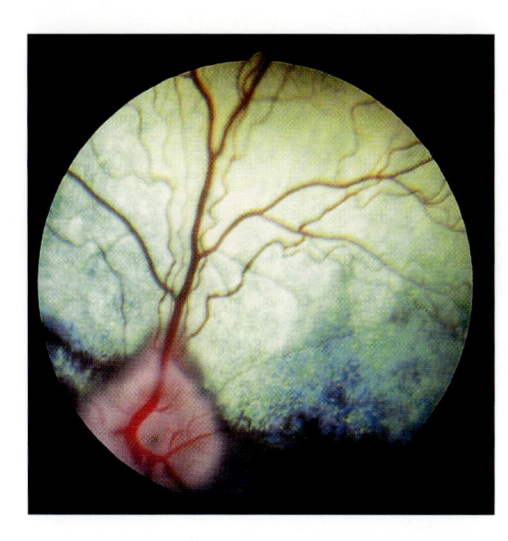

Fig. 14.90 Sudden acquired retinal degeneration in a 10-year-old West Highland White Terrier. Note early tapetal hyperreflectivity and narrowing of retinal blood vessels. This dog had been blind for a few weeks and Cushing's disease had also been diagnosed.

References

Acland GM, Blanton SH, Hershfield B, Aguirre G (1994) XLPRA: a canine retinal degeneration inherited as an x-linked trait. *American Journal of Medical Genetics* **52**: 27–33.

Ashton N, Barnett KC, Sachs DD (1968) Retinal dysplasia in the Sealyham Terrier. *Journal of Pathology and Bacteriology* **96**: 269–272.

Barnett KC, Stades FC (1979) Collie Eye Anomaly in the Shetland Sheepdog in the Netherlands. *Journal of Small Animal Practice* **20**: 321–329.

Barnett KC, Bjorck GR, Kock E (1970) Hereditary retinal dysplasia in the Labrador Retriever in England and Sweden. *Journal of Small Animal Practice* **10**: 755–759.

Bedford PGC (1984) Retinal pigment epithelial dystrophy (CPRA): A study of the disease in the Briard. *Journal of Small Animal Practice* **25**: 129–138.

Bedford PGC (1998) Collie Eye Anomaly in the Lancashire Heeler. *Veterinary Record* **143**: 354–356.

Bovee KC, Littman MP, Crabtree BJ, Aguirre G (1989) Essential hypertension in a dog. *Journal of the American Veterinary Medical Association* **195**: 81–86.

Carrig CB, MacMillan A, Brundage S, Pool RR, Morgan JP (1977) Retinal dysplasia associated with skeletal abnormalities in the Labrador Retriever. *Journal of the American Veterinary Medical Association* **170**: 49–57.

Carrig CB, Sponenberg DP, Schmidt GM, Tvedten HW (1988) Inheritance of associated ocular and skeletal dysplasia in Labrador Retrievers. *Journal of the American Veterinary Medical Association* **193**: 1269–1272.

Crispin SM, Long SE, Wheeler CA (1999) Incidence and ocular manifestations of multifocal retinal dysplasia in the golden retriever in the UK. *Veterinary Record* **145**: 669–672.

Holle DM, Stankovics ME, Sarna CS, Aguirre GD (1999) The geographic form of retinal dysplasia in dogs is not always a congenital abnormality. *Veterinary Ophthalmology* **2**: 61–66.

Keyes JEL, Goldblatt H (1937) *Archives of Ophthalmology* **17**: 1040.

Lavach TD, Murphy JM, Severin GA (1978) Retinal dysplasia in the English Springer Spaniel. *Journal of the American Animal Hospital Association* **14**: 192–199.

Lewis DG, Kelly DF, Sansom J (1986) Congenital microphthalmia and other developmental ocular anomalies in the Dobermann. *Journal of Small Animal Practice* **27**: 559–566.

Long SE, Crispin SM (1999) Inheritance of multifocal retinal dysplasia in the golden retriever in the UK. *Veterinary Record* **145**: 702–704.

MacMillan AD, Lipton DE (1978) Heritability of multifocal retinal dysplasia in American Cocker Spaniels. *Journal of the American Veterinary Medical Association* **172**: 568–572.

Magnusson H (1911) Über retinitis pigmentosa und konsanquinität beim Lunde. *Archiv für vergleichende Ophtalmologie* **2**: 147–163.

Magrane WG (1953) Congenital anomaly of the optic disc in collies. *North American Veterinarian* **34**: 646.

Meyers VNB, Jezyk PF, Aguirre GD, Patterson DF (1983) Short-limbed dwarfism and ocular defects in the Samoyed dog. *Journal of the American Veterinary Medical Association* **183**: 975–979.

Narfström K, Wrigstad A, Nilsson SEG (1989) The Briard dog: A new animal model of congenital stationary night blindness. *British Journal of Ophthalmology* **73**: 750–756.

Nelson DL, MacMillan AD (1983) Multifocal retinal dysplasia in field trial Labrador Retrievers. *Journal of the American Animal Hospital Association* **19**: 388–392.

O'Toole DO, Young S, Severin GA, Neumann S (1983) Retinal dysplasia of English Springer Spaniel dogs: Light microscopy of the postnatal lesions. *Veterinary Pathology* **20**: 298–311.

Parry HB (1954a) Degenerations of the dog retina VI. Central progressive retinal atrophy with pigment epithelial dystrophy. *British Journal of Ophthalmology* **38**: 653–688.

Parry HB (1954b) Degenerations of the dog retina IV. Retinopathies associated with dog distemper – complex virus infections. *British Journal of Ophthalmology* **38**: 295–309.

Riis R, Sheffy BE, Loe WE, Kern TJ, Smith JS (1981) Vitamin E deficiency retinopathy in dogs. *American Journal of Veterinary Research* **42**: 74–86.

Rubin LF (1963) Hereditary retinal detachment in Bedlington terriers. A preliminary report. *Small Animal Clinics* **3**: 387.

Rubin LF (1968) Heredity of retinal dysplasia in Bedlington terriers. *Journal of the American Veterinary Medical Association* **152**: 260.

Rubin LF (1974) *Atlas of Veterinary Ophthalmoscopy* p. 90 Lea & Febiger, Philadelphia.

Sansom J, Bodey A (1997) Ocular signs in four dogs with hypertension. *Veterinary Record* **140**: 593–598.

Schmidt GM, Ellersieck MR, Wheeler CA, Blanchard GL, Keller WF (1979) Inheritance of retinal dysplasia in the English Springer Spaniel. *Journal of the American Veterinary Medical Association* **174**: 1089–1090.

Stades FC (1978) Hereditary retinal dysplasia (RD) in a family of Yorkshire Terriers. *Tijdschrift voor Diergeneeskunde* **103**: 1087–1090.

Wallin-Håkanson B, Wallin-Håkanson N, Hedhammar Å (2000) Influence of selective breeding on the prevalence of chorioretinal dysplasia and coloboma in the rough collie in Sweden. *Journal of Small Animal Practice* **41**: 56–59.

Yakely WL (1972) Collie eye anomaly: Decreased prevalence through selective breeding. *Journal of the American Veterinary Medical Association* **161**: 1103–1107.

Yakely WL, Wyman M, Donovan EF, Fechkeimer NS (1968) Genetic transmission of an ocular fundus anomaly in Collies. *Journal of the American Veterinary Medical Association* **152**: 457–461.

15 Neuro-ophthalmology

Introduction

The neuro-ophthalmological examination is an important component of the general ophthalmic and neurological examination of the dog. Unique to the visual system the retina and optic disc are the only components of the nervous system directly visible in the patient. Understanding the visual pathways allows an accurate neurological localisation to be made that will greatly aid in deciding on further investigation and determining the prognosis.

Neuro-ophthalmological assessment of the canine patient

When performing the neuro-ophthalmological examination it is important first to observe the patient from a distance, the so-called 'hands-off' examination, before starting a more detailed examination. It is particularly important to ascertain the dog's interaction with the surrounding environment, to assess the dog's level of consciousness and to observe for the presence of any localising neurological signs such as circling or head tilt. A decreased level of consciousness, perceived as an altered awareness of the surrounding environment, may result in alteration of the patient's response to testing requiring conscious input, which may be erroneously interpreted as indicating a lesion within the tested pathways.

Vision

Cranial nerve (CN) II (Optic)

The optic nerve supplies sensory information for vision and the pupillary light reflex. The central visual pathways are shown in Fig. 15.1. Vision may be assessed by observing the animal moving around unfamiliar surroundings, negotiating an obstacle course and even following moving objects such as a dropped piece of cotton wool (tracking response).

The 'hands-on' tests used to assess vision include:

- The menace response: a threatening movement is made at each eye in turn (Fig. 15.2). The dog should respond by blinking or blink with aversion of the head. The visual pathways supply afferent information and the efferent response is mediated by the facial nerve. The menace response is a learned response and as such is usually absent in puppies less than 8 to 12 weeks of age. As the menace response is coordinated in the cerebellum (Fig. 15.3) it may

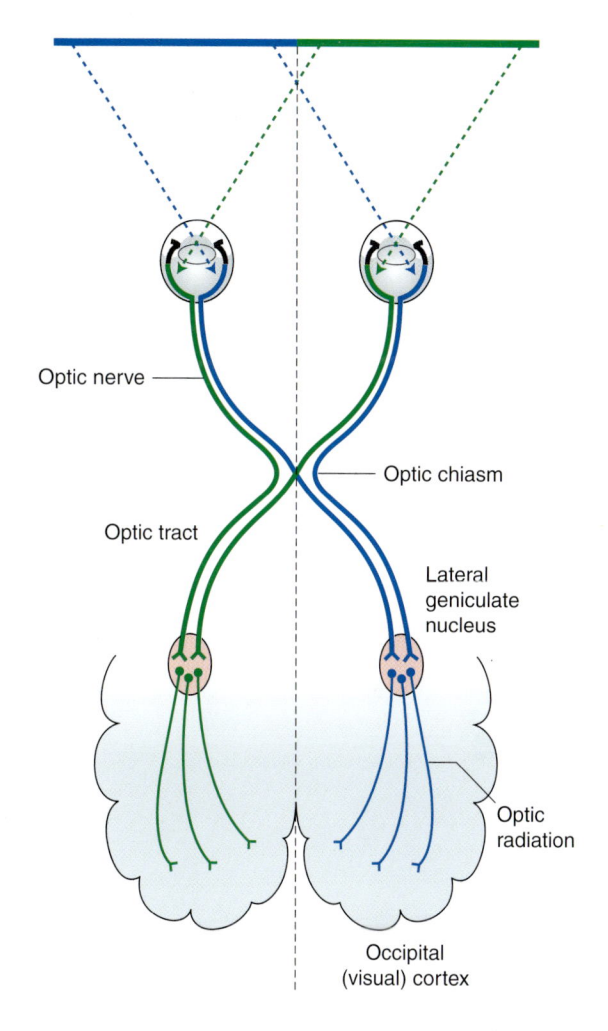

Fig. 15.1 The visual pathway and representation of the visual field within the occipital (visual) cortex of the cerebral hemispheres.

  also be absent in the presence of a diffuse cerebellar lesion and not just with a lesion affecting the visual pathways or facial nerve (Fig. 15.4) (De Lahunta, 1983).
- The pupillary light reflex.
- Visual placing response: this test combines visual sensory information with postural control of the forelimbs. The patient is supported under the thorax and the forelimbs are brought up to the table surface. The normal dog should attempt to place the forepaws on the table surface before the carpi touch the table edge (Fig. 15.5).

NEURO-OPHTHALMOLOGY

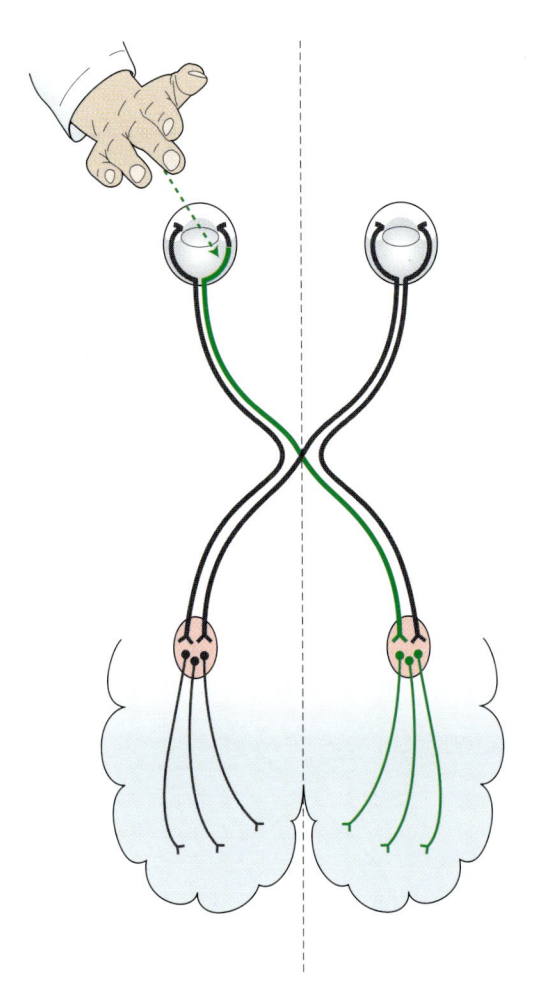

Fig. 15.2 When evaluating the menace response the visual stimulus originates in the nasal retinal field and therefore only assess the contralateral cerebral cortex.

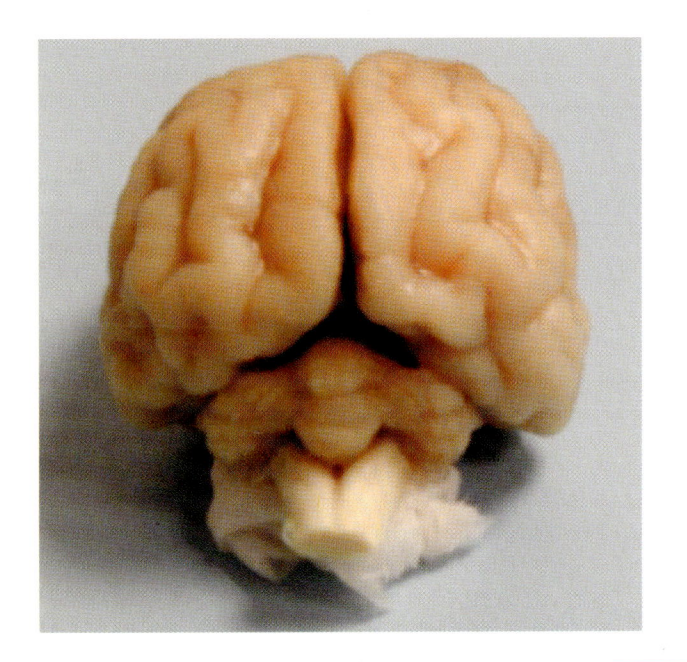

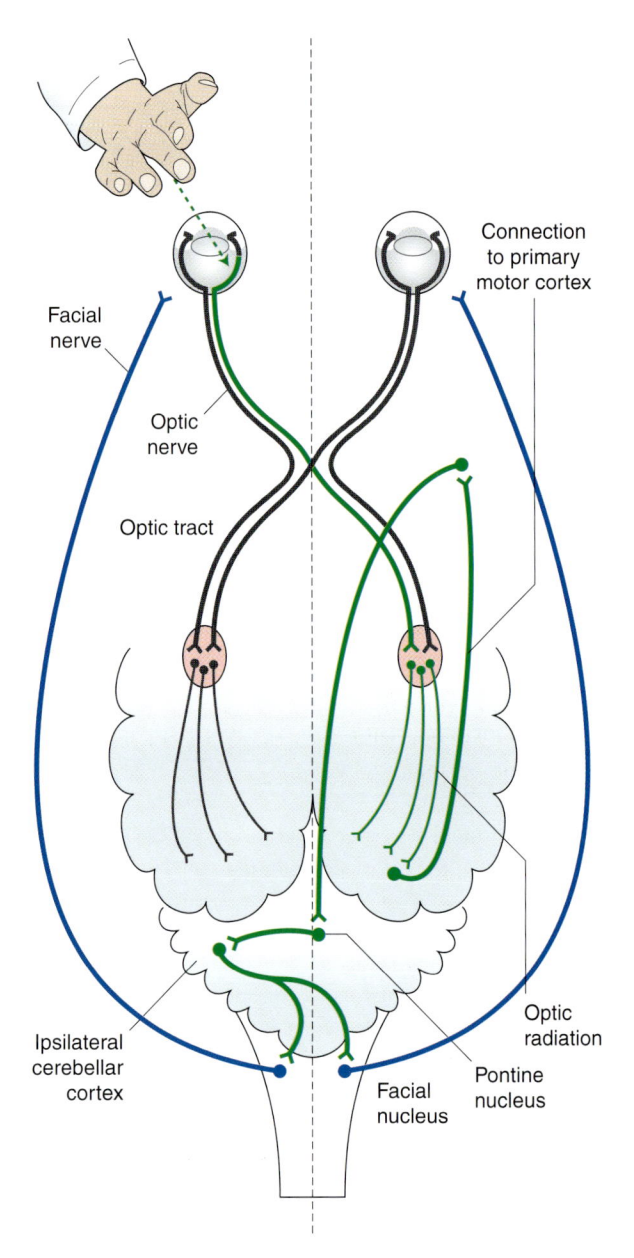

Fig. 15.3 Schematic representation of the menace pathway. The presence of a menace deficit can result from a lesion affecting any portion of the menace pathway.

Fig. 15.4 Cerebellar hypoplasia in a Dalmatian. The menace response is often absent in diffuse cerebellar lesions in the presence of normal vision and facial nerve function.

NEURO-OPHTHALMOLOGICAL ASSESSMENT

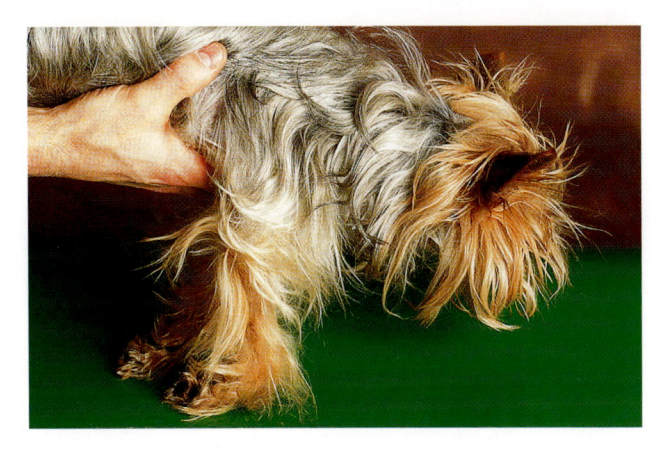

Fig. 15.5 Performing the visual placing response combines visual function and postural control of the thoracic limbs.

PUPILLARY LIGHT REFLEX

CN II (Optic) and parasympathetic portion of CN III (Oculomotor)

The pupillary light reflex (PLR) assesses the visual pathways prior to the lateral geniculate nucleus as well as the parasympathetic oculomotor nerve innervation to the pupillary constrictors (Fig. 15.6). The test is performed by shining a bright light into the eye and observing the pupil for constriction. In addition to the direct response, the contralateral pupil should also constrict (consensual response). If a direct response is present in *both* eyes then a consensual response will invariably be present and it is not necessary to observe for one.

The degree of pupillary constriction is determined by both the brightness of the light and the resting sympathetic tone. A frequent cause of apparent failure of the test is using a light that is not bright enough and testing in animals that are very afraid with high levels of sympathetic tone.

EXTRAOCULAR MUSCULAR CONTROL OF EYEBALL MOVEMENT

CN III (oculomotor), CN IV (trochlear) and CN VI (abducens)

In addition to the parasympathetic portion of CN III (iris and ciliary muscle), the oculomotor nerve supplies motor innervation to the extraocular muscles (dorsal, medial and ventral rectus muscles and the ventral oblique muscle of the eyeball) as well as to the levator palpebra muscle of the upper eyelid. The trochlear nerve innervates the dorsal oblique muscle, while the abducens nerve innervates the lateral rectus and retractor bulbi muscles.

Although these three cranial nerves can be assessed individually, this is less important as CN III is usually affected in isolation or all three nerves are affected together. Assessing eyeball movement is achieved by observing the eyes as the dog looks around voluntarily and in response to induced movements (tracking response). The eyes are assessed for the presence of any asymmetry of gaze direction (strabismus). Retraction of the globe (abducens nerve) is assessed during the corneal reflex.

The normal eye movements can further be evaluated by inducing normal vestibular eye movements (vestibulo-ocular reflex or physiological nystagmus). The head is moved from side to side or up and down at a steady rate and in the normal animal this induces nystagmus with the fast phase in the direction of the head movement. These normal vestibular eye movements are independent of vision and are normally still present in animals with acquired visual loss. The absence of normal vestibular eye movements indicates a vestibular lesion or a lesion affecting the extraocular muscles or their innervation.

VESTIBULAR CONTROL OF EYEBALL MOVEMENT

CN VIII (vestibulocochlear)

The vestibular system controls eyeball position in relation to alterations in head position. The normal vestibular function allows the dog to maintain the gaze fixed on an object while the head is moved. When the head is moved without the gaze being fixed on a particular object then the vestibular input allows the gaze to jump from object to object and follow that as the visual field moves past, instead of the visual input

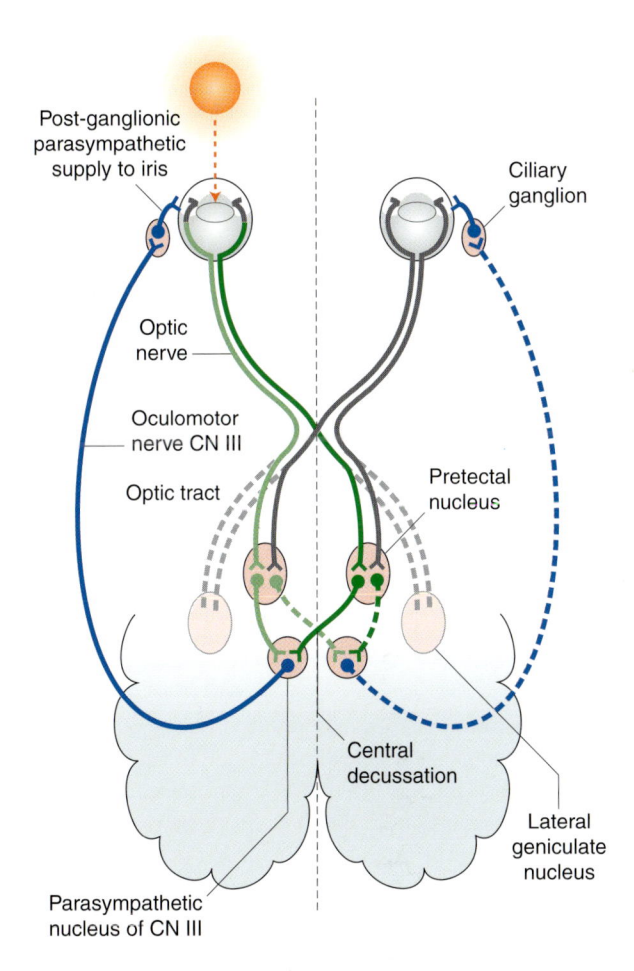

Fig. 15.6 The pupillary light reflex pathway.

recording a constant blur of passing information. An example of that is the induced physiological nystagmus or vestibulo-ocular reflex.

In contrast to normal physiological nystagmus, lesions affecting vestibular input may result in involuntary abnormal eye movements, including nystagmus and strabismus. Strabismus is a static alteration in gaze direction (squint). Nystagmus is the involuntary rhythmic movement of the eyes and may present as jerk nystagmus or pendular nystagmus. Pendular nystagmus is the constant oscillation of the eye in a single plane (ocular tremor) and is more likely due to cerebellar disorders and long-standing or congenital visual deficits. Jerk nystagmus has a slow phase in one direction (usually towards the lesion) and a rapid phase in the opposite direction and may be horizontal, vertical or rotatory. In some patients, nystagmus may only be induced by alterations in body position (for example placing the dog on its back), termed positional nystagmus (De Lahunta, 1983).

Evaluating for a strabismus or involuntary nystagmus assesses the normal vestibular control of eyeball position. This should include altering the dog's position (rolling the dog on its back), and lifting the head and holding it elevated in a horizontal plane to see if a strabismus can be induced. Other features of vestibular disease may be present and, because of the close approximation of the vestibular system to other cranial nerves, there may be concurrent ipsilateral hearing deficits, facial nerve paresis, Horner's syndrome and trigeminal nerve lesions. At the level of the vestibular nuclei in the brainstem, the ascending and descending brainstem tracts and the cerebellum may be affected.

SOMATO-SENSORY INNERVATION OF THE EYE AND EYELID

CN V (Trigeminal)

As the name suggests, the trigeminal nerve consists of three branches that originate together. The trigeminal nerve is responsible for sensory information from the entire face as well as providing motor control of the masticatory muscles. The ophthalmic branch carries sensory information from the cornea, medial canthus of the eye and the nasal mucosa. The mandibular branch carries sensory information from the mandible and lower lips and provides motor innervation to the masticatory muscles. The maxillary branch innervates the remainder of the face, including the lateral canthus of the eye.

The trigeminal innervation to the eye is tested by touching the medial canthus of the eye and observing for the presence of a blink – the palpebral reflex. The lateral canthus can also be stimulated but the response is more unreliable. The motor portion of the palpebral reflex is innervated by the facial nerve. Corneal sensation is evaluated by performing the corneal reflex, where the eyelids are held open and the cornea is lightly touched with a finger or cotton swab – if normal sensation is present the dog will retract the globe and prolapse the third eyelid.

MOTOR CONTROL OF THE EYELIDS AND LACRIMAL GLAND FUNCTION

CN VII (facial)

The facial nerve is a mixed nerve supplying, among other things, motor innervation to the muscles of facial expression, including the upper and lower eyelids, and parasympathetic innervation to the lacrimal gland.

The facial nerve control of eyelid movement is assessed by a combination of:

- observing the animal for normal blinking;
- the menace response; and
- the palpebral reflex.

The menace response consists of visual sensory input and facial nerve motor output (see Fig. 15.3). The palpebral reflex is performed by touching the medial canthus of the eye with a finger or haemostat and observing for a blink. The afferent supply for the palpebral reflex is mediated via the ophthalmic branch of the trigeminal nerve and the efferent supply through the facial nerve.

SYMPATHETIC INNERVATION OF THE EYE

The sympathetic innervation to the head and eye (Fig. 15.7) originates in the hypothalamus and rostral midbrain. From here the first order sympathetic supply travels down the spinal cord in the tectotegmental spinal tract to synapse with the second order neurones in the lateral horn of the spinal cord grey matter. The second order axons exit the spinal cord with the T1 to T3 nerve roots (the brachial plexus innervating the thoracic limb comprises nerve roots C6 to T1 and therefore part of the sympathetic supply leaving the spinal cord is closely associated with the thoracic limb innervation). These sympathetic axons leave the nerve roots as the ramus communicans to form the thoracic sympathetic trunk. The sympathetic trunk passes cranial and adjacent to the descending vagus nerve, to form the vagosympathetic trunk within the carotid sheath. The axons pass rostrally through the caudal cervical ganglion to synapse in the cranial cervical ganglion, adjacent to the tympanic bulla. The third order sympathetic axons pass into the cranial cavity in close approximation to the trigeminal nerve, before again leaving the cranial cavity to innervate the eye and adjacent structures.

POSTURAL REACTIONS

Lesions within the central nervous system (CNS) resulting in ophthalmic abnormalities may result in additional neurological abnormalities that allow localisation of these lesions to the CNS. Determining whether a lesion is localised within the CNS is important in deciding on further investigation and determining the prognosis.

The postural reactions are a useful screening test to ascertain whether there is CNS involvement as they allow evaluation of large portions of the CNS and are relatively sensitive. Postural deficits are, however, of only limited value

CLINICAL NEURO-OPHTHALMOLOGY

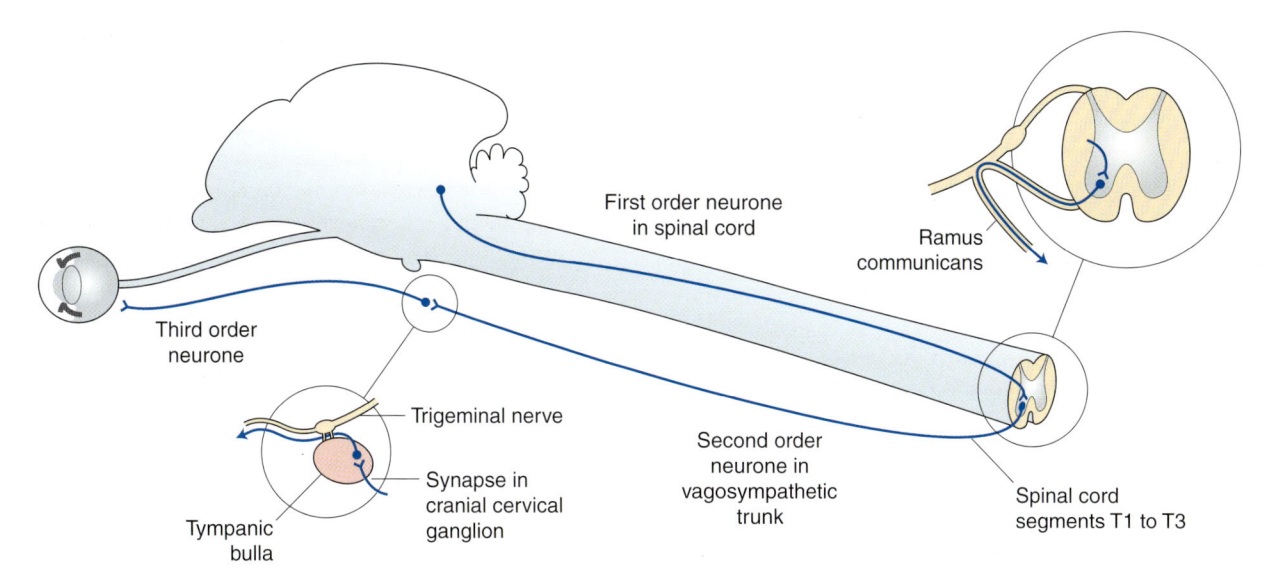

Fig. 15.7 Schematic representation of the sympathetic innervation to the eye and adjacent structures.

in accurately localising the lesion; for that a more detailed neurological examination is required. The postural reactions that are most frequently performed can roughly be divided into those that primarily assess the motor system and those that primarily assess the sensory system.

The first motor abnormality to become apparent is weakness; tests evaluating for this include:

- Hopping test: this allows each leg to be evaluated individually for weakness.
- Wheelbarrow and extensor postural thrust: compares the thoracic limbs to the pelvic limbs.
- Hemistand and hemiwalk: in lesions affecting the CNS asymmetrically this test compares one side of the body to the other.

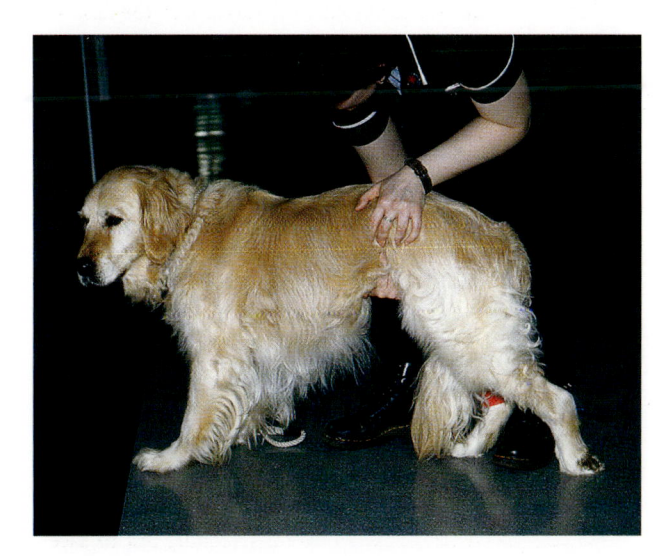

Fig. 15.8 Postural deficits, as in the demonstration of conscious proprioceptive deficits in the case with a cavernous sinus tumour, are a sensitive indicator of CNS involvement.

The first sensory deficit usually apparent is the presence of proprioceptive deficits.

- Conscious proprioceptive testing (paw-placing reflex): as the name states, the eventual endpoint of the pathway evaluated in this test is the cerebral cortex. Cerebellar lesions will not result in conscious proprioceptive deficits. The dog's weight is supported and the paw is turned over so that the dorsum rests against the ground (Fig. 15.8). The normal dog will quickly correct the paw.
- Reflex step testing: evaluates a combination of conscious and unconscious pathways. The test is performed by placing a piece of paper under the dog's paw and while supporting the dog's weight, gently trying to pull the paper laterally. The normal dog will quickly replace the paw.

CLINICAL NEURO-OPHTHALMOLOGY

DECREASED VISION WITH PLR DEFICITS

Optic disc abnormalities

Clinical signs unilateral lesions will usually result in decreased to absent vision in the affected eye (less likely with papilloedema) and decreased to absent direct and consensual PLR on stimulating the affected eye. The direct and consensual PLR should be intact on stimulating the normal eye.

Aetiology

- Sudden acquired retinal degeneration (SARD): this irreversible acute retinal degeneration presents with no ophthalmoscopic changes in the initial stages, although in the chronic stages retinal degeneration does become apparent. An electroretinogram (demonstrating abolition of the recording in SARD) is required to differentiate SARD from other causes of acute-onset blindness.

- Optic nerve hypoplasia: this may be unilateral or bilateral, is apparent on ophthalmoscopic examination and may result in decreased to absent vision. The decrease in the PLR is proportional to the decrease in vision, and extreme cases present as bilaterally blind with bilaterally dilated and unresponsive pupils. The optic discs appear small and grey in colour on examination (Peterson-Jones, 1995). This condition is seen sporadically in most breeds but has been suggested to be inherited in the Miniature Poodle (Kern and Riis, 1981).
- Optic disc atrophy: damage to the retinal ganglion cells or axonal processes between the retinal ganglion cells and the optic disc will result in Wallerian-like degeneration of the axons and surrounding myelin sheath of the optic nerve. The percentage of axons lost will ascertain the degree of atrophy of the optic disc, which is evident in its shrunken and grey appearance. This process is gradual and not immediately apparent at the time of insult and may be identified secondary to a variety of diseases including generalised retinal degeneration, glaucoma and traumatic or inflammatory lesion to the proximal optic nerve.
- Papilloedema: this is oedema of the optic disc resulting from raised intracranial pressure, optic nerve inflammation and tumours of the optic nerve (Fig. 15.9). Papilloedema needs to be differentiated from hypermyelination of the optic disc (pseudo-papilloedema) where myelination extends beyond the periphery of the optic disc as a normal feature, giving the disc margin an irregular and fluffy appearance. Hypermyelination is more evident in certain large breed dogs, including Boxers, German Shepherd Dogs and Golden Retrievers.

The presence of papilloedema (although it is inconsistently present) with evidence of CNS signs, is a reliable indicator of raised intracranial pressure (secondary to neoplasia and inflammatory disorders) and indicates an increased risk of brain herniation (Fig. 15.10). In rare cases papilloedema may occur secondary to widespread myelin oedema, for example in certain metabolic disorders. Papilloedema does not result in visual loss on its own, differentiating it from optic neuritis. However, in practice, intracranial lesions severe enough to cause papilloedema frequently interrupt the visual pathways as well (Palmer et al., 1974).

- Optic neuritis: inflammation of the optic disc is termed optic neuritis or papillitis. Optic neuritis is difficult to distinguish from papilloedema, although it invariably presents with visual loss. The optic disc appears swollen with frequent haemorrhages. The most common reported causes include granulomatous meningoencephalitis (GME) and canine distemper virus, although in many cases no underlying cause is identified. Due to the probable immune-mediated process, in many cases immunosuppressive levels of corticosteroids are often of benefit – either in controlling the underlying disease process or because of their anti-inflammatory effect. In all cases the prognosis is guarded, with relapses being likely in those cases that do respond to treatment (Peterson-Jones, 1995).

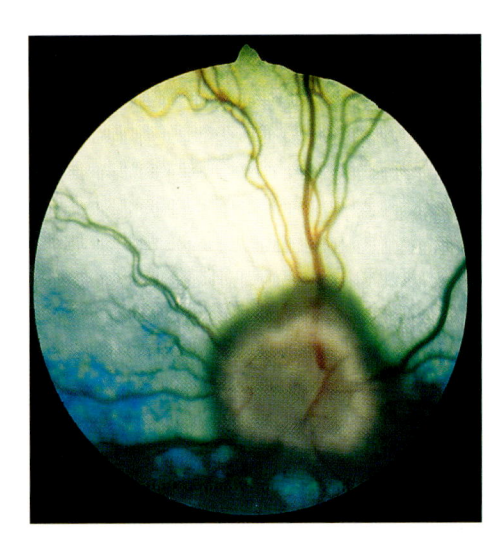

Fig. 15.9 Boxer dog demonstrating an irregular and swollen optic disc margin, the appearance of which is consistent with papilloedema. A large forebrain tumour was confirmed at post-mortem examination. (*Courtesy of J Mould.*)

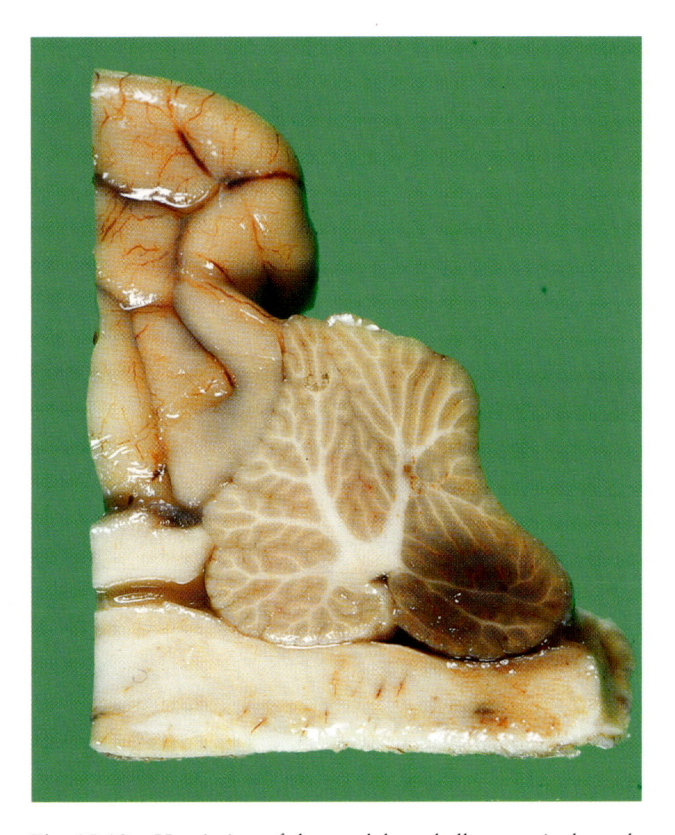

Fig. 15.10 Herniation of the caudal cerebellar vermis through the foramen magnum (secondary to a forebrain tumour with raised intracranial pressure) with resultant haemorrhage and compression of the caudal cerebellar vermis and underlying brainstem.

Optic nerve lesions

Clinical signs unilateral lesions will usually result in decreased vision in the affected eye and decreased direct and consensual PLR on stimulating the affected eye. Both the direct and consensual PLR should be intact on stimulating the normal eye.

Aetiology

- Optic nerve hypoplasia, optic neuritis and papilloedema all affect the optic disc and the optic nerve and are discussed in the preceding section.
- GME as a cause of optic neuritis may be identified on MRI examination, evidenced as a swollen optic nerve.
- Neoplastic lesions may result in primary or secondary compression of the optic nerve.
- Traumatic lesions of the orbit and eye may damage the optic nerve as a result of traction, compression or haemorrhage.
- Optic nerve compression: although hypervitaminosis A is a well-described cause of optic foramen stenosis in the calf (due to excessive bone growth), the disease is rare in companion animals (Spratling *et al.*, 1965).

Optic chiasm lesions

Clinical signs optic chiasm lesion will usually result in decreased vision in both eyes with concurrent bilateral decreased direct and consensual PLR in both eyes.

Aetiology

- Space-occupying lesions (e.g. neoplasia): the most common neoplasias resulting in compression of the optic chiasm are pituitary macroadenomas and meningiomas (Fig. 15.11).
- Vascular occlusions.
- Inflammatory lesions.

Optic tract lesions

Optic tract lesions are those from after the optic chiasm until prior to the lateral geniculate nuclei.

Clinical signs lesions of the optic tract will result in a decreased lateral visual field in the contralateral eye and a decreased medial visual field in the ipsilateral eye. The PLR will be intact in both eyes, but the degree of pupillary constriction may be slightly reduced in the contralateral eye (most evident on the swinging flashlight test).

Aetiology

- Space-occupying masses (tumours, haemorrhage and intra-arachnoid cysts).
- Inflammatory lesions (granulomatous meningoencephalitis, encephalitis and abscesses).
- Vascular occlusions.

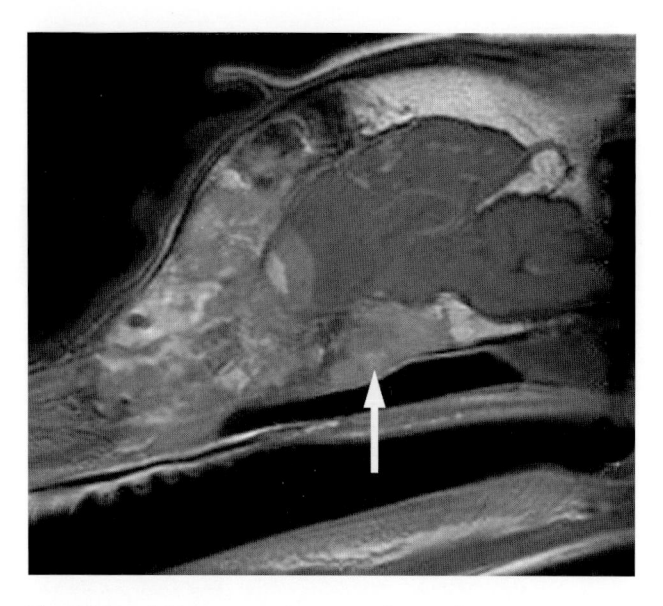

Fig. 15.11 MR image appearance of a nasal tumour extending ventral to the brain and compressing the optic chiasm (arrow). The normal air signal of the nasal cavity has been obliterated by the soft tissue mass.

DECREASED VISION WITH INTACT PLR'S

Decreased vision with intact PLRs is caused by central lesions, from the lateral geniculate nucleus to the visual cortex, affecting the optic radiations or optic cortex.

Clinical signs: unilateral lesions will result in a decreased lateral visual field in the contralateral eye and a decreased medial visual field in the ipsilateral eye.

Aetiology

- Space-occupying lesions (tumours, haemorrhage).
- Inflammatory lesions (encephalitis, granulomatous meningoencephalitis (Fig. 15.12) and abscesses).
- Hydrocephalus: one of the most consistent clinical signs of both acquired and congenital hydrocephalus is the presence of visual deficits. This is due in part to the vulnerability of the optic radiations adjacent to the lateral ventricles.
- Vascular occlusions: cerebral vascular occlusions in the dog are rare and may result in contralateral visual field loss. Cerebral vascular occlusions are usually associated with an acute onset of clinical signs and an ischaemic (or in rare cases haemorrhagic) lesion on advanced imaging.
- Trauma.
- Toxins that result in a cortical blindness are rare, with the most likely being lead poisoning (but other clinical signs are usually apparent including gastrointestinal disturbances) (Oliver *et al.*, 1997).
- Metabolic disorders (e.g. hepatic encephalopathy) may mimic a cerebral lesion, with one of the presenting clinical

NEURO-OPHTHALMOLOGY

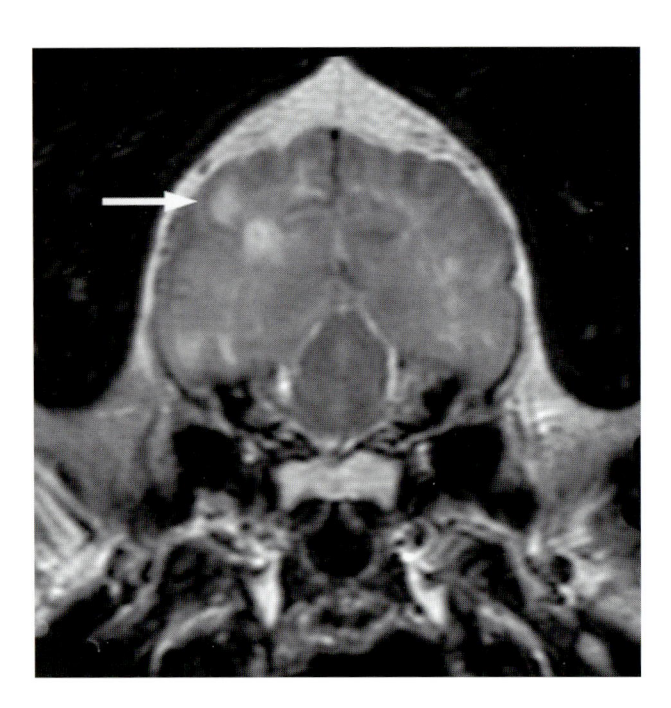

Fig. 15.12 MR image appearance of granulomatous meningoencephalitis demonstrating multifocal contrast-enhancement throughout the forebrain (arrow).

signs being apparent loss of vision with intact pupillary light reflexes.
- Degenerative disorders, particularly the lysosomal storage diseases, may have central visual disturbances as a component of their clinical presentation. Visual disturbances have been described in the gangliosidoses and in sphingomyelinosis.

DISORDERS OF PUPIL SIZE AND FUNCTION

Pharmacological evaluation of lesions affecting the PLR

Following the identification of a lesion affecting the pupillary light reflex pathway, pharmacological testing may assist in further localising the lesion (Peterson-Jones, 1995).

- Topical administration of a direct-acting parasympathomimetic (pilocarpine 1% drops) can be used to differentiate between upper motor neurone lesions (lesions situated between the pretectal nucleus and the parasympathetic nucleus of CN III) and lower motor neurone lesions (from the parasympathetic nucleus of CN III to the iris). Lower motor neurones are characterised by denervation hypersensitivity, with the iris constricting more rapidly than normal.
- Topical administration of an indirect-acting parasympathomimetic (0.5% physostigmine drops) allows differentiation between a pre- and post-ganglionic lesion (ciliary ganglion). Due to denervation hypersensitivity a pre-ganglionic lesion results in rapid pupillary constriction (the normal eye constricts in 40 to 60 minutes). The physostigmine has no effect on post-ganglionic lesions.

Pharmacological miosis and mydriasis

Although apparently obvious, but frequently overlooked, pharmacological agents accidentally or purposefully instilled into the eyes can have a profound effect on pupillary function. The most common example is the pupillary dilation observed following administration of mydriatic (e.g. tropicamide) and cycloplegic (e.g. atropine) drugs and the pupillary constriction following administration of miotic drugs (e.g. pilocarpine).

Resting anisocoria (idiopathic anisocoria)

A number of animals have a subtle resting anisocoria as a normal feature and it is of no clinical significance.

Horner's syndrome

Lesions affecting the sympathetic supply to the eye result in Horner's syndrome (Figs 15.13 and 15.14). The clinical signs of Horner's syndrome are:

- Miosis: the pupil on the affected side appears smaller than the contralateral normal pupil. In lesions affecting the brachial plexus (brachial plexus avulsions, tumours and neuritis), this is frequently the only component of Horner's syndrome that is present as only the T1 nerve root of the T1–T3 sympathetic outflow is usually affected.
- Enophthalmos: due to the loss of tone of the orbital smooth muscle the eyeball sinks back into the orbit. Enophthalmos may also be apparent in cases with severe neurogenic masticatory muscle atrophy secondary to a trigeminal nerve lesion.
- Protrusion of the third eyelid (nictitating membrane): in the dog this occurs passively secondary to the enophthalmos.
- Ptosis of the upper eyelid (drooping) and decreased tone of the lower eyelid secondary to the loss of smooth muscle tone affecting the Muller's muscle.

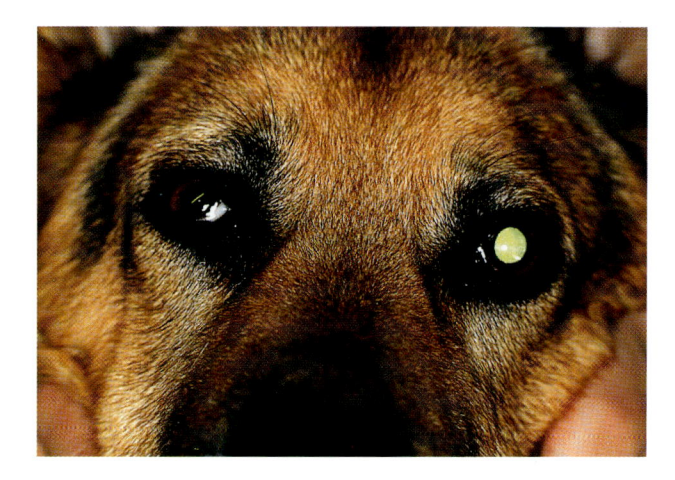

Fig. 15.13 Right Horner's syndrome in a crossbred dog demonstrating miosis, ptosis and protrusion of the third eyelid. Enophthalmos was also present in this case although this cannot be appreciated from the illustration.

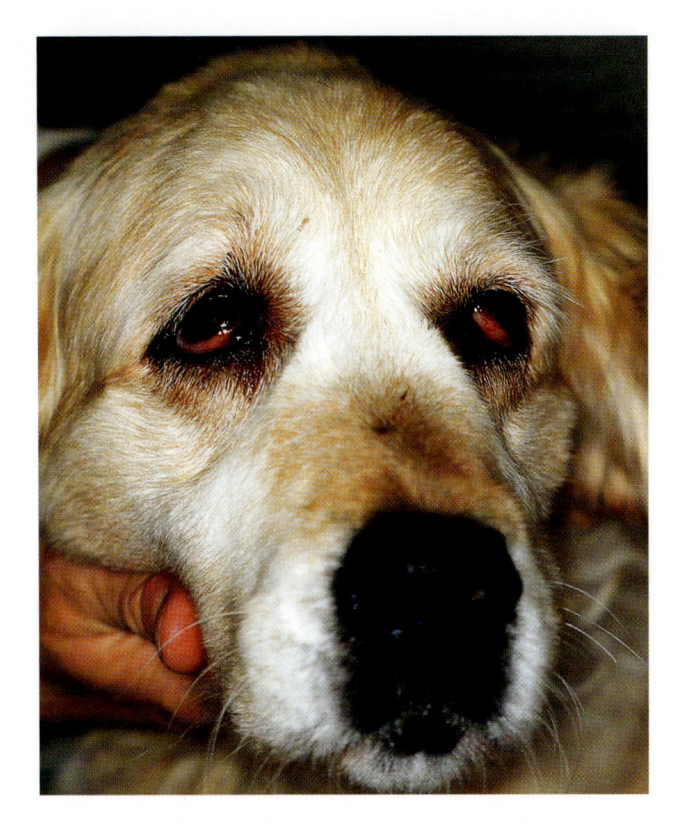

Fig. 15.14 Bilateral Horner's syndrome in a Golden Retriever. Although Horner's syndrome is mainly cosmetic, in this case the marked bilateral third eyelid protrusion has obscured both pupils and interferes with vision.

- Peripheral vasodilation occurs secondary to loss of peripheral vascular tone with resultant mild congestion of the scleral blood vessels and decrease in intraocular pressure.

In addition to the clinical signs of Horner's syndrome, if the sympathetic innervation to the head is also affected, then the dog will demonstrate loss of cutaneous vascular tone on the affected side with peripheral vasodilation. This will be clinically evident as increased cutaneous temperature (with the affected pinna being warmer than the unaffected side), hyperaemia and anhydrosis (decreased sweating on the affected side of the face – in contrast to horses where increased sweating is observed).

Horner's syndrome may result from lesions affecting the sympathetic pathway anywhere between the brain and the orbit and is usually classified as a first, second or third order Horner's syndrome (see Fig. 15.7). Pharmacological testing or other clinical signs can be used to localise further the site of the lesion. In cases with apparent third order Horner's syndrome, frequently no underlying cause can be identified and these cases have traditionally been classified as idiopathic (Boydell, 1995).

Pharmacological testing of Horner's syndrome due to the presence of denervation hypersensitivity, increased sensitivity to topical 10% phenylephrine can be used to predict the site of the lesion; 10% phenylephrine is administered topically in both eyes and the time to pupillary dilation is determined. The more rapid the pupillary dilation the less the distance between the iris and the lesion:

- less than 20 minutes implies a third order Horner's syndrome;
- 20 to 45 minutes implies a second order Horner's syndrome;
- 60 to 90 minutes implies a first order Horner's syndrome or a normal eye.

Canine dysautonomia

Although less common than feline dysautonomia, canine dysautonomia is occasionally encountered. In addition to the systemic signs of autonomic dysfunction (particularly affecting the gastrointestinal tract and urinary system) the eyes are characterised by pupillary dilation in the presence of normal vision and frequent protrusion of the third eyelid (Fig. 15.15) (Wise and Lappin, 1990).

Pupillotonia

Pupillotonia is defined as a pupil that is slow to react to light on both direct and consensual stimulation. The condition is though to be immune-mediated and is rare, only one case being reported to date.

Cerebellar disease

Contralateral mydriasis (pupillary dilation) has been described as an uncommon feature of lateralised cerebellar disease and is accompanied by other clinical signs of cerebellar disease.

Cavernous sinus syndrome

The cavernous sinuses are a paired system of venous sinuses situated on the floor of the calvarium on either side of the pituitary gland. The cavernous sinus is significant as cranial nerves III, IV and VI (innervating the extraocular muscles,

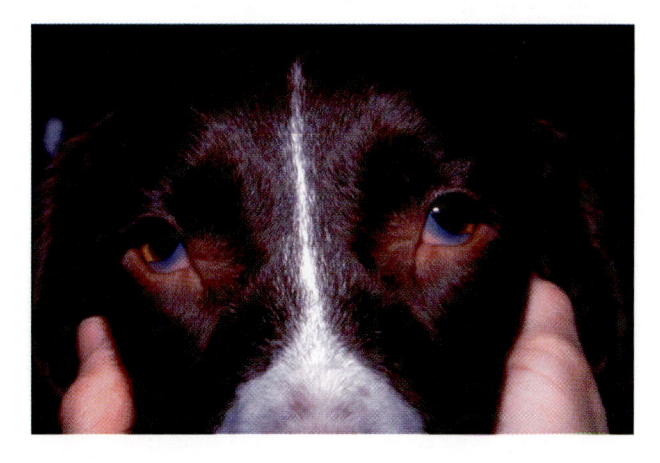

Fig. 15.15 Canine dysautonomia with pupillary dilation and protrusion of the third eyelids. (*Courtesy of the Royal (Dick) Veterinary School.*)

NEURO-OPHTHALMOLOGY

iris and ciliary muscle), as well as the trigeminal nerve (in particular the mandibular and ophthalmic branches), are situated adjacent to the cavernous sinus. Mass lesions of the cavernous sinus may therefore result in paralysis of the extraocular muscles, loss of iris and ciliary muscle function, ipsilateral sensory deficits in the ophthalmic and mandibular branches of the trigeminal nerve and atrophy of the ipsilateral masticatory muscles (innervated by the mandibular branch of the trigeminal nerve) (Fig. 15.16), or a combination of those signs. Paralysis of the extraocular muscles is termed external ophthalmoplegia, paralysis of the iris and ciliary muscle is termed internal ophthalmoplegia, and a combination of both is termed panophthalmoplegia (Fig. 15.17). In extensive lesions of the cavernous sinus, the third order sympathetic supply to the eye (where it runs adjacent to the intracranial portion of the trigeminal nerve) may be affected, resulting in an ipsilateral Horner's syndrome.

Cavernous sinus lesions are characterised by normal vision in the affected eye, however vision may be decreased in the contralateral eye if the lesion extends dorsally to affect the optic tract.

Raised intracranial pressure

Raised intracranial pressure as a result of trauma, encephalitis or intracranial neoplasia may result in transtentorial (rostral or caudal) brain herniation. In these situations the oculomotor nerve, situated ventral to the brain, is vulnerable to compression as it passes over the tentorium cerebelli. One of the early clinical signs of transtentorial brain herniation is therefore a fixed, dilated pupil ipsilateral to the side of herniation, or bilateral in more severe cases. As the oculomotor

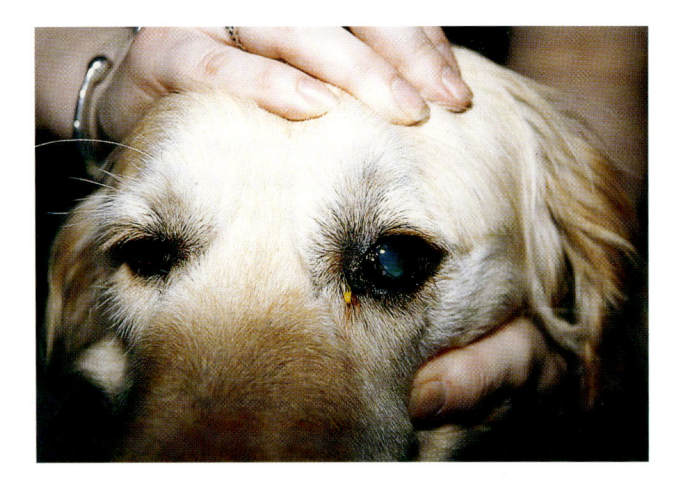

Fig. 15.17 Cavernous sinus syndrome in a dog demonstrating panophthalmoplegia with a mid-range pupil unresponsive to light and protrusion of the third eyelid.

compression becomes more pronounced, paralysis of the extraocular muscles innervated by the oculomotor nerve will develop, resulting in ventrolateral strabismus.

With progressive deterioration of the patient (or with selective midbrain to hindbrain lesions), loss of the sympathetic innervation to the pupil may occur, either on its own (resulting in small miotic, but responsive pupils) (Fig. 15.18), or in combination with the oculomotor nerve lesion (resulting in mid-position, fixed pupils). Serial evaluation of pupil size and function is an important part of the assessment of canine patients following cranial trauma or where brain herniation is suspected to have occurred, and is a reliable guide to prognosis (Oliver et al., 1997).

Organophosphate toxicity

Pupillary abnormalities are evident in a variety of toxic conditions with the most common being organophosphate toxicity, which is characterised by marked miosis, salivation, gastrointestinal disturbances, muscle twitching and possibly seizures.

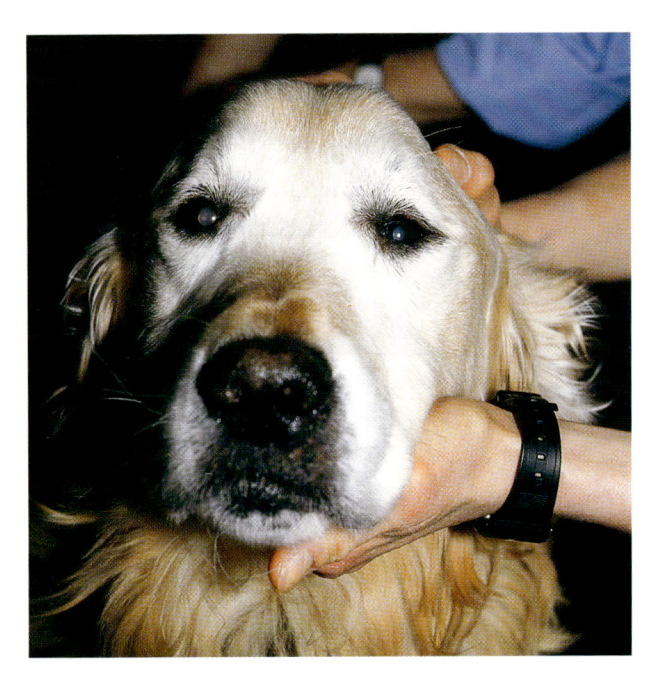

Fig. 15.16 Due to involvement of the trigeminal nerve in cavernous sinus syndrome, affected cases frequently demonstrate atrophy of the masticatory muscles on the affected side.

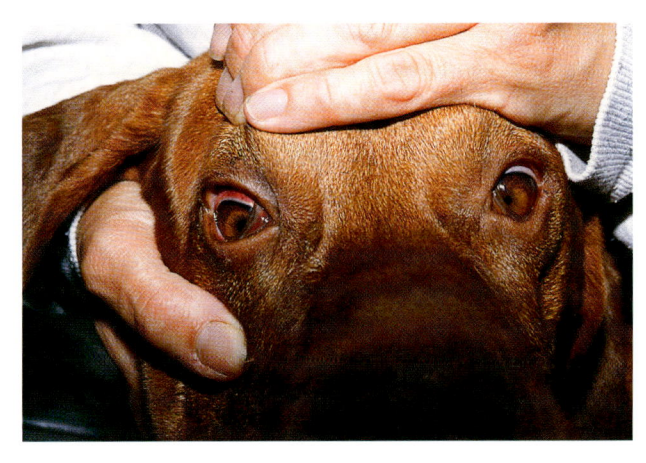

Fig. 15.18 Following CNS trauma this dog presented with a miotic left pupil and evidence of right scleral haemorrhage.

CLINICAL NEURO-OPHTHALMOLOGY

DISORDERS OF EYEBALL POSITION AND MOVEMENT

Eyeball movement is controlled by both the vestibular and saccadic systems. The vestibular system functions to maintain the visual image in a steady position on the retina in response to head movements. The vestibular system functions via the vestibulo-ocular reflex to produce eye movements that are equal but opposite to the direction and degree of head movement. An example of this is the slow phase of the eyeball movement during the vestibulo-ocular reflex (physiological nystagmus).

The function of the saccadic system is to change the line of sight to focus the visual field of interest on the retinal region with the highest visual acuity (usually the area centralis). Saccadic eye movements occur in response to startle reflexes (visual and auditory) and during the fast phase of the vestibulo-ocular reflex.

Congenital strabismus

Congenital strabismus is seen as breed normal in some of the toy breeds or may be associated with congenital vestibular disease (Fig. 15.19).

Congenital nystagmus

Congenital nystagmus in the dog is usually associated with ocular abnormalities and congenital visual deficits. The nystagmus is characterised as a continuous fine oscillation of both globes, often rotatory, or may be characterised as random eye movements, termed 'searching nystagmus'. On occasion congenital nystagmus may be evident in the absence of other ocular abnormalities (Peterson-Jones, 1995).

Vestibular disease

Disorders of the vestibular system will usually result in profound alterations in eyeball position and movement. The characteristic abnormality associated with vestibular disease is the presence of nystagmus and depending on the site of the vestibular abnormality (central or peripheral) the nystagmus may vary in nature between horizontal, rotatory, vertical and positional. Central vestibular disorders may be associated with any form of nystagmus, but positional (unless the dog is in the recovery stage of acute peripheral vestibular disease) and vertical nystagmus are not seen with peripheral vestibular disease and therefore indicate a central disorder.

Further to the presence of nystagmus the eye on the affected side may display a ventrolateral strabismus when the head is raised (Fig. 15.20). Other clinical signs of vestibular disease include the presence of an ipsilateral head tilt (Fig. 15.21), truncal deviation with loss of the righting reflex (Fig. 15.22), ataxia, occasional circling towards the side of the lesion and, in central disorders, the presence of conscious proprioceptive deficits. Involvement of the vestibular portion of the cerebellum may result in paradoxical vestibular syndrome, where due to loss of cerebellar inhibition of the vestibular nuclei, the vestibular signs are directed away from the side of the lesion. Paradoxical vestibular syndrome is associated with a central compressive lesion and usually has postural deficits or cerebellar signs on the side of the lesion (Palmer, 1970).

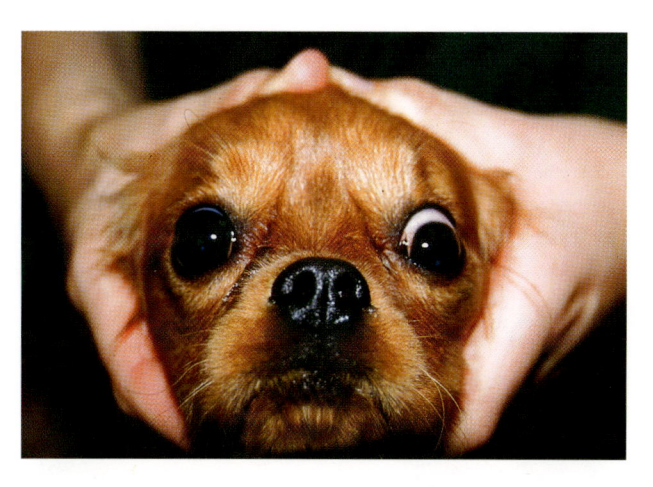

Fig. 15.20 Ventrolateral strabismus may be induced on the side of the vestibular lesion by raising the head.

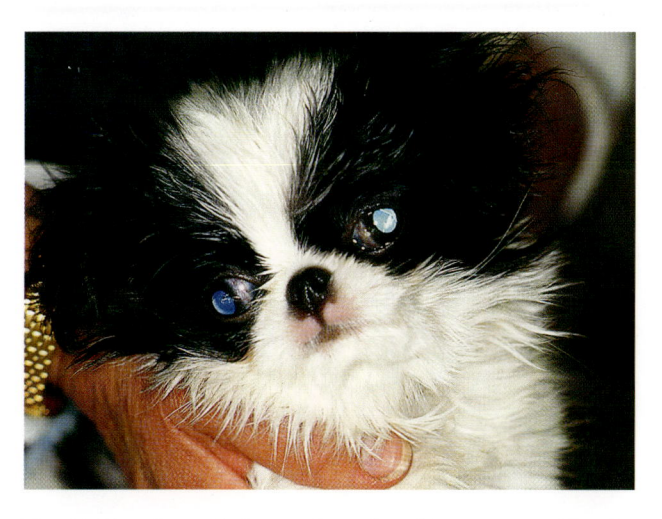

Fig. 15.19 Congenital ventrolateral strabismus was evident in this case as a component of congenital vestibular syndrome.

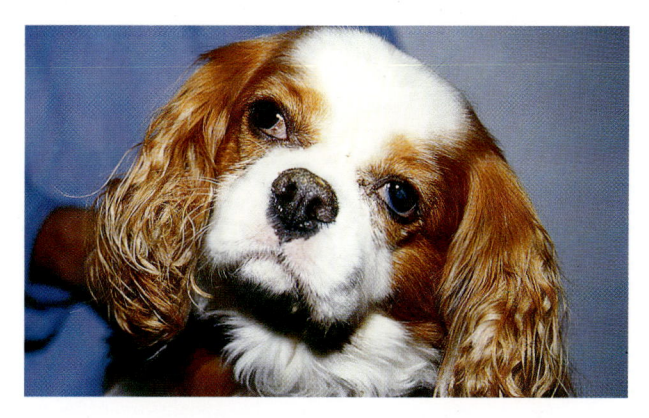

Fig. 15.21 In addition to ocular abnormalities, vestibular disease usually results in a head tilt in the direction of the lesion.

NEURO-OPHTHALMOLOGY

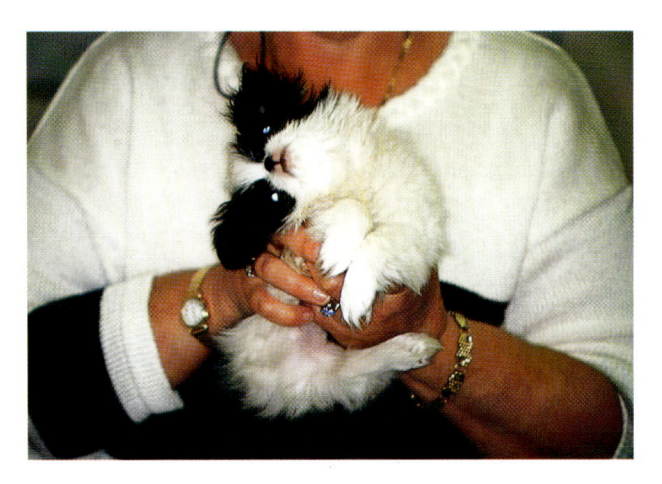

Fig. 15.22 Congenital vestibular syndrome demonstrating a dramatic truncal deviation.

Congenital hydrocephalus

Congenital hydrocephalus, due to distension of the ventricular system and the subarachnoid space with cerebrospinal fluid, is associated with an alteration in skull size and shape, with affected puppies typically developing a domed skull with open calvarial sutures (Oliver *et al.*, 1997). A prominent feature of congenital hydrocephalus is the presence of bilateral ventrolateral strabismus (Fig. 15.23), the so-called 'setting-sun sign', which may be the result of changes in bony orbit configuration caused by the enlarged skull, or due to compression of the oculomotor nerve ventral to the brain. Central blindness with normal pupillary light reflexes is a common feature of hydrocephalus due to the vulnerability of the optic radiations adjacent to the lateral ventricles.

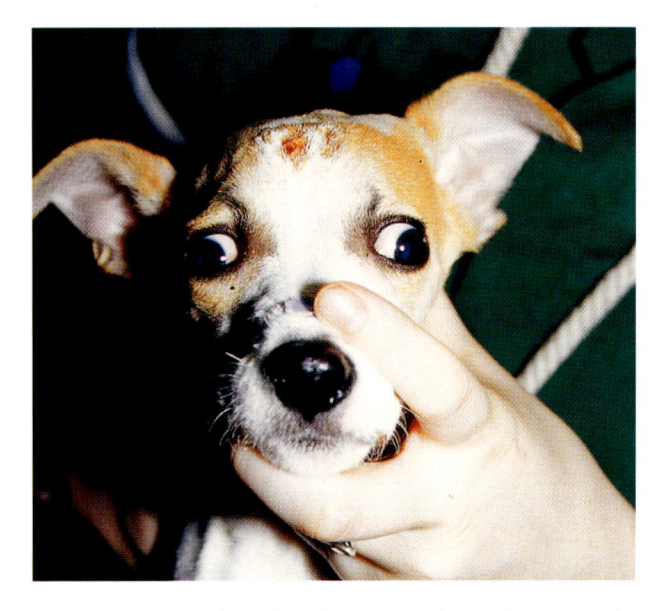

Fig. 15.23 Ventrolateral strabismus in a dog with congenital hydrocephalus. Management of the hydrocephalus by means of a ventriculo-peritoneal shunt resulted in resolution of the strabismus.

Ocular tremor secondary to cerebellar disease

Diffuse cerebellar disease is frequently characterised by a fine ocular tremor, thought to be a form of intention tremor of the extraocular muscles. This fine ocular tremor is frequently only evident on ophthalmoscopic examination.

Cavernous sinus syndrome

Cavernous sinus syndrome is the most common cause of panophthalmoplegia (total paralysis of the extraocular muscles as well as the iris and ciliary muscles). The syndrome is discussed in the section on disorders of pupil size and function.

Extraocular myositis

Bilateral extraocular myositis, presenting as exophthalmos with decreased range of eyeball movement and enlarged extraocular muscles on ultrasound examination, has been reported in a variety of dogs. The disease is thought to be similar to masticatory muscle myositis, with a presumed immune-mediated aetiology, and responds to corticosteroid therapy (Carpenter *et al.*, 1989).

Retrobulbar swelling

Any retrobulbar mass (Fig. 15.24) or swelling causing exophthalmos may interfere with normal eyeball movement and may additionally result in strabismus. Intracranial lesions may selectively affect the innervation to certain extraocular muscles resulting in a strabismus (Fig. 15.25).

DISORDERS OF BLINK

The integrity of the blink pathway is evaluated by:

- the palpebral reflex (afferent touch sensation via the trigeminal nerve and efferent motor function via the facial nerve);

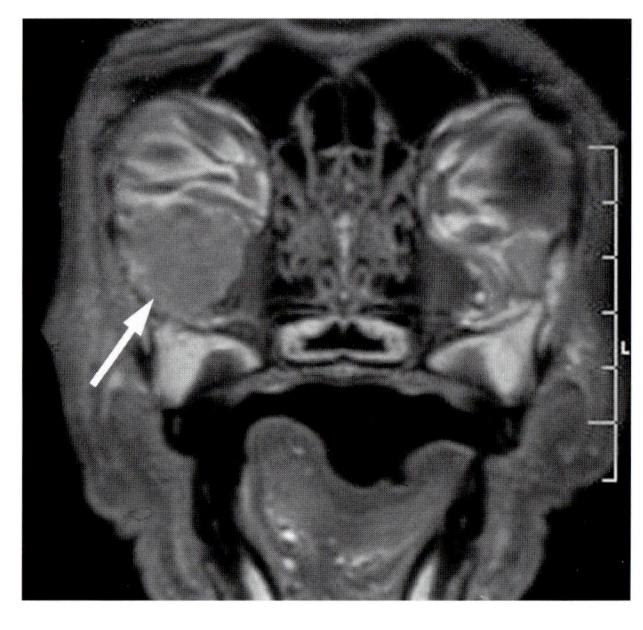

Fig. 15.24 MR image demonstrating a retrobulbar tumour (arrow) resulting in exophthalmos.

CLINICAL NEURO-OPHTHALMOLOGY

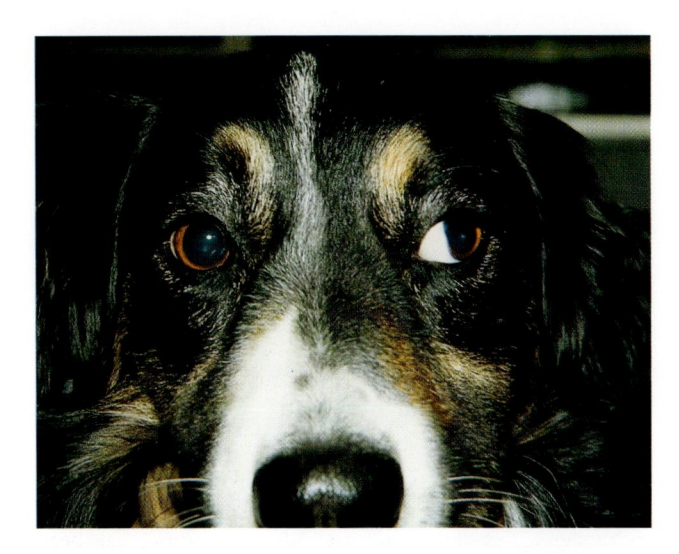

Fig. 15.25 Lateral strabismus in a dog that demonstrated seizures and neurological deficits suggestive of a progressive intracranial lesion.

- the menace response (afferent visual stimulus via the optic nerve and efferent motor function via the facial nerve).

Abnormalities of blink due to a sensory (trigeminal nerve) lesion

Lesions of the trigeminal nerve resulting in loss of sensation to the cornea and surrounding skin of the eye will lead to loss of the corneal and palpebral reflexes (Fig. 15.26). If vision and the facial nerve are preserved the menace response should still be intact. The ophthalmic branch of the trigeminal nerve is also responsible for stimulating reflex tear production following stimulation of the cornea or nasal mucosa, via the parasympathetic portion of the facial nerve. In lesions of the ophthalmic branch, reflex tear production (to corneal or nasal stimulation) is lost.

If the mandibular portion of the trigeminal nerve is affected then masticatory muscle atrophy on the affected side may become apparent (Figs 15.27 and 15.28) and the presence of denervation can be confirmed on electromyography.

Exposure keratopathy with the development of neurogenic corneal ulcers (Fig. 15.29) is a frequent complication following ophthalmic branch lesions, but is infrequently seen following facial nerve (motor) lesions.

The most common cause of trigeminal nerve lesions is neoplasia, but other possibilities include trauma, fractures of the

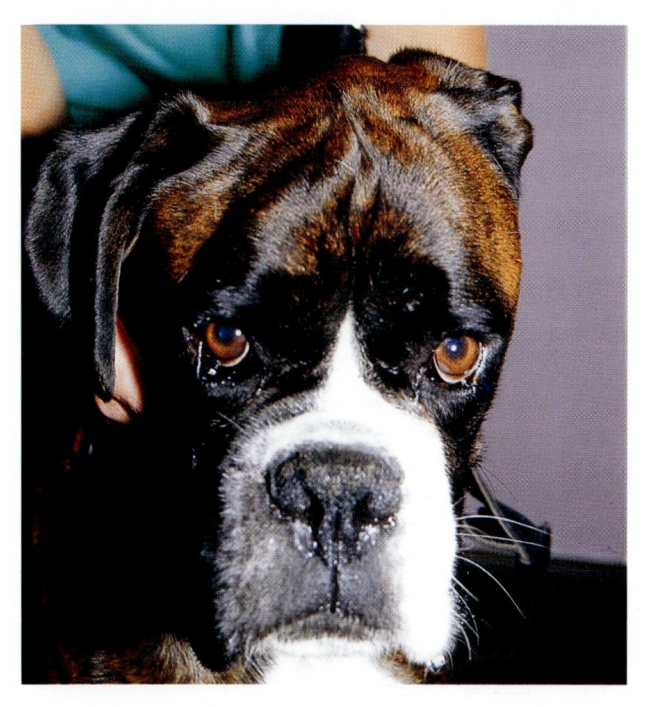

Fig. 15.27 Marked masticatory muscle atrophy in a Boxer dog indicating involvement of the mandibular branch of the trigeminal nerve.

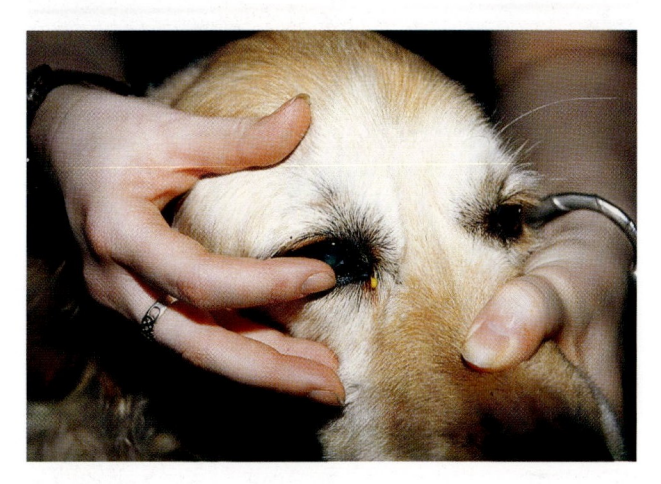

Fig. 15.26 Absent corneal sensation with loss of the corneal reflex in a Golden Retriever with a nerve root tumour affecting the ophthalmic and mandibular branches of the trigeminal nerve.

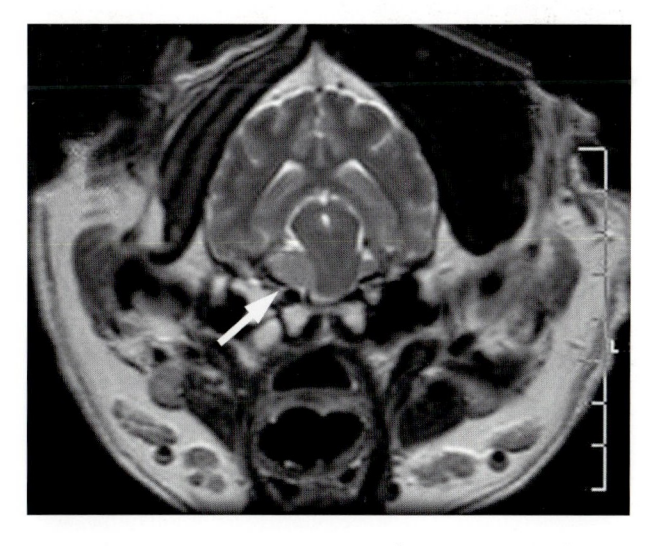

Fig. 15.28 T2 transverse MR image demonstrating an extra-axial trigeminal nerve root tumour (arrow) and resultant midbrain compression. The marked temporal muscle atrophy on the affected side is evident on the MR image.

NEURO-OPHTHALMOLOGY

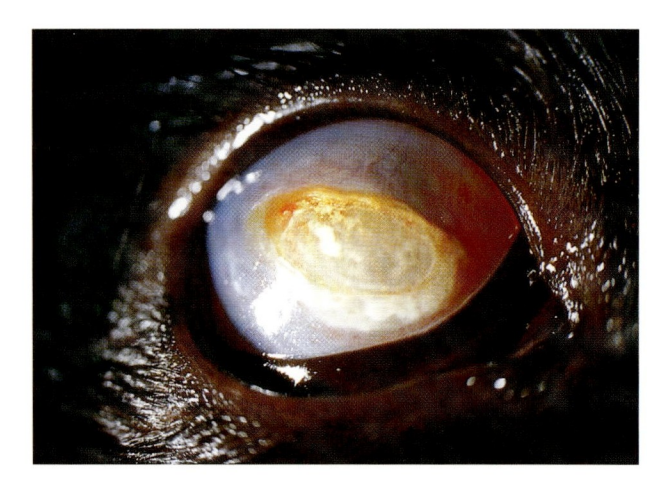

Fig. 15.29 Neurogenic corneal ulcer secondary to a tumour affecting the trigeminal nerve.

petrous temporal bone, inflammatory lesions and cranial polyneuropathies.

Abnormalities of blink due to a motor (facial nerve) lesion

Lesions affecting the facial nerve may result in decreased to absent innervation of the orbicularis oculi muscle, which is responsible for closing the eyelids. The consequence of this is loss of the menace response and palpebral reflex. As sensation to the eyeball is preserved (via the trigeminal nerve) the corneal reflex is still present. In the majority of facial nerve lesions the cause is not identified (75% in one study), followed by otitis media/interna, hypothyroidism and cerebellopontine angle lesions (neoplasia and GME) being the next most likely causes. The facial nerve may also be damaged following surgery (total ear canal ablation and bulla osteotomy) and with soft tissue tumours affecting structures adjacent to the ear. Although the parasympathetic portion of the facial nerve innervates the lacrimal gland, this is rarely affected and neurogenic keratoconjunctivitis sicca is an unusual component of a facial nerve lesion.

Besides the loss of blink, other clinical signs of a facial nerve paralysis include facial asymmetry, drooping of the lip and ear on the affected side (Figs 15.30 and 15.31), drooling of saliva on the affected side and deviation of the nasal philtrum. Due to the loss of the blink an exposure keratitis may occur, although it is more common when there is concurrent reduced tear production or trigeminal nerve damage.

Hemifacial spasm

Hemifacial spasm is a rare syndrome in dogs with blepharospasm, contraction of the upper lip, elevation of the ear and deviation of the nasal philtrum to the affected side. The condition is thought to be secondary to irritation of the facial nerve with a resultant facial neuritis and usually proceeds to facial nerve paralysis. Central lesions, with loss of upper motor neurone inhibition of the facial nucleus, may also result in hemifacial spasm.

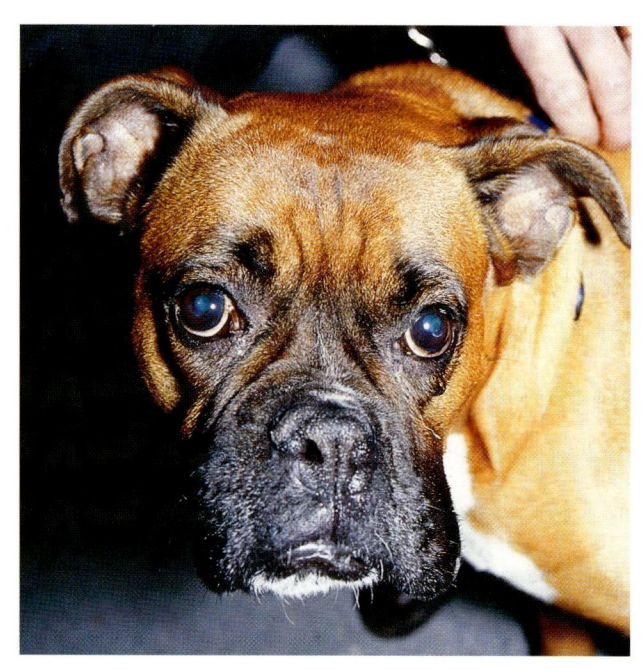

Fig. 15.30 Boxer dog with left facial nerve paralysis and vestibular syndrome demonstrating a left head tilt and drooping of the left lip.

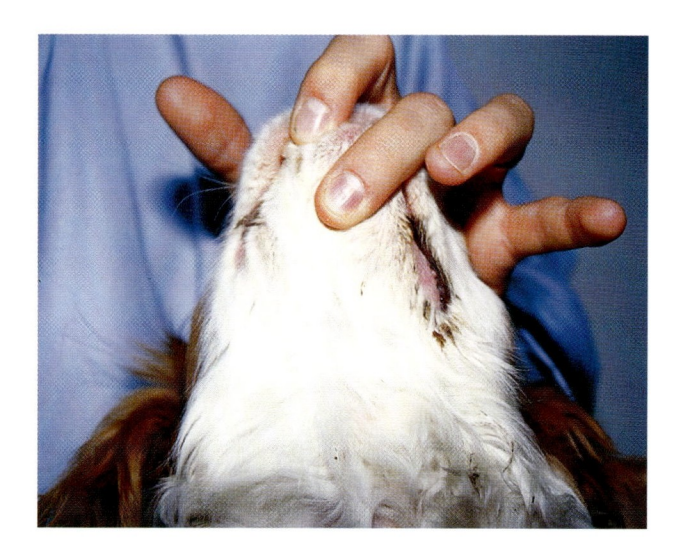

Fig. 15.31 In facial nerve paresis, due to the loss of facial muscle tone, the lip commisure on the affected side is usually lower.

DISORDERS OF EYELID OPENING

The innervation of the levator palpebra superioris muscle is mediated via the oculomotor nerve. Ptosis or drooping of the affected eyelid may be evident in lesions of the oculomotor nerve. The ptosis evident with an oculomotor nerve lesion is easily differentiated from that seen in Horner's syndrome, primarily through the difference in pupil size (miosis in Horner's syndrome and mydriasis in oculomotor nerve lesions).

REFERENCES

DISORDERS OF THE THIRD EYELID

In the dog, protrusion of the third eyelid is mediated passively by a decrease in the sympathetic tone to the orbit (in Horner's syndrome or systemic illness) or secondary to enophthalmos. Intermittent, brief protrusion of the third eyelid may occur in tetanus although the other clinical signs of tetanus are usually overwhelming (Timoney *et al.*, 1988).

DISORDERS OF LACRIMATION

The continued lubrication of the eye is provided by the basal tear production (evaluated by a Schirmer II test, following anaesthesia of the cornea) and induced tear production, following stimulation of the ophthalmic branch of the trigeminal nerve that innervates the surface of the cornea and the nasal mucosa (evaluated by a Schirmer I test).

Lesions affecting the ophthalmic branch of the trigeminal nerve will result in loss of corneal sensation and loss of reflex tearing and a decreased blink frequency, resulting in a neurogenic corneal ulcer. Lesions affecting the parasympathetic portion of the facial nerve will result in a neurogenic keratoconjunctivitis sicca, as both the basal and reflex tear production is under parasympathetic control, and an ipsilateral xeromycteria (dry nose). The presence of an ipsilateral dry nose is an important feature of a lesion of the parasympathetic portion of the facial nerve (Fig. 15.32). A dry nose would not be expected in immune-mediated keratoconjunctivitis sicca as nasal mucosa hydration is not dependent on tear production, but on parasympathetic innervation of the nasal mucosa. Parasympathetic-mediated tear production can be increased using drugs with a direct parasympathomimetic action, including pilocarpine (Scagliotti, 1998).

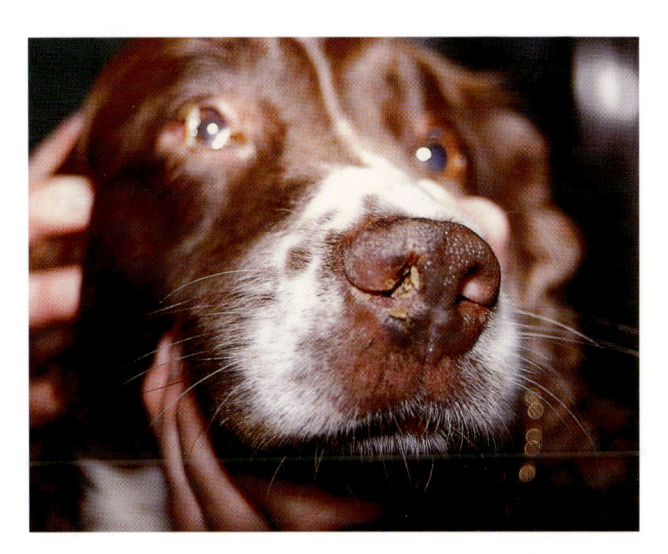

Fig. 15.32 Right facial nerve lesion with involvement of the parasympathetic portion of the facial nerve, demonstrating a dry right eye and nose.

REFERENCES

Boydell P (1995) Idiopathic Horner's syndrome in the golden retriever. *Journal of Small Animal Practice* **36**: 382–384.

Carpenter JL, Schmidt GM, Moore FM, Albert DM, Abrams KL, Elner VM (1989) Canine bilateral extraocular polymyositis. *Veterinary Pathology* **26**: 510–512.

De Lahunta A (1983) *Veterinary Neuroanatomy and Clinical Neurology*. WB Saunders, London.

Kern TJ, Riis RC (1981) Optic nerve hypoplasia in three Miniature Poodles. *Journal of the American Veterinary Medical Association* **178**: 49–54.

Oliver JE, Lorenz MD, Kornegay JN (1997) *Handbook of Veterinary Neurology*. WB Saunders, London.

Palmer AC (1970) Pathogenesis and pathology of the cerebello-vestibular syndrome. *Journal of Small Animal Practice* **11**: 167–176.

Palmer AC, Malinowski W, Barnett KC (1974) Clinical signs including papilloedema associated with brain tumours in twenty-one dogs. *Journal of Small Animal Practice* **15**: 359–386.

Peterson-Jones SM (1995) Abnormalities of eyes and vision. In: Wheeler SJ (ed.) *Manual of Small Animal Neurology*, pp. 125–142. BSAVA, Cheltenham.

Scagliotti RH (1998) Neuro-ophthalmology. *Proceedings of the Basic Science Course in Veterinary and Comparative Neurology and Neurosurgery*, Wisconsin. (Abstract).

Spratling FR, Bridge PS, Barnett KC, Abrams JT, Palmer AC, Sharman IM (1965) Experimental hypovitaminosis-A in calves. Clinical and gross post-mortem findings. *Veterinary Record* **77**: 1532–1542.

Timoney JF, Gillespie JH, Scott FW *et al.* (1988) *Hagan and Bruner's Microbiology and Infectious Diseases of Domestic Animals*. Comstock Publishing Associates, Ithaca.

Wise LA, Lappin MR (1990) Canine dysautonomia. *Seminars in Veterinary Medicine and Surgery (Small Animal)* **5**: 72–74.

Appendix I

Congenital and early onset anomalies

Chapter 4: Globe and orbit
Anophthalmos
Microphthalmos
Buphthalmos

Chapter 5: Upper and lower eyelids
Coloboma
Dermoid

Chapter 7: Lacrimal system
Imperforate puncta and micropuncta
Keratoconjunctivitis sicca
- Cavalier King Charles Spaniel

Chapter 8: Conjunctiva and sclera
Symblepharon
Dermoid
Scleral ectasia

Chapter 9: Cornea
Microcornea and megalocornea
Keratoconus
Dermoid
Infantile dystrophy
Congenital opacities

Chapter 10: Glaucoma
Congenital glaucoma

Chapter 11: Lens
Aphakia, microphakia and spherophakia
Coloboma
Lenticonus and lentiglobus
Cataract with microphthalmos
- Miniature Schnauzer
- Cavalier King Charles Spaniel

Chapter 12: Uveal tract
Aniridia
Iris hypoplasia
Coloboma
Choroidal hypoplasia
Persistent pupillary membrane
- Basenji
- Petite Basset Griffon Vendeen

Chapter 13: Vitreous
Persistent hyperplastic primary vitreous
- Staffordshire Bull Terrier
- Dobermann

Chapter 14: Fundus
Collie eye anomaly
Retinal dysplasia (multifocal and total)
Optic nerve hypoplasia
- Miniature Poodle
Coloboma

Appendix II

Hereditary eye disease

This list gives many of the hereditary eye diseases that occur in breeds in the UK and elsewhere but it is not complete. Most of these conditions have been proven to be inherited and wherever possible the mode of inheritance is given. In addition there are many conditions which show a marked breed incidence, indicating heredity but not proven. Furthermore, other hereditary eye diseases in other breeds are reported from time to time.

Chapter 4: Globe and orbit

Microphthalmos with cataract
- Miniature Schnauzer
- Cavalier King Charles Spaniel (autosomal recessive)

Microphthalmos with multiocular defects
- Dobermann

Chapter 5: Upper and lower eyelids

Entropion (inheritance not known but almost certainly multifactorial)
- many breeds, particularly Shar Pei, Chow, Golden and Labrador Retrievers

Ectropion
- many breeds

Distichiasis
- many breeds, particularly American Cocker Spaniel, Miniature Longhaired Dachshund, Miniature Poodle

Chapter 9: Cornea

Several corneal conditions show a strong breed incidence but none, to date, is proven hereditary.

Corneal dystrophies
  Basement membrane dystrophy
  - Boxer
  - Pembroke Corgi

  Corneal lipidosis
  - Rough Collie
  - Cavalier King Charles Spaniel
  - Bichon Frise
  - Shetland Sheepdog

  Endothelial dystrophy
  - Boston Terrier
  - Chihuahua
  - English Springer Spaniel

Pannus
- German Shepherd Dog and others

Superficial punctate keratitis
- Miniature Longhaired Dachshund

Keratoconjunctivitis sicca
- West Highland White Terrier

Chapter 10: Glaucoma

Primary glaucoma (goniodysgenesis)
- American Cocker Spaniel
- Basset Hound
- English Cocker Spaniel
- Welsh Springer Spaniel
- English Springer Spaniel
- Great Dane
- Flat-coated Retriever
- Siberian Husky
- Dandie Dinmont

Primary glaucoma (open angle)
- Norwegian Elkhound

Pigmentary glaucoma (ocular melanosis)
- Cairn Terrier

Chapter 11: Lens

Primary cataract
- Golden Retriever (autosomal dominant)
- Labrador Retriever (autosomal dominant)
- Chesapeake Bay Retriever (autosomal dominant)
- Large Munsterlander
- Irish Red and White Setter
- Boston Terrier: juvenile (simple autosomal recessive); late onset (inheritance not known)
- Staffordshire Bull Terrier (simple autosomal recessive)
- American Cocker Spaniel (simple autosomal recessive)
- Welsh Springer Spaniel (simple autosomal recessive)
- German Shepherd Dog (autosomal recessive)
- Miniature Schnauzer (including microphthalmos) (simple autosomal recessive)
- Cavalier King Charles Spaniel (including microphthalmos) (congenital autosomal recessive and juvenile autosomal recessive)
- Leonberger
- other breeds (Norweigan Buhund, Standard Poodle)
- suspected, but not proven, in several other breeds

Lens luxation (probable recessive)
- Terrier breeds (Wire and Smooth-haired Fox Terriers, Sealyham, Jack Russell, Tibetan, Lakeland, Welsh, Norfolk, Norwich, Miniature Bull)
- Lancashire Heeler
- Border Collie

CHAPTER 12: UVEAL TRACT

Persistent pupillary membrane
- Basenji
- Petite Bassett Griffon Vendeen
- other breeds

CHAPTER 13: VITREOUS

Persistent hyperplastic primary vitreous
- Staffordshire Bull Terrier
- Dobermann (incomplete dominant)

CHAPTER 14: FUNDUS

Collie eye anomaly
- Rough Collie
- Smooth Collie
- Shetland Sheepdog
- Border Collie
- Lancashire Heeler

Total retinal dysplasia (autosomal recessive)
- Sealyham Terrier
- Labrador Retriever
- Bedlington Terrier

Multifocal retinal dysplasia (autosomal recessive)
- English Springer Spaniel
- American Cocker Spaniel
- Golden Retriever
- Cavalier King Charles Spaniel
- and several other breeds

Generalised progressive retinal atrophy – see Table 14.1, page 170

Optic nerve hypoplasia
- Miniature Poodle

Appendix III

Neoplasia

Chapter 5: Upper and lower eyelids
Papilloma
Adenoma, adenocarcinoma
Melanoma

Chapter 6: Third eyelid
Adenocarcinoma
Melanoma
Papilloma

Chapter 8: Conjunctiva and sclera
Papilloma
Haemangioma and haemangiosarcoma
Melanoma
Squamous cell carcinoma

Chapter 9: Cornea
Squamous cell carcinoma
Fibrosarcoma
Haemangiosarcoma
Papilloma

Chapter 12: Uveal tract
Melanoma
Adenoma and adenocarcinoma
Medulloepithelioma
Lymphosarcoma (secondary)

Chapter 14: Fundus
Medulloepithelioma
Choroidal melanoma
Retrobulbar meningioma
Lymphoma (secondary)

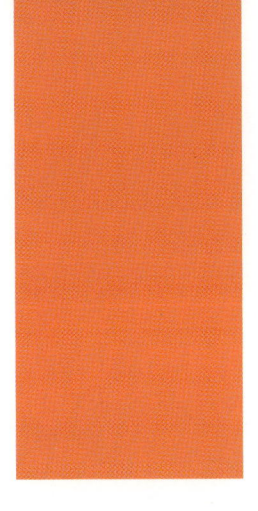

Appendix IV

Drug treatment

Chapter 10: Glaucoma

Class	Drug	Trade name	Dose	Route
Osmotic diuretics	Mannitol 10% or 20%		1–2 mg/kg over 20–30 min	Intravenous
	Glycerol syrup 50%		1–2 ml	Per os
Carbonic anhydrase inhibitors	Dorzolamide HCI 2%	Trusopt® (MSD)	Four times a day	Topical
	Brinzolamide 10 mg/ml	Azopt® (Alcon)	Three times a day	Topical
	Azetazolamide	Diamox® (Wyeth)	10–25 mg/kg twice a day	Per os
	Dichlorphenamide	Daranide®	5–10 mg/kg twice to three times a day	Per os
Prostaglandin analogues	Latanoprost	Xalatan® (Pharmacia and Upjohn)	Once to twice a day	Topical
β-adrenoceptor antagonist	Timoptol maleate	Timoptol® (MSD)	Three to four times a day	Topical

Chapter 12: Uveal tract

Nonsteroidal anti-inflammatories for systemic use

Drug	Trade name	Dose	Route
Carprofen	Rimadyl® (Pfizer)	1–2 mg/kg twice a day	Per os, subcutaneous, intravenous
Meloxicam	Metacam® (Boehringer Ingelheim Ltd)	0.1–0.2 mg/kg once a day	Per os, subcutaneous
Ketoprofen	Ketofen® (Merial Animal Health)	1 mg/kg once a day	Per os, subcutaneous

Nonsteroidal anti-inflammatories for topical use

Drug	Trade name	Dose	Route
Ketorolac	Acular® (Allergan)	4–6 hourly	Topical
Flurbiprofen	Ocufen® (Allergan)	4–6 hourly	Topical

APPENDIX IV

Steroid preparations for topical use

Drug	Trade name	Dose	Route
Dexamethasone sodium phosphate 0.1% drops	Maxidex® (Alcon)	1–2 hourly	Topical
Dexamethasone sodium phosphate 0.1% ointment	Maxitrol® (Alcon)	4–6 hourly	Topical
Prednisolone acetate 1%	Pred Forte® (Allergan)	1–2 hourly	Topical
Prednisolone sodium phosphate 0.5%	Predsol® (Evans)	1–2 hourly	Topical

Steroid preparations for systemic use

Drug	Trade name	Dose	Route
Prednisolone	Prednicare® (Millpledge)	0.5–2 mg/kg once a day	Per os
Methyl prednisolone	Medrone® (Pharmacia and Upjohn)	0.5–1 mg/kg once a day	Per os

Cycloplegics and mydriatics

Drug	Trade name	Dose	Route
Atropine sulphate 1%	Minims®, Atropine 1% (Chauvin)	Hourly to effect	Topical
Atropine sulphate 1%	Atrocare® (Animalcare)	0.1–0.2 ml	Subconjunctival
Tropicamide 1%	Mydriacyl® (Alcon)	Every 15 min to effect	Topical
Phenylephrine HCl 10%	Minims® Phenylephrine (Chauvin)	To effect, every hour	Topical

Further reading

American College of Veterinary Ophthalmology (1996) *Ocular Disorders Presumed to be Inherited in Pure Bred Dogs*, 2nd edn. American College of Veterinary Ophthalmology.

Barnett KC (1990) *A Colour Atlas of Veterinary Ophthalmology*. Wolfe Publishing, London.

Gelatt KN (ed.) (1981) *Veterinary Ophthalmology*. Lea and Febiger, Philadelphia.

Gelatt KN (ed.) (1991) *Veterinary Ophthalmology*, 2nd edn. Lea and Febiger, Philadelphia.

Gelatt KN (ed.) (1999) *Veterinary Ophthalmology*, 3rd edn. Lippincott, Williams and Wilkins, Philadelphia.

Gelatt KN (2000) *Essentials of Veterinary Ophthalmology*. Lippincott, Williams and Wilkins, Philadelphia.

Gelatt KN, Gelatt JP (1994) *Handbook of Small Animal Ophthalmic Surgery*, Vols I and II. Pergamon, Oxford.

Millichamp NJ, Dziezyc J (eds) (1990) *Veterinary Clinics of North America: Small Animal Practice* **20**(3). WB Saunders, Philadelphia.

Nasisse MP (1997) *Veterinary Clinics of North America: Small Animal Practice* **27**(5). WB Saunders, Philadelphia.

Peiffer RL (1989) *Small Animal Ophthalmology: a Problem-orientated Approach*. WB Saunders, London.

Peiffer RL (ed.) (1990) *Veterinary Clinics of North America: Small Animal Practice*. **10**(2). WB Saunders, Philadelphia.

Peiffer RL, Petersen-Jones SM (eds) (1997) *Small Animal Ophthalmology. A Problem-orientated Approach*, 2nd edn. WB Saunders, London.

Peiffer RL, Petersen-Jones SM (2001) *Small Animal Ophthalmology: A Problem-orientated Approach*, 3rd edn. WB Saunders, London.

Petersen-Jones SM, Crispin SM (eds) (1993) *Manual of Small Animal Ophthalmology*. British Small Animal Veterinary Association Publications, Cheltenham.

Prince JH, Diesem CD, Eglitis I, Ruskell GL (1960) *Anatomy and Histology of the Eye and Orbit in Domestic Animals*. Charles C Thomas, Springfield, Illinois.

Rubin LF (1974) *Atlas of Veterinary Ophthalmoscopy*. Lea and Febiger, Philadelphia.

Rubin LF (1989) *Inherited Eye Diseases in Pure bred Dogs*. Williams and Wilkins, Baltimore.

Slatter D (1990) *Fundamentals of Veterinary Ophthalmology*, 2nd edn. WB Saunders, Philadelphia.

Slatter D (ed.) (1993) *Textbook of Small Animal Surgery*, 2nd edn. WB Saunders, Philadelphia.

Stades FC, Wyman M, Boevé MH, Neumann W (1998) *Ophthalmology for the Veterinary Practitioner*. Schlutersche, Hannover.

Walde I, Schäffer EH, Kostlin RG (1990) *Atlas of Ophthalmology in Dogs and Cats*. BC Decker, Toronto, Philadelphia.

Walde I, Schäffer EH, Kostlin RG (1997) *Atlas der Augenerkrankungen bei Hund und Katz*, 2nd edn. Schattauer Stuttgart, New York.

Index

Note: The text makes comprehensive reference to the figure numbers and to the relevant material in those figures. Therefore, figures appearing on a different page to the related text have not been given an additional page reference. Only important items mentioned exclusively in figure legends have been given page references.

Abducens nerve evaluation, 183
Abscess
   corneal, 97
   retrobulbar, see Retrobulbar abscess
Acid burns, 27
Adenocarcinoma
   ciliary body, 145
   eyelid, 58
Adenoma
   ciliary body, 145
   eyelid, 58
Adnexa
   examination, 1–8
   injuries, 21–23
Age-related cataract, 120
Alkali chemicals, 27
Allergy, see Hypersensitivity and allergic reactions
Amelanotic melanoma, 144
American cocker spaniel, cataract, 114–115
Analgesia, glaucoma, 34
Anamnesis, 2–3
Angiography, fluorescein, 6
Angiokeratoma, 65, 79
Angiostrongyliasis, 139, 140
Aniridia, 128
Anisocoria, resting/idiopathic, 188
Ankyloblepharon, 55
Anophthalmos, 37, 43
Anterior chamber
   blood in, see Hyphaema
   foreign body, 30
   reformed by limbal injection, 24
   vitreous in, 104
Anterior segment
   dysgenesis (goniodysgenesis), 103, 104, 131, 199
   pain, 45
Antibiotics
   conjunctivitis, 76
   keratoconjunctivitis sicca, 73
   melting (corneal) ulcers, 26, 93
   retrobulbar abscess, 17
   traumatic globe prolapse, postoperative, 19

Anticollagenase therapy, melting ulcers, 26, 93
Aphakia, 109
   due to luxation, 121–123
Applanation tonometry, 6, 99
Aqueous (humour), 99, 128
   formation, 128
   lipid-laden, 32, 142
   outflow of, 99
   see also Blood–aqueous barrier
Arcus lipoides, 90–91
Arterioles, retinal, tortuosity, 172–174
Assessment, see Examination
Asteroid hyalosis, 151
Asthenia, cutaneous, see Ehlers–Danlos syndrome
Atopic disease
   conjunctiva, 77
   eyelids, 53–54
Atrophy
   iridal, 131
   optic, 173, 178, 186
   retinal, see Retina
   tunica vasculosa lentis, 149
Atropine, 204
   hyphaema, 32
   uveitis, 33, 204
Autoimmune disease, eyelid, 54–55
Autonomic dysfunction, 189
Avulsion lid, 22

Bacterial conjunctivitis, 76
Bacterial uveitis, 138
Barkan lens, 99
Basement membrane dystrophy, 88, 199
Biopsy, 8
Blastomycosis, 139
Blepharitis, 51
Blindness, see Night blindness; Vision, loss
Blinking, 67
   disorders, 192–194
   observing, 184
Blood
   in anterior chamber, see Hyphaema
   corneal staining with, 92
Blood–aqueous barrier, 128
   breakdown, 32, 142
Blood dyscrasias, see Haematological disorders
Blood supply
   choroid, 128
   conjunctiva, 75
   retina, see Retina
   see also specific (types of) vessels

'Blue eye'
   corneal conditions causing, 87, 96
   lipid aqueous causing, 32
Blunt trauma, orbit/globe, 15–21
Boston terrier, cataract, 113–114
Bowman's layer, 85
Breeds
   cataract predisposition, 111–117
   corneal dystrophy predisposition, 89
   generalised progressive retinal atrophy predisposition, 170
   glaucoma predisposition, 33–34
   globe size and, 37
   keratoconjunctivitis sicca predisposition, 70
   see also Hereditary conditions
Bullae, retinal, 174
Bullous keratopathy, 87–88
Buphthalmos (congenital glaucoma), 37, 44, 102–103
   megalocornea and, 85
Burns
   chemical, see Chemical injuries
   thermal, 26–27

Calcium deposits, cornea, 90, 91
Camera, retinal, 6
Canaliculi, 67
   absent, 68
Cancer, see Malignant tumours
Canine adenovirus-1, 138
Capsulopupillary vessels, persistent, 150
Carbonic anhydrase, 128
   inhibitors, 128, 203
Carcinomas
   ciliary body, 145
   conjunctiva, 80
   eyelid, 58
   limbal, 84
Cartilage, bent/deformed, 64
Cataracts (lens opacities), 110–120
   classification schemes, 110–111
   glaucoma and, 104–105, 118
   luxation of cataractous lens, 124
   microphthalmos and, see Microphthalmos
   postnatal, 12–14
   primary hereditary, 111–117, 199
   secondary, 118–120
      with multiocular defects, 119
      to non-ocular disorders, 119
      to other eye diseases, 118–119, 136, 170, 171
   treatment, 120
Caustic (alkali) chemicals, 27

INDEX

Cavalier King Charles spaniel
    cataract, 116–117
    retinal dysplasia, 166, 167
Cavernous sinus syndrome, 189–190, 192
Cellulitis
    juvenile, 51
    retrobulbar, *see* Retrobulbar cellulitis
Central nervous system lesions, 187–188
    postural reactions, 184–185
Cerebellar lesions/disease, 189
    menace response absent in, 181
    ocular tremor with, 192
Cerebral vascular occlusions, 187
Chalazion, 52
Chemical injuries/burns, 27
    cornea, 97
Chemosis, 22, 80
'Cherry eye', 64
Chesapeake Bay retriever, cataract, 112
Cholesterol, corneal deposition, 88
Chorioretinal dysplasia (CRD; choroidal hypoplasia), 12, 130, 160, 163
Chorioretinitis, 172, 173
Choristomas, 49
Choroid (posterior uveal tract)
    hypoplasia, 130
    inflammation (choroiditis), 134, 136–137
    melanoma, 143, 144
    structure/function, 128
Cilia, ectopic, 57
Ciliary body
    inflammation, *see* Uveitis, anterior
    neoplasms, 143, 145
    structure/function, 127
Clotting disorders, hyphaema, 142
Cobalt blue light, 6
Collagen disorders, eyelids in, 49
Collagenase-associated corneal ulcers, 26, 93–94
Collie eye anomaly, 159–163, 200
Coloboma
    fundal
        in collie eye anomaly, 160
        optic disc, 160, 177
    iris, 128–130
    lens, 110
    lid, 49
Colour
    iris, 128
    optic disc, 158
    tapetum lucidum, 155–157
    tapetum nigrum, 157
Computed tomography, trauma, 16, 41–42
Congenital and developmental anomalies, 197
    conjunctiva, 75
    cornea, 85–86, 197
    eyelids, 49, 55, 197
    fundus, 159–163, 176–177
    globe, 43–44, 197
    lacrimal system, 67–68, 197
    lens, 109–110, 197
    sclera, 81, 197
    uveal tract, 128–131, 197
    vitreous, 149–151, 197
Congenital glaucoma, *see* Buphthalmos

Congenital hydrocephalus, 192
Congenital keratoconjunctivitis sicca, 72
Congenital nystagmus, 191
Congenital strabismus, 191
Conjunctiva, 75–81
    congenital disorders, 75
    cysts, 62, 78
    haemorrhage, 16, 22
    hyperaemia, 71
    inflammation, *see* Conjunctivitis
    palpebral, inspection, 3
    pedicle graft/flap with descemetocoele, 25–26
    sampling, 7, 8
    structure/function, 75
    trauma, 22–23
Conjunctival sac
    cystic dilation of lacrimal duct involving, 78
    foreign body, 28
Conjunctivitis, 75–78
    canine nictitans plasmacytic, 62–63
    follicular, 62, 77
    infectious, 75–76
    ligneous, 63, 63, 77–78
    neonatal (ophthalmia neonatorum), 50
    secondary, 81
    third eyelid/nictitating membrane involvement, 62, 63
    see also Keratoconjunctivitis sicca
Contact hypersensitivity, eyelids, 53
Contact lenses
    in gonioscopy, 6, 99–100
    infection associated with, 76
Cornea, 85–97
    abscess, 97
    congenital diseases, 85–86, 197
    cyst, 97
    cytology, 7–8
    examination, 4
    foreign body, 28–30
    hereditary diseases, 199
    neoplasms, 97, 201
    oedema, *see* Oedema
    opacities, *see* Opacities
    pigmentation, 91–92
    postnatal development, 9
    size/shape changes, 85
    structure/function, 85
    trauma, 23–27, 97
    ulcer, *see* Ulcer
    see also entries under Kerat-
Corrosive agents, 27
Cortical blindness, toxins causing, 187
Corticosteroids, *see* Steroids
Cranial nerve lesions
    blink abnormalities due to, 193–194
    tests for, 181–184
    see also specific nerves
Cryptococcosis, 138–139
Cushing's syndrome, 174
Cutaneous asthenia, *see* Ehlers–Danlos syndrome
Cycloplegics, 204
Cyclosporine, keratoconjunctivitis sicca, 73
Cyst(s)
    conjunctival, 62, 78

corneal, 97
iridal, 132
uveal, 100, 153
vitreal, 153
Cystic dilatation of nasolacrimal duct, 69, 78
Cytology, 7–8

Dacryocystitis, 69
    secondary to foreign body, 27
Dacryocystorhinography, 69
Degeneration
    corneal, 91
    retinal, *see* Retina
    visual disturbances due to, 188
    vitreous, 151
Demodex canis, 51
Dermatitis, atopic, 53–54, 77
Dermatoses, zinc, 55
Dermoids, 49, 86
    cornea, 86
    eyelid, 49
Descemetocoele, 25–26, 72, 94–95
    keratoconjunctivitis sicca and, 72
Descemet's membrane, 85
    tears/rupture, 87, 102
Detergent burns, 27
Development
    disorders, *see* Congenital and developmental anomalies
    fundus, 11–14, 155
    globe, 37, 42–43
    postnatal, *see* Postnatal development
    uvea, 127
    vitreous, 149
Dexamethasone, 204
Diabetes
    cataract, 120
    fundus changes, 174
Diamond eye, 56
Dietary deficiency, cataracts, 120
Dirofilariasis, 139, 140
Discoid lupus, 54
Dislocation, lens, *see* Lens
Distemper, 172
Distichiasis, 56–57, 56
Diuretics, osmotic, 203
Doberman Pinscher, persistent hyperplastic primary vitreous, 151
'Dot and blot' type retinal haemorrhage, 174, 175
Drainage, retrobulbar abscess, 17
Drugs
    adverse reactions
        eyelids, 53
        lacrimal system, 72
        pupils, 188
    tests with
        Horner's syndrome, 189
        pupillary light reflex-affecting lesions, 188
    therapeutic use, 203–204
        glaucoma, 34, 106, 203
        uveitis, 33, 203–204
    see also Toxic substances
Dry eye (keratoconjunctivitis sicca), 70–73, 95

INDEX

Dry mouth, 70–71
Dysautonomia, 189
Dysgenesis, anterior segment
    (goniodysgenesis), 103, 104, 131,
    199
Dysplasia
  chorioretinal (CRD; choroidal
    hypoplasia), 12, 130, 160, 163
  retinal, *see* Retina
Dystrophy
  corneal, 88–89, 91, 199
    infantile, 86
  retinal, *see* Retina

Ectopic cilia, 57
Ectropion, 56, 199
EDTA, melting ulcers, 26
Ehlers–Danlos syndrome (cutaneous
    asthenia)
  cataract, 124
  eyelids in, 49
  sclera in, 81
Ehrlichia canis, 138
Emergency conditions, 15–36
Endophthalmitis, infectious, 152
Endothelium, corneal, 85
  dystrophy, 89, 199
  pigmentation, 92
English springer spaniel, retinal dysplasia,
    164, 165
Enophthalmos, 44–45
  in Horner's syndrome, 21, 45, 61, 188
  sudden onset, 20–21
  third eyelid prominence and, 61
Entropion, 55–56, 199
Enucleated eye, pathological examination,
    8
Eosinophilic myositis, 46
Epiphora, 67
Episclera, structure, 81
Episcleritis, 18, 81
  nodular, 82
  treatment, 83
Episclerokeratitis, nodular granulomatous,
    82
Epithelial neoplasms, ciliary body, 145
Epithelioma, eyelid, 58
Epithelium
  corneal, 85
    basement membrane dystrophy, 88,
      199
    recurrent erosions, 88, 92
  retinal pigment, dystrophy (central
    progressive retinal atrophy), 118,
    168, 170–172
Equipment for examination, 1–2
Ethylenediamine tetra-acetic acid, melting
    ulcers, 26
Examination/assessment, 1–8
  neuro-ophthalmological, 181–185
Exophthalmos (proptosis), 45–46
  pulsatile/intermittent, 18
  sudden onset, 17–18
  third eyelid prominence in, 61–62
Extraocular muscles
  eyeball movement control, assessment, 183
  severance, 19

Eyeball, *see* Globe
Eyelashes, extra (distichiasis), 56–57, 199
Eyelid, third (nictating membrane), 61–66
  disorders, 61–65, 78
    neoplastic, 62, 65, 201
    protrusion, 61–62, 188, 195
  injury, 22
  inspection, 3
  structure/function, 61
Eyelid, upper/lower, 49–60
  anomalies, 55–58
    congenital, 49, 55, 197
  biopsy, 8
  disorders, 50–55
    hereditary, 199
    neoplastic, 49, 58–60, 201
    of opening, 194
  fused/opening (postnatal), 9
  innervation, evaluation, 184
  ptosis, 188, 194
  structure/function, 49
  trauma, 21–22

Facial nerve, 184
  lesions
    blink abnormalities with, 194
    lacrimation disorders, 195
    tests for, 184
  menace response and, 181, 184
Fasciitis, ocular, 81
Fibrous tissue, cornea, 90
Fine needle aspirates, 8
Fluorescein
  angiography using, 6
  topical staining, 6–7
Follicular conjunctivitis, 62, 77
Folliculitis, periorbital, 51
Foreign bodies, 27–30
  MRI, 42
  third eyelid, 62
  ultrasound, 40
  vitreal, 153
Fractures, orbital, 16, 20
Freckles, iris, 131–132
Fundus, 155–179
  developing, 11–14, 155
  hereditary conditions, 159–163,
    176–177, 200
  neoplasia, 178, 201
  normal, 155–159
  see also specific parts
Fundus camera, 6
Funduscopy, *see* Ophthalmoscopy
Fungal/mycotic infections
  endophthalmic, 152
  eyelids, 51
  uvea, 138–139

Genetic disorders, *see* Hereditary
    conditions
German Shepherd, cataract, 115
Glaucoma, 33–34, 99–106
  acute-onset, 105
  cataract and, 104–105, 118
  classification, 102–106
  clinical signs, 101–102
  congenital, *see* Buphthalmos

corneal oedema in, 87, 101
drug therapy, *see* Intraocular pressure,
    drugs lowering
lens luxation and, 101–102, 104, 123
open-angle, 103–104
pathogenesis/pathophysiology, 99
primary, 103–104, 199
secondary, 104–106
treatment, 34, 106, 203
Globe (eyeball), 37–47
  blunt trauma, 15–21
  congenital anomalies, 43–44, 197
  development, 37, 42–43
  examination, 1–8
  hereditary diseases, 199
  movement abnormalities, 191–192
    tests for, 183–184
  positional abnormalities, 191–192
  prolapse, 46–47
  size
    breed and, 37
    conditions affecting, 37, 43, 44
    postnatal, ultrasound measurement, 42
Glycosaminoglycans, aqueous humour
    outflow and, 99
'Go normal' phenomenon, 160
Golden retriever
  cataract, 111–112
  retinal dysplasia, 164, 165, 168
Goniodysgenesis, 103, 104, 131, 199
Gonioscopy, 6, 99–100
Granuloma, sterile, 80
Granulomatous disease, idiopathic, 80
Granulomatous episclerokeratitis, nodular,
    82
Granulomatous meningoencephalitis, 186,
    187
'Ground glass eye', 87
Gunshot injuries, 27, 30

Haab's striae, 102
Haemangioma, conjunctival, 79
Haemangiosarcoma, conjunctival, 79
Haematogenous corneal pigmentation, 92
Haematological disorders (blood
    dyscrasias)
  conjunctival involvement, 80
  hyphaema, 142
Haematoma, orbital, 15–16
Haemorrhage
  in collie eye anomaly, 162
  conjunctival/subconjunctival, 16, 22
  corneal, 92
  retinal, *see* Retina
  retrobulbar, 46
  vitreous, 151–152
Handling of patient, 1
Head tilt, ipsilateral, 191
Helminthic infections, 139–140
Hemifacial spasm, 194
Hemistand and hemiwalk, 185
Hereditary conditions, 199–200
  cataracts, 111–117, 199
  fundic disorders, 159–163, 176–177, 200
  lens luxation, 123–124, 200
  persistent hyperplastic primary vitreous,
    151, 200

INDEX

Hereditary conditions, (contd)
　retinal dysplasia, 163–167
　see also Breeds
Herniation, vitreal, 153
Histiocytoma, eyelid, 59
Histiocytosis, systemic, 65, 80
Histoplasmosis, 139
History-taking, 2–3
Hopping test, 185
Horner's syndrome, 188–189
　enophthalmos in, 21, 45, 61, 188
　pharmacological testing, 189
　third eyelid prominence in, 61
Hyalitis, 152
Hyalocytes, 149
Hyaloid artery, persistent, 119, 150
Hyalosis, asteroid, 151
Hyaluronic acid, 149
Hydrocephalus, 187
　congenital, 192
Hydrophthalmos, 37, 44, 87, 101–102, 102
Hyperaemia, conjunctival, 71
Hypercalcaemia, cataract in, 120
Hyperlipidaemia, 32
Hypermature cataract, 110
　American cocker spaniel, 115
Hyperpigmentation, iridal, 131–132
Hyperplasia
　meibomian gland, 59
　nictitans gland, 64
Hyperplastic primary vitreous, persistent, 119, 150–151, 200
Hypersensitivity and allergic reactions
　conjunctiva, 76
　eyelids, 52
Hypertensive retinopathy, 172–174
Hypervitaminosis A, 187
Hyphaema, 31–32, 142–143
　in traumatic globe prolapse, 19
Hypoplasia
　cerebellar, 182
　choroidal (chorioretinal dysplasia; CRD), 12, 130, 160, 163
　iridal, 128
　optic nerve, 176–177, 186, 187
Hypopyon, 136
Hypotension, ocular, uveitis, 135

Imaging, 38–42
　trauma, 16
Immune-mediated uveitis, 140–141
Immunosuppressive drugs
　optic neuritis, 35
　scleritis/episcleritis, 83
Indentation tonometry, 6, 99
Infantile corneal dystrophy, 86
Infection
　conjunctival, 75–76
　　neonatal, 50
　corneal, 96
　eyelid, 51
　intraocular/endophthalmic, 152, 172
　uveal, 138–140
Inflammation
　sclera/episclera, 81–83
　third eyelid, 62–63

see also Post-inflammatory retinopathy and specific inflammatory disorders
Inherited conditions, see Hereditary conditions
Injury, see Trauma
Inspection
　close, 2–3
　distance, 2
Instruments for examination, 1–2
Interstitial keratitis, 96–97
Intraocular pressure
　drugs lowering, 106
　　in glaucoma, 34, 106, 203
　　in hyphaema, 32
　low (hypotension), uveitis in, 135
　measurement, 6, 99–100
　raised, 99, 190
　　hyphaema and, 32
Iridocorneal angle
　abnormalities, 100
　normal, 100
Iridocyclitis, see Uveitis, anterior
Iris
　absence, 128
　acquired conditions, 131–134
　colour variations, 128
　hypoplasia, 128
　melanoma, 88, 143
　prolapse, 23–24
　structure/function, 127
Iris bombé, 101, 105, 134
Irish red and white setter, cataract, 113
Iritis, cataract in, 118
　see also Uveitis, anterior

Jerk nystagmus, 184
Juvenile pyoderma and cellulitis, 51

Keratitis, 90, 95–97
　interstitial, 96–97
　superficial chronic (pannus), 95–96
　superficial diffuse, 95
　superficial punctate, 96
　see also Episclerokeratitis
Keratoconjunctivitis sicca, 70–73, 95
Keratoconus, 85
Koeppe lens, 99

Labrador retriever
　cataract, 112
　retinal dysplasia, 163, 165
　　skeletal abnormalities and, 164
Lacerations
　conjunctival, 22–23
　corneal, 23–24
　lid, 21–22
Lacrimal gland, 67
　motor control, evaluation, 184
Lacrimal (nasolacrimal) system, 67–74
　congenital anomalies, 67–68, 197
　disease, 68–73
　structure/function, 67
Lacrimation, see Tears
Large Musterlander, cataract, 112–113
Lashes, extra (distichiasis), 56–57, 199
Latanoprost, glaucoma, 34, 203
Leishmaniasis, 139

Lens, 109–125
　congenital anomalies, 109–110, 197
　foreign body, 30
　hereditary diseases, 199–200
　luxation/dislocation, 120–124
　　cataract following, 118
　　clinical signs, 121–123
　　corneal oedema/opacity with, 87, 121
　　glaucoma and, 101–102, 104, 123
　　incidence and inheritance, 123–124, 200
　　secondary, 124
　　treatment, 124
　　ultrasound, 40
　　vitreal herniation with, 153
　opacity, see Cataract
　subluxation, 101–102
　uveitis causation due to, 104, 140
　see also Contact lenses
Lenticonus, 110
　Cavalier King Charles spaniel, 116
Leonberger, cataract, 117
Lid,, see also Eyelid
Light reflex, see Pupillary light reflex
Light source, focal, 4
Ligneous conjunctivitis, 63, 77–78
Limbus
　dermoids located at, 86
　lacerations at, 24
　neoplasia, 83–84
　　melanoma, 83–84, 145
Lipid aqueous, 32, 142
Lipid deposits/infiltrates, cornea, 90, 90–91, 91
Lipid dystrophies (corneal lipidosis), 88–89, 199
Lipid keratopathy, 90
Lock jaw, see Tetanus
Lovac–Barkan lens, 99
Lupus, discoid, 54
Luxation, lens, see Lens
Lymphocytic–plasmacytic uveitis, 134, 140
Lymphoma, multicentric, 146
Lymphosarcoma
　lacrimal system, 73
　uveal, 146

Macropalpebral fissure, 55, 56
Magnetic resonance imaging, 41–42
　trauma, 16
Malignant tumours
　conjunctiva, 79–80
　exophthalmos with, 46
　eyelid, 58, 60
　uveal tract, 143–145, 145
　　secondary, 146–147
Masses
　intraocular, ultrasonography, 40
　retrobulbar, 192
　see also specific types
Mast cell tumours, 60
Medulloepithelioma, ciliary body, 145
Megalocornea, 85
Meibomian glands, 49
　hyperplasia, 59
　inflammation, 51–52
　inspection, 3
　tumours arising from, 58

INDEX

Melanoma
   conjunctiva, 79
   eyelid, 60
   limbus, 83–84, 145
   uveal tract, 143–144
      iris, 88, 143
Melanosis, 105–106
   iris, 131
Melting ulcers, 26, 93–94
Membrana nictitans, *see* Eyelid, third
Membrana pupillaris, *see* Pupillary membrane
Menace response, 181, 193
   facial nerve and, 181, 184
Meningoencephalitis, granulomatous, 186, 187
Metabolic disorders affecting vision, 187–188
Metallic foreign bodies, 30
   ultrasound, 41
   see also Gunshot injuries
Metastases, uveal, 145–146
Microcornea, 85
Micropalpebral fissure, 55
Micropapilla, 158
Microphakia, 109
Microphthalmos, 37, 43
   cataract and, 199
      Cavalier King Charles spaniel, 116
      miniature schnauzer, 116
      third eyelid prominence in, 61
Micropunctum, 67–68, 68
Miniature bull terrier, lens luxation, 123–124
Miniature schnauzer, cataract, 116
Miosis, 134–135, 188
   pharmacological, 188
Morgagnian cataract, 110
Motor control
   blink, deficits, 194
   CNS lesions affecting, tests, 185
   eyelids/lacrimal gland function, evaluation, 184
Movement, eyeball, *see* Globe
Mucinosis, 75
   focal, 49
Mucocutaneous pyoderma, 54
Mycoses, *see* Fungal infections
Mydriatics, 204
   foreign body removal, 30
   lens luxation, diagnostic value, 123
   pupillary dysfunction with, 188
   uveitis, 33, 204
Myelination, optic disc, 158
Myositis, 17–18
   eosinophilic, 46
   extraocular, 192

Nanophthalmos, 43
Nasolacrimal duct, 67
   cystic dilatation, 69, 78
   foreign body, 27
   inflammation, *see* Dacryocystitis
Nasolacrimal system, *see* Lacrimal system
Neonatal conjunctivitis (ophthalmia neonatorum), 50

Neoplasms, 201
   conjunctival, 78–80, 201
      diffuse neoplasms, 80
   corneal, 97, 201
   corneal oedema associated with, 87
   eyelids
      lower/upper, 49, 58–60, 201
      third, 62, 65, 201
   fundic, 178, 201
   lacrimal system, 73
   limbal, 83–84
   malignant, *see* Malignant tumours
   optic chiasm compression by, 187
   optic nerve compression by, 187
   orbital (in general)
      enophthalmos with, 45
      exophthalmos with, 46
      MRI, 42
      radiographs, 38
   ultrasound, 40
   uveal, 143–146, 201
   uveitis associated with, 142, 146
   vitreal, 153
Nerve supply, conjunctiva, 75
Neurogenic corneal ulcer, 193
Neurogenic dry eye, 72–73
Neuro-ophthalmology, 181–195
   assessment, 181–185
   clinical conditions, 185–195
Nictating membrane, *see* Eyelid, third
Nictitans gland, 61, 67
   disorders, 64–65
   neoplastic, 62, 65
Nictitans plasmacytic conjunctivitis, canine, 62–63
Night blindness in generalised progressive retinal atrophy, 168
Nodular episcleritis, 82
Nodular granulomatous episclerokeratitis, 82
Nonsteroidal anti-inflammatory drugs, uveitis, 33, 203
Norwegian Buhund, cataract, 117
Nuclear cataract
   Cavalier King Charles spaniel, 116
   Norwegian Buhund, 117
Nuclear sclerosis, 109
   senile, 111
Nutritional deficiency, cataracts, 120
Nystagmus, 184
   congenital, 191
   physiological, 183, 191

Oculomotor nerve lesions, 190
   tests for, 183
Oedema
   corneal, 87–88
      in infectious uveitis, 138
      postnatal (physiological), 9
   optic papilla, 177–178, 186
Opacities
   corneal, 87–91
      congenital, 85, 86
      luxated lens causing, 87, 121
      postnatal clearing of, 9
      in superficial punctate keratitis, 96
   lens, *see* Cataracts

Ophthalmia neonatorum, 50
Ophthalmic branch of trigeminal nerve, lesions, 195
Ophthalmoscopy, 4–5
   developing eye, 11–14
   direct, 4
      ophthalmoscope, 1
   indirect, 4–5
      ophthalmoscope, 2
   monocular hand-held ophthalmoscope, 5
   optic atrophy, 178
   papilloedema, 178
   retinal degeneration, 178
   retinal dysplasia, 167
   retinal dystrophies, 168, 171
Optic chiasm lesions, 187
Optic nerve, 176–178, 185–187
   atrophy, 173, 178, 186
   compression, 187
   development, 155
   head (optic papilla/disc), 158–159, 176–178, 185–186
      coloboma, 160, 177
      cupping, 102
      oedema, 177–178, 186
      pupillary light reflex deficits with abnormalities in, 185–186
   hypoplasia, 176–177, 186, 187
   tests, 181, 183
Optic neuritis, 34–35, 178, 186
Optic tract lesions, 187
Orbit
   blunt trauma, 15–21
   foreign body, 27
   hereditary diseases, 199
   neoplasia, *see* Neoplasms
Organophosphate toxicity, 190

Pain
   anterior segment, 45
   in glaucoma, 34
   ocular (in general), third eyelid prominence associated with, 61
   trigeminal, enophthalmos with, 21
Palpebral conjunctiva, inspection, 3
Palpebral fissure size/shape, 55, 56
Palpebral reflex, 184, 192
Pannus, corneal, 95–96
Papillitis (optic neuritis), 34–35, 178
Papilloedema, 177–178, 186
Papillomas, conjunctival, 79
Paradoxical vestibular syndrome, 191
Parasitic infestations, 139–140
Parasympathetic portion
   facial nerve, lesions, 195
   oculomotor nerve, tests, 183
Pars planitis, 134
Patient handling, 1
Paw-placing reflex, 185
Pemphigus foliaceus, 54
Pemphigus vulgaris, 54
Peripheral vasodilation, 189
Phacoclastic uveitis, 104, 140
Phacolytic uveitis, 118, 140
Pharmacology, *see* Drugs
Phenylephrine administration, 189
Phthisis bulbi, 44, 102

INDEX

Physostigmine, tests using, 188
Pigment epithelial dystrophy, (central progressive retinal atrophy), 118, 168, 170–172
Pigmentary uveitis, 140
Pigmentation
  corneal, 91–92
  iridal, 131–132
Pilocarpine
  hyphaema, 32
  tests using, 188
Plasmacytic conjunctivitis, canine nictitans, 62–63
Post-inflammatory retinopathy, 172
Postnatal development, 9–14
  globe, 42–43
Postural reactions, 184–185
Prednisolone
  glaucoma, 34
  melting ulcers, 26
  myositis, 18
  optic neuritis, 35
  uveitis, 33, 204
Prolapse
  globe, 19–20, 46–47
  iris, 23–24
  nictitans gland, 64
  vitreal, 153
Prominence (protrusion), third eyelid, 61–62, 188, 195
Proprioceptive testing, 185
Proptosis, see Exophthalmos
Prostaglandin analogues, glaucoma, 34, 203
Protozoal infections, 139
Protrusion, third eyelid, 61–62, 188, 195
Pseudopapilloedema, 158
Ptosis, upper eyelid, 188, 194
Puncta, lacrimal, 67
  congenital anomalies, 67–68
  obstruction, 68–69
  trauma, 69
Punctate keratitis, superficial, 96
Pupil
  dilating drugs, see Mydriatics
  functional anomalies, 188–190
  size, 188–190
    in glaucoma, 101
    in traumatic globe prolapse, 19
Pupillary light reflex, 183
  decreased vision with deficits in, 185–187
  pharmacological evaluation of lesions affecting, 188
  in traumatic globe prolapse, 19
Pupillary membrane
  development, 9
  persistent, 118, 130–131, 200
Pupillotonia, 189
Purverulent cataract, 110
Pyoderma
  juvenile, 51
  mucocutaneous, 54
Pyogranuloma, 52

Radiation-related cataract, 120
Radiography, 38–39
  obstructed puncta, 69

Radiology, see Imaging
Reflex step testing, 185
Retina, 163–176
  atrophy/dystrophy, 168–172
    central progressive atrophy, 118, 168, 170–172
    generalised progressive atrophy, 118, 168–169
  blood vessels, 159
    arteriolar tortuosity, 172–174
  classification of diseases, 155
  degeneration
    infectious causes, 172
    sudden acquired, 34, 178, 185
  detachment, 35, 162, 176
    bullous, 174
    in collie eye anomaly, 162, 176
    dysplasia and, 163–164
    in hypertensive retinopathy, 174
  development, 155
  dysplasia, 12, 118, 163–168, 200
    diagnostic difficulties, 167–168
    multifocal, 164–167, 200
    total, 118, 200
  haemorrhage, 175–176
    'dot and blot' type, 174, 175
  post-inflammatory disease, 172
Retinal camera, 6
Retrobulbar abscess, 17
  MRI, 42
  ultrasound, 40
Retrobulbar cellulitis, 17
  exophthalmos in, 46
Retrobulbar haemorrhage, 46
Retrobulbar swelling/mass, 192
Retropulsion, 4
Rickettsia, tick-borne, 138
Righting reflex, loss, 191
Rose Bengal, 7

Saccadic eye movements, 191
Salivary gland, zygomatic, inflammation, 18
Sampling techniques, 7–8
Sarcoptic mange, 51
Scabies, 51
Schiotz tonometer, 6, 99
Schirmer tear test, 3, 195
  keratoconjunctivitis sicca, 70
Sclera, 81–84
  congenital disorders, 81, 197
  structure, 81
Scleritis, 82–83
Sclerosis, nuclear, see Nuclear sclerosis
Sealyham Terrier, retinal dysplasia, 163
Sebaceous glands
  modified, see Meibomian glands
  tumours arising from, 58
Sedatives, 1
Senile cataract, 120
Senile iris atrophy, 131, 132
Senile nuclear sclerosis, 111
Sensory deficits/lesions
  blink abnormalities due to, 194–195
  CNS lesions causing, 185
Sheltie eye anomaly, 159
Sialoadenitis, 18

Sjögren's syndrome, 71
Skeletal abnormalities and retinal dysplasia, 164
Slit-lamp biomicroscope, 2, 5–6
Soap burns, 27
Somatosensory innervation, eye/eyelid, evaluation, 184
Sonography, 39–40
Spasm, hemifacial, 194
Spherophakia, 109–110
Squamous cell carcinoma
  conjunctiva, 80
  eyelid, 58
  limbal, 84
Squint, see Strabismus
Staffordshire bull terrier
  cataract, 114
  persistent hyperplastic primary vitreous, 151
Stains, topical ophthalmic, 6
Steroids (corticosteroids)
  chemical injuries, 27
  hyphaema, 32
  melting ulcers, 26
  myositis, 18
  optic neuritis, 35
  uveitis, 33, 204
Strabismus (squint), 38, 184
  congenital, 191
  ventrolateral, 191
Stroma, corneal, 85
  deposits, 90
  ulceration, 93
Subalbinotic fundus, 157
Subconjunctival haemorrhage, 16
Subluxation, lens, 101–102
Suture-line opacities, 12–14
Symblepharon, 75
Sympathetic innervation
  evaluation, 184
  lesions affecting, see Horner's syndrome
Synechiae, 132–134
  anterior, 132
  posterior, 101, 132
Systemic disease, conjunctival involvement, 80
Systemic histiocytosis, 65, 80

Tapetum (tapetal fundus; tapetum lucidum), 155–157
  development, 11–12
  islets of, in non-tapetal fundus, 158
Tapetum nigrum (non-tapetal fundus), 157–158
Tears
  film
    deficiency, 70
    excessive evaporation, 70
    overflow, 67
    production/secretion (lacrimation), 67, 195
    disorders, 195
    glands involved, see Lacrimal gland; Nictitans gland
    Schirmer test, see Schirmer tear test
  substitute preparations, 73
Telangiectasia (angiokeratoma), 65, 79

INDEX

Terrier breeds
   cataracts, 113–114
   lens luxation, 123–124
Tetanus (lock jaw), 21
   third eyelid prominence/protrusion in, 62, 195
Thermal injuries, 26–27
Tick-borne rickettsia, 138
Tigroid non-tapetal fundus, 157
Tissue plasminogen activator, hyphaema, 32, 143
Tonography, 6
Tonometry, 6
   glaucoma, 99
   uveitis, 135
TonoPen, 6, 100
Toxic substances
   cataracts with, 120
   cortical blindness with, 187
   pupillary abnormalities with, 190
   see also Drugs, adverse reactions
Toxocara canis, 139, 140
Toxoplasmosis, 139
Trauma/injury, 15–36
   cataract due to, 119
   cornea, 23–27, 97
   nasolacrimal system, 69
   optic nerve, 187
   retinal
      detachment due to, 176
      haemorrhage due to, 175
   third eyelid, 62
   uveitis due to, 137–138
Tremor, ocular, secondary to cerebellar disease, 192
Trichiasis, 57–58
Trichophyton erinacei, 52
Trigeminal nerve, 184
   enophthalmos with pain related to, 21
   lesions
      blink abnormalities, 193
      lacrimation disorders, 195
      tests for, 184
Trochlear nerve evaluation, 183
Truncal deviation, 191
Tumours, see Neoplasms

Tunica vasculosa lentis
   atrophy, 149
   persistent hyperplastic (p. h. primary vitreous), 119, 150–151, 200

Ulcer, corneal, 92–95
   melting ulcers, 26, 93–94
   neurogenic, 193
   recurrent epithelial erosions, 88, 92
   staining, 6
   superficial ulceration, 92
      chemicals causing, 27
   see also Descemetocoele
Ultrasonography, 39–40
Uvea (uveal tract), 127–148
   anterior, see Ciliary body; Iris
   congenital/development anomalies, 128–131, 197
   cysts, 100, 153
   hereditary disorders, 200
   neoplasia, 143–146, 201
   posterior, see Choroid
   structure/function, 127–128
Uveitis, 32–33, 134–142
   acute, 31, 32–33
   anterior (iris and ciliary body–iritis and iridocyclitis), 134
      cataract as sequel of, 118, 136
   corneal oedema with, 87
   glaucoma in, 101–102
   hyphaema in, 31
   immune-mediated, 140–141
   infectious, 138–140
   intermediate, 134
   lens-induced, 104, 140
   lymphocytic–plasmacytic, 134, 140
   neoplastic causes, 142, 146
   phacoclastic, 104, 140
   phacolytic, 118, 140
   posterior, 134
   traumatic, 137–138
Uveodermatologic syndrome, 140–141
Uveoscleral route, 99

Vascular occlusions, cerebral, 187
Vascular tumours, conjunctiva, 79

Vasculature, see Blood supply
Vasodilation, peripheral, 189
Vestibular system (in eyeball position/movement control), 183–184
   disorders of, 191
Vestibulocochlear nerve evaluation, 183–184
Vestibulo-ocular reflex (vestibular eye movements), 183, 191
Vision
   assessment, 181
   loss (incl. blindness)
      in generalised progressive retinal atrophy, 168
      in glaucoma, 102
      sudden, 34–35
      toxins causing cortical blindness, 187
Visual pathway, 181
Visual placing response, 181
Vitamin A excess, 187
Vitiligo, 55
Vitreous, 149–154
   in anterior chamber, 104
   congenital anomalies, 149–151, 197
   cysts, 153
   degeneration, 151
   foreign body, 153
   haemorrhage, 151–152
   inflammation, 152
   neoplasia, 153
   persistent hyperplastic primary, 119, 150–151, 200
   prolapse and herniation, 153
   structure/function/development, 149
Vogt–Koyanaga–Harada-like syndrome, 140–141

Welsh springer spaniel, cataract, 115
Wheelbarrow and extensor postural thrust, 185

X-ray radiography, see Radiography
Xerostomia, 70–71

Zinc dermatoses, 55
Zygomatic sialoadenitis, 18